Hearing
Measurement

Under the advisory editorship of
Hayes A. Newby

Hearing
Measurement

A BOOK OF READINGS

edited by

IRA M. VENTRY
TEACHERS COLLEGE
COLUMBIA UNIVERSITY

JOSEPH B. CHAIKLIN
UNIVERSITY OF MINNESOTA

RICHARD F. DIXON
THE UNIVERSITY OF NORTH CAROLINA
AT GREENSBORO

New York

APPLETON – CENTURY – CROFTS
EDUCATIONAL DIVISION
MEREDITH CORPORATION

CONTENTS

Contents vii

GENERAL INTRODUCTION

During the last twenty-five years, great strides have been made in the clinical measurement of hearing. Much of the ground traversed as well as much of the substance of audiometry today is, we hope, reflected in this collection of readings.

Our purpose is to present papers that clarify the theoretical and procedural aspects of basic measurement techniques used in clinical audiology. All aspects of audiology are not, however, covered in this book. Among the topics excluded are anatomy and physiology, hearing pathology, habilitation and rehabilitation, and pediatric audiology. The anthology's scope is limited to material that treats principles, theories, and methods of hearing measurement which the beginning and intermediate student must understand before he can do competent basic audiometry or progress to more advanced audiological procedures.

Despite the increasing number and variety of tests available to audiologists and other clinicians, the measurement of pure-tone sensitivity and speech perception still constitutes a basic and major responsibility in audiological evaluations. The information gathered during routine pure-tone and speech audiometry provides the foundation on which the clinician builds his complete evaluation, an evaluation that may then be used for differential diagnosis and/or for habilitation and rehabilitation. But the essential first step is to collect valid and reliable data about the patient's hearing for pure tones and speech.

The selections are thus organized into sections on calibration, air- and bone-conduction audiometry, speech threshold tests, speech discrimination tests, masking, identification audiometry, and special problems in measurement. Because of its focus on basic hearing measurement, this book should be of value not only to audiologists but also to otologists, speech pathologists, teachers of the deaf, nurses, and others who are confronted with the need to do routine audiometry.

In making our selections, we were guided by the conviction that good clinical practice must be based on sound research evidence. Consequently, the majority of the selections are research papers, either basic or clinical in nature. At the same time, we tried to avoid inclusion of articles that are primarily statistical exercises. Articles which appeared frequently in reference lists or bibliographies used in the major courses of training programs for audiologists throughout the United States were given favorable consideration. Some recently published articles were selected because they present new information and, at the same time, summarize data and viewpoints covered in earlier articles of comparable quality.

All of the articles in each section were selected by the three of us after considerable discussion, debate, and correspondence. Some articles were selected unanimously early in our deliberations; others were not finally agreed upon until nearly a year and a half after we started our review of the literature. In some instances a minority brief won eventual acceptance; most selections, however, were determined by a majority vote. The final table of contents reflects inevitably our collective and individual biases.

We excluded reluctantly many excellent articles because they fell beyond the scope of our project. Other fine papers were excluded because their length would have preempted space needed to include a wide variety of voices and viewpoints in the book. Some omissions are thus explainable on grounds other than our assessment of an article's intrinsic quality.

Each section of the book begins with introductory remarks placing its readings in perspective. The authors of some selections have provided additional contemporary comments, in the form of bracketed footnotes. Authors who chose to append fresh data or evaluations made valuable additions to their original work.

We gratefully acknowledge the generous cooperation of the many authors whose articles make up this collection. In a very profound sense, this volume is dedicated to their efforts in the measurement of hearing and to the hearing-impaired population that all of us endeavor to serve.

I. M. V.

J. B. C.

R. F. D.

part I

CALIBRATION

The evolution of calibration standards for pure-tone and speech audiometers reflects advances in electronics, the improvement of audiometric test environments, and audiology's growth as a scientific discipline that respects precision in clinical and research measurements. The results of pure-tone and speech audiometry are most meaningful to the clinician when he understands the calibration standards formulated for him. The articles in this section were selected to provide information on a variety of subjects related to calibration standards and procedures.

For many years there has been growing awareness of deficiencies in the 1951 American National Standard Institute (ANSI) * standard for calibration of pure-tone audiometers. This standard (ANSI Z24.5-1951) specifies more sound-pressure output at audiometric zero than young normal listeners actually require to reach the threshold of detectability for pure tones. Furthermore, the 1951 standard specifies more output at audiometric zero than do most European standards. Consequently, after many years of work and deliberation, the International Organization for Standardization (ISO) proposed a new international calibration standard for pure-tone audiometers (ISO-1964 or ISO R 389). The ISO standard specifies less pressure at audiometric zero for all frequencies so that patients appear to have higher (poorer) thresholds on the ISO standard than on the ANSI-1951 standard. The ISO standard and most European standards have been based on laboratory data, while the ANSI standard was based on survey data. Since 1964, the ISO standard has gradually replaced the 1951 American standard. In June, 1969, the ANSI finally approved a *new* American standard for pure-tone and speech audiometers. This standard, titled *American Standard Specifications for Audiometers*, S3.6-1969, was published early in 1970 and is reproduced in this book in the Appendix. This standard became effective September 1, 1970, and replaces three previous standards: one dealing with diagnostic audiometers (ANSI Z24.5-1951), one with pure-tone screening audiometers (ANSI Z24.12-1952), and a third with speech audiometers (Z24.13-1953). It is essential for the student to understand the differences between the 1951 and the 1969 standards so that he may comprehend the arbitrary aspects of standards for zero hearing level as well as the importance of specifying

* Formerly known as the American Standards Association (ASA).

reference levels for all decibel statements. Corso's early article reports a normative study in which young normal listeners were tested in an anechoic chamber; he compares his results to data from previous laboratory and survey studies. The ISO standard was eventually based on some of the laboratory data reviewed by Corso and on some of Corso's own data. Corso's article is followed by Davis and Kranz's presentation of the pros and cons of the change to ISO-1964. Davis and Kranz describe the magnitude and clinical implications of the change.

It is known that different earphones produce different sensation effects at the same sound-pressure level and that measurements in different couplers vary. Although we have not included any selections in this area, the interested reader is referred to Weissler's (1968) discussion of problems involved in transferring ISO calibration data to different types of earphones used in countries adhering to the ISO standard, and to Erber's (1968) study of variables that influence sound pressures generated in the ear canal by an audiometric earphone.

Physical calibration standards for bone-conduction receivers have not been given the energetic attention that has been directed toward earphone standards. This lag is attributable in part to instrumentation deficiencies and in part, probably, to human inertia. There is still no physical standard that is universally accepted for calibrating zero hearing level for bone-conduction audiometry. This void has been filled largely by empirical "human calibration methods" such as the one described in the next selection, the article by Roach and Carhart, which is frequently cited.

Individual manufacturers of audiometers have handled the bone-conduction calibration problem by establishing their own normative threshold voltages to apply to bone-conduction vibrators delivered with their audiometers. Recently the Hearing Aid Industry Conference (HAIC), whose membership includes the major American manufacturers of audiometers, prepared an interim bone-conduction calibration standard (Lybarger, 1966a; 1966b) to be used until a more comprehensive standard is formulated. The HAIC standard specifies input voltages and output force values. The force data were derived on a Beltone artificial mastoid (Weiss, 1960; Sanders and Olsen, 1964). The Beltone artificial mastoid, or some variant of it, appears to hold great promise as a measuring device that will permit establishment of a repeatable standard for checking the output of a bone-conduction vibrator. The article by Studebaker provides a brief description of the steps leading to the development of an acceptable artificial mastoid. Studebaker discusses the HAIC interim standard and provides some original data which demonstrate the necessity for specifying measurement method and application force before the HAIC standard, or any standard, is adopted formally. Studebaker's data, coupled with his discussion of the variables that should be specified in a bone-conduction calibration standard, provide an excellent view of the probable direction in which work will progress on establishing a bone-conduction calibration standard.

The next article, a study by Jerger, Carhart, Tillman, and Peterson, demonstrates that the differences in sound-pressure level between normal threshold for 1000 Hz and normal threshold for spondaic words is larger than some authors have indicated in the past. Jerger et al. conclude that calibration standards should establish a 12 to 13 dB difference between audiometric zero for spondees and audiometric zero for 1000 Hz. In a related article Carhart discusses the implications of selecting an appropriate calibration standard for speech audiometers. He emphasizes the effects of calibration standards on the agreement between pure-tone thresholds in the speech frequencies (500, 1000, and 2000 Hz) and spondee threshold (frequently called speech-reception threshold). The general relationship between spondee thresholds and speech-frequency thresholds is discussed in Siegenthaler and Strand's article in Part III.

Eagles and Doerfler document the distressing incidence of malfunctions and calibration defects evident in commercial audiometers. The data provided by Eagles and Doerfler underscore the importance of checking audiometer performance frequently. The same article provides information about the criteria for maximum background noise permissible for the measurement of normal hearing. Hirschorn expands on this topic and provides a more comprehensive treatment of the criteria for permissible background noise specified by ANSI in its standard, No. S3.1-1960.

This section concludes with Harford's two-part overview of factors important in the electronic calibration of an audiometer. In addition, Harford describes procedures that one can use for subjective evaluation of an audiometer's performance.

REFERENCES

1. Erber, N. P. Variables that influence sound pressure generated in the ear canal by an audiometric earphone. *J. acoust. Soc. Amer.*, **44,** pp. 555–562 (1968).

2. Lybarger, S. F. Interim bone-conduction thresholds for audiometry. *J. Speech Hearing Res.*, **9,** pp. 483–487 (1966a).

3. Lybarger, S. F. Interim bone-conduction thresholds for audiometry. *J. acoust. Soc. Amer.*, **40,** pp. 1189–1190 (1966b).

4. Sanders, J. W., and Olsen, W. O. An evaluation of a new artificial mastoid as an instrument for the calibration of audiometer bone-conduction systems. *J. Speech Hearing Dis.*, **29,** pp. 247–253 (1964).

5. *American National Standard S3.1-1960 Criteria for Background Noise in Audiometer Rooms.* New York: American National Standards Institute (1960).

6. Weiss, E. An air-damped artificial mastoid. *J. acoust. Soc. Amer.*, **32,** pp. 1582–1588 (1960).

7. Weissler, Pearl G. International standard reference zero for audiometers. *J. acoust. Soc. Amer.*, **44,** pp. 264–275 (1968).

1

Proposed Laboratory Standard of Normal Hearing

JOHN F. CORSO

JOHN F. CORSO, Ph.D., is Professor of Psychology and Chairman, Department of Psychology, State University of New York, Cortland, New York

I. INTRODUCTION[1]

The increased interest in the effects of noise on hearing[2] has recently focused attention on the American reference level of normal hearing. If the loss of sensitivity caused by prolonged or excessive noise exposure is to be separated from the loss which might be expected to accrue as the usual result of the process of aging, it is critical that normal hearing (zero reference) be appropriately defined.

It is recognized that for some purposes the specific intensity level produced at the zero-db hearing loss setting on a given audiometer is in itself of no particular significance. If the audiometer is correctly calibrated, an individual's threshold stated in terms of hearing loss can be readily converted in terms of the international reference intensity (10^{-16} w/cm², equivalent to a sound pressure level (SPL) of 0.0002 d/cm²). This is accomplished by algebraically adding the individual's hearing loss in db to the SPL in db generated by the audio-meter in a standardized closed coupler at a 0-db hearing loss setting. Thus, if an individual's threshold at 1000 cps is 20 db *re* 0.0002 d/cm², this figure will still be derived regardless of the level at which audiometric zero is set for the test. However, it has become an established clinical practice to express audiograms in terms of hearing loss since this measure is more readily interpreted. This obviates the need for the more complex notation in terms of SPL, but makes it imperative that agreement be reached internationally, if possible, on the setting for normal hearing, i.e., audiometric zero.

The present American reference for normal hearing is based upon the results of a mass survey conducted by the U.S. Public Health Service in 1935–1936.[3] Harris[4] has recently traced the history of American normal hearing and has skillfully attempted to resolve some of the discrepancies between hearing norms as collected in large clinical surveys and in laboratory studies. However, an appreciable discrepancy still exists.[5]

More recently, Glorig *et al.*[6] have provided

Reprinted by permission of the author from *J. acoust. Soc. Amer.*, **30**, pp. 14–23 (1958).

[1] This research was supported in whole or in part by the U.S. Air Force under Contract No. AF 33(038)-786 and Contract No. AF 33(616)-2626, monitored by the Bio-Acoustics Branch, Aero Medical Laboratory, Directorate of Research, Wright Air Development Center, Wright-Patterson Air Force Base, Ohio. The opinions and conclusions contained in this report are those of the author. They are not to be construed as reflecting the views or endorsements of the Department of the Air Force.

[2] Exploratory Subcommittee Z24-X-2, *The Relations of Hearing Loss to Noise Exposure* (American Standards Association, New York, 1954), pp. 5–55.

[3] National Health Survey (1935–1936): Preliminary Reports, Hearing Study Series, Bulletins, 1–7. U.S. Public Health Service, Washington, D.C., 1938.

[4] J. D. Harris, Laryngoscope **64**, 928–957 (1954).

[5] It has been suggested (see reference 4, pp. 30–31) that "the clinical-laboratory discrepancy is not due to selection of subjects, nor of familiarity of subjects with psychoacoustic judgments, but resides in features of the clinical situation which are correctable."

[6] Glorig, Quiggle, Wheeler, and Grings, J. Acoust. Soc. Am. **28**, 1110–1113 (1956).

a concise statement on the current status of the problem of normal hearing. Although the present reference was accepted by the American Medical Association [7] and the American Standards Association,[8] some uncertainty nevertheless exists as to the validity of this reference. This uncertainty is based on the general lack of agreement between the norms of the U.S. Public Health Survey (1935–1936) and the results of other studies, such as those of Sivian and White,[9] Steinberg and Gardner,[10] Dadson and King,[11] and Wheeler and Dickson.[12] The latter two studies, conducted by British investigators on about 600 selected listeners, form the basis for the proposed new standard of British normal hearing which differs markedly from the present American standard.

A review of the American standard was initiated originally in 1946 by The Committee on Hearing of the Division of Medical Sciences of the National Research Council. In 1955 it was decided by the Committee on Hearing and Bio-Acoustics of the Armed Forces-National Research Council that the present American standard was not entirely satisfactory, but no change was recommended pending the collection of additional data. Experimental studies on the problem were then in progress at the Walter Reed Army Medical Center, the National Bureau of Standards, and The Pennsylvania State University. In addition, the Research Center of the Subcommittee on Noise in Industry had completed a hearing survey on 3500 attendants at the Wisconsin State Fair in 1954 and, in 1955, initiated a detailed threshold study on 122 selected fair goers between 18 and 24 years of age.

The present paper represents the third in a series of four major studies conducted at The Pennsylvania State University on the problem of defining the normal threshold of hearing for speech and for pure tones. Data confirming both the normal threshold for speech on C.I.D. Auditory Test W-2 [13] and the normal discrimination loss for speech on C.I.D. Auditory Test W-22 [14] have already been published. The fourth paper in this series on the effects of presbycousis will be published in the near future.

II. STATEMENT OF THE PROBLEM

The present study was undertaken to determine the threshold of hearing for pure tones on a large number of carefully selected subjects tested in a standardized laboratory situation. The testing procedure was to involve three slightly different modifications of the method of limits and two different types of earphones. It was anticipated that the results of this study would aid in clarifying the problem of audiometric zero and would lead subsequently to the derivation of an acceptable laboratory standard of normal hearing for pure tones.

III. EXPERIMENTAL METHOD

The subjects in this study were obtained on a volunteer basis from classes of an introductory course in psychology at The Pennsylvania State University from 1953 to 1956. During this time, three main groups of subjects were tested: Group A, 105 subjects (75 male; 30 female); Group B, 70 subjects (33 male; 37 female); and Group C, 50 subjects (27 male; 23 female). All subjects were white and between the ages of 18 and 24 years, inclusive.

As one step in the analysis of data, the subjects in each of these groups were screened on the basis of three criteria: (1) a negative otological examination performed within 48 hr prior to the audiometric test; (2) a life

[7] Anonymous, J. Am. Med. Assoc. **146,** 255–257 (1951).

[8] Anonymous, *American Standard Specification for Audiometers for General Diagnostic Purposes, Z24.5-1951* (American Standards Association, New York, 1951), p. 9.

[9] L. J. Sivian and S. D. White, J. Acoust. Soc. Am. **4,** 288–321 (1933).

[10] J. C. Steinberg and M. B. Gardner, J. Acoust. Soc. Am. **11,** 270–277 (1940).

[11] R. S. Dadson and J. H. King, J. Laryngol. and Otol. **66,** 366–378 (1952).

[12] L. J. Wheeler and E. D. D. Dickson, J. Laryngol. and Otol. **66,** 379–395 (1952).

[13] J. F. Corso, J. Acoust. Soc. Am. **29,** 368–370 (1957).

[14] J. F. Corso, Laryngoscope **67,** 365–370 (1957).

history of minimal exposure to noise as determined from a standardized questionnaire; and (3) no period of active military service. Of the original group, 72 subjects (44 male; 28 female) in Group A, 49 subjects (22 male; 27 female) in Group B, and 39 subjects (18 male; 21 female) in Group C met these criteria. The present paper is restricted to a consideration of the data for these screened groups only.[15]

Groups A and B were tested on an ADC audiometer, Model 50-E2, equipped with ANB-H1A earphones mounted in MX-41/AR cushions. The output voltage of the audiometer was adjusted so that the calibrated sound pressure of the earphones approximated the minimum audible pressure (MAP) values of Sivian and White [16] when the hearing loss dial was set at zero db. In addition, an external attenuator with a 20-db step was provided to enable the tester to reduce the output voltage well below threshold whenever necessary in testing subjects with extremely acute hearing. Group C was tested on a Beltone audiometer, Model 10-A, which was appropriately modified with an impedance matching network to permit the use of a set of Permoflux PDR-8 earphones in place of the Telephonics TDH-39-107 earphones supplied with the audiometer. The PDR-8 earphones were mounted in cushions similar to those on the ADC audiometer. The resistive network inserted in the Beltone audiometer reduced the output voltage over the frequency range tested by approximately 15 to 30 db below the normal values of the U.S. Public Health Survey as reduced to equivalent PDR-8 pressures by the National Bureau of Standards.[17]

The sound pressure outputs of both audiometers were periodically calibrated in a National Bureau of Standards (NBS) Coupler 9-A in accordance with recommended procedures.[18] Periodic checks were also made on the frequency of the signals generated and on the characteristics of the hearing loss attenuator.

The test tones were presented to the subjects of each group by the serial order of the method of limits. For Groups A and B, the steps between successive trials were 5 db; for Group C, they were 2 db. The presentation stimuli in each group always began well above threshold with a descending series which was then alternated with an ascending series for a total of 6 series in Group A, and 4 series in Groups B and C. Also, for Groups A and B each stimulus intensity for a given series was presented to the subject only once; for Group C, it was presented three times in succession for those values near threshold. The mean of the limits at which the subject failed to respond for a descending series and made his initial response for an ascending series for Series 2 to 6 was taken as the threshold for Group A.[19] For Group B, the same technique was used on Series 2 to 4.[20] For Group C, the threshold was taken as the mean of the limits at which the subject heard two of the three tonal pulses in Series 1 to 4. All testing procedures and methods of computation were standardized and, as far as possible in an experimental situation involving human subjects, were rigidly followed.

All threshold tests were individually administered in an anechoic chamber provided with a two-way voice communication system and a closed loop television system.[21] The frequencies tested on the ADC audiometer were presented to the subjects of Group A in the following order: 1024, 512, 256, 128, 1024, 1448, 2048, 2896, 4096, 5792, 8192, and

---

[15] Data for the original groups of subjects were excluded from this report for brevity of presentation.

[16] L. J. Sivian and S. D. White, reference 9, p. 313.

[17] A. Glorig et al., reference 6, p. 1110.

[18] Anonymous, *American Standard Method for the Coupler Calibration of Earphones, Z24.9-1949.* (American Standards Association, New York, 1949), pp. 12–16.

[19] A detailed description and diagram of the procedure used for testing Group A is presented in J. F. Corso, A.M.A. Arch. Otolaryngol. **63,** 78–91 (1956).

[20] In computing the threshold values for Groups A and B, the threshold estimate of Series I was not used since the hearing loss dial was moved in 10 db steps. This trial served only to locate quickly the general region of hearing. Also, the data for each initial 1000 cps test were discarded.

[21] For a complete description of this facility, see R. L. Berger and E. Ackerman, Noise Control **2,** No. 5, 16–21, 63 (1956). The television system was not available during the testing of Group A.

11 584 cps. For Group B the same order of testing was used but the frequencies of 128, 1448, and 11 584 cps were omitted. For Group C, the frequencies of the Beltone audiometer were presented in the following order: 1000, 500, 250, 1000, 1500, 2000, 3000, 4000, 6000, and 8000 cps.[22] Threshold tests were administered by well-trained technicians on both right and left ears, with the sequence of testing alternated between subjects. A 5-min rest period was provided between the tests for the two ears. The total testing time was approximately 50-min per subject for Groups A and C, and 40-min per subject for Group B.[23]

IV. RESULTS AND CONCLUSIONS

The threshold data for the selected subjects of this study in Groups A, B, and C are presented in Tables 1-1, 1-2, and 1-3, respectively. For each frequency tested, the mean threshold in db *re* 0.0002 d/cm² is given separately for male and female subjects, and for right and left ears. The corresponding standard deviation is also given at each frequency. Notice that in each table, except for a few isolated instances, the threshold of hearing appears to be higher for the male

[22] The frequencies given for the ADC and Beltone audiometers are nominal values only. The calibrated frequencies as measured by a Hewlett-Packard electronic counter, Model 522-B, were 125, 251, 504, 1000, 1422, 1972, 2795, 3967, 5630, 7955, and 11 311 cps for the ADC audiometer and 127, 255, 505, 760, 1000, 1530, 2010, 3010, 4050, 6100, and 8000 cps for the Beltone audiometer. To simplify the task of the reader, the data of the present study are presented in terms of conventional audiometric frequencies.

[23] The subjects of Group C were given subsequently a second and a third audiometric retest following the same procedure as indicated for the group in the present paper. The results of these tests, administered at least one week apart, showed no significant differences in mean threshold values among the three tests except for 1000 cps on the right ear. Also, statistical comparisons at several selected frequencies indicated that the combined mean threshold values for Retests II and III were not significantly different from the values for Test I. Since in many clinical and laboratory situations only a single audiometric test is given, the data of the present paper are restricted to a consideration of the results of the initial audiometric test (Test I).

subjects, particularly toward the upper end of the frequency range tested. The variability of the threshold measurements also tends to be somewhat larger for male than for female subjects from about 4000 cps to 11 584 cps. For both male and female subjects, there is a general tendency for the standard deviation to increase as frequency rises. However, this

TABLE 1-1. THRESHOLD DATA FOR MEN AND WOMEN IN A SELECTED 18–24 YEAR OLD GROUP. GROUP A, THE PENNSYLVANIA STATE UNIVERSITY, 1953–1954

Nominal frequency in cps[a]	Ear	Male N[b]	mean[c]	S.D.[d]	Female N[b]	mean[c]	S.D.[d]
128	Right	44	46.18	5.74	28	43.54	5.05
	Left	44	41.01	5.24	28	39.90	6.94
256	Right	44	27.50	7.32	28	23.90	4.33
	Left	44	21.95	5.90	28	21.13	5.39
512	Right	44	15.06	7.61	28	9.41	5.78
	Left	44	10.82	8.00	28	10.79	5.84
1024	Right	44	7.68	5.00	28	2.60	5.17
	Left	44	5.69	7.17	28	4.56	5.54
1448	Right	44	6.45	7.99	28	5.29	5.32
	Left	44	4.76	7.74	28	6.83	6.95
2048	Right	44	5.13	8.51	28	4.73	6.42
	Left	44	6.50	8.92	28	7.29	9.00
2896	Right	44	9.21	9.88	28	5.36	5.65
	Left	44	3.51	11.50	28	0.63	8.52
4096	Right	44	16.86	9.70	28	12.98	7.64
	Left	44	14.68	10.52	28	8.45	12.35
5792	Right	44	16.25	13.62	27	8.58	6.42
	Left	43	15.42	13.50	25	9.24	6.76
8912	Right	44	18.10	14.26	27	9.56	9.73
	Left	41	18.24	15.40	23	14.42	6.34
11 584	Right	44	32.41	15.03	27	23.86	9.29
	Left	43	34.17	18.50	28	28.42	6.09

[a] For exact frequencies, see reference 19.

[b] The N is not constant for all frequencies as equipment difficulties or deviations from standardized testing procedures indicated that certain data should be excluded.

[c] The mean threshold value is expressed in db *re* 0.0002 d/cm² as measured in the NBS Coupler 9-A.

[d] The standard deviation (S.D.) is expressed in db.

trend is more marked for male than for female subjects.

To determine whether any statistically significant differences existed in the mean threshold values between male and female subjects, the data presented in Tables 1-1, 1-2, and 1-3 were separately analyzed. Table 1-4 presents the results of the comparisons in means and variances at each test frequency for Groups

A, B, and C. The t ratios for testing the significance of the differences in means and F ratios for testing the homogeneity of variances were computed by standard procedures.[24] The level of significance of the t ratio when the variances were unequal was computed by an

TABLE I-2. THRESHOLD DATA FOR MEN AND WOMEN IN A SELECTED 18–24 YEAR OLD GROUP. GROUP B, THE PENNSYLVANIA STATE UNIVERSITY, 1954–1955

Nominal frequency in cps[a]	Ear	Male			Female		
		N	mean	S.D.	N	mean	S.D.
256	Right	22	26.04	4.67	27	22.62	4.02
	Left	22	25.64	5.53	26	23.53	4.02
512	Right	20	11.46	6.35	26	7.68	4.13
	Left	19	12.06	6.53	26	11.83	4.72
1024	Right	21	5.97	4.42	24	4.82	5.04
	Left	21	8.23	4.82	26	7.53	5.07
2048	Right	21	5.69	6.08	27	7.48	6.47
	Left	21	10.03	4.52	26	10.95	4.83
2896	Right	21	9.65	7.88	22	7.01	7.88
	Left	21	8.96	6.60	25	3.84	8.39
4096	Right	20	15.36	8.53	25	13.10	7.49
	Left	21	14.09	8.03	23	14.29	5.47
5792	Right	20	16.07	11.87	25	8.85	5.12
	Left	22	18.74	13.89	27	12.65	5.46
8192	Right	16	20.78	14.28	21	13.50	6.85
	Left	17	18.02	8.76	24	16.67	7.02

[a] For an explanation of the column headings see footnotes, Table 1-1.

approximation method.[25] In such cases, computations were made to determine whether the obtained t ratios were significant at the 5 percent or 1 percent levels.

The data in Table 1-4 show that for Group A, there are nine mean differences which are significant at or beyond the 5 percent level (7 for right ear; 2 for left ear); for Group B, there are four (3 for right ear; 1 for left ear); and Group C, there are six (3 for right ear; 3 for left ear). Of the 19 significant differences, five occur at or below 512 cps, seven occur at or above 5792 cps, and the remaining seven occur in the midfrequency range. Since approximately 34 percent of the computed t

[24] A. L. Edwards, *Statistical Methods for the Behavioral Sciences* (Rinehart and Company, Inc., New York, 1954), pp. 246–255 and pp. 271–273.
[25] W. G. Cochran and G. M. Cox, *Experimental Designs* (John Wiley and Sons, Inc., New York, 1950), pp. 91–93.

ratios are statistically significant, it appears that real differences do exist in the auditory acuity of men and women in the 18 to 24 year old age group, particularly at the lower and higher ends of the audiometric range. In each instance where a significant difference was obtained, the mean threshold was lower for the female subjects than for the male. Likewise, in the 22 instances in which significant differences in variability were obtained, the variances were smaller for female subjects. The data in Table 1-4 provide an adequate basis for rejecting the notion that the threshold distributions for male and female subjects should be combined for normative purposes.

As the data for Groups A and B were collected under somewhat similar conditions, a comparison was made to determine whether the threshold data for these two groups given in Tables 1-1 and 1-2 could be combined for both the right and left ears. Table 1-5 presents the t ratios obtained at each frequency when the mean thresholds for male and female subjects were compared by ear across Groups A and B. For each comparison, there is also given the F ratio obtained in evaluating the

TABLE I-3. THRESHOLD DATA FOR MEN AND WOMEN IN A SELECTED 18–24 YEAR OLD GROUP. GROUP C, THE PENNSYLVANIA STATE UNIVERSITY, 1955–1956

Nominal frequency in cps[a]	Ear	Male			Female		
		N	mean	S.D.	N	mean	S.D.
250	Right	18	26.48	4.83	21	24.30	4.64
	Left	18	27.04	4.76	21	24.24	4.34
500	Right	18	11.61	6.59	21	10.53	4.75
	Left	18	10.64	4.65	21	8.73	4.92
1000	Right	18	6.62	4.65	21	5.59	4.30
	Left	18	5.22	4.05	21	3.98	4.66
1500	Right	18	8.83	4.95	20	6.39	5.05
	Left	18	5.50	4.93	20	4.09	4.33
2000	Right	18	8.89	5.60	19	5.71	5.57
	Left	18	6.42	6.56	19	3.71	3.09
3000	Right	17	13.92	7.91	20	7.75	6.54
	Left	16	11.62	6.19	16	7.74	4.20
4000	Right	17	13.19	9.11	21	11.20	6.04
	Left	18	14.68	8.18	19	8.96	4.02
6000	Right	18	29.01	13.20	20	21.18	7.10
	Left	17	31.01	12.90	20	20.97	5.66
8000	Right	18	26.86	16.56	21	17.20	6.25
	Left	17	28.41	10.55	21	21.57	9.63

[a] For an explanation of the column headings see footnotes, Table 1-1.

TABLE I-4. RESULTS OF THE COMPARISONS OF MEANS AND VARIANCES FOR MALE AND FEMALE SUBJECTS OF GROUPS A, B, AND C

Nominal frequency in cps	Ear	Group A		Group B		Nominal frequency in cps	Group C	
		t ratio	F ratio	t ratio	F ratio		t ratio	F ratio
128	Right	2.02[a]	1.28					
	Left	0.72	1.77					
256	Right	2.59[a]	2.83[c]	2.65[a]	1.36	250	1.39	1.09
	Left	0.60	1.19	1.46	1.89		1.88	1.21
512	Right	3.51[b]	1.72	2.25[a]	2.36[d]	500	0.56	1.94
	Left	0.18	1.86[d]	0.13	1.91		1.22	1.11
1024	Right	4.06[b]	1.08	0.80	1.30	1000	0.70	1.18
	Left	0.74	1.66	0.47	1.11		1.15	1.31
1448	Right	0.72	2.23[d]			1500	1.46	1.04
	Left	−1.05	1.23				0.92	1.30
2048	Right	0.61	1.76	−0.95	1.11	2000	1.68	1.01
	Left	−0.36	1.03	−0.66	1.14		1.57	4.69[c]
2896	Right	0.92	3.03[c]	1.07	1.00	3000	2.49[a]	1.46
	Left	1.20	1.80[d]	2.27[a]	1.62		2.00	2.17
4096	Right	1.87	1.60	0.91	1.30	4000	0.75	2.27[d]
	Left	2.18[a]	1.38	−0.09	2.16[d]		2.65[a]	4.14[c]
5792	Right	3.25[b]	4.50[c]	2.44[a]	5.38[c]	6000	2.18[a]	3.48[c]
	Left	2.47[a]	3.99[c]	1.95	6.53[c]		2.89[a]	5.19[c]
8192	Right	3.07[b]	2.14[d]	1.82	4.35[c]	8000	2.32[a]	7.09[c]
	Left	1.36	5.90[c]	0.51	1.56		2.07[a]	1.73
11 584	Right	2.93[b]	3.44[c]					
	Left	1.57	9.23[c]					

[a] $p < 0.05$, t ratio.　　[b] $p < 0.01$, t ratio.　　[c] $p < 0.02$, F ratio.　　[d] $p < 0.10$, F ratio.

homogeneity of variances. The data of Table I-5 indicate that none of the differences in mean threshold values for the right ear are statistically significant for either male or female subjects; for the left ear, the differences are significant at 256, 2048, and 2896 cps for the male subjects and at 4096 cps for the female subjects. The variances of threshold measures are significantly different (at or beyond the 10 percent level) on the right ear only for the male subjects at 256 cps; on the left ear, the F ratio is significant at 1024, 2048, 2896, and 8192 cps for the male subjects and at 2048 and 4096 cps for the female subjects.

As a relatively small number of mean differences were statistically significant (4 out of 32 or approximately 12 percent), it appeared justifiable to combine the data of Groups A and B by right and left ears independently for male and female subjects. The means and standard deviations of the distributions obtained by combining within ears for Groups A and B are given in Table 1-6.

In order to determine whether the threshold

TABLE I-5. RESULTS OF THE COMPARISONS OF MEANS AND VARIANCES FOR GROUPS A AND B ON RIGHT AND LEFT EARS

Nominal frequency in cps	Right ear				Left ear			
	Male		Female		Male		Female	
	t ratio	F ratio	t ratio	F ratio	t ratio	F ratio	t ratio	F ratio
256	0.97	2.39[c]	0.25	1.15	−2.44[a]	1.11	−1.83	1.80
512	1.93	1.44	1.52	1.96	−0.63	1.50	−0.71	1.53
1024	1.37	1.29	−1.71	1.05	−1.66	2.21[c]	−2.02	1.18
2048	−0.30	1.96	1.10	1.32	−2.09[a]	3.89[b]	−1.85	3.47[b]
2896	−0.19	1.57	−0.81	1.95	−2.38[a]	3.03[b]	−1.35	1.03
4096	0.61	1.29	−0.06	1.04	0.24	1.72	−2.21[a]	5.09[b]
5792	0.05	1.32	−0.17	1.57	−0.90	1.06	−1.95	1.53
8192	0.63	1.00	−1.61	2.02	0.07	3.09[b]	−1.13	1.23

[a] $p < 0.05$, t ratio.　　[b] $p < 0.02$, F ratio.　　[c] $p < 0.10$, F ratio.

TABLE 1-6. MEANS AND STANDARD DEVIATIONS OF THE THRESHOLD DATA OBTAINED BY COMBINING WITHIN EARS FOR GROUPS A AND B

| Nominal frequency in cps[a] | | Right ear | | | | | | Left ear | | | | |
| | | Male | | | Female | | | Male | | | Female | |
	N	mean	S.D.	N	mean	S.D.	N	mean	S.D.	N	mean	S.D.
256	66	27.01	6.55	55	23.27	4.07	66	23.18	5.96	54	22.28	4.86
512	64	13.94	7.31	54	8.58	5.09	63	11.19	7.60	54	11.29	5.24
1024	65	7.13	4.88	52	3.62	5.25	65	6.51	6.52	54	5.99	5.41
2048	65	5.31	7.81	55	6.08	6.57	65	7.64	7.99	54	9.05	7.46
2896	65	9.35	9.28	50	6.09	6.76	65	5.27	10.48	53	2.14	8.62
4096	64	16.40	9.09	53	13.04	7.63	65	14.49	9.77	51	11.08	10.26
5792	64	16.20	12.97	52	8.71	5.85	65	16.54	13.78	52	11.01	6.37
8192	60	18.81	13.96	48	11.28	8.79	58	18.17	13.75	47	15.56	6.72

[a] For an explanation of the column headings see footnotes, Table 1-1.

data could next be combined for right and left ears, an analysis was performed on the data given in Tables 1-3 and 1-6. The results of this analysis are given in Table 1-7. For the combined data of Groups A and B, there are nine significant mean differences (4 for male subjects; 5 for female subjects); for Group C, only one difference is significant (8000 cps for female subjects). Thus, from a statistical point of view, the data for the right and left ears of Group C can be appropriately combined into a single distribution, but the validity of combining the data for Groups A and B is open to question. However, from a practical point of view, the significant mean differences ranged only from about 2 to 4 db which indicates that no serious bias would probably be introduced if the data were combined.

TABLE 1-7. RESULTS OF THE COMPARISONS OF MEANS AND VARIANCES FOR THE RIGHT AND LEFT EARS OF COMBINED GROUPS A AND B AND OF GROUP C

| | | Combined groups A and B | | | | | Group C | | | | |
cps[a]	Sex	N	r[b]	t ratio	F ratio		cps[a]	N	r[b]	t ratio	F ratio
256	Male	66	0.70	6.38[d]	1.21		250	18	0.36	−0.43	1.03
	Female	54	0.29	1.36	1.43			21	0.44	0.06	1.14
512	Male	62	0.48	2.84[d]	1.08		500	18	0.33	0.60	2.01
	Female	53	0.48	−3.71[d]	1.06			21	0.27	1.38	1.07
1024	Male	64	0.35	0.75	1.79[f]		1000	18	0.34	1.16	1.32
	Female	52	0.65	−3.82[d]	1.06			21	0.05	1.17	1.17
							1500	18	−0.02	1.95	1.01
								20	0.23	1.72	1.36
2048	Male	64	0.80	−3.64[d]	1.05		2000	18	0.49	1.66	1.37
	Female	53	0.26	−1.35	1.33			18	0.49	1.75	3.25[e]
2896	Male	65	0.34	2.87[d]	1.28		3000	15	0.33	1.07	1.63
	Female	47	0.56	3.83[d]	1.63[f]			16	0.68	0.01	2.42[f]
4096	Male	64	0.61	1.82	1.16		4000	17	0.56	−0.74	1.24
	Female	50	0.37	1.35	1.81[f]			19	0.41	1.72	2.26[e]
5792	Male	61	0.38	−0.23	1.13		6000	17	0.73	−0.51	1.05
	Female	50	0.51	−2.74[d]	1.19			19	0.16	0.11	1.57
8192	Male	59	0.30	0.30	1.03		8000	17	0.28	−0.41	2.46[f]
	Female	44	0.48	−3.63[d]	1.71[f]			21	0.55	2.41[c]	2.37[f]

[a] Nominal frequency in cps.

[b] This r is the product moment correlation between ears based on the number of subjects shown in the N column having threshold values recorded for both right and left ears. This number is in some cases different from the N used in computing the means and standard deviations listed in Tables 1-3 and 1-6. Thus, the obtained t ratios of this table are not exact since the standard error of the difference between means is an approximation based on the computed r value. However, since the t ratios are either clearly nonsignificant or highly significant, this approximation should not alter the interpretation of the data.

[c] $p < 0.05$, t ratio.   [d] $p < 0.01$, t ratio.   [e] $p < 0.02$, F ratio.   [f] $p < 0.10$, F ratio.

TABLE 1-8. MEANS AND STANDARD DEVIATIONS OF THE THRESHOLD DATA OBTAINED BY COMBINING THE RIGHT AND LEFT EARS OF GROUPS A AND B AND OF GROUP C

Nominal frequency in cps[a]	Combined Group A and B						Nominal frequency in cps	Group C					
		Male			Female				Male			Female	
	N	mean	S.D.	N	mean	S.D.		N	mean	S.D.	N	mean	S.D.
256	132	25.10	6.53	109	22.78	4.40	250	36	26.76	4.63	42	24.27	4.33
512	127	12.58	7.54	108	9.94	5.40	500	36	11.13	5.77	42	9.63	4.98
1024	130	6.82	5.79	106	4.83	5.49	1000	36	5.92	4.44	42	4.78	4.54
							1500	36	7.16	5.16	40	5.24	4.89
2048	130	6.48	7.96	109	8.26	6.97	2000	36	7.65	6.17	38	4.71	4.62
2896	130	7.31	10.11	103	4.05	8.05	3000	33	12.80	7.23	36	7.75	5.82
4096	129	15.44	9.55	104	12.08	9.04	4000	35	13.96	8.61	40	10.41	5.37
5792	129	16.37	13.35	104	9.86	6.16	6000	35	29.98	13.05	40	21.07	6.34
8192	118	18.50	13.85	95	13.39	8.11	8000	35	27.61	14.01	42	19.38	8.37

[a] For an explanation of the column headings see footnotes, Table 1-1.

Also, the mean differences did not favor one ear consistently over the other. Thus, in the light of these considerations, the threshold data for right and left ears were combined for Groups A and B and for Group C.

Table 1-8 presents the means and standard deviations of the distributions obtained by combining the data for right and left ears of Groups A and B and of Group C. Separate values are given for male and for female subjects.

In the final attempt to combine data, an analysis was made of the data in Table 1-8 to determine whether the threshold values for Groups A and B and for Group C could be combined for male subjects and for female subjects. The results of this comparison are shown in Table 1-9. Notice that for the male subjects, there are three significant differences in means and five significant differences in variances. In other words, of the nine frequencies tested, significant differences in means or variances occurred at seven frequencies. For the female subjects, there were four significant differences in means and three in variances. Five of the nine frequencies tested produced either significant differences in means or in variances. In general, combining the data by sex for Groups A, B, and C does not appear justifiable. Reference to Table 1-8 indicates that marked differences exist in means and in standard deviations between Groups A and B and Group C for both male and female subjects, particularly at the 6000

and 8000 cps values. Thus, combining the data for all three groups would tend to obscure these differences which might be of considerable importance in medico-legal situations involving noise-induced hearing loss.

Since it did not appear appropriate to combine the data for male and for female subjects across test groups, the final set of threshold values was obtained by using only

TABLE 1-9. RESULTS OF THE COMPARISONS OF MEANS AND VARIANCES FOR COMBINED GROUPS A AND B AND FOR GROUP C

Nominal frequency in cps[a]	Male		Female	
	t ratio	F ratio	t ratio	F ratio
250	−1.73	1.93[e]	−1.89	1.01
500	1.22	1.67[e]	0.33	1.15
1000	0.98	1.67[e]	0.06	1.43
1500[b]	−1.27	2.35[d]	0.71	1.60
2000	−0.94	1.63	3.51[c]	2.23[d]
3000	−3.51[c]	1.92[e]	−2.94[c]	1.88[e]
4000	0.87	1.21	1.56	2.78[d]
6000	−5.38[c]	1.03	−9.50[c]	1.08
8000	−4.74[c]	1.04	−3.84[c]	1.09

[a] The nominal frequencies are given for Group C. Although there were differences in calibrated frequencies between the tests administered to Groups A and B and to Group C, these differences were not considered to be excessive. Of ten frequency differences, seven were less than 3 percent, two were 8 percent, and one was 11 percent as computed from the calibrated ADC frequencies as a base.

[b] The comparison at this frequency is between Groups A and C; no data were collected at 1448 cps for Group B.

[c] $p < 0.01$, t ratio.

[d] $p < 0.02$, F ratio.

[e] $p < 0.10$, F ratio.

the data of those subjects whose hearing fell within plus or minus 15 db from the mode of the distributions indicated in Table 1-8. The means, modes, and standard deviations of the truncated distributions are given in Table 1-10.

TABLE 1-10. THRESHOLD DATA FOR THE TRUNCATED DISTRIBUTIONS OF THE 18 TO 24 YR OLD GROUPS AT THE PENNSYLVANIA STATE UNIVERSITY

| | | Male | | | | | Group C | | |
cps[a]	N	Mode	Mean	S.D.	cps	N	Mode	Mean	S.D.
128[b]	86	41.0	43.6	8.4					
256	124	21.0	24.1	5.3	250	36	25.0	26.8	4.6
512	121	13.0	12.2	5.7	500	35	11.0	10.6	7.3
1024	127	11.0	6.9	5.1	1000	36	5.0	5.9	4.9
1448[b]	80	5.0	5.6	5.0	1500	35	5.0	6.7	4.7
2048	123	5.0	6.2	6.3	2000	34	5.0	6.8	5.3
2896	115	11.0	9.1	6.3	3000	30	9.0	10.4	5.1
4096	115	15.0	14.4	6.6	4000	30	9.0	11.2	6.0
5792	102	11.0	12.0	6.7	6000	25	31.0	26.8	6.5
8192	92	19.0	16.8	6.2	8000	26	19.0	19.5	7.5
11 584[b]	64	31.0	28.5	6.8					
		Female							
128[b]	55	41.0	42.3	6.1					
256	108	23.0	22.6	4.9	250	42	25.0	24.3	4.4
512	106	13.0	10.2	5.2	500	41	9.0	9.9	3.5
1024	101	1.0	4.2	4.8	1000	41	7.0	4.6	3.4
1448[b]	56	5.0	6.0	6.2	1500	40	7.0	5.2	4.9
2048	104	11.0	8.1	4.7	2000	38	7.0	4.7	4.6
2896	95	5.0	5.9	4.5	3000	40	5.0	5.9	4.6
4096	91	17.0	13.0	5.5	4000	40	9.0	10.1	5.4
5792	104	11.0	9.9	6.2	6000	39	23.0	20.0	6.9
8192	82	7.0	11.2	5.9	8000	40	17.0	18.2	6.8
11 584[b]	53	27.0	25.6	5.5					

[a] For an explanation of the column headings see footnotes, Table 1-1.
[b] Data for Group A only.

for the combined Groups A and B and for Group C. Notice that the elimination of the extreme cases has in most instances only a small effect. There is little difference between the means in Table 1-8 and those in Table 1-10. Obviously, the standard deviations of the truncated distributions should be, and are, smaller than those in Table 1-8. The most pronounced reductions occur at the higher frequencies. The data of Table 1-10 represent the threshold estimates of normal hearing for pure tones as determined at The Pennsylvania State University on a sample of otologically normal subjects ranging in age from 18 to 24 yr.

Figure 1-1 presents the results of the present study (means in Table 1-10) in graphical form for ease of comparison with the results of a selected number of other threshold studies. These include the studies of Glorig et al.,[26] Dadson and King,[27] Wheeler and

[26] A. Glorig et al., reference 6, p. 1111.
[27] R. S. Dadson and J. H. King, reference 11, p. 371.

Dickson,[28] Harris,[29] Sivian and White,[30] and the U.S. Public Health Service.[31] It is recognized that the experimental techniques and the statistical treatment of the data for these several studies are not directly comparable, but the findings are nevertheless presented in a single graph to indicate the general agreement in threshold values despite these differences. (1) It is immediately apparent that below 4000 cps the threshold values obtained in the laboratory type studies are considerably lower than those of the U.S. Public Health Service. (2) The data of the present study are in excellent agreement with those of other laboratory type studies. Notice, in particular, the effects above 4000 cps. The data obtained with the PDR-8 earphones (Group C) show the same trend as those of Glorig et al. who also used this type of earphone; the data obtained with the ANB-H1A earphones (Groups A and B) tend to follow the curves of Dadson and King, and Wheeler and Dickson who used the British type 4026A earphones. (3) The derived curve of Sivian and White which represents monaural MAP about $\frac{1}{2}$ in. from the eardrum (and is thus independent of particular earphone-coupler calibration effects) approximates in most respects a curve of best fit for the threshold data of the present study. (4) The derived curve of Harris also appears to fit the several sets of laboratory data fairly well, but is probably not low enough in the mid-frequency range. (5) There is little question that carefully controlled laboratory studies performed under somewhat similar conditions by different investigators will tend to yield essentially similar estimates of auditory thresholds.

V. DISCUSSION

The data of the present study (Table 1-4) have shown that the auditory sensitivity of male and

[28] L. J. Wheeler and E. D. D. Dickson, reference 12, p. 394.
[29] J. D. Harris, reference 4, p. 20.
[30] L. J. Sivian and S. D. White, reference 9, p. 313.
[31] National Health Survey, reference 3, Bull. 2.

female subjects in the 18 to 24 year old category differs significantly, particularly towards the lower and upper ends of the frequency range generally used in audiometry. Thus, it appears advisable to maintain a separate set of standards for male and for female populations in order to evaluate appropriately the

Although the final data of this study have been presented separately for Groups A and B and for Group C (Table 1-10), this is not intended to imply that a single set of norms cannot be derived for the 18 to 24 yr old age group. It is believed that the differences in the mean threshold data for these groups are

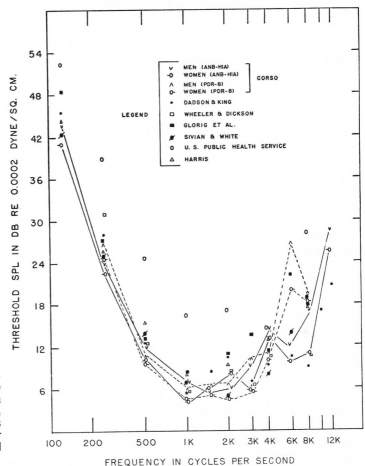

ABSOLUTE THRESHOLD OF HEARING

Figure 1-1. Auditory thresholds for subjects 18 to 24 yr of age obtained at The Pennsylvania State University, 1953–1956, compared with the values obtained in a selected number of other studies on normal hearing for pure tones.

degree of hearing loss possessed by a given individual. This is particularly relevant in the case of noise-induced hearing loss since this type of loss occurs mainly in the higher frequency range. As it also appears that the effects of presbycousis are more marked for men than for women at the higher frequencies,[32] it is recommended that any new standard of normal hearing maintain independent values for each sex.

[32] See reference 2, pp. 16–17.

primarily due to differences in earphones and possibly in procedures, rather than in inherent differences between the samples of subjects.[33] It is emphasized that the results of this study apply specifically to the types of earphones (ANB-HlA and PDR-8) which were used in the threshold tests. Although the performance

[33] In a subsequent study (Am. J. Psychol.), it was found that threshold values at frequencies below 200 cps were not affected by the differences in procedures which characterized the testing of Group A and Group C.

of a given earphone in the standard coupler approximates, in general, that in the average human ear, the standard coupler does not yield the same objective performance for earphones of different types. Nevertheless, the sound pressure produced in an approved type of coupler specifies unambiguously the normal threshold of hearing for that particular earphone when it is activated by the voltage input corresponding to the threshold excitation for a group of selected subjects. The problem of specifying normal hearing in terms of coupler calibration would be considerably reduced if loudness balance data were available for all commonly used earphones. The norms stated for one earphone could then be readily transferred to equivalent sound pressures for any other earphone.[34]

In an effort to ascertain the extent to which earphone differences were affecting the data of Table 1-8, preliminary loudness balance tests were made on eight unselected, adult subjects at 250, 6000, and 8000 cps. Threshold measurements were made on both right and left ears using the right earphone (ANB-HlA) of the ADC audiometer and the right earphone (PDR-8) of the Beltone audiometer in a counterbalanced order. These data are given in Table 1-11, together with the t ratios obtained in testing for the statistical significance of the differences in means. The discrepancy at 6000 cps is highly significant, indicating that the significant differences between the means of Groups A and B and Group C (Table 1-9) are probably the result of differences in earphones. Note that the magnitude of the differences at 6000 cps for the loudness balance group approximates that obtained for the experimental groups (Table 1-8). If an extended set of loudness balance data were to be obtained on the ANB-HlA and PDR-8 earphones, it appears likely that the differences in Table 1-8 would be essentially resolved, thus leading to a single unified curve of normal

[34] Some data are already available. See the Natl. Bur. Standards, Preliminary Results: "A comparison of sound pressures developed in earphone couplers and in the ear," Report, January 18, 1951. See also J. D. Harris, reference 4, p. 17.

hearing for men, and one for women, for this particular age group. In the absence of these data, however, as already pointed out, the specified threshold values may be taken as unambiguous normal values for that particular earphone calibrated in the NBS coupler 9-A.

The problem of selecting an appropriate reference level for audiometers for general diagnostic purposes now appears to be at least partially resolved. There is no longer any question that threshold values obtained under the usual testing conditions of large surveys vary considerably from those obtained under more carefully controlled laboratory situations. It is only of secondary interest whether these differences are brought about by sampling techniques, testing procedures, environmental conditions, naivety of subjects, motivation, etc. The question of selecting a set of sound pressure values to represent "normal" hearing now appears to involve two issues: (1) the choice between survey or laboratory data and (2) the exact specification of the threshold values in the light of the several studies currently available in the category selected.[35] The first issue is probably easier to resolve than the second.

Since the threshold values from laboratory studies are lower than those from mass surveys, it would appear that in the laboratory studies the effects of extraneous factors have been minimized and, hence, the results provide a more realistic evaluation of unimpaired hearing. From these "purer" data, the direct effects of other factors such as age and noise exposure, can be more appropriately determined. The importance of this approach has already been stressed in proposing that separate norms for male and for female populations be established.

The complexity of the solution to the second

[35] Another problem should also be mentioned, i.e., whether normal hearing should be specified in terms of SPL measured in the ear canal or in a closed acoustic coupler. Harris, reference 4, p. 7, concludes that "for a careful determination of SPL at an individual's threshold, a direct reading of threshold SPL by probe tube is preferable to an inferred reading with the intermediary of the brass coupler." The closed coupler technique, however, has certain practical advantages for routine audiometry.

TABLE I-11. PRELIMINARY LOUDNESS BALANCE DATA FOR ANB-H1A AND PERMOFLUX PDR-8 EARPHONES

Nominal frequency in cps	Right ear ($N = 8$)				Left ear ($N = 8$)			
	PDR-8	ANB-H1A	Diff.	t ratio	PDR-8	ANB-H1A	Diff.	t ratio
250	24.79[a]	23.92	0.87	0.49	22.54	23.05	−0.51	−0.45
6000	38.71	25.70	13.01	9.73[b]	41.45	31.10	10.35	8.63[b]
8000	31.16	32.40	−1.24	−0.47	37.87	34.90	2.97	2.00

[a] The primary data of this table are mean threshold values in db re 0.0002 d/cm^2 for 8 subjects tested on each earphone and on each ear.
[b] $p < 0.01$.

issue will depend entirely upon the direction and plan of attack. The simplest solution would be to select arbitrarily a set of data from among those currently available and designate that as "normal" hearing for the particular combination of earphone and coupler used in the threshold determinations. At the other extreme, the problem becomes one of attempting to obtain a common sound pressure baseline by loudness balancing different types of earphones and then resolving, statistically or otherwise, any differences which remain among the several studies. Regardless of the ultimate solution to this problem, it is now exceedingly clear that the specification of normal hearing must involve more than a statement of standard sound pressure values for a given earphone-coupler combination. Other factors such as the sex and age of the normative group, the testing procedure, and the ambient noise environment cannot be ignored.

VI. SUMMARY

1. The present study was performed to determine the normal monaural threshold of hearing (MAP) by earphone listening for three groups of otologically normal subjects ranging in age from 18 to 24 yr, inclusive. All subjects were screened for a life history of minimal exposure to noise and the absence of active military service. The study was designed to provide additional data under carefully controlled laboratory conditions which could be considered in re-establishing the standards of calibration of audiometers for general diagnostic purposes.

2. Threshold determinations were made on two types of earphones (ANB-H1A) and Permoflux PDR-8 calibrated in a National Bureau of Standards coupler 9-A. The maximal range of audiometric frequencies extended from 128 cps to 11 584 cps. For each of two groups of subjects, threshold tests were made following slightly different modifications of the method of limits with 5 db steps; the third group was tested with still another modification using 2 db steps. The results of the study showed significant differences between earphones, as well as between male and female subjects.

3. The results of the present study were compared graphically with those of several other selected studies on normal hearing. In general, excellent agreement was obtained, indicating that threshold values based on laboratory type studies are considerably lower than those for mass surveys. Some consideration was given to the problem of redefining the normal zero reference for audiometers and some tentative suggestions were made.

4. The findings of the present study are offered for consideration as proposed normal standards of hearing for pure tones for individuals, 18 to 24 yr of age, who show no evidence of otological disorders and have a life history of minimal exposure to noise.

VII. ACKNOWLEDGMENTS

The author is indebted to the many individuals who, over the several years in which this study was in progress, contributed substantially to the Human Factors Research Program of the Department of Psychology. The otological examinations were performed by Dr. H. R. Glenn, Director of the University Health Center, and Dr. E. S. Krug, Assistant University Physician. Dr. Eugene Ackerman, Associate Professor of Physics, Dr. Norton J. Brennan, Associate Professor of Engineering Research, and Mr. Walter L. Baker, Assistant Professor of Engineering Research, were primarily responsible for technical guidance in instrumentation and calibration. Mr. Donald Clark and Mr. George Mague, undergraduate majors in electrical engineering, provided the service functions of equipment maintenance and calibration. The several testers, all of whom were at one time or another graduate assistants in psychology,

included Dr. Fred L. Royer, Dr. Raymond Fowler, Dr. Bernard Guerney, Mr. Samuel Schnitzer, Mr. Jack Wilson, Mr. Peter Hanford, Mr. Anthony LoGuidice, Mr. Thomas Scott, Mr. Donald Goldstein, Mr. Donald Whalen, and Mrs. Lorraine Alderstein Low. The analysis of data was carried out primarily by Mr. Alexander Cohen, Research Associate, who was also responsible for the general integration of activities in the later phases of the study. Dr. Joseph Sataloff of the Jefferson Medical Hospital, Philadelphia, Pennsylvania, reviewed the results of all otological examinations and served generally as a consultant in otology.

2

The International Standard Reference Zero for Pure–Tone Audiometers and Its Relation to the Evaluation of Impairment of Hearing*

HALLOWELL DAVIS
FRED W. KRANZ

HALLOWELL DAVIS, M.D., is Research Associate, Central Institute for the Deaf
FRED W. KRANZ was with Otarion Electronics, Inc., when this article was prepared

For many years leading otologists and audiologists, both in the United States and in Europe, have desired a set of international standards for audiometers. One reason for this is that the present American standard reference threshold levels, embodied in the 1951 specification for Audiometers for General Diagnostic Purposes,[1] differ significantly from the corresponding British standard levels. The British standard is now employed not only in Great Britain but in most European countries as well. The American values are based on

Reprinted by permission of the authors from *J. Speech Hearing Res.*, **7**, pp. 7–16 (1964).

* In the original, this article was prefaced by the following statement prepared by the editor of the *J. Speech Hearing Res.*: "The following special article has been prepared by Davis and Kranz for simultaneous publication in all scholarly journals concerned with the evaluation of hearing impairment. It summarizes the important impact that the new ISO international zero reference levels will have on audiometric norms. *JSHR* welcomes this opportunity to join with other journals in bringing this statement to members of our profession. (Ed.)" Dr. Davis' later thinking and related developments are summarized in two subsequent articles: "Guide to the classification and evaluation of hearing handicap," *Trans. Amer. Acad. Ophthalmol. Otolaryngol.*, **69**, pp. 740–751 (1965); and "Reference levels and hearing levels in otology," *Ann. Otol. Rhinol. Laryngol.*, **75**, pp. 808–819 (1966).

[1] Z24.3-1951: American Standards Association, 10 East 40th Street, New York 16, N.Y.

determinations of the threshold of hearing in "normal" ears made in the United States National Health Survey in 1937. The British values, sometimes referred to as a "standard of normal hearing," were developed from studies carried out in England in the early nineteen-fifties. The British determinations were made fifteen years later than the American, using more modern equipment, better acoustic conditions and improved psychoacoustic techniques and they differ by about 10 dB, on the average, from the corresponding 1951 American standard values.

The International Organization for Standardization took this situation under consideration in 1955. Its writing group examined carefully and critically all of the published data on the thresholds of normal hearing. In all, fifteen different studies were found, carried out in five different countries (almost half of the studies were done in the United States), which met modern criteria of acoustic surroundings and psychoacoustic procedures. The agreement among these studies was found to be quite good; and all of them differed clearly from the 1951 American standard. After several years of calculation and discussion these data were combined to form a truly international standard reference zero for the uniform calibration of pure-tone audiometers.[2] This standard was approved by the Council of the ISO in 1963 without a dissenting vote and the recommendation is being published in 1964.

In 1959, while discussions of the international zero reference level were still in progress, the Committee on Conservation of Hearing of the American Academy of Ophthalmology and Otolaryngology endorsed the principle of such an International Standard. The Committee recognized explicitly that the international standard would probably be quite close to the British standard and significantly different from the 1951 American standard. The American Academy of Ophthalmology and Otolaryngology as a whole endorsed and accepted this principle in 1960. Similar endorsements were also voted by the American Otological Society and by the American Speech and Hearing Association. Now, in 1963, the Committee on Conservation of Hearing has reaffirmed its earlier endorsement and it expresses the strong hope that a new American Standard for Audiometers including the international zero reference level will be approved and adopted in the near future. The committee intends in any case to employ the international zero level and hopes that it will soon come into general use.

During the same period, 1958 to 1963, a writing group of the American Standards Association prepared a new American Standard for Audiometers. This draft combines in a single document and brings up to date the current American Standards entitled *Audiometers for General Diagnostic Purposes (Z24.3-1959)*, *Specification for Pure-Tone Audiometers for Screening Purposes (Z24.12-1952)* and *Specification for Speech Audiometers (Z24.13-1953)*. Most of the changes in substance are technical modifications, usually in the direction of specifying somewhat closer tolerances or making more explicit the statements of objectives and procedures. A major change, however, is the incorporation of the new ISO set of zero reference levels.

The proposed new American Standard for Audiometers was circulated in 1963 to the appropriate committee members of the American Standards Association for letter ballot. The editorial reorganization and the technical modifications met with unanimous approval, but several negative votes were cast on the basis of difficulties that might arise from the adoption of the international reference zero levels. The letter ballot has therefore been withdrawn to allow time for further consideration and explanation of the international reference levels and their implications.

ADVANTAGES

The case for the international (ISO) reference zero levels rests upon two propositions: (1) the change from the present (1951) American Standard to the new international levels is desirable, and (2) the change, although it will entail some temporary inconvenience during a transition period, can be made without jeopardy of any vital legal or financial interests.

There are three major reasons why the change in the standard reference threshold level is desirable. First, a general requirement of a standard is that it be based on measurements that can be reproduced with reasonable accuracy. It is true that results resembling the present American Standard are often obtained in tests made rather casually under so-called "clinical conditions," but the values so obtained scatter rather widely. On the other hand, threshold values obtained in all of the careful studies made under fully specified and reproducible conditions have centered quite closely around the new ISO standard. The 1951 American Standard has therefore only a limited inherent prestige, and although it has served a useful purpose it cannot possibly compete with the ISO standard for worldwide adoption.

Not only are the 1951 American Standard levels higher by about 10 dB on the average but the shape of the 1951 threshold contour

---

[2] ISO Technical Committee 43—Acoustics, No. 554, "A Standard Reference Zero for the Calibration of Pure-Tone Audiometers," American Standards Association, 10 East 40th Street, New York, N.Y.

differs significantly from that of the ISO. All of the studies on which the ISO Standard is based and also widespread clinical experience indicate that the contour of the 1951 American Standard is wrong. Our subjects' hearing thresholds regularly appear to be *relatively too good* at 250 and 500 c/s and to be *impaired* at 4 000 c/s. The so-called "4 000 cycle notch" in audiograms has been recognized for many years and has led to considerable concern on the part of otologists. At least a part of the notch is due to the faulty shape of our standard reference contour. Actually, as a numerical comparison of the two standards shows, the 1951 American Standard is relatively too lenient by about 5 dB at 250 and 500 c/s and is too stringent by about 5 dB at 4 000 c/s as compared with the middle and the two ends of the frequency scale. It is important for otologists and audiologists to correct this distortion because erroneous conclusions have been based on it in the past.

Finally, the use of a single international standard will terminate the confusion and ambiguity that now make it extremely difficult to compare audiometric measurements made in the United States with those made in Great Britain and Europe, where the British Standard is now employed. Practically speaking, it will soon be essential for any American otologist or audiologist writing for an international audience to employ the ISO Standard, and before many years the use of the ISO Standard will probably be required by most leading scientific journals.

DOUBTS AND DIFFICULTIES

Some of the arguments against adopting the ISO Standard hinge on the trouble it will cause or else on the expense of replacing or recalibrating the audiometers now in use. These arguments can be dealt with directly and briefly. Another class of objections hinges on questions of the legal status of the new and the old standards during the transition period and on possible misinterpretations of the implications of the new standard for the calculation of "percentage impairment of hearing." These doubts deserve full and careful consideration.

There is no denying that there will be some trouble and some confusion during the transition period which will follow the introduction of the ISO Standard. The difference in decibels is significant, and otologists and audiologists will have to learn to readjust their mental standards of what is within normal limits, what constitutes a significant hearing loss, etc. For several years it will be extremely important that every audiogram be clearly labelled to indicate the scale according to which it is plotted. Such difficulties always attend any significant change in a scale or reference standard. However, if the change is accepted as ultimately desirable and inevitable, the total amount of confusion and relearning is least if the change is made immediately, before any more students and technicians learn the old standards and before any more data are recorded on the old scale. Prompt and unified action represents the quickest and easiest way to the ultimate goal.

Clearly there should be no need for immediate replacement of old audiometers with new ones or even of immediate recalibration of old instruments. Recalibration to the new standard should be perfectly practical whenever an audiometer is returned to the manufacturer for recalibration, as it normally should be every year or two. Thus no great extra expense to users will be involved, nor will the facilities of the manufacturers of audiometers be taxed unduly.

The only valid reason for concern about the transition period, which will last for at least two or three years, is a doubt as to the legal status of records made during the transition period on old instruments that may not conform in all respects to the proposed new ASA Standard. To meet this difficulty, it should be easy to write into the standard itself an explicit statement concerning the transition period to the effect that, for all medico-legal purposes such as compensation, audiograms should be considered equally valid, regardless of the basis of the calibration of the audiometer, so long as the calibration is accurate by one scale or the other and provided it is clearly indicated on each audiogram *the scale according to which the hearing threshold levels are actually plotted*. As the relation between the 1951 American scale the ISO scale will be simply a matter of a difference of a few decibels at each frequency it will be easy to go from one scale to the other by simple additions or subtractions of these differences. A list of the differences and the rules for using them will be explicitly included as part of the next American Standard for Audiometers.

A POSSIBLE MISINTERPRETATION AND A CLARIFICATION

The most serious objection, which actually was the basis for most if not all of the negative votes cast against the new standard in the recent ballot of the American Standards Association, is the concern that a new zero reference level might establish automatically a new definition of "normal hearing"; and that consequently certain existing laws, rules and guides might be interpreted by lawyers or referees to mean that impairment of hearing would begin at the same number of decibels of "hearing loss" indicated on an audiometer calibrated to the new standard as it does on present audiometers. If this were done, however, the "percentage impairment" of a given listener would be significantly greater when measured with a new standard instrument than with present audiometers, and he would be entitled to greater compensation. This would be manifestly unfair and improper and would create an intolerable situation.

The term "percentage impairment of hearing" is used here, in accordance with AMA usage,[3] to designate the degree of handicap that is associated with a particular impairment of hearing. It implies a medical evaluation and is a percentage used in the calculation of compensation for industrial hearing loss. Different rules have been employed in different places and at different times to

[3] Committee on Medical Rating of Physical Impairment. Guides to the Evaluation of Permanent Impairment. *J. Am. Med. Assn.* 1958, 168: 475.

derive this "percentage impairment" from threshold measurements made with a pure-tone audiometer, but whatever rule is employed, it is perfectly obvious that the calculated percentage impairment of a listener's hearing must remain the same whether the audiometer is calibrated according to the old standard or a new one. Percentage impairment of hearing, i.e., hearing handicap, depends on a man's ability or inability to hear sounds of a certain physical intensity, but not on the scale used on the audiometer. *The proposed change in the audiometric reference zero must not be construed as altering in any way the evaluation of impairment of hearing. The only difference is to add one numerical detail of calculation.*

The American Standards Association is a voluntary organization and it has no legal authority to change, directly or indirectly, the amount of compensation that is related to a given degree of impairment. Neither can it decide what is "normal" in a medical or in a social sense. Too many shades of meaning are attached to the word "normal." We should think of a range of normal hearing, not of a single set of values. *The new reference zero levels are not designated as a "standard of normal hearing,"" either in the ISO recommendation or in the proposed American Standard.* For reference zero levels one particular set of values, one particular contour, must nevertheless be chosen. The zero contour must have the correct shape and lie at a well defined level. The ISO contour actually lies near one edge of the zone of normal hearing, and it is a more satisfactory base for audiometric measurements than the 1951 ASA levels. It is based on the hearing acuity of selected young individuals, tested by approved methods under perfect audiometric conditions.

What the adoption of the ISO standard will do is to establish a different relation between the number of decibels on the dial of an audiometer and the physical intensity of the sound that the instrument produces. But the percentage impairment of a listener must, of course, remain the same when his hearing is measured first on an audiometer with the old calibration and then on one with the new. A simple way to achieve this will be to subtract appropriate corrections, which will be given in the proposed new American Standard, from the readings made on the new scale.

The relation between the two audiometric scales and the relation of each to the range of normal hearing and to the scale of percentage impairment recommended by the American Academy of Ophthalmology and Otolaryngology (AAOO) are illustrated in the accompanying chart. Here the ISO scale is displaced upward relative to the 1951 ASA scale by 11 dB. The scale of percentage impairment may be entered from either of the audiometric scales. Note the wide range of normal hearing, which extends from the very best hearing threshold level measured under the best conditions to or nearly to the level at which impairment, in the sense of handicap, is considered to begin.

The rule for estimation of *percentage impairment* of hearing recommended by the AAOO in 1959 [4] refers to the average of the audiometric measurements made at the three frequencies 500, 1 000 and 2 000 c/s. The average of the readings for these three frequencies will be 11 dB higher if the audiometer is calibrated to the 1964 ISO values than if it is calibrated to the 1951 ASA values. Thus the appropriate correction for this average is 11 dB. *The subtraction of this correction should be regarded as a necessary and sufficient step in the technical procedure of audiometry under the new standard if the purpose of the measurement is to calculate percentage impairment of hearing under rules that were written before 1964.*

If and when a new American Standard for Audiometers incorporating the ISO zero reference level of 1964 is issued, the AAOO recommendation of 1959 should be modified to read: "For every decibel that the estimated hearing level for speech exceeds 15 dB by the American Standard of 1951 or 26 dB by the American Standard of 196–, allow one-and-one-half percent in impairment of hearing up to the maximum of 100 percent. This maximum is reached at 82 dB by the American

Standard of 1951 and at 93 dB by the American Standard of 196–." (The full titles of these standards are: "Audiometers for General Diagnostic Purposes," Z24.5-1951 and "American Standard Specifications for Audiometers," in preparation.) It will clarify the situation still further if the various states, organizations, and jurisdictions that have adopted similar rules make the corresponding amendments in due time.

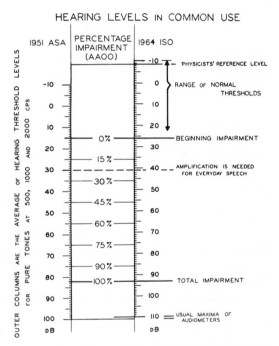

HEARING LEVELS IN COMMON USE

The center column represents percentage impairment of hearing, calculated according to the rule formulated by the Subcommittee on Noise in 1958 and adopted by the AAOO in 1959 for use in cases involving compensation. "1963 ISO" refers to the reference zero levels for pure-tone audiometers recommended by the International Organization for Standardization. (These levels were approved by that organization in 1963 but their publication will bear the date 1964.) "1951 ASA" refers to the audiometric scale defined in the American Standard for Audiometers for General Diagnostic Purposes, Z24.5-1951. The reference level for speech audiometers is the one written into the proposed (1963) revision of the American Standard for Audiometers, not yet approved. It differs by only 2 dB, however, from the present (1951) ASA standard. The reference level for speech audiometry is defined in terms of a 1 000 c/s calibration tone and therefore its relation to the scales in the figure, which represent the averages of hearing levels for three frequencies, is not exact.

[4] Report of the Committee on Conservation of Hearing. D. M. Lierle Chairman. Guide for the Evaluation of Hearing Impairment. *Trans. Amer. Acad. Ophthal. Otolaryngol.*, 1959, 63: 238.

During a transition period of several years many old audiometers already in use will still be calibrated according to the American Standard of 1951 while new instruments will be calibrated according to the proposed new standard. The basis of calibration will, of course, be clearly marked on each new instrument. "Hearing threshold level," not "hearing loss," will be the designation on the intensity dials of the new audiometers. But on each audiogram that is recorded during the transition period, it will be absolutely essential to indicate whether the hearing levels are expressed in terms of the 1951 ASA or the 1964 ISO values. Boxes for checking one or the other or an explicit statement will be printed on every audiogram blank.

PERTINENT EXCERPTS FROM THE PROPOSED NEW AMERICAN STANDARD

The proposed new American Standard for Audiometers includes a list of the exact differences in decibels at each frequency between the 1951 ASA and the 1964 ISO reference threshold levels, and also several statements which are pertinent to the problem of estimating percentage impairment of hearing. They read as follows:

"Transition to Hearing Threshold Level

"The standard reference threshold levels given in Table 2 of this standard are those adopted by the International Organization for Standardization (ISO). These values differ considerably from those which have been in use in the U.S.A. since 1939, officially adopted in 1951 and given in Table 2 of the American Standard Specification for Audiometers for General Diagnostic Purposes, Z24.5-1951. The latter may conveniently be termed the 1951 ASA values.

"The following table gives these two sets of reference threshold values, in terms of the Western Electric 705-A earphone and the 9-A coupler. The numerical values given in the 1951 specification have been shifted by 74 dB to put them on the basis of 0.0002 microbar, and have been rounded off to the nearest 0.5 dB to accord with the ISO method of presentation.

"There will inevitably be a period of time during which there are in use some audiometers calibrated to the 1951 ASA threshold levels and some calibrated to the 1964 ISO threshold levels. In order to facilitate the orderly transition from the use of the one set of reference levels to the other, it is strongly recommended that the following procedures be adopted.

1. Audiometers calibrated to the 1964 ISO values are to be identified by the designation 'Hearing Threshold Level—ISO 1964' for the attenuator dial.

2. On an audiogram form, the vertical scale is to be designated 'Hearing Threshold

| Frequency | Reference Threshold Levels | | |
	1951 ASA	1964 ISO	Differences
125	54.5 dB	45.5 dB	9 dB
250	39.5	24.5	15
500	25	11	14
1 000	16.5	6.5	10
1 500	(16.5)	6.5	(10)
2 000	17	8.5	8.5
3 000	(16.)	7.5	(8.5)
4 000	15	9.	6.
6 000	(17.5)	8.	(9.5)
8 000	21	9.5	11.5

The figures in parentheses are interpolations.

Level in dB.' During the transition period, the horizontal scale is to be labeled as follows:

Frequency, c/s

| 125 | 250 | 500 | 1 000 | 1 500 |

Difference in dB
(1964 vs. 1951)

| 9 | 15 | 14* | 10 | 10 |

Frequency, c/s *(cont.)*

| 2 000 | 3 000 | 4 000 | 6 000 | 8 000 |

Difference in dB *(cont.)*

| 8.5 | 8.5 | 6.0 | 9.5 | 11.5 |

[* Incorrectly appeared as 15 dB in the original article. HD, FWK]

3. The audiogram form is to include the following notations:

This audiogram is plotted on the basis of:

☐ 1964 ISO reference thresholds
☐ 1951 ASA reference thresholds
(Check one of these squares)

Readings obtained on an audiometer calibrated to the 1951 ASA thresholds may be converted to, and plotted as, 'Hearing Threshold Levels' based on the 1964 ISO reference thresholds by *adding* the appropriate 'Difference in dB' at each frequency. To convert readings based on the 1964 ISO reference thresholds to readings based on the 1951 ASA reference thresholds, *subtract* the 'Difference in dB.'

4. On the audiogram form, the line of 'Difference in dB' may be in smaller type than the 'Frequency' line. Also the last two sentences of 3 may be so located on the audiogram that their reproduction in a journal may be conveniently optional."

"Percentage Impairment of Hearing

"In adopting the ISO reference levels in place of the reference levels of Z24.5-1951, the American Standards Association does not intend or imply that any change should be made in other standards or rules based on the 1951 levels. In particular, *until the rules for compensation purposes have been modified by the appropriate organizations or jurisdictions to recognize specifically the new reference levels, all measurements of hearing threshold level made according to the ISO scale shall be converted to 1951 ASA values before the calculations for compensation purposes are made.* In accordance with Appendix (C), this conversion is made by subtracting the 'dB Differences' there given from the values of hearing threshold level measured with an audiometer calibrated to the 1964 ISO values."

"Relation to other Standards

"Similar conversions to 1951 ASA values shall be made before applying the specifications as to hearing loss mentioned in American Standard Method for the Measurement of Real-Ear Attenuation of Ear Protectors at Threshold, Z24.22-1957.

"The American Standard Criteria for Background Noise in Audiometer Rooms, S1.3-1960, is only indirectly involved. Its specifications are not sufficiently stringent to ensure measurement at ISO hearing threshold levels at all frequencies. The standard remains unaffected, however, until its next revision. Where reference is made therein to the zero hearing threshold level of American Standard audiometers, it shall be clearly understood that it still means the American Standards of 1951 and 1952."

APPROVAL BY THE COMMITTEE ON CONSERVATION OF HEARING [5]

As noted above, the 1963 ISO reference zero levels for pure-tone audiometers are more reproducible as to level and more accurate as to the shape of their contour than the (1951) American Standard levels. For these reasons, and in the interest of international standardization, the Committee on Conservation of Hearing of the American Academy of Ophthalmology and Otolaryngology voted, on 8 December 1963, to adopt for its own use the new ISO standard values, as of 1 January 1965. The Committee expresses the hope that the proposed revised American Standard for Audiometers, incorporating the ISO reference zero levels, will soon be approved and brought into general use.

[5] This article was prepared for and approved by the Subcommittee on Noise, and approved in principle on 8 December 1963 by the Committee on Conservation of Hearing of the American Academy of Ophthalmology and Otolaryngology. The senior author is a member of the Subcommittee on Noise of the Committee on Conservation of Hearing of the American Academy of Ophthalmology and Otolaryngology. The co-author is chairman of the Writing Group on Audiometers of the American Standards Association.

Preparation of this article was supported by Public Health Service Program Project Grant, No. B-3856, from the National Institute of Neurological Diseases and Blindness to Central Institute for the Deaf.

3

A Clinical Method for
Calibrating the Bone–Conduction Audiometer

ROBERT E. ROACH
RAYMOND CARHART

ROBERT E. ROACH, Ph.D., is Professor of Audiology and Director, Hearing Clinic, School of Medicine, University of Alabama in Birmingham

RAYMOND CARHART, Ph.D., is Professor of Audiology, Northwestern University

The clinician who wishes to make full use of pure-tone audiograms needs a valid and simple method for ensuring that the calibration for his bone-conduction system is adequate. Unfortunately, we lack a standard procedure whereby the physicist can specify for us the vibrational output representing bone-conduction norms.[1] For the time being the clinician must therefore rely upon his own efforts to assure himself that his bone measurements are acceptable. Even after a physical standard is established, the need will remain for an easy and adequate method of checking calibration in a clinical situation.

There are three calibrational methods from which the clinician can choose. The first method utilizes loudness balancing, the second is based on thresholds yielded by normal listeners, while the third relies on the responses of cases with sensorineural (or nerve-type) loss.

The loudness-balance method is advocated by Beranek as a means of transferring air-conduction norms to a bone-conduction system. However, the technique possesses three practical disadvantages. First, the equipment necessary for loudness matching is not available in all clinical situations. Second, recent studies of "on-effect" and "adaptation"[2]

clearly imply that very insightful control of the conditions must be maintained for loudness balances to be valid. Lastly, the matching of a bone-conduction sound to the loudness of a monaural air-borne stimulus will be in error because the bone-conduction stimulus will reach both ears unless the contralateral ear is effectively masked (5). Consequently, insofar as the clinical situation is concerned, there is need for a simpler yet valid procedure.

A second approach is to establish the reference values for a bone-conduction system by averaging the bone thresholds exhibited by subjects with normal hearing.[3] This approach has high face validity, and it has been widely accepted. It is, for example, the method which was specified in the American Medical Association requirements for a diagnostic pure-tone audiometer (7). These requirements define the reference threshold, at each test frequency, as the "hearing loss setting of the audiometer" representing the average of the bone thresholds obtained on six subjects with normal acuity. Only measurements on un-occluded ears are to be considered, and all tests are to be conducted ". . . in a room free from extraneous sound of sufficient intensity to vitiate the measurements" (7). Unfortunately,

---

Reprinted by permission of the authors from *Arch. Otolaryngol.*, **63,** pp. 270–279 (1956).

[1] References *1* and *2*.

[2] References *3* and *4*.

[3] Some workers prefer computing the reference values from medians or modes rather than from means (Harris *6*). The distinction probably has more theoretical than clinical importance.

there are numerous clinical situations where this last requirement cannot be easily met. Many audiometric rooms which are adequate for testing normal listeners when they have the extra protection of ear cushions possess ambient noise which is intense enough to mask these same persons when their ears are unoccluded. In other words, a room may be fully usable for air-conduction audiometry without being quiet enough to yield uncontaminated measures of normal threshold for bone. In practice, this fact means that the wise clinician will not attempt to calibrate his bone-conduction system on normal ears unless he is certain the noise level in his testing room is so low it will not influence his subjects.

The third method, which utilizes the responses of persons with hearing loss, was described by Carhart as a means of escaping the influences of unavoidable room noise (8). The method allows the clinician to take advantage of two facts. First, a moderate hearing loss offers protection against the masking effect of mild ambient noise. Second, persons with pure sensorineural loss possess the same impairment whether tested by air or by bone. The procedure involves obtaining both air- and bone-conduction thresholds, in a reasonably quiet room, on a group of ears with impairments of the sensorineural variety. The responses at each test frequency are averaged separately for air and for bone. The clinician must have assured himself in advance that his air-conduction system is in acceptable calibration. This being the case, substantial discrepancies between the two sets of averages represent the corrections required to bring the bone system into calibration. It is a simple matter, once this information is available, to apply these corrections in subsequent clinical testing. Audiometric curves incorporating these corrections should show the proper relation between a patient's loss by bone and the normal reference line on the audiogram chart.

While Carhart's method appears theoretically sound and it is adaptable to most situations, we still need to assure ourselves through appropriate experimentation that it can yield a valid reference level for bone-conduction audiometry. Here, the obvious test of validity is whether normal ears exhibit the anticipated threshold readings for bone when tested with a system calibrated on ears with sensorineural involvement. Validatory measurements must, of course, be made in an environment sufficiently quiet to avoid danger of any masking when testing by either modality. If, under these circumstances, the normal group's average audiogram for air agrees with its average audiogram for bone, Carhart's method will have been shown to be capable of yielding a valid "zero loss" level from which to estimate hearing acuity by bone conduction.[4] In other words, the final criterion for validity of a threshold reference level is that persons without hearing loss shall obtain thresholds which are labeled as normal when they are tested with the system under scrutiny.

The degree to which Carhart's proposal can satisfy this criterion was explored experimentally with a commercial audiometer. The adequacy of this instrument's air-conduction system was first assured through appropriate electroacoustic measurements. Next, a corrected calibration for its bone-conduction system was computed from the responses of 23 ears having sensorineural, or nerve-type, impairments. Thirdly, thresholds for air and bone were obtained on 127 normal ears. Finally, these data were examined statistically to ascertain the adequacy of the corrected calibration assigned to the bone-conduction system.

APPARATUS

The audiometer selected was a Maico E-2.[5] To simplify procedures, only one of the instrument's two channels was employed throughout the study. Both the air- and the bone-conduc-

---

[4] Even if the method is demonstrated to be valid in the sense that it brings the two systems into calibrational agreement, we must remember that the adequacy achieved in a given clinical situation will depend upon the accuracy with which the air-conduction system has been calibrated.

[5] The Maico Company kindly made this instrument available.

tion receivers were activated through this channel. The air-conduction receiver was a Permoflux PDR-10, in a Maico cushion. The bone-conduction receiver was of the hearing-aid variety.[6]

The physical performance of the audiometer was assessed carefully.[7] The instrument satisfied the requirements for a diagnostic audiometer (7). Test frequencies were within appropriate limits of accuracy. The attenuation system was acceptably linear. Harmonic distortion was adequately controlled. The instrument was suitably free from internal noise, and its bone oscillator did not produce excess sound radiation by air.

The acoustic output of the air-conduction system was measured, in a 6 cc. coupler of the 9A type, with a 640AA microphone. The sound pressure levels for the "zero hearing loss" settings of the audiometer were found to be within 3 db. of the correct value for the earphone involved, except for a discrepancy of 4.6 db. at 8000 cps. These values are within the limits designated for commercial audiometers (10). On this basis we can state that the air-conduction system employed in the present study was correctly calibrated within the accuracy required for clinical audiometry.

The vibrational output of the bone-conduction oscillator was investigated, in relative terms, with an artificial mastoid.[8] The performance of the bone-conduction channel proved quite satisfactory except for some excess harmonic distortion at high output levels for 250 cps.

Special precautions were taken to assure that the audiometer remained stable throughout the entire time span of the study. These precautions involved daily measurement of the acoustic and vibrational outputs of the

air and bone channels, respectively. Analysis of these measurements revealed excellent stability in physical performance.

EMPIRICAL CALIBRATION OF THE BONE-CONDUCTION SYSTEM

In order to obtain a group on which to establish an empirical calibration of the bone-conduction system, 23 persons with pure sensorineural losses of intermediate severity were chosen from the case files of the Northwestern University Hearing Clinic. All these persons had been diagnosed by staff otologists as having pure sensorineural (or nerve-type) hearing losses. There were 5 cases of presbycusis, 2 of labyrinthine hydrops, 2 with congenital impairments, and 14 due to miscellaneous or unknown causes. No attempt was made to control the sex or age distribution of the group. The group included 12 men and 11 women. The age range was from 17 to 77 years, with an average age of 50.7 years.

Each subject was given an audiometric test by both air and bone in a room with superior acoustic characteristics. The ascending method, as advocated by Hughson and Westlake (11), was employed. Only the data for each subject's better ear were used. Consequently, masking was not employed. To obtain bone measurements the oscillator was first positioned at the point on the mastoid yielding maximum sensitivity with 1000 cps as the stimulus. Thresholds for all frequencies were then determined without shifting the bone unit. Subjects were closely questioned to ascertain whether the sensation was contralateralized. Properly ipsilateralized threshold responses for bone were obtained from 23 subjects at 250 cps, 18 at 500 cps, 21 at 1000 cps, 18 at 1500 cps, 16 at 2000 cps, 13 at 3000 cps, and 19 at 4000 cps. These responses, and their comparison responses for air conduction, constitute the data from which the empirical calibration of the bone system was compiled.

Table 3-1 summarizes, in the form of means

---

[6] This bone oscillator was incorporated in the audiometer at our request. So far as we know, the Maico Company has never advocated using this type of receiver with its E-2 audiometer. Therefore, the results we report here do not indicate the performance of the instrument when equipped with the larger bone receiver, which is the standard accessory for the E-2.

[7] Details are reported in Roach (9).

[8] The Sonotone Corporation kindly supplied detailed plans for this unit.

TABLE 3-1. MEAN AUDIOMETRIC SETTINGS REPRESENTING THE AIR-CONDUCTION AND THE BONE-CONDUCTION THRESHOLDS OF TWENTY-THREE EARS WITH SENSORINEURAL IMPAIRMENT (EXPRESSED IN DECIBELS RE THE ZERO SETTING OF THE HEARING-LOSS DIAL)

Frequency	Air	Bone	Difference Between Settings
250	13.7	37.2	23.5
500	20.3	46.1	25.8
1000	39.0	41.9	2.9
1500	44.7	49.2	4.5
2000	43.4	49.7	6.3
3000	42.4	50.0	7.6
4000	42.9	43.2	0.3

for the group, the results at each frequency. The table also reports the difference, or discrepancy, at a given frequency between the mean for air thresholds and the mean for bone thresholds. These discrepancies, according to Carhart's premise, represent the approximate corrections required to equate the air- and bone-conduction systems.

Higher hearing-loss dial readings were required to reach bone-conduction thresholds than to reach air-conduction thresholds at all frequencies except 4000 cps. This fact indicates that, at a given dial reading, the bone-conduction system produced a weaker stimulus in the inner ear than did the air-conduction system at the same frequency. Since, in the present instance, the air-conduction system was found to be in satisfactory calibration, the various discrepancies were judged to reveal the amounts by which bone-conduction reading obtained with this particular audiometer should be reduced in order to yield true indications of the thresholds they represent. In other words, corrected thresholds, estimated to the nearest 5 db., should be computed by subtracting the following values from the hearing-loss dial readings when testing by bone:

> 25 db. at 250 cps
> 25 db. at 500 cps
> 5 db. at 1000 cps
> 5 db. at 1500 cps
> 5 db. at 2000 cps
> 10 db. at 3000 cps
> None at 4000 cps

Stated differently, these corrections represent the establishment of empirically revised norms for measuring bone-conduction acuity with the audiometer under study.

VALIDATORY TEST OF EMPIRICAL CALIBRATION

The question which interests us now is whether corrections established by the method just outlined are valid in the sense that they yield the same base of reference as would have been computed directly from the bone-conduction responses of normal ears. This question is easily attacked. One must first administer pure-tone tests to a group of subjects known to have normal hearing. One must then compare the estimate of the group's acuity by air with its apparent acuity by bone. Provided the two estimates of acuity are in close agreement, the bone system may be said to have essentially the same base of reference as the air-conduction system.

In the present instance, 127 college undergraduates constituted the group of normal listeners employed to make this test.[9] The age range of the group was from 17 to 27 years, with the mean age being 18.5 years. The group included 44 men and 83 women.

This phase of the study required a testing room so quiet that its ambient noise would not mask unoccluded normal ears. The room used had a noise level of less than 24 db. when measured with a sound-level meter set to the A scale.

Thresholds for both air and bone were again determined by the ascending method. It had been decided to use data on only one ear per subject. Selection of this ear was random except in those instances where the bone-conduction stimulus appeared to the subject to be contralateralized.[10] When this

[9] These cases satisfied Beasley's criterion for normal hearing by air conduction, except for a few subjects with mild high-frequency losses (Beasley *12*).
[10] Masking of the opposite ear was not employed, since Cochran has demonstrated that even a mild noise in one ear may change appreciably the threshold of the other ear (Cochran *13*).

occurred, the data for the other ear were used unless contralateralization was also evident here, in which event the subject was discarded. The 127 subjects whose thresholds were analyzed each had an ear satisfying this criterion.

The threshold responses for air conduction were recorded without modification, but audiometric readings were corrected by the values mentioned earlier, in order to obtain the estimated thresholds for bone.[11] The criterion by which the validity of the empirical calibration of the bone system was judged was the agreement to be found between the air-conduction thresholds of the 127 normal ears under study and the corrected measures of their bone-conduction acuity.

TABLE 3-2. MEAN ACUITY FOR THE BETTER EAR EXHIBITED BY 127 UNIVERSITY STUDENTS (EXPRESSED AS DECIBELS OF HEARING LOSS RE THE CORRECTED AUDIOMETRIC NORMAL)

Frequency	Air Mean	Bone Mean	Difference *	t-Ratio †
250	−7.3	−5.5	−1.8	5.43
500	−5.9	−6.9	1.0	3.49
1000	−4.8	−5.9	1.1	3.59
1500	−4.9	−6.4	1.5	3.90
2000	−3.9	−3.5	−0.4	1.04
3000	−3.9	−4.5	0.6	1.38
4000	−6.7	−4.2	−2.5	6.03

* A negative difference indicates poorer bone-conduction threshold.

† t-Ratio of 1.98 and 2.62 significant, respectively, at 5 percent and 1 percent levels.

Table 3-2 summarizes group means for air and for bone. All group means for air conduction are negative. This fact indicates that the 127 ears under study were, as a group, slightly hyperacute relative to the "average normal threshold." This result is exactly what would be expected in testing a large

[11] Actually, data from two complete tests on each subject were available. These tests, spaced about a month apart, were administered to gather information on the test-retest reliability of pure-tone audiometry. It was felt that, for present purposes, the average of a subject's two responses for a given test condition would give an improved indication of the subject's acuity. The discussion which follows is based on such an averaging of the test-retest data.

group of young college students, and it is consistent with other investigations of undergraduates at Northwestern University.

Group means for bone conduction were also negative to approximately the same degree. As is summarized in Table 3-2, the discrepancy between the means for air and bone conduction is 1.5 db. or less for five of the seven test frequencies. The differences which exceeded 1.5 db. were 1.8 db. at 250 cps and 2.5 db. at 4000 cps. Even these two latter discrepancies are small enough to be of little importance to the clinician. Moreover, the means for air conduction are not consistently higher or lower than the means for bone.

Despite the fact that the discrepancies just mentioned are too small to have much clinical meaning, most of them were statistically significant. Specifically, five of the seven t-ratios reported in Table 3-2 substantially exceed the 1 percent level of confidence. One may conclude that the discrepancies are a result of a minor yet real margin of uncertainty arising because correction values could be assigned to the bone-conduction system only to the nearest 5 db. interval. For this reason alone, any single correction might deviate by as much as 2.5 db. from the proper value. Fortunately, a systematic calibrational deviation of 2.5 db. or less does not destroy the clinical meaning of a bone-conduction measurement.

In the present instance, there is absolutely no evidence that the method employed for calibrating the bone-conduction system yielded a false base of references. The audiometer labeled normal ears as having, in the aggregate, the bone-conduction acuity which their measured acuity for air conduction required. Thus, calibration of the bone-conduction system on the basis of responses by patients with sensorineural loss has here been demonstrated to yield reference values which are clinically equivalent to those which would have been obtained had the calibration been based on the responses of normal ears.

Further confirmation of the general adequacy of the bone-conduction measurements obtained on the 127 normal ears is found in (1) comparison of population variability for the two stimulus modalities and (2) correlation between the air- and bone-conduction thresholds.

As regards population variability, the two modalities yielded threshold data which were very similar in range and distribution. This fact is illustrated in Table 3-3.

TABLE 3-3. RANGES AND STANDARD DEVIATIONS OF THRESHOLDS FOR AIR CONDUCTION AND FOR BONE CONDUCTION EXHIBITED BY 127 NORMAL EARS, EXPRESSED IN DECIBELS

| Frequency | Range | | Standard Deviation | | |
	Air	Bone	Air	Bone	Difference *
250	17.5	15.0	3.3	3.9	0.6
500	15.0	17.5	3.8	3.5	0.3
1000	17.5	17.5	3.9	4.4	−0.5
1500	22.5	15.0	4.7	4.6	0.1
2000	20.0	20.0	5.2	5.9	−0.7
3000	42.5	37.5	7.0	6.3	0.7
4000	25.0	30.0	5.1	5.6	−0.5

* A negative difference indicates that the S.D. for bone is greater than the S.D. for air.

It is particularly instructive to observe the differences between the standard deviations for air and bone which are reported in the sixth column of the table.[12] These differences are all numerically small and do not represent a clinically important distinction in the variability of air- and bone-conduction results for the 127 normal ears under consideration.

The correlation between the air- and bone-conduction thresholds exhibited by individual subjects was found to be very good, as can be seen by noting the product-moment coefficients reported in Table 3-4. The coefficients range between +0.48 and +0.76. Coefficients of this magnitude indicate a high interdependence, since they were derived from data on normal ears which encompassed relatively narrow ranges. Theoretically, such

[12] The standard deviations were found to be progressively larger as the test frequency became higher. This trend is common to both the air- and the bone-conduction data. It merely indicates that the population of "normal" ears under study possessed greater variability in acuity for higher-pitched tones.

TABLE 3-4. COEFFICIENTS OF CORRELATION BETWEEN THE THRESHOLDS FOR AIR CONDUCTION AND THE CORRECTED THRESHOLDS FOR BONE CONDUCTION

Frequency	Product-Moment r
250	0.48
500	0.57
1000	0.65
1500	0.58
2000	0.60
3000	0.76
4000	0.64

interdependence should exist if the testing environment and the testing procedures are adequate. Its manifestation in the present instance adds greatly to the confidence we may have in both the air- and bone-conduction measurements obtained on the 127 normal ears. We therefore accept these measurements with greater surety as a means of confirming the adequacy of Carhart's empirical method for establishing the zero reference level for a bone-conduction system.

COMMENT

It has often been emphasized that the median is a more accurate statement of the central tendency of data involving decibel values than the mean (14). Hence, if the primary interest in the present study had been to express the numerical values of the central tendencies with the greatest precision, medians should have been used. However, the main concern in the present instance was with the discrepancy between the central tendencies in the air- and bone-conduction measures obtained on the 23 cases with sensorineural loss. There is no reason to believe that the span between these central tendencies would have been more accurately expressed by considering medians than means. The same argument applies when comparing the threshold data yielded by the 127 normals. Hence, since tests of statistical significance are more easily applied when means are employed, the latter were chosen as the basis for the analysis reported above.

The propriety of this decision can be easily checked by ascertaining what differences would have resulted had the interpretation been based on medians.

TABLE 3-5. MEDIAN AUDIOMETRIC SETTINGS REPRESENTING THE AIR-CONDUCTION AND BONE-CONDUCTION THRESHOLDS OF TWENTY-THREE EARS WITH SENSORINEURAL IMPAIR-MENTS (EXPRESSED IN DECIBELS RE THE ZERO SETTING OF THE HEARING-LOSS DIAL)

Frequency	Air	Bone	Difference Between Settings
250	15.0	41.3	26.3
500	20.0	45.8	25.8
1000	38.7	41.2	2.5
1500	45.0	52.5	7.5
2000	46.3	53.8	7.5
3000	47.8	51.8	4.0
4000	46.3	44.4	−1.9

Table 3-5 presents the median audiometric settings for the 23 cases of sensorineural loss and reports the discrepancies between their corresponding air- and bone-conduction medians. Assuming that no correction in the reference for the bone system is necessary until the difference exceeds 2.5 db., the pattern of correction called for by Table 3-5 becomes 25 db. at 250 and 500 cps; no correction at 1000 cps; 5 db. at 1500, 2000, and 3000 cps; nothing at 4000 cps. These corrections are the same as those derived from consideration of means except at 1000 and 3000 cps, where in each instance the correction based on medians is 5 db. less than the one based on means.

These two disagreements, while not large, do raise the question as to which criterion of central tendency in this instance yielded the superior calibration. One method of examining this question is to compute the calibrations which would have been assigned to the bone system if it had been derived from the responses of the 127 normal ears. In this instance the discrepancy between the actual audiometric settings yielding air and bone thresholds of the normal group indicates the magnitude of the correction required by the bone-conduction system. This discrepancy was computed, for each test frequency separately, from the median audiometer readings for the 127 normal ears and, independently, from the mean audiometric readings. The results are reported in Table 3-6. If calibration of the bone conduction had been based on these data, the correction factors reported in Table 3-7 would have applied. Here, too, corrections are in 5 db. steps and differences of 2.5 db. or less have been disregarded. For purposes of comparison the corrections derived from the responses of the 23 cases of sensorineural are also reported in Table 3-7. A "best estimate" is also reported. This estimate is the correction most often called for at each test frequency.

Two generalizations are quickly apparent from Table 3-7.

First, there appears to have been a real discrepancy in the correction required by the two populations at 1500 cps. The normal group showed such close agreement between the median scores for air and bone, as well as between mean scores, that no correction

TABLE 3-6. DISCREPANCIES BETWEEN THE CENTRAL TENDENCIES OF THE UNCORRECTED SETTINGS OF THE HEARING-LOSS DIAL (RAW SCORES) FOR AIR AND BONE CONDUCTION REPRESENTING THRESHOLD RESPONSES OF 127 NORMAL EARS

Frequency	Group Median			Group Mean		
	Air	Bone	Difference	Air	Bone	Difference
250	−8.4	18.7	27.1	−7.3	19.1	26.4
500	−6.2	17.1	23.3	−5.9	17.3	23.2
1000	−5.0	−2.0	3.0	−4.8	−1.6	3.2
1500	−5.4	−4.2	0.8	−4.9	−3.3	1.6
2000	−4.9	−0.1	4.8	−3.9	1.1	5.0
3000	−5.3	−3.0	8.3	−3.9	4.7	8.6
4000	−8.7	−5.0	3.7	−6.7	−4.2	2.5

TABLE 3-7. THE SUMMARY OF CORRECTIONS IN THE CALIBRATION OF BONE-CONDUCTION SYSTEM REQUIRED BY VARIOUS ESTIMATES OF CENTRAL TENDENCY

Frequency	Normal Ears Median	Mean	Impaired Ears Median	Mean	Best Estimate
250	25	25	25	25	25
500	25	25	25	25	25
1000	5	5	0	5	5
1500	0	0	5	5	0 or 5
2000	5	5	5	5	5
3000	10	10	5	10	10
4000	5	0	0	0	0

appears necessary. Both sets of statistics for the hard of hearing population suggest the bone system is 5 db. weak. If one accepts the responses of the normals as the criterion of validity, then the calibration of the bone system based on responses of impaired ears proved at 1500 cycles to be 5 db. in error. Such a finding should serve as a warning to the clinician, since it indicates that errors can occur even when calibration of a bone system is based on carefully selected cases of sensorineural loss. Equally important, however, is the fact that only one such error was here observed and that it had a magnitude of only 5 db. We may retain the conclusion that a bone system can be empirically calibrated on sensorineural losses to a precision which has reasonable clinical accuracy.

Second, the corrections derived from comparison of means, whether for normals or for hard of hearing subjects, are the more defensible in the present study. It would be hazardous to presume that this situation would always apply, but in the present instance the two sets of corrections based on means were in perfect agreement at all test frequencies except 1500 cps. Concomitantly, at least one of the estimates derived from the comparison of medians was in agreement with the two estimates from means. On the other hand, if either set of medians is used as the basis for calibrating the bone system, the median response of the other population is in disagreement by one correction step (5 db.) at four of the seven test frequencies.

SUMMARY

The present study was undertaken to determine if it is possible to establish a clinically acceptable reference level for bone-conduction audiometry by comparing air- and bone-conduction responses yielded by subjects with sensorineural loss. The study has demonstrated that a clinically acceptable reference level can be achieved in this manner. A commercial audiometer whose air-conduction system met current standards for adequate calibration and performance was used. Standard audiometric tests by air and bone conduction were then administered to 23 cases diagnosed as having pure sensorineural loss. The corrections required by the bone-conduction system of the audiometer were computed to the nearest 5 db. These corrections were based on the premise that, since the air-conduction system was in calibration, any sizable discrepancy between the group's apparent acuity level by air and bone was due to incorrect calibration of the bone-conduction system.

The adequacy of these corrections was subsequently confirmed by testing 127 normal listeners in a sound-proof chamber of research caliber. Had the original calibration been based on the performance of these normal listeners, exactly the same corrections would have been obtained except at 1500 cps. Even at 1500 cps, the error in the calibration based on sensorineural losses was only 5 db.

Thus a useful set of reference values for the bone-conduction system was here achieved with an empirical procedure utilizing the responses of selected cases with hearing loss. The procedure offers the otologist, the audiologist, and the audiometrician a method for achieving a reasonable calibration of his bone-conduction system which is free from the pitfalls which plague the clinician when he tries to calibrate his bone system on normal listeners in the usual office environment.

REFERENCES

1. Carlisle, R. W., and Pearson, H. A.: A Strain-Gauge Type of Artificial Mastoid, J. Acoust. Soc. America **23**:300–302, 1951.

2. Beranek, L.: Acoustic Measurements, New York, John Wiley & Sons, Inc., 1949, p. 370.

3. Hallpike, C. S., and Hood, J. D.: Some Recent Work on Auditory Adaptation and Its Relationship to the Loudness Recruitment Problem, J. Accoust. Soc. America **23**:270–274, 1951.

4. Dix, M. R., and Hood, J. D.: Modern Development in Pure Tone Audiometry and Their Application to the Clinical Diagnosis of End-Organ Deafness, Proc. Roy. Soc. Med. **46**:992–994, 1953.

5. Zwislocki, J.: Über die Lautstärkeempfindung bei Knochenleitung, Acta oto-laryng. **37**:239–244, 1949.

6. Harris, J. D.: Normal Hearing and Its Relation to Audiometry, Laryngoscope **64**:928–957, 1954.

7. Minimum Requirement for Acceptable Pure Tone Audiometers for Diagnostic Purposes, Council on Physical Medicine and Rehabilitation, J.A.M.A. **146**: 255–257, 1951.

8. Carhart, R.: Clinical Application of Bone Conduction Audiometry, Arch. Otolaryng. **51**:789–807, 1950.

9. Roach, R. E.: A Study of the Reliability and Validity of Bone Conduction Audiometry, Dissertation, Northwestern University, 1951.

10. Audiometers for General Diagnostic Purposes, Z24:5, New York, American Standards Association, 1951.

11. Hughson, W., and Westlake, H.: Manual for Program Outline for Rehabilitation of Aural Casualties Both Military and Civilian, Tr. Am. Acad. Ophth., Supp., pp. 1-15, 1944.

12. Beasley, D.: Normal Hearing by Air and Bone Conduction, Hearing Study Series, Bulletin 4, National Health Survey, Washington, D.C., 1935–1936.

13. Cochran, M.: Masking in Audiometry, M. A. Thesis, Northwestern University, 1946.

14. Stevens, S. S.: On the Averaging of Data, Science **121**:113–116, 1955.

4

The Standardization of Bone–Conduction Thresholds

GERALD A. STUDEBAKER

GERALD A. STUDEBAKER, Ph.D., is Associate Professor, University of Oklahoma Medical Center

The need for a normal hearing reference for bone-conduction measurements has existed for many years; however, it is only within the past several years that success has seemed within reach. An artificial mastoid is now available that is immune to the effects of ageing and that can be manufactured to close tolerances permitting comparisons across individual units of the same model.

Early artificial mastoids had, as a principal component, a viscoelastic pad upon which the vibrator was placed (*1*, *2*, *3*, *4*). The pads were used to simulate the skin over the mastoid process; however, very little information about the impedance of the human mastoid was available at that time. At best, viscoelastic pads represented a first order approximation. A close evaluation reveals considerable differences in the impedance of skin and bone from that of viscoelastic pads backed by metal.

These early artificial mastoids suffered from other, equally important, limitations: first, the viscoelastic materials were susceptible to ageing effects in the form of hardening and gradual breakdown of the material; second, the transmission properties of the pads varied considerably as a function of temperature; and finally, the properties of the materials varied from sample to sample. For these reasons, readings obtained on the viscoelastic artificial mastoids varied as a function of time and temperature, and the results could be

Reprinted by permission of the author from *Laryngoscope*, **77**, pp. 823–835 (1967).

expected to differ across individual units of the mastoid (*5*).

In 1955, Corliss and Koidan (*6*) reported on their investigations of the impedance of the human mastoid and forehead. These results, with some revisions presented by Cook (*7*) in 1959, were utilized by Weiss (*5*) to develop an artificial mastoid which departed significantly from earlier designs. This bone-conduction vibrator coupler is described by Weiss as an air-damped artificial mastoid.

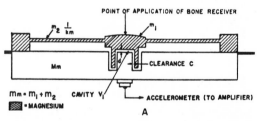

Figure 4-1. A cross-sectional drawing of the air-damped artificial mastoid. (After Weiss [5].)

Figure 4-1 shows a cross sectional drawing of the artificial mastoid. The unit consists of a small mass (Mm equals $m_1 + m_2$) and a large mass (Mm) which are in contact only at the edges. The small mass seen from above consists of a circular disc a little over one inch in diameter from which extend three "spokes" (m_2) which are clamped to the large mass at their extremities. In the center, the two major masses are constructed to form a piston and cylinder with a circular upward extension of the large mass forming the piston and a downward "skirt-like" extension of the small mass forming the cylinder wall. The dimensions, materials, and air gap within the cylinder are chosen so that the coupler presents to the bone-conduction vibrator an impedance approximately equal to that presented by the human mastoid. The viscous damping properties of the skin are simulated in this device by the behavior of air in the cavity V and the clearance C. Thereby air damping simulates viscous damping and the need for viscoelastic pads is obviated.

The device is used by placing a bone-conduction vibrator on the small mass, driving the vibrator with a suitable signal, and observing the output of an accelerometer attached to the large mass. The components of an artificial-mastoid system are in every way parallel to the instrumentation used to measure the acoustical output of earphones. The coupler is the device shown in Figure 4-1 and is analogous to a 6 cc. coupler used for earphone measurements. This is followed by an accelerometer which is analogous to a condensor microphone. The accelerometer is, in turn, followed by suitable amplification and, finally, by a read-out device such as a vacuum-tube voltmeter. A knowledge of the sensitivity of the unit permits the calculation of the acoustical force generated by the vibrator.

The output of bone-conduction vibrators is customarily expressed in decibels above a reference sound force of one dyne. It should be noted that the reference is a sound force and not a sound pressure, and that it is expressed in dynes and not dynes per square centimeter. A force scale rather than a pressure scale is used because of the difficulty of specifying the effective area of a vibrator face plate. The relationship between sound force and decibels is the same as between sound pressure and decibels, that is, a doubling of sound force is equal to 6 db and so on.

A one dyne reference is used first, because it is a convenient number with which to work, and second, because it is a level about 10 db below the most sensitive hearing by bone-conduction; thus, the normal reference values

can be expressed in positive numbers of moderate size.

While the air-damped artificial mastoid has come into general use in this country, the British have pursued a different course. In 1966, a British Standard (8) was published for an artificial mastoid utilizing a visco-elastic pad. This unit is now available commercially. Apparently, the developers feel that currently available materials are relatively immune to ageing and temperature, and that they have devised a method by which any changes that might occur can be detected.

STABILITY OF THE ARTIFICIAL MASTOID

A question of particular interest is whether the air-damped artificial mastoid is indeed stable over time. In Table 4-1 are reported the

TABLE 4-1. STANDARD DEVIATIONS OF THE CALIBRATION READINGS OF ONE EXAMINER IN DECIBELS

	Frequency in Hz				
	250	500	1000	2000	4000
Direct	.16	.33	.30	.20	.19
TDH-39; 1A	.33	.49	.47	1.49	1.43
TDH-39; 9A	.39	.46	.34	1.52	1.82
B-70-A	.54	.92	.74	1.00	.69
6-AS	.32	.51	.31	.44	.75
B-9	.88	.50	.53	.83	.66

standard deviations of 40 calibration measures carried out by one examiner over a five-month period. The upper row of figures labeled "direct" shows the standard deviations of the electrical signal that normally drives the air- and bone-conduction transducers. The variability is that of the signal generating equipment (Hewlett-Packard model 200 ABR oscillator, Grason Stadler model 162 speech audiometer) and the vacuum-tube voltmeter (Hewlett-Packard 400 H), but excluding the transducers, couplers, and associated electronic components of the calibrating equipment. As expected, these values are smaller than those obtained under other conditions. The second row records the variability of the TDH-39 earphone on an ASA Type 1 coupler, and the third row records a TDH-39 earphone with an MX/41/AR cushion on an NBS Type 9A coupler. The same Western Electric 640AA microphone and microphone complement were used with both couplers. Similar variability results are obtained with each coupler with a possible exception at 4,000 Hz where a somewhat larger value was obtained with the 9A coupler; moreover, with both couplers the variability increases with frequency. The large variability of the earphone at 2,000 and 4,000 Hz is the result of a change of about 3 db at 2,000 Hz and 4 db at 4,000 Hz which occurred suddenly midway through the measurements. The change occurred only with the earphone and only at these two frequencies. The reason for the change is not apparent but has remained for over two months. When this long term persistent change in apparent output is excluded, the variability at 2,000 and 4,000 Hz is only slightly larger than at the lower frequencies.

The next three rows of Table 4-1 show the standard deviations of the calibration readings of the three bone-conduction vibrators on the artificial mastoid. The vibrators were all driven by the same equipment which drove the earphone. The same vacuum-tube voltmeter was used to measure the output of both the air- and bone-conduction calibration systems and the measurements under all conditions were made by the same observer. The standard deviations noted in this study are of the same order of magnitude as those reported by Sanders and Olsen (9) over a three and one half month period on one vibrator.

It is concluded that the variability of the measurements made on the artificial mastoid is not larger than that associated with earphone measurements on 6 cc. couplers.

NORMAL HEARING BY BONE-CONDUCTION

The next step toward the establishment of a normal bone-conduction reference is the measurement of the bone-conduction hearing

sensitivity of a number of young adults with vibrators calibrated on the artificial mastoid. This paper is a report of an effort to determine the normal bone-conduction threshold under a variety of conditions. Among the variables studied were three vibrators (Radioear B-70-A, Sonotone 6-AS, Sonotone 9650 or B-9), two positions on the head (mastoid and forehead), two methods of applying the vibrators to the head (500 grams application force and clinical headbands), and two conditions in the opposite ear (with and without contralateral masking). One hundred and thirty-two subjects were used in the first segment of this study. The air-conduction thresholds of the test ear of these subjects are shown in Table 4-2 along with the ISO-1964

TABLE 4-2. AIR CONDUCTION THRESHOLDS OBTAINED IN THE PRESENT STUDY AND THE ISO-1964 STANDARD IN DB SPL FOR TDH-39-MX/41/AR EARPHONE AND CUSHION ON TYPE 9A COUPLER

	Frequency in Hz				
	250	500	1000	2000	4000
Present Study	25.6	10.2	5.0	5.3	7.7
ISO-1964	24.5	10.1	7.2	9.5	8.3

standard values for a TDH-39 earphone on a 9A coupler.

Figure 4-2 shows the mean bone-conduction

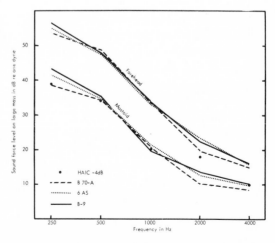

Figure 4-2. Mean bone-conduction thresholds obtained with three different vibrators at the forehead and mastoid with an application force of 500 grams.

thresholds of these same subjects under the following conditions: All subjects were tested with all three vibrators (B-70-A, 6-AS, and B-9) applied to both the mastoid and the forehead with a specially constructed, heavily-damped device. The application force was adjusted to 500 grams. A microswitch and light were used to ensure that application force remained at 500 grams throughout the measurement session. All vibrators are of the miniature hearing-aid type. There was no masking in the non-test ear. The orders in which the vibrators were used and the orders of testing at the forehead and mastoid were counterbalanced. All thresholds were obtained with a 2 db step attenuator utilizing the modified method of limits described by Corso (*10*).

Included in the figure is the Hearing Aid Industry Conference (HAIC) interim standard (*11*) normal thresholds for the mastoid position. The HAIC interim standard, as published, includes a 4 db correction for central masking on the assumption that most clinical tests are conducted with a unilateral masking noise. This 4 db has been subtracted from the HAIC interim standard in this figure in order to make the standard comparable to other results recorded.

The findings are essentially the same for all three vibrators at 500, 1,000, and 4,000 Hz although the vibrators differ slightly at 250 and 2,000 Hz. The agreement across vibrators seems better at the forehead position. The results obtained at the mastoid agree well with the HAIC standard except at 250 and 2,000 Hz. At 250 Hz the difference is not great, but at 2,000 Hz it is very substantial. The difference at 2,000 Hz is apparently caused by the method of applying the vibrator to the head used in this part of the study; it is not observed in that portion of this study in which the vibrators were applied to the head by clinical headbands.

A salient feature of Figure 4-2 is the extent of the agreement across vibrators. It is well known in air-conduction studies that normal threshold sound pressure levels, as observed on 6 cc. couplers, differ slightly from one ear-

phone to another. At low frequencies this difference is usually less than 1 db but at the highest frequencies it may be as much as 4 or 5 db. This difference occurs because a 6 cc. coupler is not an exact acoustical replica of the human ear and, therefore, earphones interact with a coupler differently than they interact with the real ear. The observed differences across vibrators, while larger than found across earphones, do not appear unreasonable considering the relative difficulties of measuring vibrator and earphone output. It appears that the artificial mastoid is a reasonably good replica of the human mastoid and forehead, at least when the behavioral thresholds are obtained with a 500-gram application force on the vibrator; further, on the basis of this criterion, it seems that the forehead is as well represented by the artificial mastoid as the human mastoid. This outcome is not unexpected because of the relatively small difference between the impedance of the forehead and mastoid (*6*).

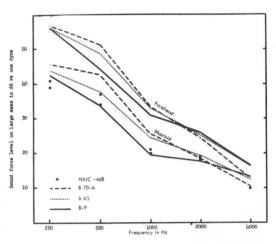

Figure 4-3. Mean bone-conduction thresholds obtained with three different vibrators at the forehead and mastoid applied with clinical headbands.

In Figure 4-3 the results were obtained in the same way as those shown in Figure 4-2 with the one exception that the vibrators were applied to both the forehead and the mastoid with standard spring steel clinical headbands. The vibrators differ considerably under this condition. The human head apparently interacts with vibrators quite differently than does the artificial mastoid when the vibrators are applied to the head by clinical headbands. The most obvious variable is application force. The clinical headbands used in this study exerted a force of about 300 grams at the mastoid and 380 grams at the forehead. The fact that the vibrators agree better at the forehead in Figure 4-3 supports application force as the significant variable; however, application force was not systematically investigated in this study and, therefore, any conclusions must be carefully limited.

It should be noted that Corliss and Koidan (6) made their measurements of mastoid and forehead impedance with 500 gram and 1,000 gram application forces. Since the Weiss artificial mastoid is based on the Corliss and Koidan results, the parameters built into it implicitly assume that the vibrators will be applied to the head with at least 500 grams of force or, alternatively, that the impedance of the human mastoid is essentially the same at 300 to 400 grams force as at 500 grams or more. The work of Barany (12) and of Franke (13) suggests that the latter assumption may be untenable.

The results of the present investigation indicate that vibrators must be applied to the head with a force greater than that supplied by clinical headbands if reasonable agreement across vibrators is to be expected.

In addition, Figure 4-3 shows that only one of the three vibrators agrees with the HAIC interim standard at 250, 500, and 1,000 Hz, while there is good agreement across vibrators and with the HAIC interim standard at 2,000 and 4,000 Hz. Notice particularly that the difference between HAIC and this study at 2,000 Hz reported in Figure 4-2 is not observed in Figure 4-3. This outcome is not unexpected, because seven of the nine studies upon which the HAIC standard is based used clinical headbands.

The method used to calculate the HAIC interim standard is pertinent to the differences between the standard and the present study at the lower frequencies. The HAIC interim standard is the arithmetic mean of nine studies, one of which is an early segment of the present investigation. The difference between the various studies range from 15 to 21 db at the various test frequencies. Inspection of the values reported by the various investigators reveals that at 250, and 500 Hz, in particular, the distribution is quite skewed with one or two investigators reporting much lower values than the others. Under these circumstances, the median is a more appropriate statistic than the mean. The median of the nine studies is shown as the upper dot on the figure. The improved agreement with the present data is apparent.

The HAIC standard is stated to be valid for both the B-70-A and B-9 vibrators, apparently on the basis that the B-70-A was used in six studies and the B-9 in two studies, and that the differences between studies using different vibrators is no larger than the differences between studies using the same vibrator. It is suggested, from the findings of the present investigation, that a single standard cannot apply to more than one type of vibrator, particularly under the testing conditions normally employed in the clinical setting.

The B-70-A is the most commonly used vibrator on audiometers today. The data reported in Figures 4-2 and 4-3 indicate that this vibrator is particularly susceptible to application force. The application force produced by the clinical headband in this study is lower than the 375 grams reported by the manufacturers for these devices; however, this headband was supplied with a new audiometer and was used only in this study. Undoubtedly many headbands with no more than 300 to 320 grams application force are in daily clinical use; further, the force applied is a function of head size and decreases over time as the headbands are used. It is apparent from this study, and from the earlier work of Konig (14), that application force significantly affects threshold, and that it acts differentially across both frequency and vibrators. It is equally apparent that a final bone-conduction standard must include application force and vibrator type as an integral part of the standard.

The effect of a unilateral noise upon threshold is of special interest, because most bone-conduction tests are performed with contralateral masking. Table 4-3 reports that extent

TABLE 4-3. THRESHOLD SHIFT PRODUCED BY A UNILATERAL 40 DB EFFECTIVE LEVEL MASKING NOISE

		Frequency in Hz				
		250	500	1000	2000	4000
Mastoid	B-70-A	4.4	2.4	3.7	3.7	1.5
	6-AS	4.2	2.1	2.9	4.2	1.8
	B-9	5.6	3.5	3.3	3.6	2.4
Forehead	B-70-A	4.4	7.5	5.4	5.9	5.6
	6-AS	4.8	5.6	5.5	6.6	5.9
	B-9	5.4	6.1	5.3	5.3	4.3

of the threshold shift produced by a 40 db effective level white noise when testing with each of the vibrators at the forehead and mastoid positions. The contralaterally masked results were obtained with vibrators applied by clinical headbands. At the mastoid position, the thresholds are elevated by 2 to 4 db at 500 through 2,000 Hz. The elevation is slightly larger at 250 Hz and slightly smaller at 4,000 Hz. The elevations produced by the noise when thresholds are measured from the forehead, are consistently greater than at the mastoid position except at 250 Hz. The larger "central masking" effect upon thresholds obtained at the forehead has been observed by several investigators (15, 16, 17, 18) in the past.

Another factor extensively studied is the difference between thresholds measured at the

mastoid and those measured at the forehead. Table 4-4 reports the difference between the two positions with each vibrator applied at 500 grams and also with clinical headbands. The difference between the thresholds obtained at the two positions generally decreases with increases in frequency. This observation is consistent with several past studies (15, 17, 19); furthermore, the differences between forehead and mastoid thresholds are smaller with the headband. This outcome is probably related to the fact that headband application force is greater at the forehead than at the mastoid, thereby reducing the apparent difference between the positions. An analysis of variance indicates that the interaction difference between head position and vibrator is not significant under the 500-gram application condition, that is, the difference between forehead and mastoid threshold is about the same with all vibrators; however, there is significant interaction with the headband, particularly involving the B-9 vibrator at the higher frequencies. This may represent another manifestation of an interaction between vibrators and application force rather than between the vibrators themselves. These results indicate that it is hazardous to use a forehead bone-conduction reference based on the sum of the difference between forehead and mastoid thresholds obtained under one set of conditions and a mastoid standard obtained under a different set of conditions.

In conclusion, considerable progress has been made toward the eventual establishment of a bone-conduction normal reference. The HAIC interim standard is a significant step in this direction; however, the interim standard is incomplete, because it specifies only normal threshold values but does not specify precisely how these thresholds are to be obtained; nor does it consider the very substantial differences that exist across bone-conduction vibrators under certain conditions.

The results of this investigation suggest that application force, in particular, must be investigated further and then made an integral part of the fully developed standard. The standard must also include a method for

TABLE 4-4. FOREHEAD VS. MASTOID THRESHOLDS. POSITIVE VALUES INDICATE THAT FOREHEAD THRESHOLDS IS HIGHER THAN MASTOID THRESHOLD

		Frequency in Hz				
		250	500	1000	2000	4000
Application Force 500 Grams	B-70-A	15.5	14.6	12.5	9.6	6.5
	6-AS	13.3	13.1	11.8	11.1	6.2
	B-9	13.0	12.4	13.6	9.1	5.9
Application By Clinical Head Band	B-70-A	11.2	8.5	8.0	6.1	2.4
	6-AS	12.2	11.1	8.6	5.6	3.7
	B-9	13.6	10.6	11.6	8.5	3.4

transferring the normal reference from one vibrator type to another, which includes application force as a part of the procedure. Finally, clinical procedures and instrumenta-

tion must be developed and refined to permit the valid application of the standard to the measurement of bone-conduction hearing level to the individual patient.

BIBLIOGRAPHY

1. Greibach, E. H.: Laboratory Method for Objective Testing of Bone Receivers and Throat Microphones. *Trans. Amer. Inst. Elect. Eng.*, 65:184, 1946.

2. Hawley, M. S.: An Artificial Mastoid for Audiphone Measurements. *Bell Lab. Rec.*, 18:73, 1939.

3. Carlisle, R. W., and Pearson, H. A.: A Strain Gauge Type Artificial Mastoid. *Jour. Acoust. Soc. of Amer.*, 23:300, 1951.

4. Carlisle, R. W., and Mundel, A. B.: Practical Hearing Aid Measurements. *Jour. Acoust. Soc. of Amer.*, 16:45, 1944.

5. Weiss, E.: An Air-Damped Artificial Mastoid. *Jour. Acoust. Soc. of Amer.*, 32:1582, 1960.

6. Corliss, E. L. R., and Koidan, W.: Mechanical Impedance of the Forehead and Mastoid. *Jour. Acoust. Soc. of Amer.*, 27:1164, 1955.

7. Cook, R. K.: Physical Standards for Bone Conduction Measurements. Paper Presented at the 1959 Annual Convention of the American Speech and Hearing Association, Nov. 14, 1959.

8. British Standard 4009:1966: An Artificial Mastoid for the Calibration of Bone Vibrators.

9. Sanders, J. W., and Oslen, W. O.: An Evaluation of a New Artificial Mastoid as an Instrument for the Calibration of Audiometer Bone-Conduction Systems. *Jour. Speech and Hearing Dis.*, 29:247, 1964.

10. Corso, J. F.: Age and Sex Differences in Pure Tone Thresholds. *Arch. Otolaryngol.*, 77:385, 1963.

11. Lybarger, S. F.: Interim Bone-Conduction Thresholds for Audiometry. *Jour. Speech and Hearing Res.*, 9:483, 1966, and *Jour. Accoust. Soc. of Amer.*, 40:1189, 1966.

12. Barany, E.: A Contribution to the Physiology of Bone-Conduction. *Acta Otolaryngol.*, 16:1, 1938.

13. Franke, E. K.: The Impedance of the Human Mastoid. *Jour. Acoust. Soc. of Amer.*, 24:410, 1952.

14. Konig, E.: Les Variations de la Conduction Osseuse en Fonction de la Force de Pression Excercee sur le Vibrateur. Presented at Ile Congress Ordinaire Societe Internationale D'Audiologie, Jan. 22, 1955 (Variations in Bone Conduction as Related to the Force of Pressure Exerted on the Vibrator). *Trans. Beltone Inst. Hearing Res.*, 6:1, 1957.

15. Dirks, D.: Bone-Conduction Measurements. *Arch. Otolaryngol.*, 79:594, 1964.

16. Dirks, D., and Malmquist, C.: Changes in Bone-Conduction Thresholds Produced by Masking in the Non-Test Ear. *Jour. Speech and Hearing Res.*, 7:271, 1964.

17. Naunton, R. F.: Clinical Bone-Conduction Audiometry. *Arch. Otolaryngol.*, 66:281, 1957.

18. Studebaker, G. A.: On Masking in Bone-Conduction Testing. *Jour. Speech and Hearing Res.*, 5:215, 1962.

19. Studebaker, G. A.: Placement of Vibrator in Bone-Conduction Testing. *Jour. Speech and Hearing Res.*, 5:321, 1962.

5

Some Relations Between
Normal Hearing for Pure Tones and for Speech

JAMES F. JERGER
RAYMOND CARHART
TOM W. TILLMAN
JOHN L. PETERSON

JAMES F. JERGER, Ph.D., is Professor of Audiology, Baylor College of Medicine
RAYMOND CARHART, Ph.D., is Professor of Audiology, Northwestern University
TOM W. TILLMAN, Ph.D., is Professor of Audiology and Associate Director, Auditory Research Laboratories, Northwestern University
JOHN L. PETERSON, Ph.D., is Dean, School of Allied Health Professions, Louisiana State University Medical Center

Serious confusion exists as to the difference between the sound pressure levels which characterize the normal threshold for a 1000-cps pure tone and the normal threshold for speech. Estimates as to the size of this discrepancy disagree by as much as 10 db. In consequence, there is need for clarification of the situation since the relationship between these two thresholds must be taken into account in establishing co-ordinated audiometric standards.[1]

The problem at hand is quickly apparent when one compares the norms as presently described by the American Standards for Audiometers with the findings of various studies reported in the literature. The American Standard Specification for Audiometers for General Diagnostic Purposes (*1*) defines the normal threshold sound pressure level for 1000 cps as 16.5 db (SPL referred to 0.0002 microbar in a National Bureau of

Reprinted by permission of the authors from *J. Speech Hearing Res.*, **2**, pp. 126–140 (1959).
[1] This study was supported by funds provided under Contract AF41(657)-185 with the USAF School of Aviation Medicine, Randolph Field, Texas.

Standards Coupler 9-A), for the Western Electric type 705-A earphone. The American Standard Specification for Speech Audiometers lists 22 db (SPL referred to 0.0002 microbar in an American Standard type-1 Coupler) as the norm for speech. Indeed, the Specification explicitly states that, ". . . the purpose of this requirement [22 db SPL] is to set the 0 hearing loss for speech at a level about *6 db* [authors' italics] above the 'normal' [sic] threshold for a pure tone of 1000 cps as defined in American Standard Audiometers for General Diagnostic Purposes . . ." (*2*, p. 9). The Specification further implies that the 6-db difference is recognized as an approximation which may require revision.

Sporadic evidence (*3, 4, 6, 9, 11*) suggests that the difference in question is considerably greater than 6 db. Davis (*6*), for example, reports the average of the thresholds for 500, 1000, and 2000 cps as 9 db (SPL) at the same time that he gives thresholds for various speech materials which range from 22 db for spondees, through 26 db for sentence material and digits, to 33 db for PB words as spoken by Rush Hughes. Lightfoot, Carhart, and Gaeth (*11*) observed a 16.5-db difference between the threshold intensities for 1000 cps and for spondee words exhibited by 31 otologically normal subjects. The most definitive finding to date, however, is derived from the 1954 Wisconsin State Fair Survey (*9*). Here, the difference between the averages of the median threshold values for a 1000-cps pure tone and for spondee words, reported for all ears in the "selected normal group" was 15 db. Discrepancies of relatively similar size characterize the results obtained in the Survey for samples (by decades) of the general population, although the data as presented must be converted to sound pressure levels before the fact is fully apparent. Most recently, there is the indirect evidence to be derived from Corso's (*4, 3*) studies of normals' thresholds for pure tones and for CID Auditory Test W-2. On relatively large groups of normal listeners, he obtained threshold SPLs of about 5 db for a 1000-cps pure tone and approximately 19 db for the W-2 spondee recording. These data imply that the difference between thresholds is on the order of 14 db.

Recent evidence (*3, 4, 7, 10*), particularly the work of Dadson and King (*5*) in England, has made it imperative to ask whether the present American norms for pure tones are correct. There is pressure in many quarters to alter these norms as a requisite step toward establishment of an international standard for pure-tone audiometers. This situation, among other things, intensifies the need to define the relation between thresholds for pure tones and for speech.

It is now clearly apparent from evidence such as that obtained in the Wisconsin State Fair Survey (*9*) that young adults yield better thresholds than a less select group of "normal" listeners derived from the population at large. Moreover, the present American norm for speech (22 db SPL) apparently represents performance of selected young adults (the so-called "laboratory ear"). The American norm for pure tones, on the other hand, is based on the responses of a less restricted sampling

(*12*). Here the "man on the street with 'normal' hearing" served as the referant. Thus, the two current American Standards seem to be in disagreement as to the category of normalcy on which they rest. If so, the situation must be rectified by relating both sets of audiometric specifications to the same criterion population.

The first step toward such a unification of audiometric standards is to define the difference in intensity between thresholds for pure tones and for speech. Particularly pressing in this respect, since the sound pressure level of a speech signal is defined in terms of the sound pressure level of an equivalent 1000-cps pure tone (*2*), is the need to know the relative acuity for speech and for 1000 cps.

The present investigation was undertaken to explore the latter need. The experimental problem was to ascertain the physical discrepancy between thresholds for a 1000-cps pure tone and for speech. The specific procedure was to measure both thresholds in the same normal-hearing subjects. Recorded spondees were employed as the speech material. Variables suspected of having a critical influence on the relationship between the two thresholds were examined. These variables included sophistication of the listener, effect of practice, method of threshold determination, order of test administration, sex, ear, and familiarity with test vocabulary. Two groups of 10 subjects each were compared in examining the first two variables, while a third group of 96 subjects was used in a counterbalanced routine designed to study the remaining five variables.

APPARATUS

Figure 5-1 shows a simplified block diagram of the experimental apparatus used to measure both pure-tone and spondee thresholds. The core of the equipment consisted of a commercially-available speech audiometer (Grason-Stadler, type 162) feeding a PDR-10 earphone mounted in an MX41/AR cushion. All spondee thresholds were obtained by playing either recorded list E or recorded list F of CID Auditory Test W-1 through this speech audiometer.

Two separate pure-tone sources were fed through the speech audiometer to the same PDR-10 earphone. One source consisted of an audio-oscillator (General Radio, type 1304A) whose output was controlled by an electronic switch (Grason-Stadler, type 829). The electronic switch was, in turn, triggered by an electronic timer (Grason-Stadler, type 471), to produce the desired temporal pattern of the pure-tone stimulus. Stability of both the oscil-

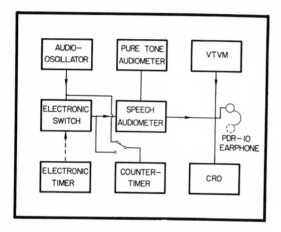

Figure 5-1. Block diagram of apparatus used to measure both pure-tone and spondee thresholds. The core of the equipment is a commercially-available speech audiometer feeding a PDR-10 earphone.

lator frequency and the duration of each short tone passed by the switch was assured by continuous monitoring of both oscillator and switch outputs with a counter-timer (Berkeley, type 5500). This pure-tone source was used to measure the 1000-cps threshold by a rigidly defined psychophysical procedure described below. The second pure-tone source was an ordinary pure-tone diagnostic audiometer (ADC, model 53C). This source was used to measure the 1000-cps threshold by the "clinical" method which was studied.

The electrical signal across the earphone was monitored with a vacuum-tube voltmeter

(Hewlett-Packard, Model 400C) and a cathode-ray oscillograph (Dumont, Model 304-A).

The acoustic output of the apparatus was calibrated by means of an ASA Type-1 coupler, calibrated condenser microphone (Western Electric, type 640AA), cathode follower (ADC, D5153) and vacuum-tube voltmeter (Hewlett-Packard, Model 400-A). All thresholds, both pure-tone and speech, are thus subsequently reported as the sound pressure level, referred to 0.0002 microbar, developed in an ASA Type-1 coupler.

The sound pressure level developed by the earphone at 1000 cps was measured daily throughout the course of the experiment. The maximum variation in output over the five-month period during which subjects were tested was 1.4 db, and the day-to-day variation exhibited no systematic trend over time. Pressure levels developed at octave frequencies from 125 to 8000 cps were measured weekly over the five-month period, and demonstrated equivalent stability.

Prior to the experiment, precautions were taken to insure that the speech audiometer conformed to all requirements listed in the American Standard Specifications for Speech Audiometers (2) with particular reference to tests of overall acoustic fidelity. The apparatus equalled or exceeded all listed specifications.

THRESHOLD MEASUREMENT TECHNIQUES

In order to evaluate the possible effect of threshold measurement technique on the relationship between pure-tone and speech threshold, two separate and distinct methods for defining each type of threshold were employed. One, the "up-and-down" method (8) was characterized by a relatively rigidly-defined set of operations. The other, hereafter called the "clinical" method, was as nearly as possible a duplication of the procedures commonly employed by audiologists within the context of the clinical situation.

Up-and-Down Method

The up-and-down method was selected in preference to any of the three classical psychophysical methods or their variants because it permitted a relatively identical stimulus temporal pattern and measurement procedure for both pure-tone and speech thresholds. The essence of the method is that the intensity level of each successive stimulus is determined by the subject's response to the previous stimulus. If the subject does not respond at a particular intensity, the next level of the stimulus is increased by a predetermined fixed amount. On the other hand, if the subject does respond at a particular intensity, the level of the next stimulus is decreased by the same amount. This simple rule, raising the intensity when the subject does not respond and lowering it when he does respond, is followed throughout the course of a predetermined number of stimulus presentations. The result is a series of response measures which oscillate about the threshold intensity. From these data the intensity level corresponding to 50 percent response may be determined by suitable arithmetic computation (8).

In the present experiment the intensity levels of successive stimuli were altered in 2-db steps over a series of 36 presentations. For the spondee threshold, the block of successive stimuli consisted of the 36 spondee words recorded as lists E or F of CID Auditory Test W-1. For the 1000-cps threshold, the stimulus sequence was a train of 36 short tones recurring at 6-sec intervals. Each short tone had a rise-decay time of 50 msec, and a duration, at maximum amplitude, of 500 msec. The 6-sec repetition rate for the pure tones was selected to match the rate at which the spondee words recur on the W-1 recordings. Thus, insofar as thresholds obtained by the up-and-down method are concerned, the experimental procedure was virtually identical for both pure-tone and spondee thresholds. The only difference was that for the spondee threshold each stimulus was a word which the subject repeated, either correctly or incorrectly, while for the 1000-cps threshold each stimulus was a pure tone to which the subject either did, or did not, respond.

Clinical Method

Devising a satisfactory analogue to so-called "clinical audiometric technique" proved to be one of the more difficult problems encountered in this investigation. Numerous sources were consulted in an attempt to find some common denominator epitomizing the basic operations to be followed in the clinical measurement of an auditory threshold. The relatively small number of even cursorily described procedures found in the literature were characterized by a certain lack of agreement on some relevant particulars (for example, the number of times a stimulus is presented at a given level, whether a pure-tone stimulus is briefly turned on or briefly turned off, whether the threshold criterion is 100 percent response, 50 percent response, 0 percent response, or some intermediate value).

Briefly, it seemed apparent that, in order to introduce some minimal degree of objectivity into the "clinical" thresholds, it was necessary for the authors to devise their own method. In so doing, the attempt was made to follow, as closely as possible, the counsel of experienced clinicians. In the final analysis the authors are able to justify the "clinical" procedures ultimately employed on the sole basis that they seemed reasonable to them.

The clinical procedure adopted for the measurement of the spondee threshold corresponded closely to the method described by Newby (13, pp. 119–120) for the W-1 records. Two or three words were initially presented at a level 20 to 30 db above the estimated threshold level. Successive blocks of two or three words were then progressively attenuated in 10-db steps until a level was reached at which two consecutive words were repeated incorrectly. At this point, the tester simply "jumped around," in no set order, from level to level in 2-db steps, presenting exactly four words per level. The spondee threshold was recorded as the lowest intensity at which the subject repeated two out of four words correctly. In the event that the subject repeated three out of four words correctly at one level, and only one out of four correctly at the next lower level, threshold was recorded as the intensity yielding three out of four responses. This problem seldom arose in actual practice.

The clinical procedure employed to measure the 1000-cps threshold closely resembled the "ascending" technique described in the 1951 revision of the "Manual for School Hearing Conservation Programs" (*14*, p. 15) prepared by the Committee on Conservation of Hearing of the American Academy of Ophthalmology and Otolaryngology. By means of the interruptor switch on the clinical audiometer, a brief tone was first presented at a level 30 db above the estimated threshold in order to familiarize the subject with the test signal. The tester then descended in 10-db steps, presenting one brief tone at each level, until the subject failed to respond. The tester next ascended in 5-db steps, presenting one brief tone at each level, until a response occurred. He then decreased the intensity by 10 or 15 db and again ascended in 5-db steps until another response occurred. This procedure was followed until the subject had responded three times at the same level. Threshold was thus defined as the lowest intensity at which the subject responded three times in ascending runs, using 5-db steps, and presenting just one stimulus per step. No attempt was made to control the duration of each tonal presentation other than to instruct the tester to keep the presentation brief. In practice, the tones were about 1 to 2 sec long.

Instructions to each subject tested by either the clinical method or the up-and-down method were as follows:

The purpose of this study is to measure your threshold for tones and for words. Two test runs will be conducted, one using tones and one using words.

During the tone test, you will hear a short burst of sound followed by intervals of silence. Each tone will be quite short. Some will be easy to hear. Others will be very faint. Whenever you hear one of these tones, no matter how faint it is, press the button. Since the tones will be very faint, it is necessary that you listen very carefully.

When I test for your word threshold, you will hear a man's voice saying two-syllable words, such as "wigwam," "therefore" or similar words. Each word will be preceded by the phrase "Say the word." It is only necessary for you to repeat the two-syllable word, not the phrase. Some of the words will be easy to hear. Others will be very faint. Whenever you hear a word, no matter how faint it is, repeat it out loud. You will have to listen carefully since the words will be very faint. At the beginning of each word test, you will hear several sentences of identifying information which you do not need to repeat.

There is no set order for the two test runs. You will be told at the beginning of each test whether it is to be a word test or a tone test.

After I have placed the phones over your ears, it is extremely important that you do not move them in any way until the tests are completed. I will tell you when you can take them off. Any questions?

SUBJECTS

All subjects were audiometrically screened at a hearing level (hearing loss dial setting) of 10 db *re* USPHS norm at octave intervals from 125 to 8000 cps, and at 1500 and 3000 cps, in order to insure that each subject had relatively normal acuity in both ears.

As already mentioned, three groups of subjects were employed. One group consisted of 10 sophisticated listeners. These individuals were selected from the staff and the graduate student population at the Audiological Laboratory. Each was highly experienced at the task of listening for very faint signals, and all were relatively familiar with the CID revised spondee word lists. They represented essentially "laboratory ears." Five subjects were male, the other five, female. They ranged in age from 20 to 31 years.

The second group was composed of 10 undergraduate students selected on the basis of having had no previous experience as listeners in auditory tests of any kind. Nine subjects were female, the other one, male. They ranged in age from 18 to 25 years.

The third group included 96 subjects, three for each of 32 separate experimental conditions. As was true of the second group, these 96 subjects were selected from the undergraduate population at Northwestern University and met the requirement that they had not had prior experience with any auditory tests. No subject was accepted who reported any history of either ear pathology or excessive noise exposure.

Prior Exposure to Spondee Words

Subjects differed in their familiarity with the spondee words. The 10 sophisticated listeners were well acquainted with these materials, while all other subjects initially were not. However, half of the 96 persons were exposed to the spondees immediately prior to the measurement of their thresholds for the words. To this end, these 48 subjects were given additional instructions as follows:

> Before the word test, I will read a series of 36 two-syllable words at a level which is easy for you to hear. You are to repeat each word. These words are the same words which you will later hear in the word test; however, they will be in a different order. Since the purpose of this initial reading of the words is to make you familiar with the words, please listen carefully.

PROCEDURE AND RESULTS

Preliminary Study

An initial investigation was conducted to determine the effects of sophistication in auditory

tests, and of practice upon the relationship between thresholds for pure tones and for speech. It was for this purpose that the first two groups of 10 subjects were formed.

Six thresholds were obtained for each subject in a single experimental session. Four of these thresholds were for pure tones of 500, 1000, 1500, and 2000 cps, respectively. The last two were spondee thresholds obtained separately with W-1 list E and with W-1 list F. All six thresholds, pure-tone and speech, were measured by the up-and-down method previously described using 2-db steps of attenuation. Subsequent comparison of the two groups yielded information on the effect of familiarity with audiological procedures.

Subjects in the sophisticated group underwent the foregoing procedure twice. The first run gave these subjects experience on the specific tasks involved. The results obtained during this session supplied the base of reference against which to estimate the effect of a practice session on thresholds measured by the up-and-down method.

Table 5-1 summarizes the findings of the preliminary investigation. The mean pure-tone threshold sound-pressure levels obtained for the sophisticated group in the first experimental session (practice session) were essentially equivalent to those obtained in the second session (test session). This was true also for the mean spondee threshold. In addition, when the mean spondee thresholds for this group are considered, no difference is noted between the first and second thresholds obtained in either the practice session or the test session.

Further inspection of Table 5-1 reveals that the pure-tone threshold sound-pressure levels are essentially equivalent for both sophisticated and unsophisticated listeners. When the spondee threshold sound-pressure levels for the two groups are compared, however, it becomes apparent that the sophisticated listeners yielded much lower thresholds than the unsophisticated listeners. Furthermore, unsophisticated listeners improved an average of about 3 db from the first threshold to the second, while sophisticated listeners did not.

TABLE 5-1. MEAN PURE-TONE AND SPONDEE (W-I) THRESHOLD SOUND PRESSURE LEVELS (DB *re*: 0.0002 MICROBAR IN ASA TYPE-I COUPLER) FOR SOPHISTICATED (N = 10) AND UNSOPHISTICATED (N = 10) LISTENERS

Threshold	Sophisticated Group		Unsophisticated Group
	Session 1	Session 2	
Pure Tone			
500 cps	12.4	12.1	10.3
1000 cps	6.8	7.3	5.7
1500 cps	7.4	6.7	7.7
2000 cps	6.6	7.1	8.8
Spondee			
First Test	17.0	16.8	24.3
Second Test	16.7	16.6	21.4
Difference	0.3	0.2	2.9
Mean	16.8	16.7	22.8
Mean Spondee Minus 1000 cps	10.0	9.4	17.1

It seemed possible that this 3-db improvement between the first and second spondee thresholds in the unsophisticated group could be due to the fact that the subjects gained knowledge of the test vocabulary during the first test. The same reasoning would account for the lack of improvement on the second spondee threshold in the sophisticated group. In other words, the sophisticated subjects probably already had the optimum degree of familiarity with the words prior to the administration of the first spondee test so that further exposure to test vocabulary had no demonstrable effect on threshold. If this interpretation is correct, one would expect the unsophisticated group to show further improvement on successive retests with spondee words until they reached a terminal level of familiarity, equivalent to that of the sophisticated group.

The foregoing results indicated the necessity of controlling, in the main experiment, both the general factor of subject sophistication in auditory tests and the specific factor of prior familiarity with the CID revised Harvard spondee words. The decision was made to restrict the main experiment to audiologically naïve listeners because such persons are more similar to the relatively unsophisticated population encountered in clinical situations. Moreover, it was deemed particularly important, since such persons showed instability of threshold with successive exposures to test material, to explore more fully the effect of familiarity with test procedure upon threshold

levels. Information on this point is essential if the variability of threshold due to retesting is to be taken into account in specifying the criterion population for audiometric norms.

Main Experiment

A five-factor design was undertaken to assess the effects on thresholds for spondee words and for a 1000-cps tone of: (a) threshold measurement technique, (b) order of test administration, (c) sex, (d) ear, and (e) prior knowledge of test vocabulary. This investigation was undertaken with the third group of subjects, 96 young adults having normal hearing but lacking prior experience with auditory tests. In order to control systematically the five factors under consideration, the group was appropriately divided. Specifically, 48 subjects were tested by the up-and-down method, the other 48 by the clinical method. Within each subgroup, the spondee test was administered first to half of the subjects, the pure-tone test first to the rest. Half of the subjects were female, and the remainder, male. The right ear was tested 50 percent of the time, and the left ear the remaining 50 percent. The 36 spondees were read to half of the subjects prior to measurement of the speech threshold, while the remaining subjects were not given this opportunity to familiarize themselves with the test items.

Each subject was seen in a single experimental session, during which two thresholds were measured, the threshold for a 1000-cps pure tone and the threshold for spondee words. The latter was obtained with recorded list E of CID Auditory Test W-1.

In order to visualize the effect of each factor separately, Tables 5-2 through 5-6 were

TABLE 5-2. MEAN 1000-CPS AND SPONDEE THRESHOLD SOUND PRESSURE LEVELS (DB *re:* 0.0002 MICROBAR IN ASA TYPE-1 COUPLER) FOR EACH METHOD OF MEASUREMENT (N = 96)

| Threshold | Method | |
	Up-and-Down	Clinical
1000 cps	8.1	9.8
Spondee	21.6	21.7

TABLE 5-3. MEAN 1000-CPS AND SPONDEE THRESHOLD SOUND PRESSURE LEVELS (DB *re:* 0.0002 MICROBAR IN ASA TYPE-1 COUPLER) FOR EACH SEX (N = 96)

| Threshold | Sex | |
	Male	Female
1000 cps	9.3	8.6
Spondee	21.3	22.0

TABLE 5-4. MEAN 1000-CPS AND SPONDEE THRESHOLD SOUND PRESSURE LEVELS (DB *re:* 0.0002 MICROBAR IN ASA TYPE-1 COUPLER) FOR EACH EAR (N = 96)

| Threshold | Ear | |
	Right	Left
1000 cps	8.3	9.6
Spondee	21.7	21.5

TABLE 5-5. MEAN 1000-CPS AND SPONDEE THRESHOLD SOUND PRESSURE LEVELS (DB *re:* 0.0002 MICROBAR IN ASA TYPE-1 COUPLER) FOR EACH TEST ORDER (N = 96)

| Threshold | Test Order | |
	Spondee First	1000 cps First
1000 cps	9.7	8.2
Spondee	22.3	21.0

TABLE 5-6. MEAN 1000-CPS AND SPONDEE THRESHOLD SOUND PRESSURE LEVELS (DB *re:* 0.0002 MICROBAR IN ASA TYPE-1 COUPLER) ACCORDING TO PRIOR KNOWLEDGE OF SPONDEE VOCABULARY (N = 96)

| Threshold | Knowledge of Spondee Vocabulary | |
	Without Prior Knowledge	With Prior Knowledge
1000 cps	8.6	9.3
Spondee	23.0	20.3

prepared to present the mean 1000-cps and spondee thresholds obtained for the two categories of each factor in turn. Table 5-2, for example, illustrates only the effect produced on each threshold by varying the method of measurement. The mean spondee threshold for subjects in the clinical method group is only 0.1 db different from the mean threshold for subjects in the up-and-down method group. There is, however, a 1.7-db difference between the two methods for the 1000-cps thresholds. This difference is almost the exact order of magnitude to be expected in view of the difference in size of intensity steps used in the two methods. For the spondee threshold 2-db steps were used for both the clinical and up-and-down methods. For the 1000-cps threshold, however, 2-db steps were used in the up-and-down method, but 5-db steps were used in the clinical method. A theoretical difference of 1.5 db, in the direction of lower threshold intensity for the method involving 2-db steps would therefore be predicted. This difference derives from the fact that, when 5-db steps are used, the mean threshold is underestimated by 2.5 db, whereas, when 2-db steps are used, the mean threshold is underestimated by only 1.0 db. The observed difference of 1.7 db appears to be in relatively good agreement with this theoretical expectation.

Thus, for both the spondee threshold and the 1000-cps threshold, after allowance has been made for differences in the size of intensity steps used, there appears to be very little difference between results obtained by a clinical versus a laboratory procedure.

Table 5-3 shows that there is no large or systematic effect of sex on the auditory acuity of young normals. Females average 0.7 db better for the 1000-cps threshold, but males are 0.7 db better for the spondee threshold. Both differences are small.

Table 5-4 reveals a slight advantage (1.3 db) for the right ear at 1000 cps. However, this effect is not maintained for the spondee threshold, so that evidence of a slight tendency for one ear to have greater acuity is lacking.

Table 5-5 suggests that the effect of test order is not critical. The 1000-cps threshold

SPL is slightly lower (1.5 db) when it is obtained first, but the spondee threshold SPL is slightly higher (1.3 db) when it is measured first.

Table 5-6 summarizes the effect of prior knowledge of the spondee vocabulary on the spondee threshold. The threshold SPL is 2.7 db lower for subjects who were read the complete list of 36 words prior to the test than for subjects not given prior knowledge. The possibility of a sampling error, such that subjects assigned to the prior knowledge group had inherently keener threshold sensitivity than subjects in the group without prior knowledge, is minimized by the fact that these same subjects did not yield a lower threshold SPL for 1000 cps. The mean 1000-cps threshold SPL for the prior knowledge group was, in fact, 0.7 db higher than the mean 1000-cps threshold SPL for subjects without prior knowledge of the spondee vocabulary.

This 2.7-db difference between spondee threshold SPL for subjects with and without prior knowledge of the spondee vocabulary was the largest effect observed over the five factors studied, and, as subsequent discussion shows, was the only effect that could be considered significant on the basis of statistical analysis.

Tables 5-7 and 5-8 summarize analyses of variance performed on the 1000-cps and spondee threshold data, respectively. Inspection of Table 5-7 shows that, for the 1000-cps threshold, none of the five factors studied

TABLE 5-7. SUMMARY OF ANALYSIS OF VARIANCE FOR 1000-CPS THRESHOLD DATA

Source		df	ms	F
Main Effects				
Method	(a)	1	63.7	3.56
Sex	(b)	1	11.1	0.62
Ear	(c)	1	42.7	2.38
Order	(d)	1	61.1	3.41
Prior Knowledge	(e)	1	8.9	0.50
Interactions				
c x e		1	255.5	14.26 *
Within Sub-Classes		64	17.9	

* Significant beyond the 1 percent level. All other interactions were nonsignificant and are not reported here.

TABLE 5-8. SUMMARY OF ANALYSIS OF VARIANCE FOR SPONDEE THRESHOLD DATA

Source	df	ms	F
Main Effects			
Method	1	0.0	0.00
Sex	1	13.3	1.21
Ear	1	0.9	0.08
Order	1	42.8	3.89
Prior Knowledge	1	169.3	15.41 *
Interactions †			
Within Sub-Classes	64	11.0	

* Exceeds value required for the 1 percent level of confidence.
† None of the interactions are reported since none exceeds value required for the 1 percent level of confidence.

appears to exert a significant effect, and there are no particular interactions worthy of note. Only one F ratio, that for the interaction between the ear tested and prior knowledge of spondee vocabulary (c x e), is significant beyond the 1 percent level ($F = 7.08$). Since it is difficult to conceive a logical basis for an actual interdependence between these two factors to exist, insofar as the threshold for 1000 cps is concerned, the authors choose to conclude that this F ratio represents that chance occurrence under the null hypothesis which will, in fact, happen 1 percent of the time in a large series of F ratios computed on the basis of pairs of samples drawn from identical populations.

Table 5-8 shows a similar, relatively negative, set of results for the spondee threshold analysis. Again, only one F ratio is significant beyond the 1 percent level. Here, however, it is a main effect, knowledge of test vocabulary, with a difference of 2.7 db between spondee thresholds for subjects with and without prior knowledge of test vocabulary, which is significant. This finding is interpreted as evidence that preliminary exposure of audiologically naïve subjects to a list of spondee words lowers the measured threshold SPL slightly (2 to 3 db). All other F ratios obtained in the analyses of variance for spondee thresholds were nonsignificant. This situation, coupled with the totally negative findings in the companion analysis of the data on acuity for 1000 cps leads

TABLE 5-9. MEAN 1000-CPS THRESHOLD SOUND PRESSURE LEVELS (DB *re:* 0.0002 MICROBAR IN ASA TYPE-I COUPLER) FOR EACH METHOD OF MEASUREMENT AND MEAN SPONDEE THRESHOLD SOUND PRESSURE LEVELS FOR EACH METHOD OF MEASUREMENT AND FOR SUBJECTS WITH AND WITHOUT PRIOR KNOWLEDGE OF SPONDEE TEST VOCABULARY

| | | Spondee Thresholds | | |
Method	1000-cps Threshold	Without Prior Knowledge	With Prior Knowledge	Combined
Up-and Down	8.1	22.3	20.9	21.6
Clinical	9.8	23.6	19.7	21.7
Combined	9.0	23.0	20.3	21.6

to the conclusion that systematic effects due to method of testing, sex, ear, and order of threshold measurement are either nonexistent or are so small that they are obscured by the uncontrollable variables in the investigation. In either event, the implication is clear. These four factors did not produce effects so large that the effects modified the measured threshold levels substantially. Hence, the influence of sex, ear, and order of test may be disregarded in examining the data at hand with the aim of assessing the relationship between acuity for 1000 cps and acuity for spondees. Technically, the same conclusion applies to the effect of method of test, but common sense argues that the size of the interval used in testing (which differed for pure tones in the two methods of test) should not be ignored completely. The rationale underlying this last statement and the bases for other general conclusions are highlighted by Tables 5-9 and 5-10.

Table 5-9 gives mean thresholds, subdivided in terms of method of test and, for the spondee thresholds, the factor of prior knowledge. Table 5-10 reports the differences, for the same breakdown of data, between the 1000-cps and the spondee thresholds. Appropriate combined values are also reported in both tables. The following conclusions seem pertinent and reasonable.

First, as seen in Table 5-9, and as mentioned earlier, the mean thesholds for 1000 cps appear essentially equivalent when allowance is made for the fact that the clinical method used a 5-db step as contrasted to the 2-db step employed in the up-and-down method. Thus, it would appear that this threshold can serve as a stable point of reference when the size of the test interval is specified.

Second, the mean thresholds for spondaic words varied appreciably. As already pointed out, the variation with method of testing can be considered random, but the variation due to familiarity with the spondees is systematic. The important point is the fact that the speech threshold is not a point of reference whose stability is comparable to that of the 1000-cps threshold. Therefore, the establishment of an audiometric norm for speech requires the designation of such additional conditions as: (a) the specific test material on which the

TABLE 5-10. DIFFERENCE BETWEEN MEAN 1000-CPS THRESHOLD SOUND PRESSURE LEVELS (DB *re:* 0.0002 MICROBAR IN ASA TYPE-I COUPLER) AND MEAN SPONDEE THRESHOLD SOUND PRESSURE LEVELS FOR EACH METHOD OF MEASUREMENT AND FOR SUBJECTS WITH AND WITHOUT PRIOR KNOWLEDGE OF TEST VOCABULARY

| | Prior Knowledge | | |
Method	Without	With	Combined
Up-and-Down	14.2	12.8	13.5
Clinical	13.8	9.9	11.9
Combined	14.0	11.3	12.6

norm is based and (b) the audiological sophistication of the subjects who are the reference group.

Third, as the foregoing conclusions imply and as Table 5-10 illustrates, the difference between the thresholds for the 1000-cps pure tone and for the W-1 spondees varies substantially. This variation is primarily the result of the instability of the spondee threshold, although the change in the size of the interval used to measure acuity for 1000 cps is thought to have exerted its influence as well. The outstanding point is that the observed differences range from 9.9 to 14.2 db, with the average for all conditions combined being 12.6 db. These differences are all substantially greater than the 6-db value currently designated in the American Standards for Speech Audiometers (2). They are in reasonable agreement with several earlier investigations (3, 4, 6), and smaller than reported by other writers (9, 11).

DISCUSSION

The practical implications of the present study have already been partially stated. These implications are: (a) that a multiplicity of conditions must be specified in order to stabilize the norm for speech audiometry, (b) that the difference between the norms for puretone audiometry and for speech is a function of the conditions chosen in specifying both but (c) that the difference between the norms for 1000 cps and for speech should be designated as substantially more than 6 db.

The magnitude of the difference which is selected as specifying the standard relation between the threshold for 1000-cps pure tone and threshold for speech must be settled by arbitrary decision of the persons responsible for establishment of standards. The present study can assist these persons only to the degree that it helps to clarify the factors to be considered.

To this end, it is instructive to examine the differences between thresholds exhibited by the 20 subjects used in the preliminary study (see Table 5-1) and to compare these results

with the findings already reported for the 96 subjects who participated in the main experiment.

It probably represents approximately the limiting range to be encountered when subjects involved have "normal" acuity. In other words, the evidence at hand leads one to the belief that, when the size of the test interval is constant for both measures, highly sophisticated listeners will detect a 1000-cps pure tone at a sound-pressure level about 10 db weaker than the level at which they correctly repeat 50 percent of the W-1 words. This difference may become as great as 17 db in consequence of complete unfamiliarity with the spondee test materials. Since the threshold for 1000 cps is but little affected by audiological sophistication, the difference may fluctuate over a range of 7 or 8 db as a result of variation in the threshold for speech.

Assuming that the foregoing analysis is correct, three choices are available in choosing a "standard" difference to be incorporated in a revision of audiometric norms.

If highly sophisticated listeners are selected as the criterion population, a difference of about 10 db must be specified. The practical consequence of such a choice will be that the naïve listener (including many a hard-of-hearing person) will yield initial thresholds which are several decibels poorer than his later ones will be, particularly if time is not taken to familiarize him with the test words prior to the initial test.

If the fully naïve listener is chosen as the standard, the reverse situation will exist. A difference of 15 or 16 db must now be specified, and any person having appreciable prior experience with the speech material will obtain thresholds which appear better by several decibels than they otherwise would.

If a difference of intermediate value (12 or 13 db) is specified, this choice would imply that a moderately sophisticated listener is the criterion, and it would keep the discrepancy small (circa 3 db) in the measurement of threshold for other types of listeners.

This choice (that is, establishing the difference between the norm for 1000 cps and the norm for speech at 12 to 13 db) would seem to be most reasonable. It represents a "middle-of-the-road" course if one is thinking in terms of spondee words as represented by W-1 recording and also if one is contemplating the array of evidence which studies other than the present one have supplied. Moreover, since the spondaic words have relatively high audibility, even audiologically sophisticated listeners will exhibit a difference between modalities of at least 12 or 13 db when the speech threshold is determined with other types of material.

SUMMARY

In order to determine the intensity difference between normal hearing for spondee words and normal hearing for a 1000-cps pure tone, both types of threshold were measured in 10 audiologically sophisticated and 106 audiologically naïve listeners.

The threshold for 1000 cps was found to be relatively independent of the sophistication factor, but prior familiarity with the spondee test vocabulary exerted a significant influence on the spondee threshold.

Results indicate that the intensity difference between normal hearing for a 1000-cps pure tone and for spondee words is considerably larger than 6 db. It ranged from 9.4 to 17.1 db depending on variations in the type of subject, the familiarity of speech materials, and aspects of the measurement procedure. A difference of 13 db is approximately medial. It represents a value which might properly be selected as the relationship to be specified for audiometric standards.

REFERENCES

1. *American Standard Sound Measurement Package, American Standard Specification for Audiometers for General Diagnostic Purposes*, appr. March 21, 1951. American Standards Association, Inc., 70 East 45th St., New York 17, N.Y.

2. *American Standard Sound Measurement Package, American Standard Specification for Speech Audiometers*, appr. July 10, 1953. American Standards Association, Inc., 70 East 45th St., New York 17, N.Y.

3. Corso, J. F., Confirmation of the normal threshold for speech on C.I.D. auditory test W-2, *J. acoust. Soc. Amer.*, 29, 1957, 368–370.

4. Corso, J. F., and Cohen, A., Methodological aspects of auditory threshold measurements. *J. exp. Psychol.*, 55, 1958, 8–12.

5. Dadson, R. S., and King, J. H., A determination of the normal threshold of hearing and its relation to the standardization of audiometers. *J. Laryngol. Otol.*, 66, 1952, 366–378.

6. Davis, H., The articulation area and the social adequacy index for hearing. *Laryngoscope*, 58, 1948, 761–778.

7. Davis, H., and Usher, J. R., What is zero hearing loss? *J. Speech Hearing Dis.*, 22, 1957, 662–690.

8. Dixon, W. J., and Massey, F. J., *Introduction To Statistical Analysis*. New York: McGraw-Hill, 1951.

9. Glorig, A., Wheeler, D., Quiggle, R., Grings, W., and Summerfield, A., *1954 Wisconsin State Fair Hearing Survey*—statistical treatment of clinical and audiometric data. American Academy of Ophthalmology and Otolaryngology, 1957, Research Center, subcomm. Noise in Industry, Los Angeles.

10. Harris, J. D., Normal hearing and its relation to audiometry. *Laryngoscope*, 64, 1954, 928–957.

11. Lightfoot, C., Carhart, R., and Gaeth, J. H., Masking of impaired ears by noise. *J. Speech Hearing Dis.*, 21, 1956, 56–70.

12. National Health Survey, 1935–1936. Preliminary reports, hearing study series, bull. 5, *Normal Hearing for Speech at Each Decade of Life*. Div. Pub. Health Methods, Nat. Inst. Health, U.S. Pub. Health Serv., Washington, 1938.

13. Newby, H. A., *Audiology, Principles and Practice*. New York: Appleton-Century Crofts, 1958.

14. Newhart, H., and Reger, S. N., (Eds.), *Manual for a School Hearing Conservation Program* (rev. 1951, for Comm. on Conservation of Hearing, C. E. Kinney, G. D. Hoople, S. R. Guild, S. N. Reger, Eds., suppl., trans. Amer. Acad. Ophth., Otolaryng., 100 First Ave. Bldg., Rochester, Minn.). Omaha: Douglas Printing Co.

6

Inconsistency Among Audiometric Zero Reference Levels

RAYMOND CARHART

RAYMOND CARHART, Ph.D., is Professor of Audiology, Northwestern University

The current American specifications for audiometers employ zero reference levels for speech and for 1 000 cps which cause the two scales to be displaced from one another by about 7 dB. Practically, this means that a person tested by audiometers perfectly calibrated to the standards will be designated as having about a 7 dB greater loss for speech than his pure-tone thresholds would indicate.

This fact is dramatically apparent in the data from the Wisconsin State Fair Survey (Glorig, 1957). This study employed pure-tone audiometers that conformed to ASA Standard Z24.5-1951 (1951) and speech audiometers using the zero reference level designated in ASA Standard Z24.13-1953 (1953). Forty-two comparisons of group data can be made from the information presented in the report on this survey. These comparisons involve the 25th percentiles, the medians, and the 75th percentiles yielded by 14 mutually exclusive groups which were determined on the basis of age and sex criteria. The threshold for speech was poorer than the threshold for 1 000 cps in all 42 comparisons. Moreover, the average difference was 7.2 dB. This systematic discrepancy between the scales for speech and for pure tones must be attributed to a disparity in reference levels for the two types of measurement, since the data were gathered with instruments that were carefully main-

Reprinted by permission of the author from *Asha*, **8,** pp. 63–66 (1966).

tained in calibration to their respective standards.

This disparity manifests itself whenever studies are done with audiometers that are monitored so as to assure that they conform to current ASA specifications. It results because equivalent criterion populations were not employed in establishing the zero reference levels for the two kinds of stimulus. The scale of hearing levels by speech audiometry was based upon performance of young adults with superior hearing. Such persons furnish a referent very similar to the criterion that underlies the ISO reference threshold levels for pure tones (I.O.S., 1964). By contrast, the current ASA standard for pure tones employs as its referent the considerably more heterogeneous group of "normal" hearers covered by the old United States National Health Survey (U.S.P.H.S., 1935–1936). As is well known, this population was characterized by about 11 dB less acute hearing in the 500–2 000 cps range than is represented by the ISO zero reference threshold levels.

A brief résumé helps one understand how this disparity arose. When the sound pressure levels (SPL's) characterizing the speech thresholds of normals were being determined in the later 1940's, the scientific community was not as fully alert as it is now to the peculiarities of the norms for pure tones derived from the United States Public Health Survey. Therefore, there seemed to be no particular problem in presuming that data on speech thresholds such as those reported by Davis (1948) could be equated to the American norms for pure tones.

Davis had designated normal threshold for spondaic words (PAL Test No. 9) at 22 dB, for connected discourse at 23 dB, and for both sentences (PAL Test No. 12) and digits (Western Electric Test 4C) at 26 dB above 0.0002 microbar. Subsequent studies on other groups of young normal hearers yielded thresholds close enough to those just reported so that differences could be attributed to such factors as the limited size of test groups, variety of speech material, diversity in method of presentation, and the like. It therefore seemed reasonable, when Z24.13-1953 was adopted in 1953 as the American Standard for Speech Audiometers, to accept 22 dB $\pm$ 4 dB above 0.0002 microbar (developed in an American Standard Type-1 coupler) as the zero reference level for speech audiometry.

It must be recalled that, as part of the Z24.5-1951 standard for pure-tone audiometers, normal threshold pressure for 1 000 cps was placed at 16.5 above 0.0002 microbar (as developed by a Western Electric 705-A earphone in an NBS 9-A coupler This value is 5.5 dB less than the level designated in Z24.13-1953 as the normal threshold pressure for speech. The following statement in Section 3.12 of Z24.13-1953 clarifies the choice of 22 dB re 0.0002 microbar as the norm for speech audiometry.

The purpose of this requirement is to set the 0 hearing loss for speech at a level about 6 dB above the "normal" threshold for a pure tone at 1 000 cps as defined in American Standard Specification for Audiometers for General Diagnostic Purposes. . . . This value is subject to future adjustment when additional experiments have been performed to evaluate the normal relation between the threshold for speech (using carefully recorded word tests) and the threshold for a 1 000 cps tone. It is believed that this adjustment will not be more than $\pm$4 dB.

It has subsequently become clear that the SPL at which a normal hearer is aware of a 1 000 cps tone and the SPL at which his speech threshold lies differ from one another by about 13 dB. Thus, the standard designated in Z24.13-1953 failed by about 7 dB in its intent to equate the hearing level scales for speech and for pure tones.

Actually, evidence was available as early as 1948 suggesting that, when expressed in SPL's, the discrepancy between the two types of threshold approximates 13 dB. Davis (1948) presents an illustration wherein he shows the normal threshold for spondees at 22 dB re 0.0002 microbar. He indicates 9 dB re 0.0002 microbar as the average of normal thresholds at 500, 1 000, and 2 000 cps. Assuming that here the threshold for 1 000 cps involved an SPL at least as low as the average for all three frequencies, and remembering that the threshold for spondees was the best of all the speech thresholds Davis reported, it is reasonable to reach the conclusion that there was a discrepancy of at least 13 dB in the SPL at which the listeners supplying these data detected 1 000 cps half the time and the level at which speech was intelligible to them half the time.

Some of the subsequent evidence pointing in the same direction has been summarized by Jerger and others (1959) as follows:

Lightfoot, Carhart, and Gaeth observed a 16.5 dB difference between the threshold intensities for 1 000 cps and for spondee words exhibited by 31 otologically normal subjects. The most definitive finding to date, however, is derived from the 1954 Wisconsin State Fair Survey. Here the difference between the averages of the median threshold for a 1 000 cps pure tone and for spondees, reported for all ears in the "selected normal group" was 15 dB. Discrepancies of relatively similar size characterize the results obtained in the Survey for samples (by decades) of the general population. . . . more recently, there is indirect evidence to be derived from Corso's studies of normals' thresholds for pure tones and for CID Auditory Test W-2. On relatively large groups of normal listeners, he obtained threshold SPL's of about 5 dB for a 1 000 cps pure tone and approximately 19 dB for the W-2 spondee recording. These data imply that the difference between thresholds is on the order of 14 dB.

These authors concluded:

The first step toward . . . a unification of audiometric standards is to define the difference in intensity between thresholds for pure tones and for speech. Particularly pressing in this respect, since the sound pressure level of a speech signal is defined in terms of the sound pressure level of an equivalent 1 000 cps pure tone, is the need to know the relative acuity for speech and for pure tones.

Jerger and others then undertook experimentation to this end. They measured the intensity differences between the threshold for recorded spondees (CID Auditory Test W-1) and for 1 000 cps as exhibited by 10 audiologically sophisticated and 106 audiologically naive listeners, all with normal hearing. The writers state:

Results indicate that the intensity difference between normal hearing for a 1 000 cps tone and for spondee words . . . ranged from 9.4 to 17.1 dB depending on variations in the type of subject, the familiarity of speech materials, and aspects of the measurement procedure. A difference of 13 dB is approximately medial. It represents a value which might properly be selected as the relationship to be specified for audiometric standards.

The main experiment performed by Jerger and others employed a five-factor design with 96 audiologically naive subjects. The five factors were (1) technique of measuring pure-tone thresholds, (2) order of test administration, (3) sex, (4) right versus left ear, and (5) prior knowledge of test vocabulary. None of these factors emerged as inducing any statistically significant variation in threshold for 1 000 cps, and only knowledge of the test vocabulary appeared to influence speech threshold levels to any noteworthy degree.

From the standpoint of the present discussion, the statistics given in Table 6-1 are the particularly pertinent ones.

TABLE 6-1. MEAN THRESHOLD SOUND PRESSURE LEVELS * OBTAINED BY JERGER AND OTHERS FOR 1 000 CPS AND FOR W-1 WORDS

Group	No. Cases	1 000 cps Threshold	W-1 Threshold	Difference
No Prior Knowledge	48	8.6	23.0	14.4
Prior Knowledge	48	9.3	20.3	11.0
Combined	96	9.0	21.6	12.6

* dB re 0.0002 microbar in ASA Type-1 coupler.

Notice, for one thing, that the grand mean of the difference between the two types of threshold emerged as 12.6 dB. This is almost 7 dB more than the 6 dB difference written into the Z24.13-1953 specification for speech audiometers.

Secondly, Jerger and others found the mean threshold for 1 000 cps to be 9.0 dB above 0.0002 microbar. This value is closer to the 6.5 dB value designated as zero reference hearing level for 1 000 cps according to the ISO standard than it is to the 16.5 dB value specified in the present American standard. Thus, the 96 subjects employed in this study may be considered to be reasonably representative (at least at this frequency) of the criterion of normal hearing embodied in the ISO standard. They certainly do not represent zero hearing level according to the 1951 ASA standard.

Third, subjects without prior knowledge of the test vocabulary obtained a mean threshold for W-1 words of 23 dB re 0.0002 microbar, while subjects with prior knowledge yielded a mean of 20.3 dB. In consequence, the mean for the entire 96 subjects was 21.6 dB. All these values are close to the 22 dB re 0.0002 microbar specified as the zero reference level by Z24.13-1953. Assuming that the population studied by Jerger and others approximated the ISO standard of zero hearing level, it would appear that the 22 dB value established in Z24.13-1953 conforms more closely to the threshold to be expected from persons representing the ISO standard for pure-tone acuity than to those representing the present American standard.

This last observation leads to the conclusion that it would have been much better if the Z24.13-1953 standard had designated a value considerably higher than 22 dB re 0.0002 microbar as the zero reference level for speech. Selecting 29 dB, for example, would have brought the hearing level scale for speech audiometry into neat conformity with the American standard for pure tones.

The rationale for this last statement is straightforward. It is based on the empirical observation that thresholds for speech are reached at intensities about 13 dB greater than are thresholds for 1 000 cps. Since Z24.5-1951 designates 16.5 dB re 0.0002 microbar as the zero reference level for 1 000 cps, the companion zero reference level for speech should have been about 13 dB higher, or at about 29 dB re 0.0002 microbar.

If 29 dB had been selected as the American zero reference level for speech instead of 22 dB, the resultant change of 7 dB in all values along the scale of hearing levels for speech would have brought the results of the Wisconsin State Fair Survey into neat agreement with one another. The 7.2 dB discrepancy which now appears in these data would have been virtually eliminated.

It is worth noting that there are clinical programs where cognizance has been taken of the foregoing factors and where speech audiometers have consistently been calibrated to a reference 7 or 8 dB higher than called for by Z24.13-1953. For example, at Northwestern University we have for years corrected our speech threshold measurements to remove the disparity in current American audiometric

references. Actually, we have found it more convenient to employ 30 dB re 0.0002 microbar as zero hearing level for speech, simply because many of our speech audiometers have attenuators with 2 dB steps and many of these instruments were calibrated to 22 dB reference level when received from the manufacturer. The minor discrepancy introduced by using 30 dB instead of 29 dB does not change the basic fact that can be abstracted from our clinical records: namely, that the adoption of this change in reference level yields clinical records wherein the scales of hearing loss for speech and for 1 000 cps are very close to one another. Stated differently, our clinical records show that retention of the 22 dB reference level for speech would have yielded a disparity between the scales of approximately 7 dB.

The validity of the foregoing statements is illustrated by the following statistical analysis of clinical records for the period from January 1960 through June 1964. Data from both Hearing Clinics maintained at Northwestern University were included. Only subjects between 10 and 80 years old, inclusive, were considered. The record for each ear was assessed separately, and the record was included in the study only if that ear exhibited pure-tone responses which did not vary in hearing level by more than 10 dB across the 500–2 000 cps range.[1] In addition the hearing level at 1 000 cps must have been between 10 dB and 70 dB, and a speech reception threshold must have been recorded for that ear. All the above requirements were satisfied by 703 ears. The mean hearing loss for the entire 703 ears was 39.0 dB for 1 000 cps and 37.2 dB for spondee words. The difference between the two means was 1.8 dB. If, instead of 30 dB, 29 dB re 0.0002 microbar had been used as the zero reference level for speech, the mean hearing loss for spondee words would have emerged as 38.2 dB, in which event the difference between means would have been only 0.8 dB.

---

[1] This requirement was imposed to assure that each loss included was relatively uniform, since irregularities in the pure-tone audiogram would have contaminated the relations under investigation.

Of course, the important point is that we have here a view of the relation which emerged from a clinical situation where careful calibration was maintained but where the speech scale had been shifted 8 dB for the purpose of bringing it into close parallelism with the pure-tone scale. The correction thus achieved was fully adequate for clinical purposes and, in retrospect, it is clear that more precise interlocking would have emerged had the reference level for speech been set at 29 dB re 0.0002 microbar. In fact, from these statistics it would appear that 28 dB re 0.0002 microbar might have been the best value to have selected. Be that as it may, these data confirm the contention that a sizeable inconsistency exists between the present American standard for pure-tone audiometers and the standard for speech audiometers.

The existence of this inconsistency poses a problem for each clinician the moment he makes the transition to the ISO standard for pure-tone audiometers (I.O.S., 1964), a change which ASHA has endorsed. The change shifts the zero reference level by 10 dB at 1 000 cps, and by an average of 10.8 dB across the 500–2 000 cps range. The end result is about a 10 dB realignment in the relationship which the clinician will observe between the pure-tone and speech thresholds that his patients yield. For example, if the clinician has previously been using the American standard for speech audiometers (22 dB re 0.0002 microbar), and if he retains this standard after shifting to ISO for pure tones, an original discrepancy of 7 dB in one direction will be replaced by a 3 dB disparity in the other. By contrast, if the clinician has previously been using a higher zero reference level for speech, say 29 dB re 0.0002 microbar, so as to eliminate the 7 dB discrepancy imposed by the current American standards, he now faces the prospect of a 10 dB disagreement. Unless he shifts his reference for speech as well as for pure tones by 10 dB (to 19 dB in this example) he will introduce a major disparity between the two scales.

These examples illustrate the question which is before the clinician. There would be no problem if the forthcoming revision of the American standards were already available, since it is to be expected that these standards will include the ISO levels for pure tones and will set the reference level for speech at about 19 dB re 0.0002 microbar. However, it may be some time before the new American standards are finalized and approved. Meanwhile, most clinicians in the speech and hearing profession will have adopted the ISO reference for their pure-tone audiometry. What reference for speech should they adopt in the interim so as to eliminate inconsistencies and furnish scales for speech and for pure tones whose reference levels are in reasonable coordination?

Two courses of action suggest themselves. The first course is to use a zero reference level for speech approximately 13 dB above the ISO reference level of 6.5 dB for 1 000 cps. This procedure would set the speech reference at about 19 dB re 0.0002 microbar. It would bring the two scales into close agreement. Moreover, there is good probability that both the ISO standard for speech, when it is selected, and the forthcoming revision of the American standard for audiometers will specify a level fairly close to 19 dB. Of course, one can not know now what the final decisions in this matter will be.

The second alternative is to use the present American standard for speech (22 dB re 0.0002 microbar) as an interim reference level. This interim level would bring the speech scale within 3 dB of what it would be if 19 dB were used as the reference. This amount of disparity is not large enough to cause serious clinical difficulty in routine audiometric evaluations.

This second alternative is the one which the Committee on Conservation of Hearing of the American Academy of Ophthalmology and Otolaryngology recommends (Davis, 1965): to wit,

Inasmuch as the next action of the American Standards Association is uncertain both [as] to timing and as to substance and inasmuch as a working group of the ISO is also considering the question, the Committee on Conservation of Hearing *recommends that users of speech audiometers make* NO CHANGE *at the present time in their zero reference levels.* The speech thresholds that they measure in this way should agree with predictions from ISO pure-tone audiometry at least as well as and probably much better than they did with ASA-1951 pure-tone audiometry.

The other action is suggested for the future. It can prove a great help and can be adopted now. Specifically,

the Committee also recommends that, to avoid ambiguity in the future when a new standard is issued and establishes a new ASA or an ISO reference zero level, all users of speech audiometers henceforth indicate specifically on all records and in publications the sound pressure level that they employ as their reference, presumably either "re 29 dB" or "re 22 dB" or "re 19 dB."

In view of all the considerations involved, it would certainly seem wise to follow this recommendation. Fortunately, even the minor inconsistency in audiometric scales which this procedure imposes should not be with us too long. We may expect the new American standards for audiometers to bring the two scales into as good agreement as can be expected in view of the many variables which affect threshold responses to pure tones and speech stimuli.

SUMMARY

Both experimental and clinical evidence indicate that a difference of about 13 dB exists between the SPL at which a normal hearer is aware of a 1 000 cps tone and the SPL at which his speech threshold lies. The present American standards set the zero hearing level for speech at an SPL which is only 5.5 dB above the zero hearing level for 1 000 cps. In consequence, the current American scales of hearing level for speech and for pure tones are displaced from one another by approximately 7 dB. Some clinicians have adjusted their speech audiometers to eliminate this discrepancy. The implications of the foregoing facts must be borne in mind in the transition to use of the ISO reference levels for pure tones. A reasonable interim procedure is to retain the present American standard for speech audiometers, since only a minor displacement between the speech scale and the ISO scale for pure tones will result. In any event, each clinician should include the reference level he uses for speech audiometry in any report of speech thresholds he makes to others. In due time, the forthcoming American standards for audiometers should rectify even this minor discrepancy.[2]

[2] Preparation of this paper was supported by Public Health Service Research Grant No. K6 NB 16224 from the National Institute of Neurological Diseases and Blindness.

REFERENCES

American Standard Specification for Audiometers for General Diagnostic Purposes. Z24.5-1951, American Standards Association, March 21 (1951).

American Standard Specification for Speech Audiometers. Z.24.13-1953, American Standards Association, July 10, 1953.

Davis, H., The articulation area and the social adequacy index for hearing. *Laryngoscope,* **58,** 761–778 (1948).

Davis, H., Guide for the classification and evaluation of hearing handicap in relation to the international audiometric zero. *Trans. Amer. Acad. Ophthal. Otolaryng.,* 69, 740–751 (1965).

Davis, H., and Kranz, F. W. The international standard reference zero for pure-tone audiometers and its relations to the evaluation of impairment of hearing.

J. Speech Hearing Res. **7,** 7–16 (1964).

Glorig, A., Wheeler, D., Quiggle, R., Grings, W., and Summerfield, A., 1954 Wisconsin state fair survey. *Amer. Acad. Ophthal. Otolaryng.* (1957).

Jerger, J. F., Carhart, R., Tillman, T. W., and Peterson, J. L., Some relations between normal hearing for pure tones and for speech. *J. Speech Hearing Res.,* **2,** 126–140 (1959).

U.S. Public Health Service, *Preliminary Reports of the National Health Survey Hearing Study Series.* U.S. Public Health Service, Bull. No. 5 (1935–1936).

I.O.S., International Organization for Standardization. *Standard Reference Zero for Calibration of Pure-Tone Audiometers,* ISO/R 389-1964, International Organization for Standarization.

7

Hearing in Children:
Acoustic Environment and Audiometer Performance

ELDON L. EAGLES
LEO G. DOERFLER

ELDON L. EAGLES, M.D., is Deputy Director, National Institute of Neurological Diseases and Blindness
LEO G. DOERFLER, Ph.D., is Professor of Audiology and Director, Department of Audiology, Eye and Ear Hospital, and Doctoral Program in Bioacoustics, School of Medicine, University of Pittsburgh

For several years, the American Academy of Ophthalmology and Otolaryngology, through its Subcommittee on Hearing in Children of the Committee on Conservation of Hearing, has been concerned with a long-term, nationwide study of hearing problems in children. An initial study is being conducted in Pittsburgh, through the cooperation of the Subcommittee with the Maternal and Child Health Section of the University of Pittsburgh's Graduate School of Public Health, to evaluate methods for the testing of hearing in children in order to decide which are more efficient, economical, and valid in terms of time and manpower, and. to evaluate and define medical signs and symptoms which may indicate danger of hearing impairment. A significant outcome of the study will be the development of the methods and techniques for the Subcommittee's national studies.[1]

The initial study, which is planned for a five-year period, is being conducted on a population of approximately 5 000 children ranging in age from three to 15 years. The school-age portion of this population is 97.5 percent of the enrollment of four public schools. The preschool children are those who are expected eventually to attend the four study schools. The four schools were chosen to be representative, as a group, of the general Pittsburgh public school population from a socioeconomic standpoint.

Individual air-conduction hearing levels are being determined and otological examinations made on the children at varying intervals. Medical histories have been obtained. The relation among otological findings, medi-

Reprinted by permission of the authors from J. Speech Hearing Res., 4, pp. 149–163 (1961).
[1] Financial support is provided by grant number B2375 (C3) from the National Institute of Neurological Diseases and Blindness, and by funds from the American Academy of Ophthalmology and Otolaryngology to the Subcommittee on Hearing in Children. Members of the Subcommittee on Hearing in Children are Raymond E. Jordan, M.D., Chairman, Clinical Professor of Otology, University of Pittsburgh School of Medicine; John E. Bordley, M.D., Professor of Otolaryngology, Johns

Hopkins University School of Medicine, and Adjunct Professor of Environmental Medicine, Johns Hopkins University School of Hygiene and Public Health; Victor Goodhill, M.D., Professor of Surgery (Otology), University of Southern California, and Consultant, John Tracy Clinic; Hollie E. McHugh, M.D., Associate Professor of Otolaryngology, McGill University; and S. Richard Silverman, Ph.D., Director, Central Institute for the Deaf, and Professor of Audiology, Washington University. Financial support in addition to that of the Subcommittee on Hearing in Children is provided by a grant from the Children's Bureau through the Commonwealth of Pennsylvania Department of Health to the University of Pittsburgh.

cal histories, air-conduction hearing levels, academic achievement, and other aspects of child development are being studied.

A prime objective of the Study of Hearing in Children is to obtain information on hearing levels by determining individual air-conduction hearing levels. It was felt that these hearing levels were substantially better than adult norms, and to measure them accurately it was necessary to have both the proper acoustic environment and audiometers which would test with linearity to 30 db below the American Standard audiometric zero. This paper presents the solutions to problems encountered in connection with the acoustic environment and with the audiometers.

ACOUSTIC ENVIRONMENT

The choice of audiometric test rooms was made after an investigation of the various types of rooms commercially available and after a study of their construction and attenuation characteristics. Double-wall rooms were selected because single-wall rooms did not provide sufficient attenuation of ambient noise, particularly for testing at low frequencies.

The audiometric test rooms used in the Pittsburgh Study are prefabricated, portable rooms [2] which were erected in rooms set aside for this purpose in Pittsburgh schools, after acoustic surveys showed that the sites were relatively quiet areas. Each test room is actually a room within a room with an air space between two separate housings; the inner room rests on rubber vibration insulators while the outer room rests on the area floor. Walls and ceilings of both inner and outer rooms are constructed of 4″ thick acoustic panels. The test rooms have two adjacent separately hinged doors that open in opposite directions. Each room contains a double-glazed window, is lighted by an incandescent light and has continuous ventilation. The inside measure-

ments of the rooms are 72 in. by 64 in. Outside measurements are 96 in. by 88 in. The weight is approximately 6 225 lb.

Before the audiometric test rooms were chosen, advice was sought regarding the sound pressure levels which must not be exceeded in the audiometric test rooms if hearing levels of children well below audiometric zero (American Standard) were to be determined without masking. The maximum allowable sound pressure levels in order to test at 30 db below the American Standard audiometric zero (1, 2) are listed by octave band in Table 7-1.

Acoustic surveys were made at the sites chosen in the four study schools, both before and at periodic intervals after the erection of the audiometric test rooms. In Table 7-1, the results of a recent survey in one school are summarized. The findings in this survey, which was made after the rooms had been in use over a year, are typical of the conditions found at the remaining three study sites. During the acoustic surveys, sound pressure levels were recorded both inside and outside the audiometric test rooms. The sound pressure levels recorded in Table 7-1 were the highest noted during test periods which were chosen to include periods of peak noise during the school day. The 150 to 300 cps octave band was of particular concern, since the lowest test frequency was 250 cps. When the attenuating effect of the earphones is added, it can be seen that there is a margin of safety even in the 150 to 300 cps octave band, which allows the determination of hearing levels to 30 db below audiometric zero.[3]

AUDIOMETERS

Two methods were considered for dealing with the problem of determining hearing

[2] Model 1202, by Industrial Acoustics Co., 341 Jackson Ave., New York 54, N.Y.

[3] Sound level measurements were made by a General Radio Octave Band Analyzer, type number 1550-A, used in conjunction with a General Radio Sound Level Meter, type number 1551-A. Both instruments were calibrated in the Acoustics Laboratory of the Graduate School of Public Health and were found to meet the American Standard Specification for instruments of this type.

TABLE 7-1. SOUND PRESSURE LEVELS (IN DECIBELS RE 0.0002 DYNE/CM^2 AS MEASURED IN OCTAVE BANDS LISTED) RECORDED DURING ACOUSTIC SURVEY AT H. C. FRICK SCHOOL, SEPTEMBER 15, 1959. RECORDING WAS DONE BOTH OUTSIDE AND INSIDE THE AUDIOMETRIC TEST ROOM AND UNDER VARYING NOISE CONDITIONS: WITH HALL DOOR CLOSED AND OPEN, WITH TEST ROOM VENTILATOR ON AND OFF, WITH AND WITHOUT CONVERSATION IN THE ROOM, DURING LUNCH PERIOD, AND DURING CHANGE OF CLASSES. GIVEN BELOW ALSO, FOR PURPOSES OF COMPARISON, ARE THE MAXIMUM ALLOWABLE SOUND PRESSURE LEVELS (SPL) TO DETERMINE HEARING LEVELS AT 30 DECIBELS BELOW AUDIOMETRIC ZERO WITH NO MASKING

Octave Bands (in cps)								
20 to 10 000	20 to 75	75 to 150	150 to 300	300 to 600	600 to 1 200	1 200 to 2 400	2 400 to 4 800	4 800 to 10 000
Outside Test Room								
62	58	54	54	48	42	38	34	28
(hall door closed, ventilator on, conversation)								
58	55	54	48	43	33	36	32	30
(hall door closed, ventilator on, no conversation)								
58	54	52	50	52	46	50	48	30
(hall door closed, ventilator on, lunch hour)								
58	50	55	54	54	51	44	38	36
(hall door open, ventilator off, conversation)								
Inside Test Room, Test Room Door Closed								
43	44	30	11	8	8	9	9	13
(hall door open, ventilator on)								
46	44	24	7	8	8	9	10	13
(hall door closed, ventilator off, classes changing)								
48	49	38	11	9	8	8	9	13
(hall door closed, ventilator off, lunch hour)								
44	46	29	10	8	7	8	9	14
(hall door closed, ventilator off)								
Maximum Allowable SPL								
		10	10	10	10	12	22	32

levels with linearity below audiometric zero. The first was to construct audiometers which would test to the required levels. Highly accurate laboratory type audiometers could be built, but this would be costly and time consuming. In addition, there was the question of whether a commercially available audiometer could be made to serve the purposes of the study. A plan for building special audiometers was, therefore, not developed. The second method considered, and adopted, was to obtain five commercially available audiometers constructed with auxiliary 40 db precision attenuators placed in the earphone lines. These attenuators could be switched in or out of the circuit and would be switched in on the linear portion of the attenuator scale so that low hearing levels could be measured accurately.

An audiometer manufacturing company, which constructed audiometers as described, guaranteed them to meet the American Standard Specification. A significant feature of the audiometers was their Western Electric 705-A earphones for which the threshold characteristics are known. The audiometers were not required to provide masking or bone conduction. The frequencies supplied were 250, 500, 1 000, 2 000, 4 000, 6 000, and 8 000 cps. The hearing level dials were graduated in 5 db steps from zero to 60 db. The audiometers were of a type that is widely used throughout the country and are produced by a company that cooperated to the fullest extent in complying with its guarantee that the audiometers meet the American Standard Specification. It is emphasized that the experience with audiometer performance, as described on the following pages, is not unique to the make of audiometer used in the study.

AUDIOMETER PERFORMANCE

Performance at Initial Calibration

First attempts to check the calibration data supplied by the manufacturer against the physical performance of the audiometers were unsuccessful. At this time, the Acoustics Laboratory at the University of Pittsburgh was in the process of development and not able to calibrate the audiometers. A portable artificial ear, which is available commercially, was used instead. The artificial ear was found to have an unstable microphone and not to meet the American Standard Specification. Advice and help was then obtained from the Sound Section of the National Bureau of Standards.

The audiometers failed to meet the American Standard Specification in the following aspects:

> interrupter click on termination of tone; acoustic radiation from audiometer chassis; intensity and frequency changes at onset and termination of signal tone; extraneous signals at certain frequencies; erratic earphone response; frequencies outside the 5% tolerance of the American Standard Specification; rms sound pressure errors of certain earphones greater than the tolerance limits of 4.0 db at the test frequency of 2 000 cps and lower, and 5.0 db at the test frequencies above 2 000 cps; variation in the sound pressure output greater than 2 db as specified in the American Standard Specification when line voltage was varied from 105 to 125 volts; tone interrupter showing rise and decay times of tones outside of specifications; overshoot of tone outside specifications; attenuator linearity outside the tolerance limit of plus or minus 1.5 db at 10 to 5, and 5 to 0 steps; and tests of purity of test tones showing the sound pressure levels of the fundamental to be less than 25 db above any harmonic at certain frequencies

Not all of these faults were found in each audiometer. However, none of the five met all specifications at the first calibration, and were returned to the manufacturer for repair or correction or for replacement of unstable earphones. After correction, the audiometers were sent to the Bureau of Standards for their second calibration. At this time, one audiometer was found to be within specifications and went into use in the study in Pittsburgh. The remaining four audiometers were again returned to the manufacturer for further changes and then were sent to the Bureau of Standards for the third calibration. Three audiometers met specifications at the third calibration. The fifth audiometer was again returned to the manufacturer for correction and was finally received in June 1958 and was found to meet the American Standard Specification. A sixth audiometer was purchased later as a spare.

The difficulties experienced in getting the audiometers to meet the American Standard Specification involved a period of five months, and demonstrated the need for comprehensive calibration and repair facilities which would be easily and quickly available. The Department of Occupational Health of the Graduate School of Public Health expanded its Acoustics Laboratory so that by the time the audiometers were ready for use the laboratory was fully equipped to carry out artificial ear calibration of audiometers. Periodic calibration of the hearing study audiometers was then established.

Performance Following Initial Calibration

The audiometers were calibrated as often as possible until sufficient information was available to judge their stability. Beginning in July 1958, 45 complete calibrations were done on six audiometers through July, August, and September. During this period, two of the audiometers were out of operation for several weeks at a time while unstable earphones were replaced. Therefore, an average of three calibrations per month was performed on each audiometer in operation during the three months. In October the interval between calibrations was lengthened to two weeks, and in November to one month. As a result of this experience, the interval between calibrations was set not to exceed one month unless the performance of the audiometer indicated the need for more frequent calibration. Necessary servicing of the audiometers was carried out at the time of calibration so that the American Standard Specification was consistently maintained at all times when the audiometers were in use.

In addition to the monthly acoustic calibration, the audiometers received daily checks by the technicians. Beginning in January 1959, a weekly measurement of the voltage output of the audiometers at the terminals of the earphones was instituted. This measurement is carried out at the site where the audiometer is used. A series of measurements established a baseline of output readings for each frequency. Variation of plus or minus 2 db from this baseline on two successive days was taken to indicate the need for an acoustic calibration.

Problems in Tone Presentation. The most serious problem in performance of the audiometers was delay in rise and decay times of the tone presentation, and overshoot and undershoot of tone. The difficulty arose from the fact that the tone in the audiometers was interrupted by the starting and stopping of a Wien bridge oscillator. All of the audiometers met the American Standard Specification at the start of the study but were close to the tolerance limit in respect to rise time of tone presentation. Overshoot of tone beyond the required plus or minus 1 db of the required sound pressure was sufficient to place one audiometer out of operation early in the study. The remaining audiometers showed overshoot which tended to increase with the passage of time.

The problem of delay in tone presentation, and of overshoot and undershoot was finally solved by the staff of the Acoustics Laboratory. To correct the difficulty, the audiometers were modified by introducing tone interruption through a separate electronic switch placed between the oscillator and the output. By this method the oscillator is left on all the time that the audiometer is turned on and interruption is accomplished by the electronic switch. The need to operate the oscillator continuously introduced a number of electronic problems which did not exist when the tone was interrupted by stopping the oscillator. These problems were associated with a strong leakthrough of tone due to stray wiring capacitance, and with the location of the audiometer components. This last was eliminated only after modification of the audiometer circuits to the extent that the output transformer was removed from its location and mounted elsewhere on the chassis.

These changes have resulted in a smooth tone where the duration of onset is approximately 0.3 sec. Furthermore, there is no discernible overshoot or undershoot. Tracings of the tone presentation before and after tone modification are shown in Figure 7-1.

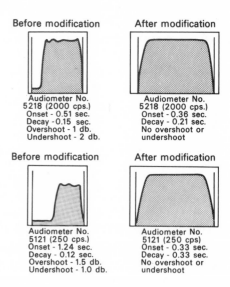

Figure 7-1. Tracings of tone representation in audiometers before and after modification with specially constructed electronic switches to control tone presentation.

Other Major Defects. The major defects in performance of the six audiometers, occurring during the 21-month period from July 1,

1958, to March 31, 1960, in addition to that of tone presentation, are listed below:

Defect in Performance	Number of Times of Occurrence
Sound Pressure Output Approaching or Exceeding Tolerance Limits	45
Faulty Earphone Performance	10
Earphones Replaced Due to Performance	6
Frequency Outside 5% Tolerance	8
Harmonic Distortion	7
Extraneous Instrument Noise	4
Worn Interrupter Switch	2
Defect in 40 db Attenuator	4
Defect in Electronic Switch	1

From this tabulation it can be seen that the most common defect in performance was the tendency of the audiometers to produce sound pressure errors greater than the tolerance limits of 4.0 db at the test frequency of 2 000 cps and lower, and 5.0 db at the frequencies above 2 000 cps. This defect occurred 45 times in all six audiometers. The smallest number of occasions on which it occurred in any one audiometer was three times, and the greatest, 13 times.

The sound pressure output of one audiometer is illustrated in Figure 7-2, for the period July 1, 1958, to May 30, 1959, during which time it was necessary to readjust the audiometer on seven occasions. In the figure, each break in the lines representing the output of the earphones indicates one of the occasions on which readjustment or repair was made at one or more frequencies. In this connection, it should be mentioned that the audiometers were brought into specifications when the sound pressure errors drifted close to the tolerance limits. It is not known how far they would have drifted outside the tolerance limits if the audiometers had not been readjusted.

Not all audiometers behaved in the same manner in respect to output. During the 21-month period previously mentioned, the longest continuous periods each audiometer remained within specifications were: one for eight months, one for five months, one for

four months, two for three months, and the sixth audiometer stayed within the specification at no time longer than two months.

Faulty earphone performance necessitating the replacement of earphones on six occasions was the next most frequent problem. On eight occasions, frequencies were outside the 5 percent tolerance in two of the audiometers. Excessive harmonic distortion occurred on one occasion in each audiometer and on two occasions in one audiometer at 500 and 8 000 cps. These occasions followed closely after the previously described modification of the audio-

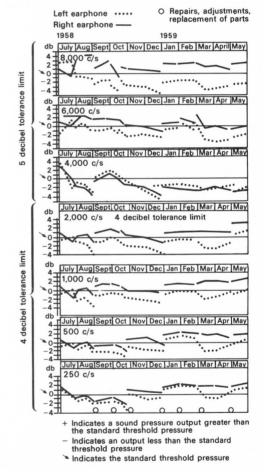

Figure 7-2. Sound pressure errors determined during acoustic calibrations of audiometer number 5 211, showing variation from standard threshold pressures, by earphone, by frequency, and by time. Each break in the output lines indicates one of the occasions on which readjustment or repair was made at one or more frequencies.

meters to correct the defects in tone presentation.

The audiometers remained relatively stable in respect to the 5 db hearing loss intervals or attenuator steps, varying not more than plus or minus 1.5 db at each interval. The cumulative tendency in each audiometer was for the intervals to be less than the 5 db step so that the range from 0 to 60 db was actually not 60 db but usually closer to 55 db.

The 40 db attenuators also remained relatively constant, although each of the six actually attenuated 39 db or slightly less. With the use of these attenuators switched into the circuit at an attenuator dial reading of zero, the audiometers had a range of attenuation from 60 db above audiometric zero to 40 db below, as far as dial settings were concerned, but actually the ranges were 6 to 8 db less than this.

In summary, the following audiometer components produced variations or errors which influenced the hearing levels recorded at each threshold determination: (a) the 40 db attenuators in the earphone lines, a relatively constant variation; (b) the 5 db attenuator steps, relatively constant variations; and (c) the sound pressure output at the various frequencies, errors which varied with time, frequency, earphone, and with audiometer.

Following are examples of the magnitude of errors in these three components for two adjacent calibrations in one audiometer: the average error in the 40 db attenuator equalled 1.6 db; the average error at the 5 db attenuator steps varied at each respective step and ranged from 0.0 db to 1.4 db; the sound pressure output showed average errors by frequency ranging from —1.0 db to +3.8 db in the right earphone and from —4.1 db to +1.4 db in the left earphone.

When these three variations or errors were added algebraically to the results obtained in hearing level determinations, it was found that in some instances as much as a 5 or 10 db shift was obtained in a reading at a particular frequency. In other instances, no change occurred in a recorded reading. Table 7-2 is presented to show an example of the magnitude and direction of the combined errors when the average errors in the 40 db attenuator, attenuator (hearing-level dial) steps, and the sound pressure output of each earphone are added algebraically. The variations by hearing level, frequency, and by earphone, in this instance, have a range of approximately 10 db.

CORRECTION OF READINGS

Because of the magnitude of error as shown in Table 7-2, the readings obtained in hearing level determinations were corrected first by the appropriate exact numerical error. However, this involved adding an "exact" error to a relatively gross measurement of hearing level obtained in 5 db steps. Thus, individuals who hear a particular frequency at 10 db and who do not hear at 5 db are recorded as having thresholds of 10 db but actually they may be able to hear at the 6, 7, 8, or 9 db level. If it is assumed that of all individuals with hearing levels recorded as 10 db an equal number begins to hear at each point between 5 and 10 db, then the whole group, although recorded as having a hearing level of 10 db, actually had an average hearing level of 7.5 db. Thus the hearing levels, as determined, may underestimate the hearing levels for the group by 2.5 db. Because of this, it was felt that the hearing levels could be made more exact, although still approximations, by subtracting 2.5 db from each hearing level determination. With this second adjustment, the addition of the exact numerical error as described above becomes more realistic. A further adjustment was the rounding off of the resultant hearing level value to the nearest whole number.

Tables of adjusted and corrected values were computed for each month of the study, for both earphones of each audiometer, by frequency, and for each possible attenuator dial reading. The computation of adjusted and corrected values for a particular month is made by averaging the total error obtained from the calibration at the start of that month with the error obtained at the start of the fol-

TABLE 7-2. COMBINED AVERAGE ERRORS FROM THE 40 DB ATTENUATOR, THE 5 DB ATTENUATOR STEPS, AND SOUND PRESSURE OUTPUT FOR EACH EARPHONE FOR THE PERIOD MARCH 16 TO 30, 1959, FOR AUDIOMETER #5 121

Hearing Level (in db)	Frequency						
	250	500	1000	2000	4000	6000	8000
Right Earphone							
−20	4.6	4.9	6.6	2.0	5.6	4.4	1.9
−15	4.6	4.9	6.6	2.0	5.6	4.4	1.9
−10	4.2	4.5	6.2	1.6	5.2	4.0	1.5
− 5	4.4	4.7	6.4	1.8	5.4	4.2	1.7
0	4.0	4.4	6.1	1.5	5.0	3.8	1.4
5	4.2	4.5	6.2	1.6	5.2	4.0	1.5
10	3.8	4.2	6.0	1.4	4.8	3.6	1.2
15	3.8	4.2	5.9	1.3	4.8	3.6	1.2
20	3.2	3.5	5.2	0.6	4.2	3.0	0.5
25	3.0	3.4	5.1	0.5	4.0	2.8	0.4
30	2.6	3.0	4.7	0.1	3.6	2.4	0.0
35	2.8	3.2	4.9	0.3	3.8	2.6	0.2
40	2.4	2.8	4.6	0.0	3.4	2.2	−0.2
45	2.6	3.0	4.7	0.1	3.6	2.4	0.0
50	2.3	2.6	4.4	−0.2	3.3	2.1	−0.4
55	2.2	2.6	4.4	−0.2	3.2	2.0	−0.4
60	1.6	2.0	3.7	−0.9	2.6	1.4	−1.0
Left Earphone							
−20	0.6	1.4	3.4	0.0	4.4	3.5	−1.2
−15	0.6	1.4	3.4	0.0	4.4	3.5	−1.2
−10	0.2	1.0	3.0	−0.4	4.0	3.1	−1.6
− 5	0.4	1.2	3.2	−0.2	4.2	3.3	−1.4
0	0.1	0.9	2.8	−0.6	3.8	3.0	−1.7
5	0.2	1.0	3.0	−0.4	4.0	3.1	−1.6
10	0.0	0.8	2.6	−0.7	3.6	2.8	−1.8
15	−0.1	0.7	2.6	−0.8	3.6	2.8	−1.9
20	−0.8	0.0	2.0	−1.4	3.0	2.8	−2.6
25	−0.9	−0.1	1.8	−1.6	2.8	2.1	−2.7
30	−1.3	−0.5	1.4	−2.0	2.4	1.6	−3.1
35	−1.1	−0.3	1.6	−1.8	2.6	1.8	−2.9
40	−1.4	−0.6	1.2	−2.1	2.2	1.4	−3.2
45	−1.3	−0.5	1.4	−2.0	2.4	1.6	−3.1
50	−1.6	−0.8	1.1	−2.2	2.1	1.2	−3.4
55	−1.6	−0.8	−1.0	−2.3	2.0	1.2	−3.4
60	−2.3	−1.5	0.4	−3.0	1.4	0.6	−4.1

lowing month. In those months in which there were calibrations in addition to the monthly calibration, a weighted average is calculated. In computing this average, adjacent calibration results are averaged and weighted by the number of days between the calibrations.

Tables 7-3, 7-4, and 7-5 are presented to show the differences between the readings obtained by correcting the hearing levels as described, and what the readings would have been if they had remained uncorrected. These differences in mean hearing levels have been computed for selected frequencies of 250, 1 000, 4 000, and 8 000 cps.

In Table 7-3, for the right ear it can be seen that the differences in hearing levels measured by audiometer number 5 040 range by frequency from 0.5 to 1.3 db, and by audiometer number 5 211 from 0.7 to 4.5 db. The differences, therefore, vary in magnitude from audiometer to audiometer. It is also seen that there is an additional variation between right and left ears by audiometer and by frequency.

In Tables 7-4 and 7-5, it can be seen that the

TABLE 7-3. DIFFERENCE (IN DB RE AUDIOMETRIC ZERO) BETWEEN CORRECTED AND UNCORRECTED MEAN HEARING LEVELS (MEAN HEARING LEVELS BASED UPON RESULTS OF ALL RELIABLE AUDIOMETRIC TESTS CONDUCTED DURING THE GIVEN TIME PERIOD) FOR RIGHT AND LEFT EARS AT SELECTED FREQUENCIES FOR EACH AUDIOMETER USED BETWEEN JUNE 1958 AND JUNE 1959. "UNCORRECTED" HEARING LEVELS ARE THOSE OBTAINED FROM THE DIAL READINGS OF THE 5 DB ATTENUATOR IN THE NORMAL COURSE OF TESTING. "CORRECTED" HEARING LEVELS ARE OBTAINED BY ADDING, TO THE "UNCORRECTED" RESULT, THE SUM OF THE ERRORS INHERENT IN THE OUTPUT OF THE EARPHONE, THE 5 DB ATTENUATOR STEPS, AND THE 40 DB ATTENUATOR

| Audiometer | Ears | Number of Ears Tested | | | | Corrected, Uncorrected Diff | | | |
		250 cps	1000 cps	4000 cps	8000 cps	250 cps	1000 cps	4000 cps	8000 cps
All	Right	6340	6740	6739	6285	2.3	1.8	2.1	1.8
	Left	6338	6741	6739	6285	3.2	2.8	2.2	2.0
#5 040	Right	623	671	671	615	1.0	1.0	1.3	0.5
	Left	624	671	671	615	1.8	3.4	1.9	0.5
#5 121	Right	1011	1058	1056	1003	3.9	2.7	4.2	4.0
	Left	1011	1058	1057	1003	3.7	3.6	2.2	0.7
#5 148	Right	1159	1300	1300	1147	1.7	1.7	3.1	0.7
	Left	1157	1300	1299	1147	3.6	3.3	2.7	4.0
#5 211	Right	1193	1218	1219	1191	3.9	3.9	0.7	4.5
	Left	1193	1219	1219	1191	2.3	3.5	1.3	0.3
#5 218	Right	1063	1152	1152	1053	1.3	1.3	1.8	0.9
	Left	1062	1152	1152	1053	2.6	2.4	2.8	3.5
#5 226	Right	1291	1341	1341	1276	1.6	0.1	1.2	−0.2
	Left	1291	1341	1341	1276	4.1	1.0	2.4	2.4

differences between corrected and uncorrected mean hearing levels vary from month to month. For example, the differences in hearing levels in the right ear range at 250 cps from +1.1 to +4.8 db; at 1 000 cps from +0.8 to +3.7 db; at 4 000 cps from +0.2 to +4.9 db, and at 8 000 cps from −0.8 to +5.9 db. Table 7-5 shows similar ranges of differences for the left ear and again there is seen a variation between right and left ears.

TABLE 7-4. DIFFERENCE (IN DB RE AUDIOMETRIC ZERO) BETWEEN CORRECTED AND UNCORRECTED MEAN HEARING LEVELS (MEAN HEARING LEVELS ARE BASED UPON THE RESULTS OF ALL RELIABLE AUDIOMETRIC TESTS CONDUCTED DURING THE GIVEN TIME PERIOD) FOR RIGHT EARS AT SELECTED FREQUENCIES FOR EACH MONTH BETWEEN JUNE 1958 AND JUNE 1959. "UNCORRECTED" HEARING LEVELS ARE THOSE OBTAINED FROM THE DIAL READINGS OF THE 5 DB ATTENUATOR IN THE NORMAL COURSE OF TESTING. "CORRECTED" HEARING LEVELS ARE OBTAINED BY ADDING, TO THE "UNCORRECTED" RESULTS, THE SUM OF THE ERRORS INHERENT IN THE OUTPUT OF THE EARPHONE, THE 5 DB ATTENUATOR STEPS, AND THE 40 DB ATTENUATOR

| Period of Time | Number of Ears Tested | | | | Corrected, Uncorrected Diff | | | |
	250 cps	1000 cps	4000 cps	8000 cps	250 cps	1000 cps	4000 cps	8000 cps
June 1958 to June 1959	6340	6740	6739	6285	2.3	1.8	2.1	1.8
June 1958	390	470	470	390	2.5	1.3	3.4	5.9
July 1958	443	587	587	440	1.6	0.8	2.6	4.5
August 1958	514	640	640	513	1.2	0.6	1.2	3.6
September 1958	389	394	394	388	1.1	1.5	1.7	1.8
October 1958	408	408	408	408	1.6	1.9	2.5	1.5
November 1958	367	368	368	367	1.4	1.1	0.8	0.7
December 1958	561	561	561	561	1.4	1.2	0.2	0.3
January 1959	547	561	561	532	2.8	2.3	0.4	2.2
February 1959	614	618	618	600	2.1	1.5	0.8	1.2
March 1959	302	304	303	300	1.6	2.2	1.9	−0.8
April 1959	767	778	779	761	2.4	2.4	2.4	1.0
May 1959	636	642	641	626	4.6	3.4	4.9	0.8
June 1959	402	409	409	399	4.8	3.7	3.7	1.2

TABLE 7-5. DIFFERENCE (IN DB RE AUDIOMETRIC ZERO) BETWEEN CORRECTED AND UNCORRECTED MEAN HEARING LEVELS (MEAN HEARING LEVELS ARE BASED UPON THE RESULTS OF ALL RELIABLE AUDIOMETRIC TESTS CONDUCTED DURING THE GIVEN TIME PERIOD) FOR LEFT EARS AT SELECTED FREQUENCIES FOR EACH MONTH BETWEEN JUNE 1958 AND JUNE 1959. "UNCORRECTED" HEARING LEVELS ARE THOSE OBTAINED FROM THE DIAL READINGS OF THE 5 DB ATTENUATOR IN THE NORMAL COURSE OF TESTING. "CORRECTED" HEARING LEVELS ARE OBTAINED BY ADDING, TO THE "UNCORRECTED" RESULTS, THE SUM OF THE ERRORS INHERENT IN THE OUTPUT OF THE EARPHONE, THE 5 DB ATTENUATOR STEPS, AND THE 40 DB ATTENUATOR

	Number of Ears Tested				Corrected, Uncorrected Diff			
Period of Time	250 cps	1000 cps	4000 cps	8000 cps	250 cps	1000 cps	4000 cps	8000 cps
June 1958–June 1959	6338	6741	6739	6285	3.2	2.8	2.2	2.0
June 1958	390	470	469	389	2.6	3.6	3.4	5.5
July 1958	443	587	587	441	3.1	3.6	2.4	4.4
August 1958	514	640	640	513	3.6	3.9	1.8	4.1
September 1958	389	394	394	388	3.5	2.6	2.7	3.0
October 1958	408	408	408	408	4.2	3.1	2.7	2.3
November 1958	367	368	368	367	4.2	3.8	1.1	2.5
December 1958	561	561	561	561	4.9	2.4	0.0	0.7
January 1959	546	561	561	532	3.5	3.2	0.4	1.1
February 1959	614	618	618	600	3.7	3.5	1.0	1.0
March 1959	302	304	303	300	3.1	2.3	2.4	0.2
April 1959	767	779	779	761	3.3	2.4	2.8	0.6
May 1959	635	642	642	626	1.0	0.9	4.7	1.3
June 1959	402	409	409	399	0.6	0.4	4.3	2.0

For research purposes it was important to adjust the hearing level determinations in this study, despite the relatively small differences in some instances. When attempting to obtain normative data a shift of a few decibels will change a child from one category of hearing to another at certain hearing levels, and when such a shift is applied generally it will affect thousands of children.

DISCUSSION

As has been stated earlier, it was felt that hearing levels in children are substantially better than adult norms, and to measure them accurately it is necessary to have both the proper acoustic environment and audiometers which will test with linearity to 30 db below the American Standard audiometric zero. To demonstrate that this is so and that children in this study had hearing levels measured well below audiometric zero without masking, the findings on hearing levels determined between June 1, 1958, and June 30, 1959, are summarized in the following paragraphs. The detailed findings are being published elsewhere (3).

During the above mentioned period, 2 175 children, evenly distributed between 5 and 14 years of age, had no otological abnormalities on physical examination. Those children with demonstrable otological abnormalities numbered 457.

The mean and median hearing levels, and the standard deviations for the two groups of children, are shown in Table 7-6. Both the means and medians of the otologically abnormal group are higher, or less sensitive, than those for the normal children. It is to be noted that these measures of central tendency in both groups of children are significantly lower than the audiometric zero in current use.

Figures 7-3 and 7-4 are presented to show the percentage distribution of hearing levels by ear and frequency for the otologically normal and the otologically abnormal groups of children. Of the otologically normal group, 92 percent had hearing levels lower or more sensitive than the American Standard audiometric zero at 250 cps. This percentage falls progressively as frequencies increase, until at 8 000 cps 65 percent of the children without abnormalities have hearing levels below audiometric zero. Of 457 children with demonstrable otological abnormalities, 80 percent have

TABLE 7-6. MEAN AND MEDIAN HEARING LEVELS (HL), IN DB RE AUDIOMETRIC ZERO, AND STANDARD DEVIATIONS FOR CHILDREN IN OTOLOGICALLY "NORMAL" AND "ABNORMAL" POPULATIONS TESTED BETWEEN JUNE 1958 AND JUNE 1959

Frequency (cps)	Number Tested		Mean HL		Median HL		SD	
	Norm	Abnorm	Norm	Abnorm	Norm	Abnorm	Norm	Abnorm
Right Ear								
250	2 029	412	−9.8	−5.2	−10.6	−6.9	7.7	12.2
500	2 175	457	−7.2	−2.2	−7.4	−4.5	7.6	12.3
1 000	2 175	457	−5.3	−0.3	−5.8	−2.7	7.6	12.7
2 000	2 174	456	−4.4	−0.1	−4.7	−2.9	8.0	13.0
4 000	2 026	411	−3.6	+2.3	−4.1	−1.4	9.2	15.2
6 000	2 040	420	−1.8	+4.4	−3.0	+0.7	10.1	15.5
8 000	2 017	407	−3.0	+3.4	−3.9	0.0	11.0	17.8
Left Ear								
250	2 029	413	−10.6	−6.8	−11.1	−8.9	7.1	10.7
500	2 175	457	−7.4	−3.0	−7.8	−4.8	7.3	11.4
1 000	2 175	457	−5.2	−0.2	−5.6	−2.8	7.4	12.7
2 000	2 175	456	−4.5	−0.7	−4.8	−2.8	8.2	12.6
4000	2 026	410	−3.1	+1.2	−3.7	−2.2	9.1	12.0
6 000	2 040	419	−1.4	+3.7	−2.4	+0.7	10.3	15.7
8 000	2 018	406	−3.0	+3.0	−3.8	−0.5	11.1	16.7

hearing levels below audiometric zero at 250 cps. This percentage also falls as frequencies increase, to 50 percent at 8 000 cps. These data indicate the high percentages of children with otological abnormalities as well as those without these defects who have hearing levels substantially better than audiometric zero. A study of the distribution in Figure 7-3 indicates no evidence of masking.

There can be no question as to whether or not audiometers need to be properly maintained within the American Standard Specification if hearing measurement with these instruments is to be done with accuracy. This study demonstrated that at least one commercially available audiometer can be made to meet the American Standard Specification and that it can be modified to test with linearity below audiometric zero, but to accomplish this, proper calibration and repair facilities are needed.

Information obtained from reputable acoustics laboratories in the United States indicates that the experience with audiometers and audiometer performance in this study is not unique to the make of audiometer used. Recent studies (4, 5) on the output and general condition of audiometers in use in clinical situations in Scotland provide further evidence of the instability of these instruments and the need for better construction, better maintenance, and more frequent calibration.

A distinction should be made between the steps taken for the research purposes of this study, such as the adjustment of hearing level determination readings, and the necessary precautions taken in regard to maintenance of acoustic environment and audiometer calibration. These latter must be made an integral part of any hearing measurement program whether of a school population, a clinical case load, or an industrial program.

SUMMARY

Preliminary to a long-term nationwide study of children's hearing problems, an experiment was conducted in acoustic environment control and audiometer modification and performance. It is concluded that rigid criteria for control of acoustic environment can be met in the field; that audiometers can be modified to test accurately levels well below the American Standard audiometric zero; that precautions taken to control acoustic environment and to check audiometer calibration before and during use should be an integral part of any measurement hearing program.

Mean and median values of hearing levels

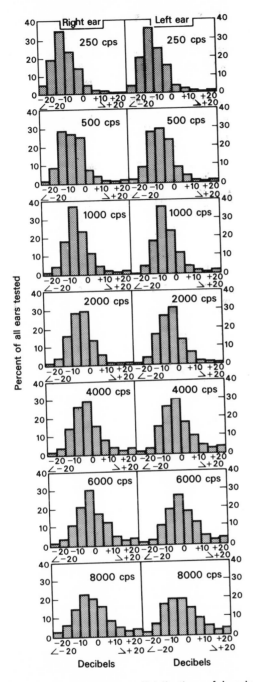

Figure 7-3. Percentage distribution of hearing levels (in db re American Standard audiometric zero) of 2 175 children in an otologically "normal" population tested between June 1958 and June 1959, each frequency by ear.

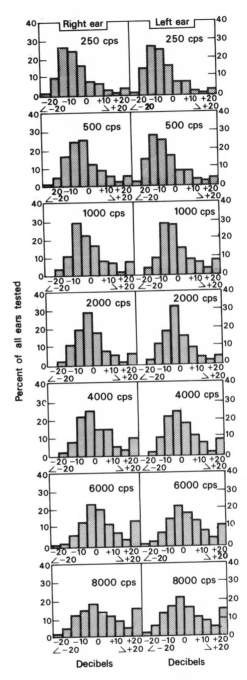

Figure 7-4. Percentage distribution of hearing levels (in db re American Standard audiometric zero) of 457 children in an otologically "abnormal" population tested between June 1958 and June 1959, each frequency by ear.

of children in this study vary with frequency and are more sensitive than the American Standard audiometric zero. A substantial number of otoscopically abnormal ears do not show hearing loss and conversely many ears with hearing loss show no observable otologic abnormality. It is concluded that audiometric testing alone cannot identify physical abnormalities of the ear which may have predictive value.

ACKNOWLEDGEMENT

Consultants to the study from the University of Pittsburgh include: Isidore Altman, Ph.D., Professor of Medical Care Statistics; Raymond E. Jordan, M.D., Clinical Professor of Otology; Samuel M. Wishik, M.D., M.P.H., Professor of Maternal and Child Health. The excellent work of the staff of the study is gratefully acknowledged, in particular that of Herbert S. Levine, M.Sc. (Hyg.), Biostatistician; William Melnick, Ph.D., Audiologist; and Mrs. Shirley J. Bakker, Administrative Assistant. The assistance of the Department of Occupational Health in the University of Pittsburgh's Graduate School of Public Health, and in particular of Assistant Professor Kenneth Stewart, Director of its Acoustic Laboratory, is also gratefully acknowledged.

REFERENCES

1. American Standards Association, *American Standard Criteria for Background Noise in Audiometer Rooms*, S3.1-1960. New York: Am. Standards Ass.

2. Cox. J. R., Jr., How quiet must it be to measure normal hearing? *Noise Control*, 1, 1, 1955, 25–29.

3. Eagles, E. L., and Wishik, S. M., A study of hearing in children: objectives and preliminary findings. *Trans. Amer. Acad. Ophthal. Otolaryngol.*, May–June, 1961.

4. Hinchcliffe, R., and Littler, T. S., Methodology of air-conduction audiometry for hearing surveys. *Ann. occup. Hyg.*, 1, 1958, 114–133.

5. Lenihan, J. M. A., *Scottish Audiometer Calibration Service Annual Report*. Glasgow: Dept. Health Scotland, West. Regional Hosp. Bd., 1957.

8

Acoustical Environment
for Industrial Audiometric Programs

MARTIN HIRSCHORN

MARTIN HIRSCHORN is President, Industrial Acoustics Company, Inc., New York City

The investment in good test equipment for an effective industrial audiometric program is not significant relative to operating costs and potential benefits. Satisfactory acoustical environments for testing purposes have become more critical due to the introduction of the 1964 ISO zero hearing level reference values in the United States.

In considering instrumentation and acoustical environment required for an audiometric testing program, it will be assumed that the decision to institute or improve an existing audiometric examination program has already been taken as part of a comprehensive hearing conservation program. The need for such

This article has been revised from the original and is reprinted by permission of the author from *Sound Vibration*, **1**, pp. 8–15 (1967).

Please note that this article refers to three standards.

1. ASA 1960 . . . sets criteria for background noise in audiometric rooms.

2. ASA 1951 . . . sets standard reference threshold hearing levels for audiometers for general diagnostic purposes.

3. ISO 1964 . . . sets standard reference threshold hearing levels adopted by the International Organization for Standardization. The values given differ considerably from ASA 1951 but have been made part of a proposed new American Standard for Audiometers now under consideration.

4. This article also includes a discussion regarding a possible amendment to ASA 1960 for audiometric rooms to conform with ISO 1964 and the proposed new American Standard for Audiometers.

5. ASA, the American Standards Association, became the U.S.A. Standards Institute in 1966, and all ASA standards are now known as USASI standards.

programs is being increasingly accepted, and reviews of legislative and claims activity related to noise-induced deafness have been published (*1*).

One reason for this emphasis is that the initial capital investment for an audiometric testing room and audiometers is usually much less than the cost of maintaining and administering such a program over a period of a few years.

A good audiometric testing program must be under medical supervision and will require the services of nurses and technicians. In addition, of course, the necessary space and administrative services, such as secretarial work and record keeping, must be provided. Though many variables will affect the cost of an industrial audiometric examination program, an annual operating expense of $6000 for a plant of 1000 employees would be reasonable. Such an expense can readily be offset if one considers that recent settlements, according to the chief industrial hygienist of a large corporation, have ranged from $1500 to $2000 per claim.

For a program of this size, a manual audiometer can be purchased for approximately $300, whereas an automatic audiometer would cost approximately $1500. A one-man audiometric examination room—designed for occupancy by the subject only—complete with ventilation system and installed, would cost about $1800. Therefore, basic equipment cost

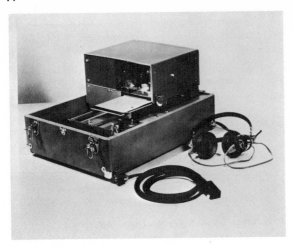

Figure 8-1.
An automatic self-recording audiometer for pure tone screening in an industrial audiometric program. The test subject uses a push button switch to control the level of the test tone. Hearing loss is automatically recorded as a function of frequency.

may range from $2100 to about $3600. As this constitutes a relatively small investment in relation to running costs and potential savings, it obviously makes sense to install testing equipment that will assure valid audiograms at all times.

If the validity of an audiogram can be questioned because of improperly calibrated instrumentation, because the noise levels in the testing area are too high, or because of poor medical supervision or poor record keeping, then the whole objective of the program will have been defeated. This objective is the hearing conservation of all employees and the protection of management against unjust compensation claims.

Proper instrumentation is, therefore, a major consideration. Any discussion of instrumentation requirements, moreover, has to cover not only the audiometer, but the testing environment as well.

THE AUDIOMETER

The time is long over when hearing-testing in industry and elsewhere was performed chiefly by the use of a conversational voice, a tuning fork, watch-tick tests, and similar procedures, which at best could provide only a cursory estimate of a person's hearing ability.

For an industrial hearing-testing program, however, all that is really required is a properly calibrated and maintained pure-tone air conduction screening instrument, made in accordance with ASA Standards and preferably listed by the American Academy of Ophthalmology and Otolaryngology (AAOO). Audiometers with provisions for bone-conduction and speech tests are unnecessary and may be needlessly expensive for industrial programs.

An industrial, screening audiometer should have test frequencies at 500, 1000, 2000, 3000, 4000, and 6000 c/s. These are the frequencies recommended by the "Guide for Conservation of Hearing in Noise" (2).

Manual and Self-Recording Audiometers

In selecting an audiometer there is a choice between a *manual* and an *automatic* or *self-recording* audiometer (Figure 8-1) plus a manual audiometer. The reason for including the manual audiometer when an automatic instrument is available is that, in the experience of some otologists and audiometricians, approximately 12 per cent of all subjects are unsuitable for automatic audiometry.

With a self-recording instrument, the subject controls the test and in effect makes his own hearing threshold determination. With a manually operated instrument, this is the responsibility of the nurse or technician, who must be in constant attendance. The operation of a self-recording audiometer, therefore, has the advantage of saving time, personnel, and expense. Because it is less demanding and tiring on the technician, it also tends to reduce errors.

The self-recording audiometer has its greatest usefulness when a large number of employees have to be tested or when the person in charge of the instrument is expected to perform other functions as well. Up to four instruments and test rooms can be used simultaneously, and one technician can supervise

for many years, that correction factors for background noise can be applied is completely false and misleading. This subject is discussed in detail in "How Quiet Must it Be to Measure Normal Hearing?" (3). The large volume of work done in this field has culminated in the American Standard Criteria for Background Noise in Audiometer Rooms (4).

An Acceptable Acoustical Environment for Audiometric Testing

The maximum permissible background sound-pressure levels that would not mask the test

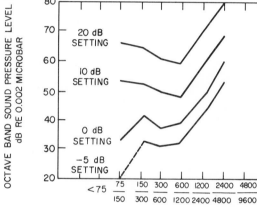

Figure 8-2.
Ambient noise levels in the audiometric testing environment that will just mask the audiometer test tones at given settings of the hearing-loss dial. The data are presented in terms of sound pressure levels within octave bands applied to a subject wearing a properly fitting binaural head set.

the entire operation. Experts in the field do not consider group testing, using a single audiometer with multiple earphones, to be practical, and therefore it is not recommended for threshold audiometry in industry.

THE TESTING ENVIRONMENT

Regardless of whether the instrument is manually operated or self-recording, a calibrated acoustical environment is required. This can be defined as a room with an ambient sound level that will permit the determination of a subject's threshold of hearing (Figure 8-2). It has been demonstrated that in the presence of extraneous ambient sounds incorrect audiograms will be obtained. The assumption, held

tone can be defined in terms of octave bands and for narrow-band sound whose center frequency is nearly that of the test tone (Tables 8-1 and 8-3). Substantially lower sound-pressure levels are required if the masking frequencies are close to those of the test tone itself. The type of narrow-band noise that could create such a high degree of masking could come from the screech of a machine part or the burbling of a peanut whistle.

The ASA Standard and the Guide do not set any levels for the first octave; in addition, the Guide does not set any levels for the second and third octaves, because the ambient noise in these bands has little or no effect at the recommended test frequencies, if audiograms begin at 500 c/s.

The possible effects of vibration on the test

TABLE 8-1. MAXIMUM ALLOWABLE BACKGROUND SOUND PRESSURE LEVELS FOR NO MASKING ABOVE THE ZERO HEARING LOSS SETTING ON A STANDARD AUDIOMETER (DECIBELS RE 0.0002 MICROBAR), AS PER ASA STANDARD S3.1-1960 (4)

Audiometric Test Frequency (c/s)	Octave Band Cut-off Frequencies (c/s)*	Sound-Pressure Level (dB)	Spectrum Level of Narrow-Band Sound (dB)
125	75– 150	40	21
250	150– 300	40	18
500	300– 600	40	15
1000	600– 1200	40	12
2000	1200– 2400	47	16
4000	2400– 4800	57	23
6000	4800– 9600	62	25
8000	4800– 9600	67	30

* Which has a center frequency nearly that of the test tone.

environment must also be borne in mind. For instance, vibration transmitted through a subject's chair or through the table on which he may lean may cause interference.

The Effect of the International Standard Reference Zero

In considering the maximum background noise levels, an important, relatively recent development must be discussed. When the original reference threshold hearing levels were established in 1935 by the U.S. Public Health Service, they were definitely higher than those obtained later in more careful field studies (5). It is therefore considered today that the zero hearing level reference used in the United States is approximately 10 dB higher than the equivalent levels used in Western Europe. In 1964 the International Organization for Standardization, of which the United States is a member, accepted zero hearing level reference values that meet the most rigid standards possible and therefore are suitable as a worldwide standard. Accordingly, if the ISO Standard is also adopted in the United States, threshold levels that are approximately 10 dB lower than the present American Standard will result.

Currently, neither the ASA nor the Industrial Medical Association have accepted the ISO recommendations, though the American Academy of Ophthalmology and Otolaryngology, the American Speech and Hearing Association, and other groups of specialists are already using them, and at least one major manufacturing company has adopted the ISO Standard for industrial screening. Consequently, two separate audiometric reference levels are used in this country. To differentiate between the two, it is necessary to define the reference levels very clearly in each case.

A comparison can be made between the hearing levels of the American Standard Specification for Audiometers for General Diagnostic Purposes (Z24.5-1951) and those adopted by the International Organization for Standardization (ISO) (2). It will be seen that the adoption of the ISO Standards would result in threshold levels approximately 9 to 15 dB lower than presently used (Table 8-2).

TABLE 8-2. 1951 ASA AND 1964 ISO REFERENCE THRESHOLD LEVELS (2)

Frequency (c/s)	Reference Threshold Levels		
	1951 ASA (dB)	1964 ISO (dB)	Differences (dB)
125	54.5	45.5	9
250	39.5	24.5	15
500	25	11	14
1000	16.5	6.5	10
1500	(16.5)*	6.5	(10)
2000	17	8.5	8.5
3000	(16)	7.5	(8.5)
4000	15	9	6
6000	(17.5)	8	(9.5)
8000	21	9.5	11.5

* The figures in parentheses are interpolations.

As already indicated, opposition has developed in this country against adopting the ISO Standard because it is feared that higher compensation awards might be payable through a misunderstanding of the new ISO scale. In the determination of hearing loss, a so-called low fence or upper limit of normal hearing is employed, which under the ISO values would be increased by 11 dB. The low fence, or point where hearing impairment is considered to begin, lies at 15 dB relative to ASA 1951 and 26 dB relative to ISO 1964 (5). A simple comparison of the two scales can

TABLE 8-3. MAXIMUM ALLOWABLE BACKGROUND SOUND PRESSURE LEVELS IN DB FOR NO MASKING ABOVE THE ZERO HEARING LOSS SETTING ON A STANDARD AUDIOMETER (DECIBELS RE 0.0002 MICROBAR). THE PROPOSED STANDARD DATA WERE DEVELOPED BY SUBTRACTING THE DIFFERENCE BETWEEN THE ASA AND ISO REFERENCE THRESHOLD VALUES FROM THE ASA BACKGROUND NOISE DATA

Audiometric Test Frequency (c/s)	Octave Band Sound-Pressure Level (dB)			Spectrum Level of Narrow-Band Sound (dB)		
	Octaves	ASA 1960	Proposed Standard	c/s	ASA 1960	Proposed Standard
125	75/150	40	31	125	21	12
250	150/300	40	25	250	18	3
500	300/600	40	26	500	15	1
1000	600/1200	40	30	1000	12	2
2000	1200/2400	47	38	2000	16	7
4000	2400/4800	57	51	4000	23	17
6000	4800/9600	62	51	6000	25	15
8000	4800/9600	67	56	8000	30	18

readily prevent any misunderstandings on the part of compensation officials (Figure 8-3).

SELECTION OF AN AUDIOMETRIC TESTING ROOM

Sound isolated testing rooms must be provided to obtain satisfactory levels for audiometric testing. Such a room can either be construc-

ted on the *do-it-yourself principle* or be purchased in accordance with time-proven performance specifications. The latter method is much to be preferred and in fact constitutes a widely accepted method for providing an adequate audiometric testing environment.

In selecting an audiometric testing room one must first decide on the required *dimensions*. If only one person is to be tested at any one time, a relatively small room can be

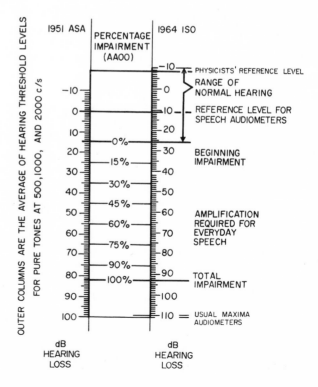

Figure 8-3.
Comparison between the ASA 1951 and ISO 1964 scales and the AAOO percentage impairment scale. Most audiometric test instrumentation can be calibrated to either ASA or ISO standards and both are in common use throughout the United States. An approximate comparison of ASA and ISO audiograms can be made for the 500, 1000, and 2000 c/s test tones with the above chart (2). Physical reference values are also indicated.

selected; a frequently used standard measures 48 in. × 44 in. × 90 in. high. Such a room could be located inside another room having approximately 150 to 200 sq ft of floor area. This would provide space for the technician outside the testing room and also for storage of pertinent records and other reference materials. If, of course, two persons are to be tested simultaneously, two audiometric test rooms would be required and a correspondingly larger area.

After a *location* for the test facility has been selected, which may be influenced by its proximity to the medical or personnel department, an acoustical survey will have to be made. Depending on the results obtained, a decision must be made on the acoustical structure to be employed to obtain a satisfactory audiometric testing environment. Rarely can this ever be obtained without the provision of a sound-isolated room.

Often, the first thought that occurs to those providing such a facility is to apply acoustical treatment to the walls and ceiling of an existing room. Absorptive walls are, of course, a prime prerequisite for any room that is to be used for audiometry, because testing in a reverberant environment is likely to result in inaccurate audiograms. Nevertheless, acoustical treatment alone is rarely adequate to obtain the degree of sound isolation required. The amount of noise reduction inside a room obtainable with heavy acoustical lining on the walls is about 5 dB. The figure 10 dB is often mentioned, but in practice this is unrealizable and represents a theoretical maximum.

Instead, sound isolation, as distinct from sound absorption, is required. A sound-isolating wall must be impervious, solid, and usually of substantial weight. A sound-absorptive material does not have to be heavy and can be acoustically transparent; it usually consists of fibrous porous material. Thus, in considering the use of absorptive material, its sound isolation or sound transmission loss values can usually be neglected.

Up to the early 1950's sound-isolated rooms were often built with common construction materials. These may have involved 2-in. ×

4-in. studs with gypsum board or plywood on both sides; other constructions involved 4-in. cinder or concrete block with one or both sides plastered, or alternatively 8-in. brick walls, and other structures. Although the theoretical sound transmission loss values of some of these constructions are good, the end results were often unsatisfactory.

Good design, alone, for a sound-isolated room is not enough. The end results depend on continuous supervision of the construction details. Because this is generally impractical, many shortcuts are likely to be taken, and the end result will be quite unsatisfactory. Further-

TABLE 8-4. TYPICAL NOISE REDUCTION VALUES FOR IAC PREFABRICATED AUDIOMETRIC ROOMS

Octave Band Cut-Off Frequencies (c/s)	Single 4-in. Wall Transmission Loss (dB)	Double 4-in. Wall Transmission Loss (dB)
75–150	28	48
150–300	36	64
300–600	46	79
600–1200	53	81
1200–2400	58	79
2400–4800	61	83
4800–9600	63	80

more, the cost of such construction is likely to be very high, and it cannot be recovered if a facility has to be relocated.

During the last twelve years, well over 80 percent of all sound-isolated audiometric testing rooms have been constructed using completely prefabricated structures. Rooms are available in two basic forms of construction, with single 4-in.-thick walls, and double 4-in.-thick walls with a 4-in. air space. Such rooms can be provided with their own floors, which rest on rubber in shear vibration isolators.

MAXIMUM PERMISSIBLE OUTSIDE-NOISE FIELDS

The maximum allowable noise levels outside of both single and double wall audiometric test rooms can be calculated based on the ASA

TABLE 8-5. MAXIMUM ALLOWABLE OUTSIDE NOISE LEVELS FOR SINGLE AND DOUBLE-WALLED ROOMS. NOTE THAT A SAFETY FACTOR OF 10 DB HAS BEEN ADDED TO ACCOUNT FOR FLUCTUATING AMBIENT NOISE CONDITIONS. EITHER THE ASA OR PROPOSED STANDARD AMBIENT DATA SHOULD BE SELECTED BASED ON CALIBRATION OF THE AUDIOMETER TO BE USED WITH THE ROOM. (COURTESY INDUSTRIAL ACOUSTICS COMPANY.)

Frequencies (c/s)	125	250	500	1000	2000	4000	6000	8000
Octave band cut-off frequencies (c/s)	$\frac{75}{150}$	$\frac{150}{300}$	$\frac{300}{600}$	$\frac{600}{1200}$	$\frac{1200}{2400}$	$\frac{2400}{4800}$	$\frac{4800}{9600}$	$\frac{4800}{9600}$
Permissible octave-band levels ASA 1960 (dB)	40	40	40	40	47	57	62	67
Single-walled Room								
Room attenuation (+)	28	36	46	53	58	61	63	63
Uncorrected ambient levels	68	76	86	93	105	118	125	130
Safety factor (−)	10	10	10	10	10	10	10	10
Maximum allowable ambient levels ASA 1960 (dB)	58	66	76	83	95	108	115	120
Correction factors (−)	9	15	14	10	8.5	6	9.5	11.5
Maximum allowable ambient levels for proposed standard (dB)	49	51	62	73	86.5	102	105.5	108.5
Double-walled Room								
Room attenuation (+)	48	64	79	81	79	83	80	80
Uncorrected ambient levels	88	104	119	121	126	140	142	147
Safety factor (−)	10	10	10	10	10	10	10	10
Maximum allowable ambient levels ASA 1960 (dB)	78	94	109	111	116	130	132	137
Correction factors (−)	9	15	14	10	8.5	6	9.5	11.5
Maximum allowable ambient levels for proposed standard (dB)	69	79	95	101	107.5	124	122.5	125.5

background noise data, the attenuation of the room, and the ISO threshold data (Tables 8-4 and 8-5). A minimum safety factor of 10 dB and perhaps even 15 dB should be used in determining these levels. Frequently, the ambient conditions that have been measured in an area fluctuate; moreover, they may increase with time. Therefore the use of such a safety factor is good planning and will assure long-term adequacy of the audiometric testing facility.

The noise reduction or attenuation values of a room increase rapidly with frequency, whereas a typical industrial spectrum may go the other way. This means that the high-frequency noise levels are often considerably lower than the low-frequency noise levels.

TABLE 8-6. COMPARISON OF NC40 CRITERION WITH ASA 1960 AND PROPOSED STANDARD ALLOWABLE BACKGROUND SOUND-PRESSURE LEVELS

Octave Band Cut-Off Frequencies (c/s)	$\frac{75}{150}$	$\frac{150}{300}$	$\frac{300}{600}$	$\frac{600}{1200}$	$\frac{1200}{2400}$	$\frac{2400}{4800}$	$\frac{4800}{9600}$
NC40 (dB)	59	52	46	42	40	38	37
ASA 1960 (dB)	40	40	40	49	47	57	62
Proposed Standard (dB)	31	25	26	30	38	51	51

The most critical octaves generally are the 75–150, 150–300, and 300–600 c/s bands. Once the criteria for these have been met, the higher bands are generally of less consequence.

EARPHONE/EARMUFF COMBINATIONS

The use of audiometer earphones mounted inside earmuffs has been suggested to save

tions of the nurse or technician who administers the test. It is obvious that the maximum allowable levels previously tabulated are too high for comfort; indeed, they could seriously endanger hearing. A reasonably quiet environment for the technician is a noise criterion of NC 40. This data should be compared with the allowable background sound-pressure levels under ASA 1960 and for the proposed modified levels taking into account ISO 1964 reference levels (Table 8-6).

It can readily be seen that in the high fre-

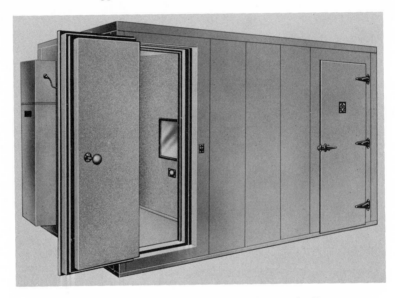

Figure 8-4. A combined control/audiometric examination room.

the cost of an audiometric room. Adaptation of such an apparent low-cost solution cannot be recommended. Results would not be in accordance with required standards and, in any case, would be rather unreliable because earphone attenuation may vary with each individual—the fit in each application may be different.

A QUIET ENVIRONMENT FOR THE TECHNICIAN

It is considered best for the subject to sit inside the audiometric examination room, thus some thought must be given to the working condi-

quencies the conditions for a quiet environment for the technician are more severe than those required for audiometric testing. It may therefore also be necessary to provide a sound-isolated area for the technician.

Such a requirement can be met by placing the test room in an area that meets NC 40 data or by procuring a combination control and test room. These are also available in different sizes (Figure 8-4).

CONCLUSIONS

An examination room with sufficient isolation for existing ambient noise levels and a precision audiometer are required for valid audiograms in an industrial audiometric program. Sufficient isolation must be at least 10 dB better than specified in ASA standards if the audiometric measurements are to be made relative to the ISO 1964 zero hearing level reference values.

It appears very likely that for the next several years both standards will be used in this country; many doctors, schools, and clinics, and at least one large manufacturing plant have already adopted ISO 1964. Which one to use must be decided by each company or organization, in conjunction with its advisers. In the meantime, however, prefabricated audiometric testing rooms and audiometers are available to meet both the ASA and the ISO Standards.

ACKNOWLEDGMENT

The author is pleased to acknowledge Mr. Ellis Singer's many helpful suggestions, including the provision of reference materials.

REFERENCES

1. Martin Hirschorn, "Industrial Noise—Economic Considerations, Legal Trends, and Abatement Techniques," *National Safety News*, June 1965.

2. "Guide for Conservation of Hearing In Noise," Subcommittee on Noise of the Committee on Conservation of Hearing and Research Subcommittee on Noise, American Academy of Ophthalmology and Otolaryngology.

3. Jerome R. Cox, Jr., "How Quiet Must It Be to Measure Normal Hearing?" *Noise Control*, January 1955, pp. 25–29.

4. American Standard Criteria for Background Noise in Audiometer Rooms, S3.1-1960, American Standards Association.

5. Aram Glorig, "Audiometric Reference Levels," *The Laryngoscope*, LXXVI, 5 (May 1960).

9

Audiometer Calibration

EARL R. HARFORD

EARL R. HARFORD, Ph.D., is Professor of Audiology, Northwestern University

PART I

Accuracy in audiometry is based upon three important requisites: a competent tester, a controlled acoustic test environment, and accurate test equipment. Too often attention is directed mainly toward these first two requisites, whereas little or no attention is given to the strict calibration and periodic maintenance of test equipment. Satisfaction of these three prime ingredients is as important to the conduct of clinical audiometry as it is to research. It is understandable that the clinician might be inclined to sacrifice rigor in his instrumentation in the face of challenging and difficult clinical problems and a burdensome case load. Yet, as we shall attempt to point out, such neglect is most undesirable and, in fact, a prelude to clinical folly. The word *clinical*, as it is used here, implies any setting where one finds applied audiometry, which includes hearing conservation programs as well as clinics or physicians' offices.

Undoubtedly there are some individuals using audiometers regularly who have little understanding and appreciation for the meaning of the term *calibration*. Consequently, it may be appropriate to begin our discussion of this topic with a brief working definition of this term. A calibrated audiometer is simply one which: (1) emits the signal at the level and frequency it claims to be producing, (2) de-

livers the signal only to the place (i.e. a specific earphone) it is directed, (3) produces the signal free from contamination by extraneous noises or unwanted by-products of the test signal. For example, when the audiometer is set to deliver a 1000 cps pure tone signal at 40 dB, re: zero hearing level, to the right earphone, it should do precisely this; instead of, for example, delivering a signal of 1170 cps at 55 dB to the right earphone with a portion of the same signal to the left phone as well.

Of course, there are recognized tolerances for the important physical characteristics of pure-tone audiometric signals and these should be taken into account in any critical evaluation of the output of one of these units.

The American Standards Association (1) has a published pamphlet of these specifications including tolerance allowances. These specifications are in the process of revision and a new set should be available in the foreseeable future. Further, there are separate specifications for diagnostic and screening audiometers, which do not, however, differ greatly. We will refer to the diagnostic specifications here.

On the whole, audiometer manufacturers are careful to design and produce audiometers which meet the specifications quoted by the ASA. Unfortunately, once an audiometer is set to these standards of performance, there is no assurance that it will remain in calibration. As a matter of fact, this equipment is sensitive and highly susceptible to

Reprinted by permission of the author from *Maico Audiological Library Series*, **3**, Reports 5 and 6 (1965).

unintentional abuse that can result in faulty operation. Recommendations by audiometer manufacturers, personal experience, and published reports (3) attest to the importance of periodic calibration to assure accuracy of the signal and an overall high level of performance by the audiometer.

The Problem

There are some 50,000 audiometers extant in the United States and probably in excess of 10,000 in active service. The majority are being used in the armed forces, school hearing conservation programs, doctors' offices, industry, speech and hearing centers, and hearing aid dealers' offices. The operators of these audiometers are doctors, nurses, speech clinicians, audiologists, technicians, teachers, parents, high school seniors, and businessmen.

Provided a facility does not conduct its own calibrations, the major source for this service is through the manufacturer or one of his local or regional representatives. A check with two of the leading audiometer manufacturers clearly supports the suspicion that a very small percentage of audiometers receive periodic calibration. In fact, most calibrations are done only after an audiometer has stopped operating completely, or after it becomes noticeably unusable.

One reason for this neglect may be the result of the inconvenience of packing and shipping the instrument as well as parting with a unit that seems to be operating adequately. Regardless of the cause, there appears to be a serious need for a vigorous educational program to draw attention to the importance and value of periodic audiometer calibration.

There are numerous reasons for an audiometer to lose its precision; such as, dropping earphones, overheating (leaving the audiometer turned on after covering it with a dust protector), exposure to excessive dust (transporting an audiometer in the trunk of an automobile over dusty roads), exposure to high humidity and salt-air, excessive jarring, and normal aging of the electrical components. Whenever it is known that an audiometer or the earphones have been subjected to abuse, it should be suspect until proven otherwise.

Let us now examine the nature of inaccurate calibration and the possible sources of error in the signal which an audiometer produces.

Frequency. Most audiometers have little difficulty meeting the ASA ±5 percent specified tolerance for frequency. (The new specifications call for a ±3 percent error.) For example, on the basis of the current standards, this means that an audiometer can produce a signal from 950 to 1050 cycles per second when set at 1000 cps or 3800 to 4200 cycles when set at 4000 cps. Of course, the lower the frequency, the less tolerable variance in cycles per second (i.e. 120 to 130 for 125 cps). Even though these tolerances are established, one should strive to maintain as accurate a frequency output as possible. It is obvious what would result if a person with a sharp drop in hearing starting at precisely 1000 cps would show on two audiometers with considerable variance in frequency output. On one that produces 950 cps at the 1000 cps setting, threshold could be close to normal, but on another that produces 1200 cps at the same setting, threshold could conceivably be much poorer than normal. Inaccurate frequency output is a problem chiefly in clinical or diagnostic audiometry. It is of minimal consequence in "field" audiometry.

Harmonics. Even though we are allegedly using pure tones in the basic measurement of hearing, it is possible to have harmonics of the fundamental (test frequency) present in the earphones. The ASA specifications call for the fundamental to be at least 25 dB (30 dB in the new specifications) above the sound pressure level of any harmonic.

A person with a hearing loss in the lower frequencies, with better hearing in the higher frequencies could present optimistic thresholds in the lows if the harmonics are not well below the fundamental. That is, threshold would be obtained for the harmonic instead of the fundamental.

Intensity. In this category we can encounter two problems which may or may not be related. First, the intensity output can be generally too strong or too weak. The ASA standard allows for a ±4 dB variance in intensity over the full range from −10 to maximum output at the test frequency of 2000 cps and lower, and ±5 dB at the test frequencies above 2000 cps. It also specifies a ±1.5 dB variation in any 5-dB step throughout the intensity range. The ASA standard notwithstanding, it is important to know whether your audiometer is producing the intensity it claims to be producing on the dial, or if, in fact, it is producing more or less than this reading. For example, if one audiometer is 10–15 dB weak, every person tested on it will show a greater hearing loss than on an accurate audiometer. This can cause such results as an overly optimistic air-bone gap, atypical audiometric configurations in otherwise typical clinical cases (where one or two frequencies are off) and an apparent greater need for amplification or middle-ear surgery than otherwise is the actual case. Further, a person's hearing might be classified as progressive in a case where an audiometer developed

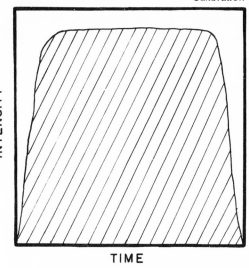

Figure 9-2. An illustration of uniform rise (on) and decay (off) times of a pure tone test signal with an absence of undesirable overshoot and uneven plateau.

this problem between an initial test and follow-up testing. An audiometer that is too strong, however, can present problems similar to those just described, but in an opposite direction.

This problem is probably even more critical in identification audiometry where 5–10 dB one way or the other (strong or weak) can mean the difference between effective screening or an almost complete waste of time. The screening audiometer that is too strong will pass cases that should not have passed. A strong audiometer is a real hazard in an identification audiometry program.

The second problem with intensity is nonlinearity. Figure 9-1 illustrates what happens when an audiometer fails to attenuate (decrease output) uniformly below 10 dB. Anyone with an actual threshold of 0 or 5 dB will report hearing a tone when the dial is set at −10 dB. This may be an insignificant problem so far as diagnostic audiometry is concerned, but it does present serious problems in identification audiometry. Audiometers that are non-linear below 15 dB are virtually useless in identification audiometry.

Tone Interruption. Figure 9-2 illustrates the upper-half of a signal on an oscilloscope when

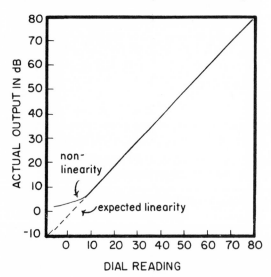

Figure 9-1. A graphic illustration of an example of a non-linear auditory test signal. Note, as the dial reading is decreased below 10 dB, the actual output of the signal fails to decrease as the dial reading indicates and then remains constant. In other words, a decrease of the dial does not decrease the output of the signal.

it is turned on and then turned off. According to the 1951 ASA specifications, it should rise to its peak within 100 to 500 milliseconds and go off in the same period of time. Actually, it is undesirable to have a rise-decay time more than 200 milliseconds. The audiometer should not present an unusually long rise and decay time (Figure 9-3) and there should be an absence of overshoot in the tone (Figure 9-4). The precision of the signal presentation can be very critical for accuracy in audiometry. The physiological rationale and clinical implications for this are clearly presented by Carhart and Jerger (2). Briefly a slow rise time may fail to elicit maximum on-effect of the auditory mechanism and result in a poorer threshold than, in fact, is present. On the other hand, overshoot may result in the establishment of better thresholds than are present. Finally, if the rise time is too brief and overshoot is present (Figure 9-5) the result could be an audible click in the pure tone signal, thus encouraging a threshold for clicks and not for pure tones.

Isolation Between Earphones. Perhaps one of the more subtle and least recognized problems in accurate pure tone instrumentation is a lack of complete isolation between earphones.

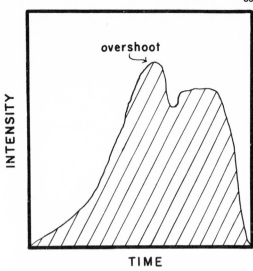

Figure 9-4. An illustration of unwanted overshoot in the presentation of a pure-tone test signal.

Ideally, in threshold measurements, when a test signal is delivered to one earphone, nothing should be going to the opposite phone, except, of course, a masking stimulus when desired. Figure 9-6 illustrates what sometimes occurs in an audiometer when complete isolation is neglected. This leakage or cross-talk can be so low in intensity that the average adult ear and even delicate laboratory measuring equipment may not detect the problem. However, we know that children and young adults typically have thresholds somewhat better than −10 dB, re: the USPH norms. Therefore, one could obtain absolutely normal thresholds for both ears in a case where one ear actually has a mild to moderate loss in acuity, because the good ear could have been stimulated when the test tone was delivered to the poorer ear. A quick check of this possibility would be the introduction of masking to the good ear, or disconnecting the earphone cord to the good ear, or slipping the non-test earphone away from the ear. Unfortunately, even the alert clinician can err in this situation because children, where slight cross-talk presents the greatest problem, are often unaware of a hearing imbalance between ears. Often, it is not until speech audiometry or other tests are employed that this situation is revealed.

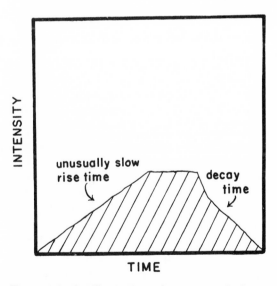

Figure 9-3. An illustration of an unusually long rise time and a decay which is unequal to the rise time. A desirable rise and decay time is approximately 100 milliseconds.

Nevertheless, clinicians should be constantly alert to the possibility of cross-talk and double check clinical cases where bilateral super-normal thresholds are obtained by using low levels of masking in the non-test phone or one of the other two techniques mentioned above.

Other problems. At least the more common shortcomings in audiometer calibration have been discussed above. There certainly are other problems, which are simply listed:

Audible click in earphone when changing frequency (especially undesirable in screening audiometers).

Acoustic radiation from audiometer chassis (a serious problem when testing persons with one normal ear or an ear with normal thresholds for a portion of the test frequency range, especially when attempting to establish bone conduction thresholds).

Erratic earphone response.

Static or scratching noise with change of hearing level dial.

External or mechanical click in tone interruptor.

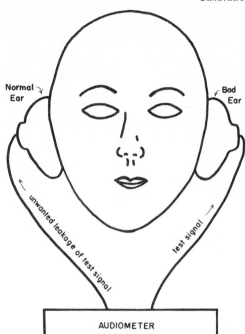

Figure 9-6. A schematic showing cross talk or leakage of a test signal from the intended earphone to the opposite phone. This situation could result in an audiogram showing two normal ears, where, in fact, one ear has a hearing loss.

Noise from other sources (line or power hum) than test signal in earphones. The new ASA specifications state that no noise should be present when audiometer is turned to 50 dB. Above this level, the noise should be 60 dB below the test signal.

Conclusion

Attention to the precision of an audiometer cannot be over-emphasized. Well documented evidence and personal experience attests to the fact that an audiometer can easily fall short of the physical characteristics required as basic requisites to the accurate assessment of auditory function. Audiometers should receive periodic rigorous maintenance and calibration. Methods and procedures of both laboratory and field calibrations for air conduction and bone conduction receivers will appear in the following Report.

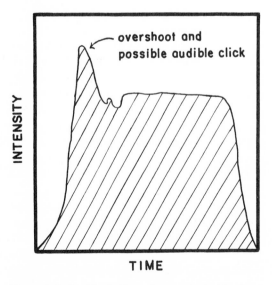

Figure 9-5. An illustration of an undesirably short rise time with overshoot. This situation can lead to an audible click as the tone is presented.

PART II

The previous Report in this two-part series discussed some of the inaccuracies which can affect the precision of an audiometer and stressed the importance of careful periodic maintenance and checks on the calibration of these electroacoustical instruments. This second part of the series will deal with procedures for checking the pure tone signals, both for air and bone conduction. Emphasis will be on non-laboratory procedures, the assumption being that the majority of audiometer users do not have immediate access to specialized technical knowledge and costly measuring equipment.

Accessibility to expensive equipment and special technical knowledge notwithstanding, it is worthwhile to mention at least the equipment necessary to conduct a thorough check on the characteristics of a pure tone signal which were described in Part I of this series. The following is a list and approximate value of the components involved in a laboratory calibration of a pure tone audiometer:

Equipment	Approximate Cost
Condenser microphone	$ 275.00
Microphone complement	875.00
Wave analyzer	1,275.00
Attenuators	200.00
Power amplifier	200.00
Vacuum tube Voltmeter	225.00
Sweep-frequency Oscillator	680.00
Graphic recorder	1,085.00
Oscilloscope	1,000.00
Events per Unit Time Meter	650.00
Total	$6,465.00

Competent assemblage and operation of this equipment is vital to achieve valid measurements and interpretation; consequently, the services of a person well-versed in electro-acoustics is essential.

Obviously this array of equipment is more than one could expect to maintain for a small number of audiometers such as often found in the typical school hearing conservation program, a modest speech and hearing center, a doctor's office, or hearing aid dealer's office.

Even so, the absence of such skilled personnel and special equipment is no excuse for neglect of the accuracy of audiometric equipment. It behooves the user to pay strict attention to the operating condition of his unit. Although in some areas laboratory facilities may be readily accessible for periodic calibrations, the operator of the audiometer should be aware of techniques for "spot checks" during those periods between laboratory checks.

The prime objective of this Report will be to discuss procedures and methods for checking accuracy of an audiometer in the absence of special laboratory measuring equipment similar to that listed above. Obviously, precise calibration is not intended, for only sensitive measuring equipment will provide this, but if one follows suggestions cited below he should at least be capable of determining when a laboratory calibration is indicated.

Gross Physical Check and Trouble Shooting

At the start of each day, the operator of an audiometer should examine his unit, both visually and auditorily. He should inspect the earphone cords (the weakest link, incidentally) for worn or cracked insulation, and straighten twisted cords. He should inspect the earphone cushions to be sure they are not cracked or marked with crevices due to shrinkage. The face of the audiometer should be inspected to insure against loose or slipped dials which may have gone out of alignment. Manipulation of the controls will offer a check on mechanical clicks in the attenuators, frequency selector, and interruptor switch. It is wise to vacuum carefully the dust from the inside of an audiometer periodically as it accumulates. Audiometers used in the field are more frequently subject to this need than those used in sound-isolated rooms. Let us now discuss in some detail several problems for which to listen in a gross check.

Following the visual check and after the power on the audiometer has been on for 10–15 minutes, the tester should place the earphones over his ears and listen to the signals as he manipulates the controls on the audiometer.

While the pure tone is on continuously in first one phone and then the other at a hearing level high enough to be heard with ease, one should twist first one earphone cord and then the other back and forth a half-turn and jiggle the cord at a place close to the earphone. If the tone goes off and on, either the cord is defective or one or both of the small screws holding the cord plug in the earphone is loose. A small jeweler's type screwdriver should be kept close at hand to tighten these screws periodically. If this does not rectify the problem, chances are good that the earphone cord needs replacement. It is wise always to keep a supply of cords, as well as earphone cushions. Defective cords and earphones are the most frequent cause of faulty operating equipment.

Next, with the pure tone signal at a high intensity level, one should listen for a change in the quality of the sound. An earphone which is distorting will frequently be detected by the human ear at high levels whereas such distortion may be inaudible at lower levels of intensity. With the hearing level set high one should interrupt the tone several times and listen for a "click" or "splat" sound just as the tone is turned on followed by the expected pure tone signal. If this is present, there is a good chance of undesirable overshoot or a transient in the rise-time of the signal (refer to Part I of this Series for more details relative to the consequences of this problem).

With the hearing level set at −10 dB and the signal on continuously, the intensity should gradually be increased in steps of 5 dB up to a high level. Each increment must be listened to carefully for a uniform increase in the intensity of the tone. It is not necessary to check this at more than one frequency or for more than one earphone. This provides a gross check on the linearity or uniformity of the attenuator (hearing level control). If a signal does not change in loudness with an increase of the dial, or if it appears to change drastically, it is a clue to a non-linear attenuator.

With the masking signal on in one earphone and the opposite earphone over the cheekbone, one should interrupt the pure tone several times at various intensity levels and listen for a "click" in the masking phone. Such a condition is undesirable for competent testing and can prove to be highly distracting for the person under test when masking is used.

To determine if the loudness varies from presentation to presentation, one should set the hearing level to a comfortable loudness and interrupt the pure tone several times. An audiometer may develop an inconsistency in the actual level of the pure tone signal when it is held at a constant intensity level and interrupted several times.

With the audiometer hearing level control set at about 40 dB, *without presenting the pure tone*, one should increase the intensity to its maximum and listen for the introduction of a hum or any other type of constant random signal. This is especially common in the speech circuit of combination pure tone and speech audiometers. A check for this same noise in the speech network, if it is not found to be present in the pure tone setting, is necessary. If this noise is detected, it is frequently alleviated by running a piece of hook-up wire from a screw on the back of the audiometer chassis to the screw which holds the face plate over a duplex wall power receptacle.

Simultaneously with a check for hum at high intensity levels, it is wise to listen for a static or scratching sound as the hearing level dial is varied. This suggests presence of dust or foreign particles in the attenuator and should be cleaned by a qualified technician if it cannot be alleviated by "working" the hearing level dial back and forth several dozen times.

The frequency selector should be moved through the frequency range with special attention to extraneous noises, such as clicks in the earphones when changing from one frequency to the next. Many audiometers make some noise when changing frequency, but these are external and do not occur in the earphones. Neither mechanical nor electrical noises present a serious problem except in screening audiometers where the frequency is changed more than the hearing level. In this latter case the noises should be alleviated.

"Cross-talk" between earphones can be a very serious problem, as we pointed out in Part I of the Report. Moreover, a couple of methods for checking the presence of "cross-talk" were given in the previous Report. As a last and important step, one earphone should be disconnected and the pure tone signal presented to it with the opposite phone at the ear of the examiner. For example, with the right earphone disconnected and the earphone-selector set to the Right Earphone, the left phone may be placed over the ear of a person with hearing well within normal limits and the pure tone presented. If, under these circumstances, a pure tone signal is heard in the left earphone, there is "cross-talk" in the system. This does not present a problem if the cross-talk occurs only at higher hearing levels starting at 50 or 60 dB because masking is used on the ear of a unilateral under these circumstances (i.e. if the subject has normal hearing in the good ear). It does, however, present a serious problem when the cross-talk is present at lower hearing levels, below 40 dB. Under these circumstances masking is usually not used because the difference between ears is within the interaural attenuation rate. Nevertheless, cross-talk at low hearing levels should be alleviated as soon as possible after detection.

To summarize, in this section various ways of detecting undesirable elements in the operating characteristics of an audiometer have been discussed. Our comments were limited primarily to the pure tone audiometer. Care should be taken that the person checking the audiometer has normal hearing, at least in one ear. The following section will deal with empirical methods for the calibration of the output level of a pure tone audiometer, both for air and bone conduction.

"Calibration" of the Output Level

We will now address ourselves to the empirical calibration of the accuracy in the output level of the audiometer. That is, is there agreement between what the hearing level dial says is coming out of the earphone and what the earphone *actually* emits? A method for deter-

mining this without accessibility to precision measuring equipment will be discussed.

Perhaps the quickest and easiest method is for the operator of the audiometer to keep a record of his own thresholds. He can then check his thresholds with the audiometer in question to determine its accuracy. The shortcomings of this approach are obvious. For one thing, threshold is not a fixed point. Threshold of acuity can be expected to vary within a range of 10 dB from day to day. Slight inconsistency in the location of earphone placement will also have an effect upon the obtained threshold and can cause as much as a 10 dB variance in threshold, especially in the low frequencies. Further, many operators of audiometers have thresholds at or better than −10 dB on our present audiometric scale. Thus, if an audiometer is emitting a signal which is too strong, the person with very acute hearing will have trouble detecting this problem. If the operator has a hearing loss, then this problem does not prevail, however, the possibility of a progressive hearing loss or one which fluctuates must be considered.

Another method was advocated several years ago before some of the valuable research had been reported on age and hearing level. In recent years we have come to appreciate some of the shortcomings in the 1951 ASA audiometric standard for threshold and the strong influence of age upon the average thresholds of groups.

The method advocated was to run threshold measurements on 10 or so young persons with "healthy normal ears." The persons in the group should be chosen carefully to avoid a history of familial hearing loss, ear problems, or noise exposure. The idea was to take an average of the thresholds obtained from the group and correct the audiometer to the amount which this average at each frequency deviated from zero. The problem with this approach is that a young healthy group of normal ears will present an average threshold at most frequencies of −10 dB on an audiometer with accurate output calibration. Unfortunately, they will also present a −10 dB average threshold if the audiometer is emitting a signal which is too strong. This method will isolate the audiometer which is too weak, provided the interpretation takes into account the 10 dB better sensitivity of young healthy ears. In brief, this method of employing a "group of normals" can be very risky.

If it is used, one should insert an attenuator in the line of the earphone which will decrease the output of the pure tone a known amount at each frequency. This will avoid the problem of obtaining a −10 dB average and the amount of this intended attenuation can be subtracted from the mean thresholds for the corrected value. However, the final interpretation will still have to take into account the 10 dB better sensitivity of the young normal group.

An approach which seems to be practical and void of serious shortcomings is a loudness balance method. In this case, the output from an audiometer known to be accurate is matched against an audiometer under question of accuracy. The mechanics of this procedure are simple, as illustrated in Figure 9-7. One earphone is detached from the headband of the accurate audiometer and placed on the headband of the "unknown" audio-

meter after removing one of its phones. The earphones should be placed on the ears of a young listener with healthy normal ears and with negligible difference in sensitivity between ears. Each audiometer is then set to the same frequency and the known audiometer is set to present a 40 dB interrupted-train of signals from 1 to $1\frac{1}{2}$ seconds duration for each toneburst. When the signal is off in the "known" earphone, it should be presented in the unknown earphone. While this presentation of signals continues, the hearing level of the unknown audiometer is varied until the point is reached where the signals in each earphone are equal in loudness. Simultaneous presentation of the signals from both audiometers should be carefully avoided.

At least three observers should be used when checking an audiometer with this method. It is worthwhile to balance at three hearing levels (20, 40 and 60 dB) at each frequency. Also, an average of three judgements should be obtained at each level for each frequency. A loudness-matching procedure can be very accurate, provided the subject is careful and well trained. Further, this approach is not nearly as time consuming as it may appear. Three subjects could be run through this procedure in one hour.

If a well-calibrated audiometer is available, this loudness balance procedure need not be used. Instead, thresholds can be obtained for ten hearing-impaired ears (one ear per subject) with both the "known" and "unknown" audiometers. The average threshold obtained at each frequency with the "unknown" audiometer can be compared with the "known" audiometer. Any difference between mean thresholds is probably due to an error in the unknown audiometer and can be corrected by this amount. That is, if a mean threshold of 40 dB is obtained with the accurate audiometer at a particular frequency, and a 50 dB mean threshold with the suspected audiometer at the same frequency, it might be assumed that the suspected audiometer is weak by 10 dB.

At least one obvious problem with these procedures is accessibility of the "known"

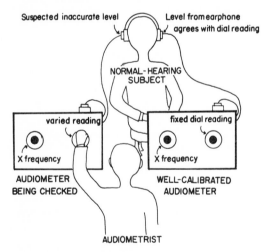

Figure 9-7. An illustration of a loudness balance method for checking an audiometer suspected of being inaccurate with one that is well-calibrated. The "tester" alternately operates the interruptor switches manually by first depressing one and then the other. At the same time, he varies the hearing level of the "unknown" audiometer until the subject reports that the signals delivered to each ear are equal in loudness.

audiometer. If one is available, it can certainly be used to check others that are unknown. When errors are found, it is not necessary to retire the audiometer until it is correctly adjusted at the source of trouble.

Instead, a simple correction notation can be attached to control panel in view of the tester. A sample of such a correction chart is shown in Figure 9-8. This chart can be used until the audiometer is calibrated by a service laboratory.

If funds are available it is wise to procure a simplified "artificial ear." A variety of these instruments are usually exhibited at the national meetings of the American Speech and Hearing Association and the American Academy of Ophthalmology and Otolaryngology. An accurate and a stable artificial ear is a valuable asset to a facility engaged in the measurement of hearing.

Let us now turn our attention to the calibration of the bone conduction system on an audiometer.

There is an artificial mastoid now commercially available for approximately $3000.00 which is stable and has very promising potential. Unfortunately, at the time of this writing, there is no standard bone threshold, thus this mastoid has limitations for clinical application. Moreover, the cost is rather high so that most clinicians are left with empirical bone calibration for the present time. Because of the problems of isolating a bone-conducted signal to a specific ear, loudness matching is perforce an undesirable technique for calibrating a bone vibrator.

Over the years, the method which has probably best stood the test of time as the most accurate approach is the one advocated by Roach and Carhart (4). Their method utilizes a group (ten persons will suffice) of individuals with otologically-diagnosed sensorineural hearing impairment. From our present-day experiences, the hearing loss should be of moderate degree and bilaterally symmetrical, but persons with presbycusis should be avoided.

Only one ear from each subject should be used; and masking should not be necessary if air thresholds are nearly identical in both

Corrections					date:				
	125	250	500	1K	2K	3K	4K	6K	8K
right									
left									
bone									
Red: make hearing poorer by above amounts									
Black: make hearing better by above amounts									

Figure 9-8. An example of a calibration correction card which can be mounted on the control panel of an audiometer. A color code reduces the confusion created by + or − signs. For example, black numbers could mean, "make hearing level better by the designated amount," and red numbers could mean, "make hearing level poorer by the designated amount." These corrections can be posted for b/c as well as a/c and can be changed when necessary.

ears. Of course, the ears should be unoccluded when making the bone measurements. The subjects should first have their hearing tested with a well-calibrated air conduction system. Then the bone conduction thresholds are obtained using the vibrator in question. Average air and bone thresholds are obtained for each frequency. The bone threshold is corrected to the air threshold at each frequency. For example, if the average air conduction threshold is found to be 40 dB at 1000 cps and the average of the bone thresholds for the group is 30 dB, one can assume that the bone system is too strong and optimistic bone thresholds are being obtained at this frequency. Therefore, a notation should be made on the correction card indicating that obtained bone thresholds at 1000 cps should be made 10 dB poorer. The reverse situation exists when the average bone threshold is found to be greater (poorer) than the air threshold. In this case, the correction should instruct the tester to make the obtained bone threshold better by a specified amount.

These empirical calibration checks should be made if an earphone or bone vibrator is dropped or receives a hard blow. There is a good chance that other problems, such as distortion, also are present. Under current conditions, it is not uncommon to find a bone vibrator to deviate 10 to 20 dB from air conduction "norms." Such deviations in the bone system do not necessarily suggest other problems. Consequently, it is probably safe simply to be aware of the deviation in the bone system and make the necessary corrections when recording the audiometric results.

Replacing the bone vibrator with a new one of the same make may not alleviate the error. However, in the air conduction channel, if it is discovered that rather large (more than 5 dB) corrections are necessary for an earphone at more than one or two frequencies, the earphone should be replaced.

Summary

Consistent attention to the accuracy of an audiometer should not be taken lightly.

Validity and reliability of hearing tests rest heavily upon the accuracy of the audiometer being used. Part I of this Series describes the problems which can develop in an audiometer. Part II offers suggestions for checking some of these problems in the absence of costly laboratory measuring equipment and specialized technical knowledge. Errors in the intensity level of pure tone signals can be noted on the face of an audiometer and be made in the recording of audiometric thresholds. However, when other problems are detected, arrangements for competent service should be made to correct the situation as quickly as possible. It is important that the operators of audiometric equipment should recognize that these units cannot be used ad infinitum without service.

REFERENCES

1. American Standards Association, Z24.5-1951, approved March 21, 1951. See Hirsh, I., *The Measurement of Hearing*. McGraw-Hill, New York, 1952, pp. 321–327.
2. Carhart, R., and Jerger, J. F., Preferred Method for Clinical Determination of Pure-Tone Thresholds. *Journal of Speech and Hearing Disorders*, **24**, 1959, 330–345
3. Eagles, E., and Doerfler, L. G., A Study of Hearing

in Children: Acoustic Environment and Audiometer Performance. *Transactions of the American Academy of Ophthalmology and Otolaryngology*, May–June, 1961, 283–296.
4. Roach, R., and Carhart, R., A method for calibrating a bone-conduction audiometer, *AMA Archives of Otolaryngology*, **63**, 1956, 270–278.

MEASUREMENT OF PURE-TONE THRESHOLDS

Comparison of air- and bone-conduction thresholds is still the most definitive method for determining the degree and type of hearing loss. Other assessments of auditory function, with few exceptions, must be interpreted with the audiogram in mind. The papers presented here are concerned primarily with techniques for insuring reliable threshold measurements and consideration of physiological factors affecting threshold estimation.

Although the first two papers are concerned with air-conduction measurements, their recommendations apply as well to bone-conduction threshold estimations. Carhart and Jerger propose a particular method for clinical measurement of auditory threshold. They present theoretical as well as experimental arguments for universal acceptance of the Hughson-Westlake technique. The technique includes the use of an "ascending" approach to threshold with relatively short tone-pulses presented at 5-dB intervals. Most clinicians have responded favorably to the suggestions of Carhart and Jerger, and this article is undoubtedly one of the most frequently cited in the audiological literature.

Lloyd discusses operant conditioning and its importance in clinical measurement, particularly with the difficult patient. He reviews a number of techniques designed to elicit threshold measurements in cases in which simple verbal instructions to the subject, as described by Carhart and Jerger, are not effective.

Comparison of bone-conduction sensitivity with air-conduction thresholds is still the most acceptable method for determining the relative contributions of conductive and sensorineural elements to a particular hearing problem. The clinical audiologist, however, must be aware of non-sensorineural changes which may affect bone-conduction transmission. These "mechanical" influences, peripheral to the cochlea, may result in improvement or depression of bone-conduction sensitivity and are generally caused by differential effects of pathology of the middle or external ear although they may be induced by the test procedure itself. While it might be desirable that bone conduction be independent of conditions peripheral to the cochlea, such is clearly not the case. The remaining papers in this section consider alterations of bone conduction due to mechanical factors and to the effects of these influences on the clinical measurement of bone conduction.

Obtaining bone-conduction thresholds presents difficulties not inherent in the measurement of air-conduction sensitivity. Some of these difficulties are caused by the virtual lack of interaural attenuation for bone-conducted stimuli; masking of the non-test ear is frequently necessary. Furthermore, bone-conduction thresholds will change depending upon the place and force of application of the vibrator, and will be affected by occlusion of one or both ears by an earphone.

Pathology of the conductive mechanism of the ear often alters bone-conduction thresholds, with the amount and direction of the change depending upon the type of lesion. Carhart, whose article is concerned primarily with the mechanical effects on bone conduction associated with otosclerosis, describes the characteristic configuration of the "Carhart notch" and reviews the evidence that the loss is mechanical rather than sensorineural. He discusses the disagreement among some theorists concerning the reasons for this mechanical change in bone-conduction transmission. Even though conductive hearing losses alter transmission of sound through the skull, the effects are probably different for various pathologies in the middle ear; Carhart uses otitis media and otosclerosis as examples to demonstrate differences for two types of conductive lesions. Knowledge of the expected mechanical loss in otosclerosis enables one to predict, with reasonable certainty, post-surgical hearing levels. Finally, Carhart identifies some problems encountered in the accurate assessment of bone conduction and describes briefly other methods of determining cochlear function.

The effects of the middle and external ear on bone-conduction sensitivity have been extensively studied by Tonndorf (1966). We present a summary version of his longer paper to demonstrate the complexity of the problem and to show that different conductive lesions affect bone conduction for different reasons. Various tuning fork tests are discussed in the light of his experimental results. In a subsequent paper (1968), Tonndorf presents a theory of bone conduction that is based, to a large degree, on his animal studies.

The reliability of bone-conduction measurements has been an important concern of audiologists and other investigators. Under carefully-controlled conditions, Dirks assessed the repeatability of bone-conduction measurements with different vibrators under a number of different conditions. He found that with reasonable care in adjusting vibrator pressure the clinician can expect good reliability. The reader is also referred to Weston, Gengel, and Hirsh (1967) for more information concerning the effects of type of vibrator and vibrator placement on reliability.

The two papers that follow concern the results of occlusion of the external ear on bone conduction. As is well known, such occlusion results in improved bone-conduction thresholds, particularly for lower frequencies, unless a conductive lesion is present. The occlusive effect can be related to increased sound pressure in the external auditory meatus. Goldstein and Hayes furnish data concerning the magnitude of this increase and then make comparisons between these measurements and the observed threshold shift for mastoid vs. forehead placement of the vibrator. Although positive relationships are found, the increase in sound-pressure level (SPL) in the occluded canal appears to be larger than the corresponding threshold shift. The authors discuss some possible explanations for the SPL increase. In a later study, Tyszka and Goldstein (1968) attempt to explain the discrepancy between the SPL increase and the threshold shift.

Dirks and Swindeman find that occlusion itself seems not to increase bone-conduction variability. They demonstrate this point with two occluding devices and with two groups of subjects having different levels of sophistication.

The commonly-held notion that bone conduction cannot be poorer than air conduction is discussed in a theoretical paper by Studebaker. He also indicates the danger inherent in attributing every AC–BC difference to conductive pathology. Because of normal variability, bone conduction will be better or poorer than air conduction in a certain percentage of cases.

The paper by Tillman evaluates SAL audiometry after audiologists in the United States had used this technique for approximately four years. He presents evidence that use of the SAL test produces two types of "errors": (1) unexpectedly low thresholds for high-frequency signals in sensorineural ears; and (2) unexpectedly high thresholds for low frequencies in ears with clinical otosclerosis, which is a finding in agreement with results of previous investigators. Later, Jerger and Jerger performed an additional study of the effects described by Tillman, as well as others involved in SAL audiometry. They found that differential consequences of occlusion on normal and conductively-deafened ears seem to account for the relatively poor low-frequency thresholds in otosclerotic ears unless occlusion factors are somehow eliminated or compensated for in the normal calibration group. The Tillman results concerning sensorineural ears were, generally, not found by Jerger and Jerger. More investigation of SAL results seems to be needed in such cases. The Jerger and Jerger paper contains descriptions of a number of variables related to bone-conduction audiometry which should be of interest to the student.

REFERENCES

1. Tonndorf, J. Bone-conduction: Studies in experimental animals. *Acta Otolaryngol.*, Suppl. 213 (1966).
2. Tonndorf, J. A new concept of bone conduction. *Arch. Otolaryngol.*, **87,** pp. 595–600 (1968).
3. Tyszka, F. A., and Goldstein, D. P. Occlusion effect: Unilateral sensorineural hearing loss. *J. acoust. Soc. Amer.*, **43,** pp. 324–327 (1968).
4. Weston, P. B., Gengel, R. W., and Hirsh, I. J. Effects of vibrator types and their placement on bone-conduction threshold measurements. *J. acoust. Soc. Amer.*, **41,** pp. 788–792 (1967).

10

Preferred Method for Clinical Determination of Pure-Tone Thresholds

RAYMOND CARHART
JAMES F. JERGER

RAYMOND CARHART, Ph.D., is Professor of Audiology, Northwestern University
JAMES F. JERGER, Ph.D., is Professor of Audiology, Baylor College of Medicine

Confusion and disagreement exist as to the preferred method for clinical determination of pure-tone thresholds. The procedures described in the literature are contradictory and sometimes quite complicated (*1, 7, 18, 27*). Moreover, as Hirsh emphasizes, "Since there is still no accepted standard technique, the clinician must be warned that the differences among these techniques may be responsible for differences among the thresholds that result from their use" (*8*). Not only does this uncertainty distress the conscientious audiometrist, but he often feels uneasy because necessary simplifications of routine cause him to deviate from full adherence to recognized methods for psychophysical measurement.

The purpose of the present paper is to urge that clinicians standardize their practices by adopting the basic features of the Hughson-Westlake (*10*) technique.[1] Both theoretical and practical considerations make this procedure logical for routine use when testing is done with a conventional pure-tone audiometer. This technique was accepted in 1944 by the Committee on Conservation of Hearing of the American Academy of Ophthalmology and Otolaryngology. In slightly revised form, it has since been advocated in various publications sponsored by the Committee (*19, 20*). Clinicians who have used the method have found it to be straightforward and satisfactory.

The discussion which follows (1) gives a brief description of an improved version of the Hughson-Westlake technique, (2) reviews those features of auditory behavior which determine the suitability of this method and (3) reports an experimental comparison between this method and two other procedures.

HUGHSON-WESTLAKE METHOD

The fundamental feature of the Hughson-Westlake procedure is that *minimum audibility is measured only by progressively increasing the stimulus intensity*. In other words, presentations always progress from levels where the sound is inaudible to the first level where perception of the stimulus occurs. As soon as the stimulus is heard, a new ascent is initiated. When using this procedure, *the clinical threshold is defined as the minimal level at which perception is achieved in more than half of the ascents*. In consequence, the Hughson-Westlake technique is sometimes called "the ascending method."

Obviously, the specific exploratory proce-

Reprinted by permission of the authors from *J. Speech Hearing Dis.*, **24**, pp. 330–345 (1959).

[1] This research was supported by the United States Air Force under Contract AF 41(657)-185, monitored by the School of Aviation Medicine, USAF, Randolph Air Force Base, Texas.

dure just described cannot be undertaken until the subject has been appropriately prepared for it. Consequently, the total process of administering an audiometric test is more involved than the preceding paragraph implies. The important thing, from the clinician's standpoint, is to keep the preparatory phases clearly separate in his own thinking from the procedures of threshold exploration *per se.*

The first step in preparation is to assure that the subject is fully aware of the experience for which he is to listen. The audiometrist, therefore, begins by presenting to the subject a tone of sufficient intensity to evoke a clear and concise response. This tonal presentation, as is also true of all subsequent ones, should be one or two seconds in duration. A particularly easy way of evaluating the subject's response is to have him raise his finger whenever he hears the stimulus. The audiometrist must, of course, estimate the presentation level which is required and must be prepared to use more intense levels if a clear and concise response is not evoked at the outset. The only purpose here is to be certain that the subject understands fully the task expected of him.

It has proved practical, when testing by air conduction, to administer the first tonal presentation at a hearing level of 30 to 40 db if the subject appears to have approximately normal acuity, and at a hearing level of 70 db if only a moderate impairment seems to be present. Provided these levels are inadequate, subsequent presentations are increased in steps of 15 db until the subject's response is positive. In any event, at least one definitive practice response should be elicited before proceeding to the next step in the procedure.

The second step is to decrease the tonal level until the stimulus is definitely inaudible. The only purpose here is to prepare for the first exploratory ascent. An efficient method for reaching the level of inaudibility is to drop the intensity of successive presentations in steps of 10 or 15 db. This sequence is carried through rapidly. A single response at one level is the cue to decrease to the next lower level. The advantage of such a sequence, in contrast to the process of dropping immediately to a

hearing level of zero db or weaker, is that the subsequent ascent will usually be started closer to the level at which the threshold lies. The saving in time is important to the clinician.

Once the level of inaudibility has been reached, the exploration for threshold begins. This exploration is carried out with a series of short tonal presentations. So long as the subject does not respond, each presentation is made five decibels stronger than its predecessor. However, as soon as a response occurs, the level of the next stimulus is dropped 10 to 15 db and another ascent in five-decibel steps is begun. The clinician keeps track of the levels at which responses occur. He designates the intensity at which the majority of responses appear as the threshold level for the test tone. Experience has shown that a practical criterion is to accept three responses at a single intensity as the threshold. This criterion is often achieved in three or four ascents.

The clinician must remember always to present successive stimuli as discrete events separated by completely toneless intervals. Moreover, each tonal burst should be not less than one second and not more than two seconds in duration. This requirement is easily achieved. The clinician merely adjusts the audiometer while the instrument is set so that no signal is being emitted. He then presses the "tone-on" switch to produce the next stimulus presentation.

All other details of procedure, such as the choice of the ear to be tested and of the progression of frequencies to be employed, are flexible. Moreover, the revised Hughson-Westlake technique is applicable to both air-conduction and bone-conduction explorations. The only restrictions in the latter instances are those imposed by the reduced range of hearing levels which are testable through bone conduction.

In summary, the critical features of the revised Hughson-Westlake technique are (1) that only ascending series of tonal stimuli are used, (2) that successive stimuli are separated by toneless intervals and (3) that each ascending run is terminated as soon as the subject responds. The technique is easy to employ when the subject is properly indoctrinated. The question which remains to be answered is whether the Hughson-Westlake technique is defensible from the standpoint of audiological theory.

ADAPTATION AND ON-EFFECT

It is a fundamental fact, as the statement quoted earlier from Hirsh implies, that an individual's auditory sensitivity can be modified substantially by the conditions of stimulus presentation. This fact imposes a responsibility on the clinician to select test conditions which encourage consistency in the subject's momentary acuity and which explore a precise boundary of sensitivity. In other words, since arbitrary decisions regarding procedure are unavoidable, it is the clinician's duty to choose reasonable stimulus conditions and to understand why he has chosen them.

Our knowledge of two auditory phenomena, on-effect and adaptation, makes it possible to state categorically that relatively brief tonal presentations must be used in conventional pure-tone audiometry. Such presentations enhance the reliability of the measured threshold. They also encourage response at the minimal intensity level to which the subject is ordinarily sensitive, thus giving an estimate of his best practical acuity. Stated conversely, continuous stimuli are clinically unacceptable because they induce variability in the intensity levels at which responses occur. This problem arises because prolonged stimuli produce temporary and progressive desensitization of the auditory system. Such desensitization becomes particularly pronounced with some kinds of hearing impairment.

To explain: the initial response of the auditory system at the onset of stimulation is its most vigorous response. This initial reaction is termed the on-effect. When the stimulus is sustained, the on-effect is followed by a reduction in responsiveness even though the stimulus is too weak to produce fatigue. This change is known as auditory adaptation.

On-effect and adaptation have been demon-strated through animal experimentation. Derbyshire and Davis (2) observed the two phenomena of on-effect and equilibration in the action potentials recorded from the eighth nerve of the cat. Galambos and Davis (4) found both rate-adaptation and amplitude-adaptation in the impulse trains carried by second order neurons of the cat's auditory system, while Tasaki (24) noted gradual decrease in the frequency of impulses elicited in response to sustained tones within first-order nerve fibers of the guinea pig.

The features of on-effect and adaptation, as exhibited by both subjects with normal hearing and with auditory impairments, were discussed by Hood (9) when he reported his studies on perstimulatory fatigue. Normal adaptation has subsequently been explored extensively (3, 11). However, it was Hallpike and Hood (5) who highlighted the clinical implications of the two phenomena by their suggestion that "on-effect normality" may be combined with susceptibility to extreme adaptation, called relapse. This combination, they claim, characterizes not only the adapted normal ear, but also the "recruiting sense organ of Ménière's disease." In both instances, there is an initial burst of auditory response at the onset of stimulation, provided, of course, that the threshold intensity is exceeded. This state is manifest to the listener as an initial maximal loudness. It is followed, if the stimulus is sustained, by a rapid deterioration in the response. This deterioration is the manifestation of relapse. Hallpike and Hood emphasize that recovery occurs quickly. The full on-effect may be elicited anew provided the listener is allowed a brief respite from stimulation.

The existence of individuals who undergo relapse and yet preserve the capacity for strong on-effect responses has been demonstrated repeatedly and in various ways (12, 13, 14, 21). One must now recognize that relapse at threshold is not restricted to cases with cochlear lesion, but that this phenomenon can at times be encountered with neural lesions. One must also recognize that details such as the speed of relapse, the rapidity of recovery, and the variation of effect with frequency differ from one case to another. The unescapable fact, from the standpoint of deciding on a routine for clinical audiometry, is that subjects are encountered whose momentary responsiveness is radically affected by exposure to sustained tones.

A critical point here is that both the normally adapted auditory system and the relapsed auditory system regain responsiveness after a brief resting period. Full recovery ordinarily occurs in a second or two. Consequently, the audiometrist may have confidence that he is exploring his subject's maximal acuity at each test frequency if every stimulus is preceded by a toneless interval of several seconds. Moreover, since the on-effect will be elicited at the outset of stimulation, there is no value in prolonging any tonal presentation more than a couple of seconds. When the audiometrist does prolong the tone, he merely initiates a process of normal adaptation or one of relapse, depending upon the case being tested.

The foregoing considerations lead to the conclusion that, provided one wishes to measure the subject's unadapted threshold (his on-effect responsiveness) by conventional audiometry,[2] each audiometric stimulus should be one or two seconds long and should follow a silent interval of at least three seconds. One is not justified in conducting a routine clinical test by presenting a clearly audible tone and then decreasing its intensity without interruption until the tone becomes inaudible. Such a procedure produces an unknown amount of adaptation. The amount depends upon the speed of stimulus transitions, upon the susceptibility of the subject to abnormal adaptation and, since higher intensities produce greater adaptation, upon the starting level of the sequence. The only thing one can be certain about is that such a procedure will usually give a pessimistic impression of the subject's acuity.

Evidence supporting this last statement

[2] Various techniques of pulse-tone audiometry are justifiable in terms of the considerations reviewed here. However, discussion of these techniques is beyond the scope of the present paper, which is concerned exclusively with an analysis of the traditional audiometric methodology.

was obtained by Miller and Rosenblith. These investigators, according to Hirsh (8), found that "descending" thresholds obtained on normal hearers with continuous tones of 4000 cps required as much as 15 db more sound pressure than did the analogous "ascending" thresholds. They also found that the magnitude of the discrepancy increased as the starting level of the descending sequence was raised. Only when the descending sequence was begun essentially at threshold was acuity as good with it as with the ascending progression. Furthermore, Rosenblith and Miller obtained better thresholds for both ascending and descending progressions when the 4000-cps stimulus was interrupted than either progression yielded when the stimulus was continuous. One would expect the differences to be more dramatic in cases where relapse operates.

The clinician must recognize one further characteristic of any procedure which uses discrete tonal presentations separated by substantial intervals of time. Such a test situation is not even analogous to one wherein a train of successive pulses is changing continuously in intensity. In the former case each tonal presentation is an event sufficiently isolated in time so that it is independent of its neighbors. The subject will respond if his momentary sensitivity in relation to the stimulus intensity is sufficient for the on-effect to be evoked. Since each event is independent, it is theoretically irrelevant whether the clinician has patterned the succession of stimuli in a descending, in an ascending, or in a combined sequence. One is not justified in thinking of this procedure as constituting a form of the method of limits simply because he decides to vary presentation levels progressively. Therefore, one need not feel any responsibility to combine sequences of ascending and descending "crossings" of the threshold. Instead, the audiometrist may choose whichever sequence has the greatest practical advantage. Hence, it is legitimate to adopt the revised Hughson-Westlake technique. This method has the practical advantages of simplicity and of high economy in clinical effort.

FIVE-DECIBEL STEP

The traditional concept of a threshold rests on the premise that the subject is continually undergoing fluctuations in sensitivity (23). According to this view, the subject's minimal response level at any given instant is determined by his status at that instant. Therefore, a series of measurements must be made in order to obtain a statistical estimate of his threshold, which is usually defined as the stimulus value at which there is a 50 percent chance that he will perceive the stimulus. This estimate is derived from a finite series of measurements. The series is obtained according to one of the standard psychophysical methods.

A critical requirement, which applies to all psychophysical methods, is that it must be possible to present a reasonable array of stimulus values which actually lie within the subject's range of moment-to-moment variability. Stated conversely, if the steps between stimulus levels are too large, a precise estimate of the threshold will be impossible because information which contributes to the estimate is not obtainable at enough levels. Under such circumstances, some levels will be useless in threshold computation because they always evoke response, whereas others will be analogously useless because they never evoke response. The most extreme case, of course, is the situation where the size of the interval between successive stimulus levels is greater than the range of the subject's moment-to-moment variability. When this situation exists, all that can usually be determined is that response never occurs at one presentation level and always occurs at the next higher level. Here, even in those fortuitous instances where one stimulus level happens to probe the subject's moment-to-moment variability, the none-and-all pattern will characterize responses at the two flanking levels. Again, a precise estimate of threshold is impossible, and the investigator must still be satisfied with designating one presentation level at which responses seldom or never occur and a second level, immediately higher, at which responses usually occur. Such information may be highly useful, but it is not

threshold determination according to the traditional premises of psychophysical exploration.

There exists substantial evidence, some of which is reviewed below, that moment-to-moment fluctuations in auditory sensitivity are often encompassed within a range which is less than the five-decibel step used in conventional audiometry. Since such is the case, the audiometrist should recognize that he cannot define an individual's threshold in precise statistical fashion so long as he varies stimulus intensity in five-decibel steps. Hence, the audiometrist need not feel impelled to structure his testing technique according to one of the classical methods of psychophysics, and he need not feel guilty if he does not do so. Instead, the clinician should choose his audiometric technique to take advantage of the high consistency of response which may be expected from most subjects during single tests when the five-decibel step is used. He should adopt a procedure which quickly gives the dichotomous information to which the five-decibel step restricts him.

Several studies supply evidence supporting the premise that the moment-to-moment variability of the individual is not large in relation to the five-decibel step of conventional audiometry. These studies help one answer the question, "What is the moment-to-moment stability in the auditory sensitivity in the ordinary listener?"

Ward (25, 26), while developing his technique of "single descent" group audiometry, obtained two kinds of information which are pertinent. For one thing, Ward tested 12 enlisted men repeatedly at both 500 and 4000 cps. The stimulus was a continuously changing train of pulses. Ward combined two pulse rates (1.5 and 2.25 pps) with two attenuation speeds (1.5 and 3.0 db). Each of the four resulting conditions was presented five times to every subject. Subjects were instructed to report "just when the beats disappeared." Ward found his four parameters of stimulus descent to be essentially equivalent in reliability as gauged by the standard deviation of repeat judgments. Moreover, he comments,

". . . the standard deviation of repeat judgments (earphones not moved) is 1.7 db . . ." (*26*).

Secondly, Ward used his 2.25 pps and 3 db/sec. parameter of descent to study the test-retest consistency exhibited at 2000 and 8000 cps by 1200 naval personnel. He remarks, "The median difference, disregarding sign, is 2.4 db for both 2000 and 8000 cps. This implies that the median SD of repeat judgments is 1.7 db" (*25*). It is also evident from Ward's data that almost 50 percent of the test-retest discrepancies were less than 2.5 db and about 80 percent were smaller than five db.

One may interpret Ward's findings as indirect evidence that the short-term physiological fluctuations in the auditory acuity of ordinary listeners (as exemplified by Ward's subjects) are generally of the same order of magnitude as the five-decibel step employed in clinical audiometry. If this had not been the case, test-retest differences would have emerged as much larger in Ward's study— since physiological fluctuations constitute only one of several factors contributing to the variability he observed.

Of course, since Ward used only descending series of pulses, one wonders whether the consistency he found in repeat judgment was thereby spuriously improved. In one sense it is irrelevant to raise this question, because any method which induces consistency in human response demonstrates the reliability which it is possible to achieve if one structures the test situation properly. In another sense, however, the question is highly pertinent when one is inquiring into the moment-to-moment fluctuations of human listeners. Hence, the findings of other workers are *apropos*.

Wertheimer (*28*) investigated the stability of the threshold for 80-msec. clicks by the method of constant stimuli. Three subjects were used. Wertheimer found ". . . that the average sigma of measurement of the auditory threshold within one session was .69 db. . . ." This value is astonishingly small, and it indicates short term stability in auditory acuity which is much better than clinicians usually assume. Interestingly, Wertheimer found that the average sigma of 10 thresholds obtained within a single day was only .87 db, while the sigma of thresholds obtained daily over a period of 23 successive days was only 1.22 db. Hence, he demonstrated that consistency of auditory acuity can persist over relatively long periods of time.

Munson and Wiener (*15*) investigated the differences between successive thresholds at 1000 and 6000 cps as obtained by the "ABX" method. They reason, "Within the framework of the limited tests reported here, it can be concluded that the variance σ^2 of the threshold determinations . . . is about 1.5 (db)^2 if a good method is used for measuring the stimulus. This variance is believed to be primarily a measure of the variability of the observers' sensory system." Harris and Myers (*6*) add the comment that each threshold obtained by Munson and Wiener was roughly an average of the status of sensitivity over a five-minute interval. Even as such, the Munson-Wiener findings bespeak greater stability of auditory sensitivity than many would expect.

The investigation conducted by Myers and Harris (*17*) on the inherent stability of auditory thresholds is a most provocative exploration of short-term fluctuations in auditory sensitivity. Myers and Harris measured the auditory acuity of three young men at each of 11 frequencies. The procedure used was the serial method of limits. Five descents and five ascents were employed at each test frequency. Stimuli were presented at five-sec. intervals. Every stimulus was a .75-sec. pulse of the test tone. Successive pulses differed in intensity by one db. A point of "threshold crossing" was computed independently for each descent and for each ascent. The exploration was conducted not only by air conduction but, in duplicate, by bone conduction. Myers and Harris summarize their basic finding as follows, "The typical short-term threshold fluctuation was of the order of less than a decibel. This is the total fluctuation as the result of instability in the subject's attending and responding systems as well as in his auditory system proper."

The minimum standard deviation exhibited

by a single subject for a single frequency is .34 db and the maximum is 1.68 db. Considering individual subjects and each frequency separately, the standard deviation is under one db in exactly half of the instances. Moreover, Myers and Harris (*17*) conclude that, "There is no difference in threshold fluctuation between air and bone conduction or among frequencies." They also state, "Inexperienced subjects are not troubled with the 'zone of detectability,' a region within which an experienced subject is uncertain whether the stimulus is an indefinite noise or is actually a pure tone."

Two further points are important:

1. Myers and Harris (*17*) report, "There is a tendency for a descending series to yield a somewhat better threshold than an ascending series." They add, however, "No completely reliable difference (between the two sequences) exists at any frequency for any subject . . . At most . . . (the difference) . . . amounts to little more than one decibel . . ." Actually, the average superiority of the descending thresholds over the ascending thresholds is .16 db when computed for all subjects at all frequencies by both air and bone conduction. Obviously, from the practical point of view, .16 db is an infinitesimal difference which is completely negligible. Hence, the Myers and Harris data support the expectation, which derives from recognition of on-effect, that a single tone of short duration is a sufficiently discrete entity that the listener's response to each presentation is essentially independent of the sequence in which it is placed.

2. Myers and Harris (*16*) found, "Four crossings of the threshold (two ascending and two descending) are a sufficient number to produce a reliable threshold." Actually, in only five comparisons out of 66 does the threshold as estimated from the first four crossings differ by a decibel or more from the threshold as estimated from all 10 crossings. Furthermore, the mean difference for all 66 comparisons is .35 db. Such results are encouraging to the clinician because they add to the assurance with which he can accept a threshold based on a few trials, provided, of course, he employs a method which has the requisite inherent reliability.

All the foregoing findings give one confidence in the validity of the Hughson-Westlake technique as a method for assessing the maximal acuity of clinical subjects. The moment-to-moment variability which typifies the normal hearing subject is sufficiently small so that the five-decibel step employed in conventional audiometry is too large to allow effective exploration of this variability. In other words, when the five-decibel step is used, any technique which excites on-effect may be expected to yield essentially equivalent findings for subjects with normal hearing. All that one can do under such circumstances is to ascertain the five-decibel step which separates the minimum hearing level at which responses always or usually occur from the maximum level at which responses are evoked only occasionally or not at all. Moreover, one is restricted to the same kind of information when testing cases with conductive impairments, since these people possess normal sensori-neural systems and hence will exhibit moment-to-moment variability similar to that of persons without hearing impairment.

The situation is less certain when dealing with sensori-neural losses. Many such cases, particularly those whose involvements have stabilized, probably also undergo restricted fluctuations in acuity. True, this expectation awaits experimental test. The important point, for the moment, is that the Hughson-Westlake method is justified even in instances where this expectation is not realized. To explain: when testing patients who undergo abnormal moment-to-moment variability in acuity, it is particularly important to use a technique which evokes on-effect, because many, if not all, of these patients will be prone to relapse. Testing such patients with sustained stimuli will increase their variabilities by evoking responses while they are in various stages of relapse. Exploration with short-duration tones will counteract this difficulty by eliciting on-effect. Such exploration has the further advantage of yielding estimates of unadapted acuity. These estimates are more valid criteria of each subject's capacity to react to transient sounds, like speech, than are measures of their sensitivities while relapsed. Therefore, the Hughson-Westlake method is appropriate even when testing subjects whose transient fluctuations in acuity are abnormally large. The method's simplicity recommends it over other procedures which evoke on-effects but which embody more complicated explora- tory sequences.

EXPERIMENTAL COMPARISON

Theoretically, the Hughson-Westlake method will yield thresholds which are equivalent to those obtained with other clinical techniques that also excite on-effect responses. This pre- mise required experimental scrutiny. There- fore, the investigation reported below was undertaken. Its purpose was to evaluate the extent to which different sequences of stimulus presentation affect the level that is designated as threshold. Specifically, thresholds were obtained by the ascending method of Hughson- Westlake, by an analogous descending se- quence of isolated tones, and by a combined ascending-descending sequence.

All testing was done with a commercial audiometer (ADC-50-E) which activated a PDR-1 earphone mounted in an MX41/AR cushion. An auxiliary 20-db pad was inserted between the audiometer and the earphone to provide the range of low intensities required to test normal hearing subjects, some of whom could be expected to exhibit hyperacute audi- tory sensitivity.

The acoustic output of the audiometer was measured daily by means of a 6-cc coupler (ASA Type 1), a calibrated condenser microphone (Western Electric, 640 AA), a cathode follower (ADC, D5153) and a vacu- um-tube voltmeter (Hewlett-Packard, Model 400A). The pure-tone thresholds obtained during the study could consequently be re- ported in terms of the sound pressure level developed in the ASA Type 1 coupler.

The clinical room employed was one con- structed for psychoacoustic research. The ambient noise level in the room was 30 db, as measured on the C scale of a sound level meter (General Radio, Type 759).

The subjects used in the study were 36 students at Northwestern University. Their ages ranged from 18 to 24 years. Half were males and the other half females. Each was re- quired to exhibit normal hearing as evidenced by the ability to pass an audiometric screen at a hearing level of 10 db re the USPHS norm. This screening test was administered at the octave frequencies from 125 through 8000 cps. In addition, only subjects whose history indicated freedom from ear pathology and from excessive noise exposure were ac- cepted.

Each subject was seen for a single experi- mental session, during which thresholds at 250, 1000 and 4000 cps were established by each of the three clinical methods under in- vestigation. The order of presentation of these three frequencies was counter-balanced with the three testing methods through the use of a Graeco-Latin Square design. One ear per subject was tested and the earphone was not moved once the test sequence had begun.

The following instructions were read to each subject at the outset of the experimental ses- sion:

The purpose of this test is to see how well you can hear some faint tones. Each tone will be quite short. Some will be easy to hear. Others will be very faint. When- ever you hear one of these tones, no matter how faint it is, raise your finger. As soon as the tone goes off, lower your finger.

The experimenter assured himself that these instructions were understood and then the threshold testing was begun.

The three methods of threshold determina- tion were designed to be as parallel as possible except for the progression of intensity changes:

1. The ascending method was the Hughson- Westlake procedure. Specifically, the follow- ing sequence was employed. The pure-tone stimulus was first presented 30 db above the

subject's presumed threshold. The purpose was to obtain a positive and decisive response. Attenuation was next introduced in 10-decibel steps until the subject failed to react. Only one stimulus per level was presented. Both during this downward progression and in subsequent ascents, each stimulus was a tonal pulse lasting between one and two seconds. After the subject failed to respond, the first ascent was initiated. Successive increments were in five-decibel steps. The first ascent was stopped as soon as the subject reacted to a stimulus. The signal was next attenuated 10 to 15 db, and a new ascent was begun at this latter level. Ascending trials were continued until the subject had responded three times at one level. It was not required that these three responses be consecutive. The level eliciting these three reactions was recorded as the threshold.

2. The descending method was patterned analogously. Again, the exploration was initiated by presenting the pure-tone stimulus 30 db above the subject's presumed threshold. Again, too, all stimuli were tonal pulses of a second or two, and only one stimulus was presented per audiometric level. Here, however, the second step was to descend in five-decibel intervals until the subject failed to respond. The level was then increased 10 to 15 db and a new descent was initiated. This process was repeated until three failures to respond were obtained at a single audiometric level. The next higher hearing level, *i.e.*, the last level at which response was noted in these three instances, was designated as the threshold.

3. The third method combined descending and ascending progressions. After an initial presentation at approximately 30 db above the subject's threshold, a descent like those just described was performed. The lowest intensity at which response persisted was recorded. Next, an additional attenuation of 10 to 15 db was introduced and then an ascent such as used in the Hughson-Westlake method was initiated. The level at which reaction first appeared was recorded. The hearing level was increased 10 or 15 db and a second descent was conducted, following which a second ascent was, in turn, completed. After a third descent and a third ascent, the average for the six measures of minimum audible levels was computed as representing threshold.

Table 10-1 summarizes the results obtained when the foregoing methods were administered to the 36 university students. The table reports both mean thresholds and standard deviations for the group. One notes that the mean threshold for the descending method is slightly better at every frequency than for either of the other two methods. Its maximum superiority occurred at 1000 cps where the mean threshold for the combined method was 1.7 db higher. The means of descending thresholds were .6, 1.5 and 1.3 db better than the means of ascending thresholds at 250, 1000 and 4000 cps, respectively. Interestingly enough, the combined method yielded poorer mean thresholds than did the ascending method at 250 and 1000 cps.

The superiority of the descending method over the other two methods might be argued from the results reported in Table 10-1. However, the magnitude of the mean advantage achieved by the descending thresholds over the ascending thresholds falls far short of the 10 to 15 db differential which clinicians

TABLE 10-1. MEANS AND STANDARD DEVIATIONS OF THRESHOLD SOUND PRESSURE LEVELS *
YIELDED BY 36 NORMAL HEARING SUBJECTS UNDER THREE MEASUREMENT TECHNIQUES

Technique	250 cps		1000 cps		4000 cps	
	Mean	S.D.	Mean	S.D.	Mean	S.D.
Ascending	24.7	4.0	9.3	4.6	16.8	7.2
Descending	24.1	4.3	7.8	4.8	15.5	8.4
Ascending-Descending	25.1	4.0	9.5	4.0	16.4	7.5

* db re: .0002 microbar in ASA Type 1 Coupler.

often assume to exist. Moreover, the present results fail to confirm the commonly held hypothesis that a combination of ascending and descending series will yield threshold values intermediate between those which either type of run will yield if employed alone. Thus, as one contemplates the present results, he is impressed by the fact that the mean thresholds obtained here by the three methods are indistinguishable, from the practical point of view.

Further confidence in the general equivalence of the three methods is found in the standard deviations reported in Table 10-1. Considering each test frequency separately, the three standard deviations were highly similar. Thus, one concludes that the variability among subjects remained the same from one method to another.

The data at hand may be summarized in another way. One may ask how closely each subject agreed with himself when tested by the three methods. Such a comparison gives a particularly provocative picture of the findings because it highlights the practical equivalence which the three test methods exhibit.

The procedure for making the comparison was simple. All thresholds first had to be designated on a five-decibel scale. The original data from both ascending and descending techniques were already aligned in five-decibel intervals. It was therefore only necessary to assign each origiual threshold for the combined sequence to the closest five-decibel step on the audiometric scale. When the original measure was equidistant between steps, the better hearing level was selected. In other words, the data for the combined method were recast in the form that would logically be used in recording routine findings on an audiogram.

Differences among thresholds obtained by the three test procedures were then compared for each subject separately. Tables 10-2, 10-3, and 10-4 summarize the tabulations of these differences. One notes that within each table the distribution of differences is sufficiently similar for the three test frequencies so that only the totals of differences for all frequencies need be discussed in comparing methods. There is *no* difference between the individual thresholds in 74 (68.5 percent) out of the 108 comparisons involving the ascending and descending methods. In all but one of the remaining comparisons the difference in threshold is a single audiometric step (five db). The agreement is even better between ascending and combined methods. Here, 83 subjects (76.9 percent) yielded identical thresholds; all of the 25 differences (23.1 percent) were discrepancies of only five db. Finally, the parallelism between descending and combined methods was almost identical to the parallelism between descending and ascending procedures. Again, 74 (68.5 percent) of the comparisons represented complete equivalence. All of the remaining 34 comparisons yielded a discrepancy of one audiometric step. Thus, Tables 10-2, 10-3, and 10-4 may be summarized by the statement that in approximately seven out of every 10 comparisons, audiometric results were identical when designated in a conventional clinical manner, and (with only one exception in the 318 comparisons) the remainder yielded differences of only one interval on the recording scale.

Two further factual items have some interest: (1) Identical thresholds for a single subject were obtained by all three methods in 62

TABLE 10-2. DISTRIBUTION OF DIFFERENCES IN CLINICAL THRESHOLDS YIELDED BY 36 NORMAL HEARING SUBJECTS WHEN TESTED BY ASCENDING AND BY DESCENDING SEQUENCES

Ascending Minus Descending	Test Frequency			Total	
	250	1000	4000	N	%
−5	3	0	2	5	4.6
0	25	26	23	74	68.5
5	8	9	11	28	25.9
10	0	1	0	1	.9
Total	36	36	36	108	

TABLE 10-3. DISTRIBUTION OF DIFFERENCES IN CLINICAL THRESHOLDS YIELDED BY 36 NORMAL HEARING SUBJECTS WHEN TESTED BY ASCENDING AND BY COMBINED ASCENDING-DESCENDING * SEQUENCES

Ascending Minus Combined	Test Frequency			Total	
	250	1000	4000	N	%
−5	5	2	2	9	8.3
0	24	31	28	83	76.9
5	7	3	6	16	14.8
Total	36	36	36	108	

* Nearest 5-db step designated as clinical threshold for combined sequences with better level selected when the mean of six runs was equidistant between two audiometric levels.

TABLE 10-4. DISTRIBUTION OF DIFFERENCES IN CLINICAL THRESHOLDS YIELDED BY 36 NORMAL HEARING SUBJECTS WHEN TESTED BY DESCENDING AND BY COMBINED ASCENDING-DESCENDING * SEQUENCES

Descending Minus Combined	Test Frequency			Total	
	250	1000	4000	N	%
−5	6	10	10	26	24.2
0	27	26	21	74	68.4
5	3	0	5	8	7.4
Total	36	36	36	108	

* Nearest 5-db step designated as clinical threshold for combined sequences, with better level selected when the mean of six runs was equidistant between two audiometric levels.

(57.4 percent) out of a possible 108 instances. Thus, more than half the time there was absolutely no deviation of one method from the other two. (2) In 45 of the 46 remaining instances, two of the three thresholds were the same. Here the distribution was as follows: the descending and the ascending thresholds were alike 12 times, the descending and the combined 13 times, while the ascending and the combined thresholds were equal 20 times. Thus, if one were using the results for the combined method as a criterion, he would observe that the ascending thresholds agree with this criterion better than do the descending ones. However, since there is really no way in the present instance of selecting a particular threshold as the more valid in each specific incident of discrepancy, one must reach the conclusion that the three methods under study emerge as clinically indistinguishable when the five-decibel step is the unit of testing and of threshold recording. Therefore, the choice among methods may rest on practical considerations rather than theoretical imperatives.

DISCUSSION

The failure of the present study to demonstrate clinically important differences between procedures is merely evidence that the five-decibel step employed in routine pure-tone audiometry is too large to yield measurements which distinguish the subtleties of the listener's auditory variability. This outcome is to be expected when one remembers the nature of the on-effect and the small range of momentary fluctuations in auditory sensitivity which normal hearers undergo.

The clinician must be clear on the implications of these facts. He must distinguish between the reliability of reaction he may expect from an individual subject during a single audiometric test and the day-to-day consistency he may assume for re-tests performed in the clinical situation. The reliability of the former can be very good, as the foregoing discussion has demonstrated, while the repeatability of measurement from one clinical examination to the next can be relatively poor. The latter fact has been amply demonstrated in many studies, ranging from the investigation by Hughson and Witting (29) to the one by Roach and Carhart (22). These studies supply the clinician with information on the precision with which he may accept any particular test as illustrative of the audiometric level which characterizes the patient's everyday hearing. These studies do not tell the clinician anything about the precision of measurement within a single test. In other words, such factors as difference in adjusting the earphones, other changes in the test situation, and true shifts in the hearing of the patient are responsible for the discrepancies which appear from one day's test to another. The clinician must make allowances for the unreliability which such factors produce, but he must not make the mistake of presuming that comparable variability is inherent in the patient's acuity from one moment to the next.

The alert clinician will bear in mind Hirsh's comment, "The sources of . . . threshold variability are numerous and are not necessarily related to the variability of the observer's physiological threshold" (8). He will choose a technique for testing which is parsimonious of his own effort, which is simple for the subject and which gives an estimate of the observer's physiological threshold that satisfies clinical requirements for intra-test reliability.

The Hughson-Westlake technique meets these three criteria. Clinicians who have used it found it to be highly satisfactory because of the rapidity with which a skilled tester can obtain threshold and because of the easy task it imposes on the subject. Moreover, as demonstrated above, the Hughson-Westlake technique is equivalent, within reasonable clinical margin, to other techniques which also excite on-effect and which also employ the five-decibel step of traditional pure-tone audiometry. The procedure has the added merit of having been recommended for many years to audiometrists by the Committee on Conservation of Hearing of the American Academy of Ophthalmology and Otolaryngology. Therefore, the Hughson-Westlake method can quite properly be adopted by clinicians throughout the world as the preferred technique for determining thresholds for pure tones when using the conventional audiometer.

One thing must be remembered by the reader as he contemplates the recommendation, which is here renewed, that he use the Hughson-Westlake method. Every clinician has habituated a procedure which is now so comfortable for him that he finds it hard to believe another method could be as good. Despite his feelings of comfortableness with it, his technique has theoretical and practical limitations if it does not elicit on-effect. However, if he uses a technique which does elicit on-effect, his method is as good in seeking out the unadapted physiological threshold as is the Hughson-Westlake technique. Under such circumstances, choice between methods cannot be resolved by the criteria of simplicity and of parsimony. For one thing, habituation regarding these matters influences belief. In addition, there are other methods, such as the analogous descending exploration, which are equally fast and precise. The only way of choosing between clinical procedures which are fundamentally equivalent in seeking out the unadapted threshold is to make an arbitrary selection. In the writers' opinion, the reason favoring arbitrary selection of the Hughson-Westlake technique is found in the long-term sponsorship which has been given to the method by the Committee on Conservation of Hearing. This sponsorship should encourage clinicians to adopt the method for the purpose of achieving widespread uniformity of routine audiometric procedures. Obviously, there will continue to be specific instances in which other audiometric methods are preferable, but audiology will achieve new maturity if clinicians employ these other techniques as conscious variations from a standardized practice.

SUMMARY

The Hughson-Westlake ascending method for establishing pure-tone auditory threshold is recommended for general clinical use when audiometry is performed with a five-decibel intensity interval. The procedure, which presents stimuli for a second or two so as to elicit on-effect responses from the subject, encourages stability of reactions and yields measurement of the unadapted level of acuity. According to the theory of on-effect, the Hughson-Westlake method should yield thresholds which are clinically equivalent to those obtained by similar short tonal presentations patterned in descending or "threshold crossing" sequences. Experimental exploration with 36 normal hearing subjects confirmed this expectation. Adoption of the Hughson-Westlake method is recommended over the other methods which also elicit on-effect for the purpose of gaining uniformity of procedure throughout the field of clinical audiometry.

ACKNOWLEDGMENTS

The authors acknowledge the helpful assistance of Earl R. Harford, Bud D. Kimball and Robert J. Harrison in the successful completion of this study.

REFERENCES

1. Bunch, C. C., *Clinical Audiometry*. St. Louis: Mosby, 1943.

2. Derbyshire, A. J., and Davis, H., The action potentials of the auditory nerve. *Amer. J. Physiol.*, 113, 1935, 476–504.

3. Egan, J. P., and Thwing, E. J., Further studies on perstimulatory fatigue. *J. acoust. Soc. Amer.*, 27, 1955, 1225–1226.

4. Galambos, R., and Davis, H., The response of single auditory nerve fibers to acoustic stimulation. *J. Neurophysiol.*, 6, 1943, 39–57.

5. Hallpike, C. S., and Hood, J. D., Some recent work on auditory adaptation and its relationship to the loudness recruitment phenomenon. *J. acoust. Soc. Amer.*, 23, 1951, 270–274.

6. Harris, J. D., and Myers, C. K., Experiments on fluctuation of auditory acuity. U.S. Navy Med. Res. Lab. Rep. No. 196, 1952, 2–29.

7. Heller, M. F., *Functional Otology*. New York: Springer, 1955.

8. Hirsh, I. J., *Measurement of Hearing*. New York: McGraw-Hill, 1952.

9. Hood, J. D., Studies in auditory fatigue and adaptation. *Acta Otolaryng., Stockh., Suppl.*, 92, 1950, 1–57.

10. Hughson, W., and Westlake, H., Manual for program outline for rehabilitation of aural casualties both military and civilian. *Trans. Amer. Acad. Ophthal. Oto-laryng. Suppl.*, 48, 1944, 1–15.

11. Jerger, J. F., Auditory adaptation. *J. acoust. Soc. Amer.*, 29, 1957, 357–363.

12. Jerger, J. F., Carhart, R., and Lassman, J., Clinical observations on excessive threshold adaptation. *Arch. Otolaryng., Chicago*, 68, 1958, 617–623.

13. Jerger, J. F., Differential intensity sensitivity in the ear with loudness recruitment. *J. Speech Hearing Dis.*, 20, 1955, 183–193.

14. Lierle, D. M., and Reger, S. N., Experimentally induced temporary threshold shifts in ears with impaired hearing. *Ann. Otol., etc., St Louis*, 64, 1955, 263–277.

15. Munson, W. A., and Wiener, F. M., Sound measurement for psychophysical tests. *J. acoust. Soc. Amer.*, 22, 1950, 382–386.

16. Myers, C. K., and Harris, J. D., Variability of the auditory threshold with time. U.S. Navy Med. Res. Lab. Rep. No. 165, 1950, 230–257.

17. Myers, C. K., and Harris, J. D., The inherent stability of the auditory threshold. U.S. Naval Med. Res. Lab. Progress Rep. No. 3, Bu Med Project NM-003-021, April, 1949.

18. Newby, H., *Audiology*. New York: Appleton-Century-Crofts, 1958.

19. Newhart, H., and Reger, S., Manual for a school hearing conservation program (revised 1951, C. E. Kinney, G. D. Hoople, S. R. Guild and S. N. Reger, eds., for Committee on Conservation of Hearing). *Trans. Amer. Acad. Ophthal. Otolaryng. Suppl.*, 1951.

20. Newhart, H., and Reger, S. N. (eds.), Syllabus of audiometric procedures in the administration of a program for the conservation of hearing of school children. *Trans. Amer. Acad. Ophthal. Oto-laryng. Suppl.*, April, 1945, 1–28.

21. Palva, T., Studies on per-stimulatory adaptation in various groups of deafness. *Laryngoscope, St Louis*, 65, 1955, 829–847.

22. Roach, R. E., and Carhart, R., A clinical method for calibrating the bone-conduction audiometer. *Arch. Otolaryng., Chicago*, 63, 1956, 270–278.

23. Stevens, S. S. (ed.), *Handbook of Experimental Psychology*. New York: John Wiley and Sons, 1951.

24. Tasaki, I., Nerve impulses in individual auditory nerve fibers of guinea pig. *J. Neurophysiol.*, 17, 1954, 97–122.

25. Ward, W. D., Method of "single descent" in group audiometry. *J. acoust. Soc. Amer.*, 29, 1957, 371–376.

26. Ward, W. D., The single-descent group audiometer. *Noise Control*, 3, 1957, No. 3, 15–18.

27. Watson, L. A., and Tolan, T., *Hearing Tests and Hearing Instruments*. Baltimore: Williams and Wilkins, 1949.

28. Wertheimer, M., The variability of auditory and visual absolute thresholds in time. *J. gen. Psychol.*, 52, 1955, 111–147.

29. Witting, E. G., and Hughson, W., Inherent accuracy of a series of repeated clinical audiograms. *Laryngoscope, St Louis*, 50, 1940, 259–269.

11

Behavioral Audiometry Viewed as an Operant Procedure

LYLE L. LLOYD

LYLE L. LLOYD, Ph.D., is Executive Secretary, Mental Retardation Research and Training Committee, National Institute of Child Health and Human Development, National Institutes of Health

Behavioral audiometry as defined by Frisina (1963, p. 137) is based on the principle of reinforcement. The essence of behavioral audiometry is to bring operant responses of the subject under stimulus control and then use such responses to obtain a reliable index of some aspect of the subject's hearing. This generalization is true in the case of both threshold and suprathreshold measures. The purpose of this paper is to discuss the more frequently used forms of pure-tone behavioral audiometry in terms of reinforcement and other operant principles.

THE CONVENTIONAL OR STANDARD METHODS

Conventional or standard pure-tone audiometry, where the subject is asked to raise his hand or press a signal button when he hears a sound, uses verbal reinforcement. Frequently the subject's first appropriate response is followed by the examiner's statement of "good," "that's fine," or some other statement which serves as social reinforcement. The verbal forms of social reinforcement are usually paired with, or in some cases supplemented by, other forms of social reinforcement such as a smile or nod of the head. Throughout the testing session the astute examiner administers addi-

Reprinted by permission of the author from *J. Speech Hearing Dis.*, **31**, pp. 128–136 (1966).

tional social reinforcement as frequently as he thinks is appropriate. For example, when testing an intelligent, motivated, and cooperative adult, verbal reinforcement may be provided after the first appropriate response and then only an additional time or two throughout the testing session. However, when testing a suspicious, uncooperative, or poorly motivated young child, the examiner will initially follow each of the child's appropriate responses with social reinforcement. With a child of this type the social reinforcement will probably include a "pat on the back," "hand clapping," or some other animated actions indicating approval and fun. Actually such overt behavior by the clinician is the main form of social reinforcement paired with verbal forms of social reinforcement. As the child's response is strengthened, e.g., it has shorter latency and is more decisive, the examiner will reduce the reinforcement schedule from 100 percent reinforcement. Although the schedule may be reduced, the frequency, either variable ratio or fixed ratio, will probably be higher at the end of the test session in the latter case than in the previous case of the adult.

Once the pattern of responding to sound is established, the clinician usually reduces frequency and amount of reinforcement. This reduction during the testing session results in greater testing efficiency. The skilled audiologist attempts to apply a sufficient schedule and amount of reinforcement to maintain a high rate of responding but does not waste time administering excessive reinforcement, which is not only inefficient in terms of measurements per unit of test time but which also increases the chances that the subject will become satiated and cease responding.

A typical example of the intrasession reduction in reinforcement may be observed in the example mentioned above of the doubtful, suspicious child. The clinician reduces the schedule from reinforcement once every appropriate response to every several responses. In addition to this reduction in the schedule of reinforcement, the clinician would probably reduce the amount of time and energy in the reinforcement. Initially, the reinforcement which includes overt, animated approval behavior paired with verbal praise is reduced to less overt behavior and verbal output. On the basis of clinical observation the reinforcement with such a child is frequently reduced to an occasional nod of the head or smile.

Since reinforcement increases the frequency of the subject's responses, the audiologist makes the reinforcement contingent upon the desired behavior or responses, usually raising a hand or pressing a button when the auditory signal is heard. The audiologist knows only when the signal is presented, not when the subject hears the signal. Therefore, the initial signal presentations are usually at levels assumed, upon the bases of clinical observation and case history data, to be above the subject's threshold. These suprathreshold presentations afford the opportunity to administer reinforcement for appropriate responses. When reinforcement principles are applied in behavioral audiometry the primarily descending, and the descending-ascending or bracketing, methods over the ascending methods are apparently advantageous. The threshold searching methods that include suprathreshold presentation offer more opportunity to administer reinforcement when the subject has met the appropriate response contingency. Although such methods do not automatically eliminate the possible error of reinforcing a subject for responding when he did not hear the sound, they do reduce such errors. The primarily descending methods allow the audiologist better control of the delivery of reinforcement under the appropriate contingencies.

One minor problem in the use of reinforcement with a primarily descending threshold searching method is the danger of administering reinforcement only at suprathreshold levels, and thereby training the subject to respond at these levels but not near threshold. This danger is reduced by the instructions and demonstrations given to the subject. The effectiveness of typical instructions depends primarily upon the subject's ability to understand the audiologist's verbal communication system. Dependence on the subject's understanding of verbal instructions is reduced by demonstration of the task. By using reinforcement principles the subject is taught to respond to lower and lower signals during the instruction and demonstration phase of the test session. During the threshold searching phase the reinforcement of responses to various levels of signal presentations further strengthens the response to signal at any level.

The use of partial reinforcement schedules was discussed as a testing efficiency measure, but partial reinforcement is also useful in maintaining response patterns. In general, partial reinforcement schedules may result in learning a given task more slowly, but when a task is learned the use of partial reinforcement tends to result in a response more resistant to extinction. The use of partial reinforcement is one of the clinician's best safeguards against failure of the subject to respond to the signal control as a result of satiation.

EAR CHOICE METHODS

Once the most conventional forms of behavioral audiometry, use of standard hand raising or button pressing response, are viewed as operant procedures, the application of these principles in other forms of behavioral audiometry becomes apparent. In the original Curry and Kurtzrock (1951) ear choice technique and the modified ear choice technique (Lloyd, 1965a), the application of reinforcement is almost identical to that described above for the conventional or standard method. The same forms of verbal and nonverbal social reinforcement are used in the same schedules for reinforcing appropriate responses. In applying reinforcement principles to the ear choice methods the only thing that has changed is what is considered an appropriate response. In the standard methods either raising a hand or finger or pressing a signal button is defined as the response. In the ear choice methods the appropriate response is pointing to the ear in which the signal is presented.

PLAY METHODS

When confronted with young children, especially those between 2 and 6 years of age, many audiologists employ various forms of play audiometry (e.g., Barr, 1955; Donnelly, 1965; Frisina, 1962; Lloyd, 1965a; Lowell and others, 1956; O'Neill and others, 1961; Utley, 1949). Play audiometry has involved a number of responses such as putting rings on a peg, putting pegs in holes, hitting a peg board, hitting a drum, stacking blocks, putting marbles in a box, and putting blocks in a box. In this paper the block dropping, putting blocks in a box, response will be used to illustrate the various play audiometry techniques. The child is taught through verbal instruction and demonstration to drop a block in a box when and only when the auditory signal is presented.

It is assumed that the child's play activity is of interest to him and that completion of the response is rewarding. The child's block dropping behavior may be considered as high probability behavior, and the proper structuring of such as a play activity is an extremely useful operant technique. High probability behavior may be used to increase low probability behavior. However, in the typical application of play audiometry the clinician simply uses the child's high probability behavior by structuring the contingencies which allow the child to respond with such behavior.

Although the child's block dropping response may in itself be reinforcing, the skilled

clinician usually pairs the inherent reinforcement of the play response with considerable social reinforcement. Actually with some children the play activity may be of only limited interest; it may be a relatively weak reinforcer. In such cases, the verbal and nonverbal behavior of the clinician may be the more powerful reinforcer and the block dropping response a secondary reinforcer. In some cases the game played alone is not reinforcing but with a partner, such as a lively clinician, it is extremely reinforcing. The social reinforcement used in play audiometry is similar to the verbal and nonverbal reinforcement discussed above for other forms of behavioral audiometry. The clinical application of a variation in the amount and schedule of social reinforcement is also similar.

In general, a combination of the high probability behavior of the child and the social behavior of the clinician provides a powerful reinforcer for testing most young children, although obviously what is reinforcing for one subject may not be for another. The novice clinician frequently makes the mistake of assuming that because a given method or procedure was successful with several subjects, it is infallible. The experienced clinician recognizes individual differences and exercises ingenuity in finding an appropriate reinforcer for each subject.

What may be reinforcing for a subject at the beginning of the test session may be a relatively weak reinforcer by the end of the session. Such subject satiation can be extremely perplexing to the audiologist. It is easy to observe satiation in experimental animals when food is the reinforcer, but it takes a keenly observant clinician to recognize the early signs of a client's satiation in the audiometric testing session.

The individuality of reinforcers and the problem of satiation in play audiometry can be illustrated by the following two cases. The first is a relatively negative and extremely aggressive six year old boy seen in a university out-patient clinic. During the day he failed to cooperate on the psychological tests and in the speech and language examination. He showed no interest in several forms of play audiometry using blocks, rings on a peg, or various toys, but did indicate interest in playing with a drum. High probability drum beating behavior was therefore structured into the test. The boy's drum beating was put under stimulus control. Approximately fifteen minutes and two broken drumsticks later an entire air conduction threshold test was completed.

The second example is a relatively cooperative five year old girl, who quickly conditioned to play audiometry using a block dropping response paired with a social reinforcer. She responded quickly while the first three frequencies were tested, but when the fourth frequency test was begun her responses were slower. When this change in response pattern was observed, the clinician increased his verbal and nonverbal behavior in an attempt to increase social reinforcement. The girl's responses again were sharp and quick. Four additional frequencies were tested with short latency responses but again the responses slowed down; consequently, the clinician increased his verbal and nonverbal behavior to increase the reinforcement. This change in the clinician's behavior did not, however, bring the girl's block dropping under sharp stimulus control as it did earlier. Therefore, the clinician, enthusiastically changed the game and had the girl stack the blocks as a response to the auditory stimulus, which, once more brought the response under good stimulus control. Before the test was completed two additional responses—putting rings on a peg and hitting a toy xylophone—were used. Although the reinforcer varied slightly during the test, it was basically the same reinforcer; namely, a combination of some form of high probability play behavior of the girl and the social reinforcer of the clinician's contingent behavior.

VISUAL REINFORCER METHODS

Since the successful use of audiometric tests with visual reinforcers was first described

(Evans, 1943; Dix and Hallpike, 1947), numerous variations of these instrumental or operant conditioning methods have been employed to test young children. Basically, the child's responses to auditory signals are increased by reinforcing his pressing of a button when the signal is presented and not reinforcing his button pressing when no signal is presented. The multitude of visual reinforcement methods previously described by audiologists are enumerated below under the five main types of visual reinforcers utilized.

1. *Pictures* (Dix and Hallpike, 1947; Evans, 1943; Kaplin, 1957; Lloyd, 1965a, 1965b; Miller, 1962; Miller, 1963; Shimizu and Nakamura, 1957; Weaver, 1965).
2. *Miniature Scenes* (Statten and Wishart, 1956).
3. *Animated Toy Animals or Puppets* (Cotton and Hall, 1939; Green, 1958; Guilford and Haug, 1952; Miller, 1962; Sullivan and others, 1962; Waldrop, 1953).
4. *Toy Trains* (Ewing, 1930; Gaines, 1961; Ishisawa, 1962; Keaster, 1951).
5. *Other Mechanical Toys* (Denmark, 1950; MacPherson, 1960; Schwartz, 1952).

Typically, the visual reinforcers are presented on a 100 percent reinforcement schedule. In the clinical application of these visual reinforcer methods, social reinforcers are also employed. In most behavioral audiometry methods, regardless of response method and the kind of reinforcer, verbal and nonverbal social reinforcers are important. The prominent role may be related to the universality of this type of verbal and nonverbal behavior as a positive reinforcer. The generalized reinforcement value of much of the clinician's behavior is apparent when one considers that a smile is usually associated with pleasurable experiences. The same is true of many other types of clinical behavior such as a nod of the head, a pat on the back, clapping of hands, the word "good," or even the expression "oh boy!" Such behavior is a powerful tool when used with proper contingencies, i.e., when it occurs immediately after the child's appropriate response.

Two findings are of interest in the literature on visual reinforcement audiometric methods. First, the study by Statten and Wishart (1956) demonstrated superiority of the operant conditioning procedure with visual reinforcers over the classical conditioning psychogalvanic skin response (GSR) procedure. A second finding was the relative lack of success with the early use of the tunnel test (Ewing, 1930, p. 51) and the toy dog test (Cotton and Hall, 1939). The reinforcers were strong in these two unsuccessful attempts to use visual reinforcement. The children engaged in high probability behavior of playing with the objects intended as reinforcers and did not attend to the listening task because the contingencies were not properly structured. The children were allowed considerable access to the reinforcers for a minimal amount of responding. By restructuring the contingencies later investigations have eliminated the difficulty and have found the test quite useful. Gaines (1961) has even reported success in using the train test with institutionalized moderately retarded subjects. More recently Lloyd (1965a, 1965b) and Weaver (1965) have reported the successful use of the slide show type of visual reinforcers with institutionalized retardates.

A variation of the button pressing procedure is the conditioned orientation reflex (COR) previously described by Suzuki and Ogiba (1960, 1961). The COR reinforces a localization response and does not require the child to make a button pressing response to receive visual reinforcement. If the child looks at the appropriate loudspeaker when an auditory signal is presented, a doll located near that speaker is illuminated as a form of visual reinforcement. MacPherson (1960) and Fulton (1962) in their doctoral dissertations reported on the use of COR procedures with severely retarded subjects. Fulton's (1962) data indicated greater success with the behavioral conditioning (COR) procedure than with the classical conditioning (GSR) procedure. This basic procedure of reinforcing the location of the signal has been modified by several audio-logists who use lights rather than an illuminated doll (Houston Speech and Hearing Center, 1964; Kimball, 1964; MacPherson, 1960).

TANGIBLE REINFORCER METHODS

Relatively intangible reinforcers have been used in the forms of behavioral audiometry mentioned above. Such intangible reinforcers as the word "good," a smile, a pat on the back, or the opportunity to see a picture function as reinforcers for many children, but for some subjects such behavior or consequences are relatively ineffective. More tangible reinforcers have been used with operant conditioning procedures to obtain audiometric data on retardates (Meyerson and Michael, 1960; LaCrosse and Bidlake, 1964; Spradlin and Lloyd, 1965).* Edible items such as candy, popcorn, sugar coated cereal, crackers, dietary supplements, and various fluids as well as nonedible objects such as miniature toys or trinkets have been used in various forms of tangible reinforcement operant conditioning audiometry (TROCA).

In some cases the examiner decided that a single tangible item would be given to each subject. In other cases each subject was given a variety of these tangible items as selected by the examiner. With others, the experimenter has attempted to determine which items are

[* Spradlin and Lloyd (1965) made their preliminary report of the TROCA procedure developed at Parsons in a monograph publication of limited printing. However, Lloyd, Spradlin, and Reid have recently published a more complete description of the TROCA procedure in *J. Speech Hearing Dis.*, **33**, 236–245 (1968). Lloyd *et al* (1968) describe the TROCA procedure in five interrelated phases: (1) determining the reinforcer, (2) initial training, (3) stimulus generalization, (4) sound field screening, and (5) bilateral screening and threshold testing. They report the results of the first fifty (50) profoundly retarded patients they attempted to test with TROCA and the initial results obtained from three normal infants (5, 15, and 18 mos. old) to demonstrate some of the potential of this procedure with non verbal and difficult-to-test-patients. The validity of the procedure was demonstrated by reasonable audiometric configurations, agreement with other data, and three cases of unilateral hearing impairment. Masking and bone-conduction testing were briefly considered.—LLL]

effective reinforcers before starting the audiometric test; then that reinforcer is used during the test. Spradlin and Lloyd (1965) have described one procedure for determining which tangible items are effective reinforcers for a given subject. Since the only reason for using tangible reinforcers is that the other more conventional forms of reinforcement were not effective, it would seem that the audiologist using TROCA should attempt to determine an effective, tangible reinforcer for each subject rather than use an arbitrarily determined reinforcer. It should be noted that a reinforcer is defined in terms of its functional relationship to the behavior being reinforced and is not some item or event that the experimenter or clinician has predesignated as a reinforcer.

One of the TROCA reports (LaCrosse and Bidlake, 1964) did not give details on their procedure; however, the other two (Meyerson and Michael, 1960; Spradlin and Lloyd, 1965) did describe their procedures. These investigations were designed to test the retarded child who did not respond to verbal instructions. After using a variety of procedures Meyerson and Michael (1960) concluded by suggesting that the most effective procedure involved two responses. When there was no auditory signal present, the response of pressing one button was reinforced on a partial schedule, and when the signal was present the response of pushing a second button was reinforced on a similar schedule. They also provided extra reinforcement for appropriate quick switches.

Spradlin and Lloyd (1965) also tried various procedures, but they reported that a single response system which reinforced pressing the button when the auditory signal was present was the most efficient for clinical testing. They used a 100 percent reinforcement schedule with the single response system. This TROCA procedure is similar to the operant audiometry procedures which use visual reinforcers. The primary difference is in the reinforcers.

Both investigations (Meyerson and Michael, 1960; Spradlin and Lloyd, 1965) used automated programs of signal presentation. The programming equipment also reduced the latency of reinforcement delivery. Some of the visual reinforcer operant procedures involved immediate (automated) reinforcement, but most of the behavior audiometry procedures considered were not automated for reinforcement delivery. In the typical audiometric test an extremely small latency in reinforcement delivery is of relatively little consequence, but in some cases the reinforcement latency may be an extremely critical factor. With the more difficult cases special attention should be afforded the reinforcement timing. The reinforcement should be presented immediately after an appropriate response.

SUMMARY AND CONCLUSIONS

Several behavioral audiometry methods are reviewed in terms of operant conditioning principles. A primary focus of the paper is upon reinforcement principles. The importance of stimulus control is obvious in all forms of audiometry. The obtaining of stimulus control is related to factors such as simplicity of response, selection of an appropriate reinforcer, reinforcement contingencies, immediate reinforcement, reinforcement schedules, and reinforcement shifting. Sensitivity in the use of these variables frequently marks the difference between the skilled and the unskilled clinician. Many of the rather vague clinical qualities considered under the term "rapport" may also be analyzed in terms of operant principles.

ACKNOWLEDGMENTS

Preparation of this paper was partially supported by a National Institute of Mental Health Grant No. MH-01127. The author is grateful to his friend and colleague Joseph E. Spradlin, Coordinator of Research, Bureau of Child Research, University of Kansas and Parsons State Hospital and Training Center, for his review and constructive criticism of the manuscript.

REFERENCES

Barr, B., Pure tone audiometry for pre-school children. *Acta-Otolaryng.*, Suppl. 121 (1955).

Cotton, J. C., and Hall, Jayne, Administration of the 6-A audiometer test to kindergarten and first grade children. *Volta Rev.*, **41**, 291 (1939).

Denmark, F. G. W., A development of the peep-show audiometer. *J. Laryng. Otol.*, **64**, 357–360 (1950).

Curry, E. T., and Kurtzrock, G. H., A preliminary investigation of the ear-choice technique in threshold audiometry. *J. Speech Hearing Dis.*, **16**, 340–345 (1951).

Dix, Mary R., and Hallpike, C. S., The peep show: a new technique for pure tone audiometry in young children. *Brit. Med. J.*, **2**, 719–723 (1947).

Donnelly, K. G., A vibro-tactile method of conditioning young children for hearing tests. In Lloyd, L. L., and Frisina, D. R. (Ed.), *The Audiologic Assessment of the Mentally Retarded: Proceedings of a National Conference*, Parsons, Kansas: Speech and Hearing Dept., PSH&TC (1965).

Evans, Mary L., An adaptation of the audiometric technique for use with small children. Masters thesis, Univ. Illinois (1943).

Ewing, A. W. G., *Aphasia in Children*. London: Oxford Medical Publication (1930).

Frisina, D. R., Audiometric evaluation and its relation to habilitation and rehabilitation of the deaf. *Amer. Ann. Deaf*, **107**, 478–481 (1962).

Frisina, D. R., Measurement of hearing in children. In Jerger, J. (Ed.), *Modern Developments in Audiology*, N.Y.: Academic Press (1963).

Fulton, R. T., Psychogalvanic skin response and conditioned orientation reflex audiometry with mentally retarded children. Doctoral dissertation, Purdue Univ. (1962).

Gaines, Judy A. L., A comparison of two audiometric tests administered to a group of mentally retarded children. Masters thesis, Univ. of Nebraska (1961).

Green, D. S., The pup-show: a simple, inexpensive modification of the peep-show. *J. Speech Hearing Dis.*, **23**, 118–120 (1958).

Guilford, R., and Haug, O., Diagnosis of deafness in the very young child. *Arch. Otolaryng.*, **55**, 101–106 (1952).

Houston Speech and Hearing Center, Audiometric assessment technique. *Asha*, **6**, 261 (1964).

Ishisawa, H., A study on play audiometry. (Japanese text) *Otol. Fukuoka*, 6 (Supp. 7), 397–415 (1960). From: *dsh Abst.*, **2**, 201 (1962).

Kaplin, Harriet, A comparison of picture response and hand raising technique for pure tone audiometry with young children. Masters thesis, Penn. State Univ. (1957).

Keaster, Marjorie J., A pure-tone audiometric test for preschool children. Masters thesis, Univ. of Wisc. (1951).

Kimball, B. D., Addendum to previous article. *Asha*, **6**, 500 (1964).

LaCrosse, E. L., and Bidlake, H., A method to test the hearing of mentally retarded children. *Volta Rev.*, **66**, 27–30 (1964).

Lloyd, L. L., A comparison of selected auditory measures on normal hearing mentally retarded children. Doctoral dissertation, Univ. of Iowa (1965a).

Lloyd, L. L., Use of the slide show audiometric technique with mentally retarded children. *Exceptional Children*, **32**, 93–98 (1965b).

Lowell, E., Rushford, Georgina, Hoversten, Gloria, and Stoner, Marguerite, Evaluation of pure tone audiometry with pre-school age children. *J. Speech Hearing Dis.*, **21**, 292–302 (1956).

MacPherson, J. B., The evaluation and development of techniques for testing the auditory acuity of trainable mentally retarded children. Doctoral dissertation, Univ. of Texas (1960).

Meyerson, L., and Michael, J. L., *The Measurement of Sensory Thresholds in Exceptional Children: An Experimental Approach to Some Problems of Differential Diagnosis and Education with Special Reference to Hearing*. U.S. Office of Education, Cooperative Research Project No. 418, Univ. of Houston, Houston, Texas (1960).

Miller, A. L., The use of reward techniques in testing young children's hearing. *Hear. News*, **30**, 5–7 (1962).

Miller, A. L., The use of slide projectors in pure tone audiometric testing. *J. Speech Hearing Dis.*, **28**, 94–96 (1963).

O'Neill, J., Oyer, H., and Hillis, J., Audiometric procedures used with children. *J. Speech Hearing Dis.*, **26**, 61–66 (1961).

Shimizu, H., and Nakamura, F., Pure-tone audiometry in children: lantern-slides test. *Ann. Oto. Rhino. Laryng.*, **66**, 392–398 (1957).

Spradlin, J. E., and Lloyd, L. L., Operant conditioning audiometry (OCA) with low level retardates: a preliminary report. In Lloyd, L. L., and Frisina, D. R. (Ed.), *The Audiologic Assessment of the Mentally Retarded: The Proceedings of a National Conference*, Parsons, Kansas: Speech and Hearing Dept., PSH&TC (1965).

Statten, P., and Wishart, D. E. S., Pure tone audiometry in young children: Psychogalvanic-skin-resistance and peep-show. *Ann. Oto. Rhino. Laryng.*, **65**, 511–534 (1956).

Schwartz, A., Supplementary pure tone audiometric screening test for pre-school children. Masters thesis, Univ. of Wisconsin (1952).

Sullivan, R., Miller, M. H., and Polisar, I. A., The portable pup-show: A further modification of the pup-show. *Arch Otolaryng.*, **76**, 49–51 (1962).

Suzuki, T., and Ogiba, Y., A technique of pure tone audiometry for children under three years of age: Conditioned orientation reflex (COR) audiometry. *Rev. Laryng.*, Paris, **1**, 33–45 (1960).

Suzuki, T., and Ogiba, Y., Conditioned orientation reflex audiometry. *Arch. Otolaryng.*, **74**, 192–198 (1961).

Utley, J., Suggestive procedures for determining auditory acuity in very young acoustically handicapped children. *Eye, Ear, Nose, Thr., Mon.*, **28**, 590–595 (1949).

Waldrop, W., A puppet show hearing test. *Volta Rev.*, **55**, 488–489 (1953).

Weaver, R. M., The use of filmstrip audiometry in assessing the auditory sensitivity of mentally retarded children. In Lloyd, L. L., and Frisina, D. R. (Ed.), *The Audiologic Assessment of the Mentally Retarded: The Proceedings of a National Conference*, Parsons, Kansas: Speech and Hearing Dept., PSH&TC (1965).

12

Effects of Stapes Fixation on Bone–Conduction Response

RAYMOND CARHART

RAYMOND CARHART, Ph.D., is Professor of Audiology, Northwestern University

MECHANICAL MODIFICATION OF THE BONE CONDUCTION RESPONSE

For more than a decade it has been known that careful bone conduction audiometry reveals distinctive configurations in the threshold curves of persons with stapes fixation (3). Obviously, this effect is most frequently observed as a consequence of otosclerosis, although it will also occur as the result of any other lesion, whether acquired or congenital, whose primary influence is reduction in stapedial mobility. Moreover, the characteristic shift in bone conduction response caused by stapes fixation is strictly mechanical, that is, stapes fixation changes the efficiency with which skull vibration reaches the hair cell mechanism. The end result is that the bone conduction curve is not an uncontaminated indication of the patient's sensorineural reserve. Instead, the patient's cochlear and neural adequacy determines the general level of his responses to bone conduction, but the mechanical factor also affects his bone thresholds noticeably. The clinician who desires to estimate sensorineural capacity may do so by making allowance for this mechanical factor as he interprets the patient's bone conduction audiogram.

The Typical Mechanical Configuration

It is common clinical practice to measure bone

Reprinted by permission of the author from *Otosclerosis*. Boston, Mass.: Little, Brown, 1962. Pp. 175–197.

conduction thresholds in the frequency range from 250 cps through 4000 cps, usually only at octave intervals. Considering only the effect at these intervals, the typical mechanical shift resulting from stapes fixation is a decrease in bone conduction acuity at the four highest test frequencies. More specifically, the work of both Carhart (3) and McConnell (18) suggest that the typical reductions in sensitivity are 5 db at 500 cps, 10 db at 1000 cps, 15 db at 2000 cps and 5 db at 4000 cps. This shift has frequently been called the Carhart notch. Sonday (24) obtained very similar values for this mechanical shift when he tested patients with otosclerosis by conventional audiometry, but the data he gathered by automatic audiometry yielded estimates of mechanical enhancement in bone conduction acuity in the range from 250 cps through 500 cps. Thus, it would appear that the method of measurement may have an effect on the values which characterize the typical distortion in bone conduction responsiveness caused by stapes fixation.

Whether or not this proves to be the case, the configuration which typically emerges when patients with otosclerosis are tested by conventional discrete frequency technique is approximately as described by Carhart and McConnell (19). This configuration is illustrated in Figure 12-1, which presents two bone conduction curves. The figure also shows the estimated level of sensorineural reserve. This sensorineural level is derived by assuming that each bone conduction curve includes a mechanical distortion of the magnitude described above. Case A is characteristic of clinical otosclerosis without secondary nerve degeneration. It is a bone conduction audiogram commonly encountered when stapes fixation occurs in conjunction with a normal sensorineural system. The second bone conduction audiogram (case B) illustrates the result which emerges when the idealized mechanical shift is superimposed upon a sensorineural impairment. In the present example, this sensorineural impairment is 20 db at 250 cps, and it increases for higher frequencies at the rate of 5 db per octave. A different sensorineural deficit would change the configuration and level of the bone conduction curve, but this curve would still include the mechanical component.

Evidence that the Modification is Mechanical

There are four facts which demonstrate clearly that stapes fixation induces mechanical modifications in bone conduction response.

Before examining these facts, it is well to remember that physical changes in the conduction system of the ear affect bone conduction thresholds in various ways. Occlusion of the external auditory canal (25), loading of the drum membrane (21), and change of pressure in either the external canal or the middle ear (11) are among the factors which have been shown to shift temporarily the bone conduction thresholds of normal-hearing persons. The Gellé test and the Bing test are among the clinical tools which seek to discover whether or not the ear under test possesses a lesion in the transmissional system by noting whether responsiveness to bone conduction stimuli can still be changed by such mechanical factors. The patient whose responsiveness is unchanged during these tests is the patient with a conduction lesion.

In view of the foregoing it is safe to generalize that only the exceptional case of conduction hearing loss will not show some mechanical modification in bone conduction acuity. Of course, not all conduction lesions cause the same pattern of mechanical distortion, and

differences in configuration can be of great help to the diagnostician. The task before us at the moment is one of reviewing the four facts which demonstrate that stapes fixation is one of the factors producing mechanical shift in bone conduction thresholds, and that the configuration of this shift has the pattern previously described.

First, there is the observation that patients with clinical otosclerosis do not experience the shift in loudness of bone-conducted stimuli which both normal persons and patients with sensorineural loss experience when the external

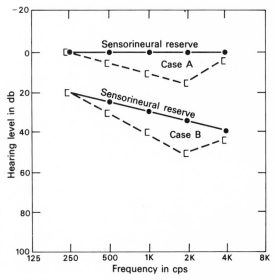

Figure 12-1. Two bone conduction audiograms illustrating the typical distortion in the measurement of sensorineural reserve which results from the mechanical reduction in cochlear efficiency induced by stapes fixation. Case A shows the pattern when there is no sensorineural impairment and case B shows the result of sensorineural deficit combined with the mechanical distortion.

meatus is occluded (Bing's test) or when pressure is varied in the external canal (Gellé's test). One may reason from this that stapes fixation has disturbed the status of the conduction mechanism so that the peripheral variations no longer have a mechanical influence on the efficiency with which skull vibration reaches the organ of Corti, that is, stapes fixation inhibits susceptibility to other mechanical influences on bone conduction acuity. It must be noted, of course, that this observation per se does not tell us whether or not stapes fixation modifies a patient's bone conduction threshold, since it merely states that phenomena which are normally induced by varying conditions in the middle ear or in the external ear do not occur when the stapes is fixed.

Secondly, and here we have one evidence that stapes fixation does modify bone conduction thresholds, it is unusual to find a patient with otosclerosis whose bone conduction thresholds are fully normal, and it is even rarer to find such a patient with bone conduction thresholds which are better than normal. This situation exists even when we restrict ourselves to patients who are free from any sensorineural impairment. In other words, patients with otosclerosis who possess normal cochlear and neural function do not yield completely normal bone conduction audiograms. The situation is illustrated by the work of Sonday (24), who carefully measured the bone conduction acuity of 24 patients with otosclerosis who possessed normal cochlear function according to Jerger's DL Difference technique. The mean bone conduction thresholds for these 24 cases, as derived by conventional audiometry, were at hearing levels of +4.6 db at 250 cps, +6.8 db at 500 cps, +10.6 db at 1000 cps, +15.9 db at 2000 cps, and +4.1 db at 4000 cps. Since measures of the cochlear reserve for this group should have averaged essentially zero hearing loss, the group's systematic deficit in bone conduction acuity indicates that this measure is contaminated when stapes fixation is present. Furthermore, the direction of this discrepancy indicates that the mechanical effect of stapes fixation on bone thresholds is mainly detrimental, i.e., the efficiency of energy transmission to the organ of Corti is reduced.[1]

Thirdly, endaural surgery can improve

[1] Various facts, including Sonday's findings with automatic bone conduction audiometry, lead one to suspect that this generalization may be valid only for frequencies from 600 cps or 700 cps upward.

bone conduction thresholds. In 1948 both Juers (15) and Woods (27) reported postoperative improvement in the bone conduction thresholds of fenestrated ears. Different observers have varied somewhat in the magnitude they assign to this improvement. An illustrative set of values are those obtained by McConnell (18), who performed the first meticulous audiometric exploration of this phenomenon. His series of cases showed improvement in bone acuity, following fenestration, which averaged 6.5 db at 1000 cps, 7.4 db at 1500 cps, 8.5 db at 2000 cps, 6.4 db at 3000 cps, and 4.2 db at 4000 cps. Sonday (24) obtained fairly similar results by automatic audiometry. In interpreting his findings, McConnell stressed that a fenestrated ear is not equivalent to an ear with a normal conductive mechanism. Hence, the postoperative improvement in bone acuity resulting from fenestration should not be expected to reverse completely the mechanical shift in threshold caused by stapes fixation. The validity of this interpretation is supported by more recent experiences with other techniques for the surgical management of otosclerosis. Findings vary, probably at least partly because different surgical procedures result in mechanically different revisions of the middle ear system. Shambaugh (22), for example, reports cases of complete reversal of the Carhart notch after stapes mobilization. By contrast, Rosen et al. (20) did not find improvement in the mean bone conduction acuity of one hundred and fifty-five ears after stapes mobilization. The critical point to remember is that such discrepancies do not negate two basic facts: (a) persons with stapes fixation do not usually have normal bone conduction even though their cochlear function is perfect; and (b) when such persons exhibit changes in bone conduction acuity after successful endaural surgery, these changes are in the direction of improved acuity. In other words, the postsurgical bone conduction thresholds of such cases are in closer agreement than are their presurgical ones to the status of their cochlear sensitivity as estimated from other forms of evidence. Hence, one may reason (from the fact that surgery designed to counteract otosclerosis often changes the patient's bone conduction acuity) that the presence of a change in bone conduction responsiveness resulting from stapes fixation has been demonstrated. The alternative would be to conclude that stapes fixation has a detrimental influence on the sensitivity of the organ of Corti and that surgical revision restricted to the conduction mechanism revives the cochlear structures. The fallacy of such a conclusion is immediately obvious.

Fourthly, experimentally produced stapes fixation causes bone conduction thresholds to become poorer. Smith (23) demonstrated this effect by measuring cochlear microphonics in the cat. He found that experimental fixation of the stapes decreased response to bone-conducted stimuli at all frequencies except those in the extremely high range. He observed an effect at low frequencies which is not paralleled in clinical otosclerosis, but this discrepancy is not basic. The fact that bone conduction sensitivity can be changed by mechanical interference with the stapes is inescapable from Smith's work.

Progression of the Mechanical Shift

Survey of the clinical records of the otosclerotic population supplies information regarding the point in the progression of stapes fixation at which the mechanical shift in bone conduction acuity appears. The shift seems to occur rather abruptly and to reach its full magnitude quickly when stapes fixation has progressed to the stage where it causes a mild air conduction loss.

More explicitly, the preclinical stage of stapes fixation does not appear to be characterized by mechanical notching of the bone conduction curve, although there is minor modification of the air conduction audiogram at this stage. Figure 12-2, illustrating this situation, shows the audiogram of a patient with preclinical otosclerosis and normal sensorineural reserve. Note that the bone conduction audiogram is completely normal, i.e., lies along the zero-hearing-level contour; whereas

the air conduction audiogram shows minor depression in response to low frequencies with hyperacuity at 4000 cps and 8000 cps. In other words, the air conduction curve manifests a tilt resulting from an increased stiffness of the conduction system which is caused by early ankylosis. At this stage the physical change is still small enough so that it has caused neither a generalized air conduction loss nor a

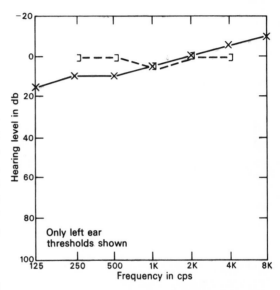

Figure 12-2. Audiogram of a patient with preclinical otosclerosis and a normal sensorineural reserve. Early stapes fixation has here induced a slight stiffness tilt in the air conduction audiogram without affecting responsiveness to bone conduction stimuli. X—X: Air conduction;]- - -]: bone conduction.

noticeable shift in transmission of skull-borne vibration within the inner ear.

Graham's (7) work leads to the belief that this first stage does not persist long. As stapes fixation progresses, a notching of the bone conduction audiogram soon appears. This second stage is illustrated in Figure 12-3, which presents the test results on a patient with incomplete stapes ankylosis and normal cochleoneural function. This patient exhibited only mild clinical otosclerosis. As compared with the case in Figure 12-2, the additional impairment for air conduction is slight; yet

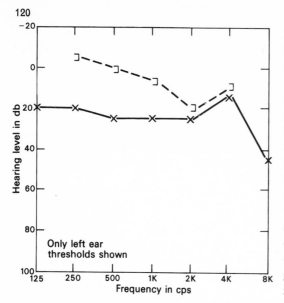

Figure 12-3. Incomplete stapes fixation in an ear free from sensorineural impairment induces mild generalized loss for air-conducted tones and typical mechanical distortion of the bone conduction audiogram. The sharp air conduction loss at 8000 cps is probably a temporary effect of progressive stapes fixation which appears soon after the stage represented by Figure 12-2 and disappears soon after the stage depicted above. X—X: Air conduction;]‐ ‐ ‐]: bone conduction.

now there is a fully developed depression of the bone conduction curve.

The transition to an audiogram characteristic of complete stapes fixation (still with normal sensorineural reserve) is illustrated in Figure 12-4. This patient suffered a much greater air conduction loss at all frequencies without noticeable further depression in the bone conduction curve. The audiogram illustrates the principle that the mechanical change in bone acuity does not increase with progressively greater stapes fixation, as does impairment for air-conducted sounds.

RELATION TO THEORY OF BONE CONDUCTION

No theory of bone conduction can be considered adequate unless it can account for the effect of stapes fixation on bone conduction thresholds. Unfortunately, a fully satisfactory description has not yet been expounded.

However, the present status of thinking can be illustrated by brief comments on four contemporary views.

It is sometimes suggested that stapes fixation eliminates inertial (translatory) bone conduction as an important factor in stimulating the inner ear. According to this view, the resultant threshold is the residue of response due to compressional bone conduction alone (26). The major deterrent to this explanation, as both Fournier (6) and Huizing (11) have pointed out, is that stapes fixation should cause reduced bone conduction efficiency at low frequencies since inertial bone conduction is traditionally considered to be greatest for low frequencies. There should be improvement for high frequencies due to an enhanced compressional factor at these frequencies. This prediction goes counter to clinical observation, which demonstrates that stapes fixation causes negligible change in acuity for low frequencies, with maximal

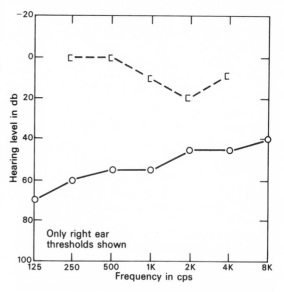

Figure 12-4. Complete stapes fixation in an ear free from sensorineural impairment induces marked loss for air-conducted tone and typical mechanical distortion of the bone conduction audiogram. Note that the transition from the incomplete stapes fixation, as represented in Figure 12-3, to the stage depicted above produces a marked effect on air conduction response but no noticeable effect on bone conduction response. O—O: Air conduction;]‐ ‐ ‐]: bone conduction.

reduction in acuity between 1000 cps and 2000 cps. Therefore, the explanation that stapes fixation eliminates inertial bone conduction is questionable.

A different theory is propounded by Huizing (*11*), who believes that bone conduction efficiency depends on interaction among various vibratory systems which are intricately coupled within the ear. He feels that the findings after various clinical and experimental modifications which can be produced in bone conduction may be explained by changes in one or more of these vibratory systems. Such changes, Huizing says, affect the impedance relationships and couplings of the auditory system. The vibration within the cochlear fluid is thereby affected. When it comes to accounting for the effect of stapes fixation, Huizing believes there is elimination of a reinforcement to the cochlear oscillation which is normally supplied by vibrations of the ossicular chain. Thus, while discounting inertial bone conduction in accounting for the phenomenon, Huizing is satisfied with a generalized postulation of an alternative mechanism.

A third theory is developed by Allen and Fernández (*2*), who argue that bone conduction stimulation is due exclusively to a compressional mechanism. They then attribute all mechanically induced changes in bone conduction threshold to two factors which are simultaneously affected by the physical state of the external and middle ear. These two factors are (*a*) the efficiency with which sound energy escapes from the cochlea via the ossicular path and (*b*) the impedance match between the skull and the inner ear. Changes in these factors modify the agitation which occurs at the basilar membrane. Allen (*1*) says that otosclerosis affects these two factors so that the changes ". . . tend to cancel each other at low tones. The resultant effect on bone conduction is that low tones remain nearly unchanged but the higher tones are somewhat impaired, the picture seen with the typical Carhart notch." Stated differently, Allen and Fernández (*2*) theorize that in otosclerosis the predominant effect is one

where transmission of vibratory energy from skull to inner ear is reduced because stapes fixation increases the impedance mismatch at the boundary between bone and labyrinthine fluid. This view has the advantage of parsimony, but it, too, is restricted to generalities.

Groen has a fourth point of view, which he has just presented to this symposium (Chapter 13). Tonndorf takes issue with some aspects of the theory it outlines.

The conflicting opinions which we have heard these two competent researchers express clearly illustrate the current uncertainty. Each of the several theorists mentioned above is satisfied that his conception integrates the evidence at hand with the principles of physics. To the rest of us, however, this divergence of views regarding the cause of the Carhart notch requires more definitive explanation.

EFFECT OF SIMULTANEOUS CONDUCTION LESIONS

One feature of the mechanical phenomena under consideration is that the effect produced by stapes fixation supersedes other effects which more peripheral lesions of the conduction mechanism would produce if they occurred alone. Rytzner (*21*) illustrated this feature experimentally when he demonstrated that loading the eardrum of patients with otosclerosis produced no change in their bone conduction thresholds, whereas similar loading in normal persons increased bone conduction responsiveness 16.5 db at 250 cps, 12 db at 500 cps, and almost 7 db at 1000 cps. The effect is also found in clinical cases where stapes fixation is combined with other disturbances of the conduction mechanism. The following two cases illustrate this situation.

The audiogram shown in Figure 12-5 is the record from a patient with hearing loss resulting from chronic suppurative otitis media only. Here the outstanding feature is a bone conduction curve which is better than normal at low frequencies and poorer than normal at high frequencies. Lierle and Reger (*17*)

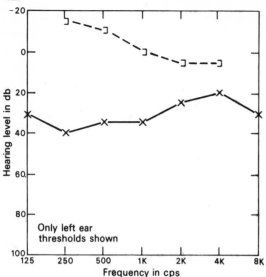

Figure 12-5. Case where chronic suppurative otitis media in an ear free from sensorineural impairment has caused both a definite air conduction loss and a mechanical distortion of the bone conduction audiogram. The latter is clearly different from the distortion of the bone conduction curve characteristic of stapes fixation. X—X: Air conduction;]- - -]: bone conduction.

pointed out years ago that a configuration of this type is common in middle ear disease. The important thing to realize is that bone conduction patterns of this variety are obtained from patients with normal sensorineural function (as confirmed by other evidence). In such instances, both the improved bone acuity for low frequencies and the reduced acuity for high frequencies are the result of mechanical modification in the responsiveness of the auditory system. In other words, Figure 12-5 illustrates that otitis media commonly produces a mechanical distortion in the bone conduction curve. Moreover, its configuration is entirely different from the pattern which characterizes stapes fixation.

By contrast, Figure 12-6 records the audiometric results yielded by a patient having a pure conduction loss resulting from both chronic suppurative otitis media and stapes fixation. One notes that the bone conduction audiogram in this case exhibits only the Carhart notch, which is attributable to the

stapes fixation. In this instance, the more peripheral pathological changes exerted no influence on bone conduction sensitivity; i.e., the otitis media here ceased to affect the vibratory efficiency of the inner ear system as it would have done had the stapes been normally mobile. There is no hint in the bone conduction curve of an improved responsiveness at low frequencies arising from the patient's chronic middle ear disease. Thus, this case illustrates the principle that stapes fixation obscures the effects which more peripheral lesions produce when these lesions occur by themselves.

CLINICAL VALUE OF BONE CONDUCTION AUDIOMETRY

The bone conduction audiogram helps the otologist in two important ways as he deals with the problem of otosclerosis.

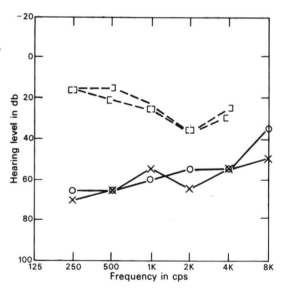

Figure 12-6. Record of a case where complete stapes fixation bilaterally was complicated by chronic suppurative otitis media in left ear. Equivalence of the audiometric curves for the two sides illustrates that stapes fixation obscures the mechanical influence on bone conduction responsiveness (Figure 12-5) which would otherwise be expected because of the otitis media. X—X: Air conduction in left ear; O—O: air conduction in right ear;]- - -]: bone conduction in left ear; [- - -[: bone conduction in right ear.

In the first place, the knowledge that a specific configuration of bone conduction typifies stapes fixation, whereas different configurations characterize other conduction lesions, can aid the otologist in the differential diagnosis of conduction hearing losses. This knowledge is also helpful in identifying the conduction element in a mixed loss. Here the sensorineural component will determine the general level and slope of the bone conduction audiogram, but the mechanical configuration which results from the conduction lesion will modify the details of this curve.

estimates are particularly important when evaluating the patient's suitability for otological surgery, because they form a base from which to predict the benefit which a successful operation should bring him.

For example, Shambaugh (22) used this approach in the system he developed a decade ago for predicting the outcome of fenestration surgery. The Shambaugh system is based on two generalizations: (a) a reasonable estimate of a patient's cochlear reserve is obtained by correcting his bone conduction audiogram for the idealized Carhart notch,

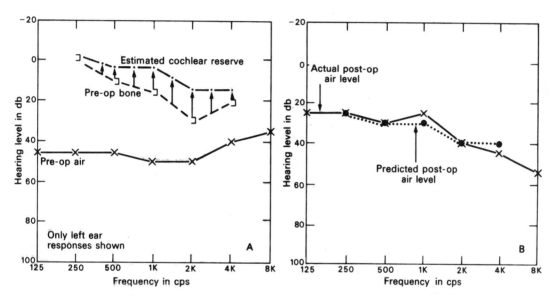

Figure 12-7. Record of a case of stapes fixation with minimal sensorineural impairment which illustrates Shambaugh's method for prediction of air conduction acuity after fenestration. The method assumes that the postoperative air level will be 25 db poorer than the estimated cochlear reserve, which is computed by correcting the preoperative bone conduction audiogram for the average mechanical distortion due to stapes fixation. (A) Preoperative audiogram; (B) prediction and postoperative outcome.

In the second place, the otologist can estimate with added accuracy the sensorineural reserve which a patient with otosclerosis retains by correcting the patient's bone conduction audiogram for mechanical distortion due to stapes fixation. Stated conversely, the otologist can more precisely determine a patient's hearing impairment due to secondary nerve degeneration by making allowance for the Carhart notch when interpreting the patient's bone conduction thresholds. Such

i.e., cochlear sensitivity is presumed to be better than his bone conduction thresholds by 5 db at 500 cps, 10 db at 1000 cps, 15 db at 2000 cps, and 5 db at 4000 cps; and (b) a successful fenestration, as Davis and Walsh (5) first emphasized, usually leaves the patient with a deficit of about 25 db in air conduction threshold in the speech range. This deficit is a residual conduction loss due to surgical disruption of the ossicular chain. On the basis of these two generalizations the surgeon may predict that successful fenestration will yield a postoperative air conduction audiogram which is 25 db poorer than the level which results when the patient's preoperative bone conduction audiogram has been corrected for the idealized Carhart notch.[2] Figure 12-7 illustrates the application of the Shambaugh method in a representative case where the prediction was good. Figure 12-7A presents the preoperative audiogram of an ear scheduled for surgery and the estimate of sensorineural reserve derived from the preoperative bone conduction findings. Figure 12-7B records the prediction of postoperative level, which is drawn 25 db below the aforementioned estimate of sensorineural reserve, and shows the actual air conduction thresholds obtained 3 months after surgery. The agreement between the prediction and the postsurgical audiogram is very close.

Similar techniques for prediction can be employed in estimating results to be expected from the various stapes operations. Some early work, such as that of Guilford and Haug (8), suggested that Shambaugh's original method might also serve in predicting the outcome of stapes mobilization. However, there are many instances where stapes surgery eliminates the conduction impairment almost entirely. At present the important consideration for the surgeon is the estimation of the patient's level of sensorineural reserve, since it is the surgeon's hope that the patient will approximate this level postoperatively.

Of course, the surgeon must bear in mind, as he uses bone conduction measurements in the prediction of postoperative hearing level, that there are factors which will reduce the accuracy of his judgment. Three of these factors [3] must concern us here: (a) the success of the surgery itself depends on the multitude of variables which differentiate one otosclerotic lesion from another as well as one operation

from the next; (b) the mechanical shift in bone conduction response differs from patient to patient, so that use of an average correction for the Carhart notch can be significantly inaccurate; and (c) important errors in measuring bone conduction threshold can arise from limitations in the test procedure itself. Since the variables determining surgical success are beyond the scope of the present discussion, only the second and third sources of error are discussed below.

Variability in the Mechanical Configuration

The amount and detail of shift in bone conduction thresholds due to stapes fixation fluctuates sufficiently from patient to patient so that these variations are of practical significance. The causes of these fluctuations are not yet identifiable. However, as clinical experience clearly attests, there are instances in which the mechanical shift is very different from the average values usually encountered. Obviously, when this is the situation any prediction of postoperative hearing levels derived from the average correction will be in serious error. In the case where the mechanical shift is unusually large, the average correction leads the surgeon to assume that the patient has poorer sensorineural reserve than he actually possesses which may discourage a good prospect for surgical aid. The reverse error occurs when the actual mechanical shift is very slight, the sensorineural reserve being not as good as one would assume on the basis of the average correction, with a disappointing outcome the result if surgery is undertaken. The problem for the surgeon, obviously, is to determine whether the patient with stapes fixation he is examining at the moment exhibits an atypical or a normal mechanical modification in responsiveness to bone-conducted stimuli.

There are two ways of estimating whether or not the mechanical notching in the bone conduction audiogram of a patient with otosclerosis is unusual.

One way is to compare the configurations of his air and bone conduction curves. If the bone curve shows an irregularity or pecu-

---

[2] The postoperative deficit at 4000 cps is so often greater than 25 db that the above system for predicting postoperative air conduction acuity is not satisfactory at 4000 cps.

[3] The limitations in procedure which concern us here are those which remain after the clinician has taken the precautions which insure that his audiometer is in calibration, his testing environment is acceptable, and his testing technique is both correct and careful.

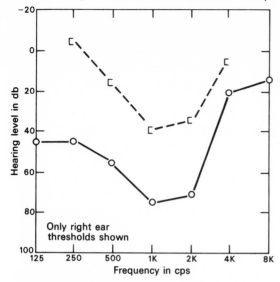

Figure 12-8. Parallel irregularities in air and bone conduction configurations of a patient with otosclerosis. This parallelism indicates that the unusual notching of the bone conduction audiogram is not an atypical mechanical distortion due to stapes fixation but instead is a composite of a fairly typical mechanical distortion and a sensorineural impairment restricted to the middle frequency range. O—O: Air conduction; [- - - [: bone conduction.

concomitant irregularities in the bone conduction curve are properly interpreted as an unusual mechanical notching. In other words, here is a patient with otosclerosis who exhibited a mechanical notch of abnormal severity, i.e., it is as great as the whole depression in the bone conduction audiogram.

A second way to identify the patient with otosclerosis whose bone conduction curve is atypical is to determine his sensorineural reserve with a technique that does not depend upon conventional audiometry. Unfortunately, very little attention has been given to the development of such alternatives, even though they have the advantage of bypassing the mechanical artifacts which occur in bone conduction audiometry. Alternative techniques, however, can be employed to obtain quantitative estimates of sensorineural efficiency. A very good example is Jerger's use of the DL test (12). By studying the responses of patients with pure sensorineural losses, Jerger derived a set of values for converting

liarity which the air conduction curve duplicates, this peculiarity should be attributed to sensorineural impairment. Conversely, when the air conduction curve fails to exhibit the peculiarity, the audiogram should be viewed as incorporating an unusual mechanical modification in the bone conduction response. Figures 12-8 and 12-9 illustrate these principles. Figure 12-8 is the record of a patient with otosclerosis who exhibited similar irregularities in his air and bone conduction audiograms. The parallelism of the two curves reveals that in this instance the bone conduction curve is the product of two factors: (a) a sensorineural abnormality and (b) a fairly typical mechanical distortion revealed by an approximately conventional Carhart notch. By contrast, the air conduction curve reproduced in Figure 12-9 lacks irregularity. Instead it has the relatively flat and slightly rising pattern which is characteristic of complete stapes fixation without the complication of secondary nerve degeneration. Hence, the

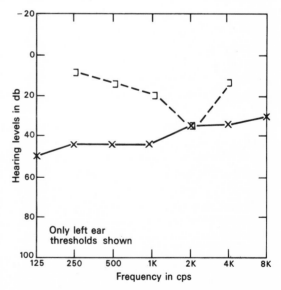

Figure 12-9. Unusual notching of the bone conduction audiogram without parallel irregularity in the air conduction curve. This lack of parallelism indicates an atypical distortion in the bone conduction curve due to stapes fixation. In this case the absence of any sensorineural impairment was subsequently confirmed by the excellent hearing level achieved through stapes mobilization. X—X: Air conduction;] - - -]: bone conduction.

DL scores into amount of sensorineural impairment. He next administered the DL test to 55 patients with otosclerosis and estimated their sensorineural reserves from the results. He could then predict the air conduction levels which these patients should achieve following fenestration by merely assuming that each patient's postoperative air thresholds would be 25 db poorer than the level of sensorineural reserve as gauged from the DL results. In other words, Jerger's method was identical with Shambaugh's technique for prediction except for the manner in which the estimate of sensorineural level was obtained. The following findings emerged: In 30 of the 55 patients Jerger's prediction and the prediction by Shambaugh's system were both within 5 db of the average postoperative outcome for the 500 to 2000 cps range, i.e., both methods were effective; in 22 of the remaining patients Jerger's estimate was closer to the surgical result. These latter not only were the patients for whom there was discrepancy between predictions, but they were also the patients for whom the Shambaugh method proved relatively unprecise. Certainly it would seem that Jerger's method, by avoiding the bone conduction modality, gave the more accurate estimates of sensorineural reserve in these latter cases. Thus, even though we need more research before the DL scores can be used confidently in this way by the clinician, Jerger's use of the method is a good illustration of an alternative technique which can help identify the patient with otosclerosis who exhibits an unusual Carhart notch. Here is an area worthy of renewed attention.

Limitations in Bone Conduction Audiometry

Finally, even when bone conduction audiometry is meticulously performed, it possesses three defects which sometimes cause serious error in threshold measurement when testing patients with otosclerosis (as well as when testing patients with other types of lesions).

One cause of error is false lateralization of the auditory experience. False lateralization occurs for the patient with otosclerosis when he has the impression of hearing in the poorer ear because of phase differences in the bone conduction responses on the two sides. This error is common when bone conduction audiometry is performed without masking. Under these circumstances the bone threshold in the poorer ear, to which the sensation is referred, may seem to the tester to be better than it really is by 10 db or more. Sonday (24) demonstrated the severity of this problem when he obtained preoperative and postoperative thresholds for bone conduction by von Békésy automatic audiometry. Sonday concludes that when patients with otosclerosis are tested without masking ". . . the subject's report of the location of the bone-conducted stimulus is not a reliable indication of the ear which is responding to the test signal" (24).

It is traditional to use masking to counteract false lateralization and to eliminate other shadow responses. Unfortunately, there are instances where the introduction of a masking sound creates serious interference with the response in the ear under test, even though the sound is not strong enough to produce masking in this ear. It is hazardous to speculate on the reason for this difficulty, but, as Cochran (4) demonstrated years ago, there are some persons whose thresholds are significantly disturbed by moderate noise levels in the contralateral ear. Such patients do poorly even though the noise is too weak to be causing any true masking in the test ear. Such hyperdistractibility is a second cause of error in bone conduction audiometry. An example of this, involving a patient with unilateral stapes fixation, was recently reported by Jerger and Wertz (14). The patient yielded a record of equal loss by air and bone conduction in his otosclerotic ear provided his opposite ear, which was essentially normal in acuity, was masked. The resultant audiogram, with its interweaving air and bone conduction curves, would conventionally be interpreted as indicating a pure sensorineural impairment rather than a conduction loss, yet such an interpretation is fallacious in the present case. Confirmation of this statement was obtained by experimental exploration of the patient's middle ear, which revealed a fixation so solid that the stapes could not be mobilized with extensive palpation and percussion. Interestingly enough, when masking was omitted, the bone conduction thresholds obtained for the patient's otosclerotic ear showed a fairly typical Carhart notch. This finding was originally discounted as a shadow response because bone conduction thresholds became so poor when masking was applied to the contralateral ear.

The third factor which complicates bone conduction audiometry is that many patients have hearing losses so great that efforts to mask the contralateral ear are ineffective. This difficulty is poorly recognized by many clinicians even though its *raison d'être* has been clearly expounded by several writers, including Leden *et al.* (*16*) and Hood (*10*). The situation arises because effective masking is reduced at each test frequency by the amount of the air conduction loss in the masked ear at that frequency. For example, a masking noise which causes 50 db of threshold shift in a normal ear will produce only about 10 db of shift in an ear with a hearing loss of 40 db. This same noise will not cause any threshold shift in an ear where the air conduction loss exceeds 50 db.

In applying these considerations to the present discussion, remember that many commercial audiometers do not produce more than 50 db of effective masking at any test frequency. It is useless to employ masking from such an audiometer when trying temporarily to deactivate an ear having severe hearing loss, such as an ear with 50 to 60 db of impairment due to stapes fixation. Shadow responses will be evoked in this ear as readily when the masking sound is present as when this noise is absent. Figure 12-10 reports the kind of audiometric configuration that can emerge when a patient with a marked conduction loss in his right ear caused by otosclerosis and with a profoundly deaf left ear is tested with a typical commercial audiometer. In this example, the audiogram for the right ear is accurate. By contrast, the thresholds here attributed to the left ear for both air and

bone conduction are shadow responses. Full masking applied to the right ear fails to eliminate these shadow responses because both the bone and air conduction stimuli reach the right ear via skull vibration,[4] whereas the masking sound cannot penetrate the impaired right ear sufficiently to reduce its sensitivity for skull-borne vibration. The tragic feature here is that the results falsely attributed to the

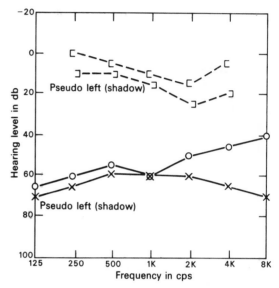

Figure 12-10. Example of the manner in which shadow responses for both air and bone conduction can create the impression of marked stapes fixation in a profoundly deaf (left) ear because complete stapes fixation in the other (right) ear induces so great an air conduction impairment that 50 db of masking applied to that ear (right) is ineffectual. X—X: Air conduction in left ear; O—O: air conduction in right ear;]---]: bone conduction in left ear; [---[: bone conduction in right ear.

left ear give the impression that there is very good sensorineural function with a large air-bone gap in that ear. Here is an audiogram which indicates, in this case incorrectly, a left ear highly suitable for surgery, whereas, of course, the right ear actually is. If, on the basis of these audiometric findings, the left ear is chosen for surgery, failure is inescapable.

The foregoing pitfalls in bone conduction

---

[4] An audiometer earphone will initiate a skull-borne stimulus when the air signal becomes strong enough, i.e., a hearing level of about 60 db.

audiometry are fundamental. They mean that, even though good bone conduction audiometry is valid in the majority of cases, highly erroneous results will be obtained with some patients despite the care with which the traditional precautions of audiometry are followed. The prospect of making a surgical decision based on an erroneous audiometric picture is an eventuality which the endaural surgeon cannot tolerate. His great need is for an alternative method for estimating sensorineural reserve. It must be a method which avoids the pitfalls we have been discussing. Jerger's DL test offers such a technique, but it awaits better standardization. Moreover, since it is a hard procedure to use with some cases, a simpler alternative is desirable. Another alternative is the SAL test (sensorineural acuity level test) which is described below. This test is especially valuable to the surgeon as a check on his findings by conventional bone conduction audiometry.

THE SAL TEST

The SAL (sensorineural acuity level) technique was developed by Jerger and Tillman (*13*). It has features which are reminiscent of Rainville's procedure of masking by bone conduction (*6*). The method is simple. A bone conduction vibrator is centered on the forehead and an air conduction headphone is placed over each ear. Pure tone thresholds are measured twice in each ear. The first set of thresholds is obtained while the bone conduction vibrator is inactive. The second set of thresholds is measured while the bone unit is emitting white noise to the skull at a standardized level. The white noise constitutes a mechanical disturbance which reaches both cochleae. It produces masking in each ear separately provided the sensorineural efficiency of that ear remains sufficiently good. Stated differently, this masking effect will be maximal when the sensorineural system is normal. The effect decreases in exact proportion to the degree of sensorineural impairment; i.e., an impairment of 20 db reduces by 20 db the masking which the bone-conduc-

ted disturbance causes. The magnitude of the masking effect for each frequency can be easily computed by noting the differences between the two air conduction thresholds obtained at that test frequency. Each difference measures the threshold shifts which the introduction of the masking noise evoked. The question to be answered is whether or not each shift is as great as a listener with normal hearing would experience. Broadly speaking, any deficit in amount of shift represents a decrease in sensorineural acuity. This deficit may be plotted on an audiogram as a deviation (in the direction of impaired response) from o-db hearing level, just as bone conduction thresholds are now plotted. Hence, the resultant curve is interpreted in the same manner as a bone conduction audiogram would be.

The clinician must remember that mechanical factors affect SAL measurements much as these factors affect bone conduction measurements. In other words, the SAL technique does not free the clinician from responsibility to make allowance for the changes which conduction lesions impose on the efficiency with which skull-borne vibrations reach the organ of Corti, i.e., the counterpart of the Carhart notch appears in SAL test results.[5] The advantage of the SAL technique is that it eliminates danger of ignoring unsuspected shadow responses. Thus, the SAL test not only gives usable information on sensorineural acuity level, but also, as a major merit, it identifies as bad surgical prospects those ears which on the basis of unrecognized shadow responses during conventional audiometry would be falsely classified as good surgical prospects.

SUMMARY

Stapes fixation produces a change in response to bone-conducted stimuli. The change ordinarily appears during routine audiometry as reduction in bone sensitivity of 5 db at 500

[5] The pattern of this counterpart is somewhat different because norms for the SAL test are based on responses of occluded normal ears. Description of the detail of difference is outside the scope of the present paper, which is concerned with bone conduction audiometry.

cps, 10 db at 1000 cps, 15 db at 2000 cps and 5 db at 4000 cps. The mechanical nature of the phenomenon is demonstrated by several types of fact, including the observation that fenestration surgery partially reverses the shift. The shift first comes into existence when stapes fixation reaches the stage where it causes mild air conduction loss. The configuration of the shift does not change much thereafter despite increase in the air conduction loss. Contemporary theories of bone conduction do not account in detail for the phenomenon. An interesting clinical observation is that the mechanical change due to stapes fixation takes precedence and, thus, obscures other patterns of bone conduction shift which more peripheral lesions evoke alone. Knowledge of the foregoing matters aids the otologist in reaching the diagnosis of otosclerosis and in predicting the outcome of endaural surgery. Care must be taken, however, to allow for those cases in which patients with otosclerosis exhibit atypical mechanical shifts. Moreover, the clinician must recognize that bone conduction audiometry can be in serious error for some patients because of false lateralization, hyperdistractibility in the presence of masking noise, and the fact that masking noise becomes ineffective when applied to an ear with substantial hearing impairment. In view of these pitfalls, alternative methods for estimating sensorineural reserve (such as the DL Difference and SAL tests) can supplement bone conduction audiometry most helpfully in the clinical evaluation of otosclerosis.

REFERENCES

1. Allen, G. W. Some clinical implications of recent research on bone conduction. *Quart. Bull. Northwestern Univ. M. School* 34 101 1960.

2. Allen, G. W., and Fernández, C. The mechanism of bone conduction. *Ann. Otol. Rhin. & Laryng.* 69 5 1960.

3. Carhart, R. Clinical application of bone conduction audiometry. *Arch. Otolaryng.* 51 798 1950.

4. Cochran, M. W. Masking in audiometry. Northwestern University M.A. Thesis 1946.

5. Davis, H., and Walsh, T. E. The limits of improvement of hearing following the fenestration operation. *Laryngoscope* 60 273 1950.

6. Fournier, J. E. Bone conduction. In Kobrak, H., *The Middle Ear*. Chicago: University of Chicago Press, 1959, p. 92.

7. Graham, A. B. An audiological and otological investigation of normal hearing individuals with a family history of clinical otosclerosis. Northwestern University Ph.D. Thesis 1953.

8. Guilford, F. R., and Haug, C. O. The Carhart-Shambaugh formula used for stapes mobilization prediction. *Laryngoscope* 68 637 1958.

9. Hirsh, I. J. *The Measurement of Hearing*. New York: McGraw-Hill Co., 1952.

10. Hood, J. D. The principles and practice of bone conduction audiometry. *Laryngoscope* 70 1211 1960.

11. Huizing, E. H. Bone conduction: the influence of the middle ear. *Acta oto-laryng.* Suppl. 155 1 1960.

12. Jerger, J. F. A new test for cochlear reserve in the selection of patients for fenestration surgery. *Ann. Otol. Rhin. & Laryng.* 62 724 1953.

13. Jerger, J., and Tillman, T. A new method for the clinical determination of sensorineural acuity level (SAL). *A.M.A. Arch. Otolaryng.* 71 948 1960.

14. Jerger, J., and Wertz, M. The indiscriminate use of masking in bone-conduction audiometry. *A.M.A. Arch. Otolaryng.* 70 419 1959.

15. Juers, A. L. Observations on bone conduction in fenestration cases. *Ann. Otol. Rhin. & Laryng.* 57 28 1948.

16. Leden, G., Nilsson, G., and Anderson, H. Masking in clinical audiometry. *Acta oto-laryng.* 50 125 1959.

17. Lierle, D., and Reger, S. Correlations between bone and air conduction acuity measurements over wide frequency ranges in different types of hearing impairments. *Laryngoscope* 56 187 1946.

18. McConnell, F. E. Influence of fenestration surgery on bone conduction acuity. Northwestern University Ph.D. Thesis 1950.

19. McConnell, F., and Carhart, R. Influence of fenestration surgery on bone conduction measurements. *Laryngoscope* 62 1267 1952.

20. Rosen, S., Bergman, M., and Grossman, I. Bone conduction thresholds in stapes surgery. *A.M.A. Arch. Otolaryng.* 70 365 1959.

21. Rytzner, C. Sound transmission in clinical otosclerosis. *Acta oto-laryng.* Suppl. 117 1 1954.

22. Shambaugh, G. E., Jr. *Surgery of the Ear*. Philadelphia: W. B. Saunders Co., 1959.

23. Smith, K. R. Bone conduction during experimental fixation of the stapes. *J. Exper. Psycho.* 33 96 1943.

24. Sonday, F. L. Measurement of fenestration results by automatic audiometry. Northwestern University Ph.D. Thesis (1957).

25. Watson, N. A., and Gales, R. S. Bone-conduction threshold measurements: effects of occlusion, enclosures, and masking devices. *J. Acoust. Soc. Am.* 14 207 1943.

26. Wever, G. E., and Lawrence, M. *Physiological Acoustics*. Princeton, N. J.: Princeton University Press, 1954.

27. Woods, R. R. Some observations on bone conduction following the fenestration operation. *J. Laryng. & Otol.* 62 22 1948.

13

Animal Experiments in Bone Conduction: Clinical Conclusions

JUERGEN TONNDORF

JUERGEN TONNDORF, M.D., is Professor of Otolaryngology, College of Physicians and Surgeons, Columbia University

The clinical testing of bone conduction (BC) is one of the most important audiological tools for the differentiation of conductive and sensorineural hearing losses. To distinguish it from other forms (e.g. skull vibrations induced by aerial sounds of large amplitude), Békésy (*5*) once suggested the term "*clinical bone conduction.*" This paper is only concerned with the latter form. Over the years, innumerable theories have been proposed which cannot possibly be mentioned here. An excellent recent summary is that of Hood (*14*). Some of the earlier history is well described in Politzer's *Geschichte der Ohrenheilkunde* (*22*).

The present experiments were begun in 1960. Most of them were conducted on experimental animals (cats, dogs, guinea pigs, and rats). Some additional studies were carried out in mechanical cochlear models of the Békésy type and still some others in cadaver heads of cats. Over the years, a number of people have participated in this work. Their names are listed as co-authors on a series of detailed reports published (*28*) or now in preparation (*30–34*).

The list of topics studied, to which solutions or explanations can now be offered, include the following:

1. Role of the cochlear aqueduct with respect to BC responses.

Reprinted by permission of the author from *Trans. Amer. Otol. Soc.*, **52,** pp. 22–41 (1964) and from *Ann. Otol. Rhinol. Laryngol.*, **73,** pp. 659–678 (1964).

2. Compressional BC responses of the cochlea in the absence of any cochlear openings.

3. Traveling-wave mechanism in compressional BC responses.

4. Loading of the tympanic membrane.

5. Stapedial loading.

6. Quantitative analysis of BC components.

7. Quantitative comparison of AC and BC responses in terms of stimulus magnitude.

8. Carhart's notch.

9. Occlusion effect of the external ear canal.

10. Direct evidence against the "outflow" theory of Mach.

11. Evidence for the osseotympanic component of BC.

All of these points will be discussed in detail in the papers just mentioned (*28–34*). Very few of the concepts which evolved from these studies are really new. The classical hypotheses of Herzog and Krainz (*15*) (compressional mode of BC, 1926), of Bárány (*2*) (ossicular inertial mode of BC, 1938), of Békésy (*3*) (identical mechanism of excitation due to AC and BC stimulation, 1932), as well as Groen's (*12*) mathematical derivation of various BC components, were largely confirmed and in some instances expanded. However, there is a large series of notions which in some form or another were also proposed over the years. Many of them, according to the present findings, contained some truths. The reason why they often failed to become generally accepted was that their authors had tried to explain *all* BC phenomena on the basis of one unifying simple concept, which they, more often than not, had developed from studying only *one* partial aspect of BC. To show that this is not possible and that BC is really quite a complex phenomenon is one of the purposes of the present paper.

This paper will be confined to those aspects of the present experiments which have direct bearings upon clinical BC testing. Among the above listed topics, discussion will be limited to:

I. Stapedial loading.
II. Simultaneous occlusion of both cochlear windows.
III. Carhart's notch.
IV. The occlusion effect of the external ear canal.

(In connection with the last named effect, reference will be made to the clinical tests of Bing, Runge, Weber, and Gelle.)

PROCEDURE

Suffice it to mention here that in living animals registration of cochlear microphonics (CM) served as indicator of the degree of response of the inner ear. The BC input was monitored by an accelerometer, rigidly fastened to the head, much in the same manner as a probe microphone in the external canal is utilized to monitor the input of air conduction (AC) signals. In the earlier experiments, in which only relative changes were studied, the accelerometer was independent of the BC vibrator. Later, it was made an integral part of the BC driving system. The head and the driving system were then rigidly connected. In some experiments, a probe microphone with a small probe diameter (1 mm) was inserted into the short osseous ear canal, according to a method suggested by Pfalz (*21*). Its opening was less than 1 mm from the drum membrane, facing a direction normal to that of the axis of the ear canal.

(Reference numbers attached to the section headings in the following refer to the papers in which the particular subject is treated in greater detail.)

RESULTS

I. Stapedial Loading (*28, 30*)

This comment is based upon a chance finding in the present series of investigations. Experimental occlusion of the cochlear windows by means of dental cement is by no means easily accomplished. Figure 13-1 shows that the first attempts in this respect produced very

Figure 13-1. BC losses for various frequencies due to different attempts to immobilize the oval window. Curves A through C represent several stages in which stapedial fixation by means of dental cement was gradually improved (cf. text). Each curve represents an average of five to six animals (Results from [*28,30*]).

Also included in the graph are results of K. R. Smith (J. Exper. Psychol. 33:96, 1943) who had "immobilized" the stapes by means of a string slung around one stapedial crus.— Note that the differences in amplitude change between the four methods are confined to frequencies around and below the resonant point of the ossicular system (600 c/s).

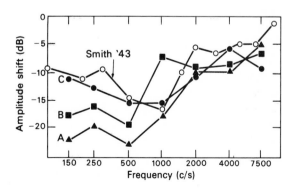

pronounced BC losses (curve A). Ordinary zinc oxide cement had been used. Micro-dissection at the termination of the experiments revealed that in each case a large glob of cement had been deposited around the crura and sometimes also around the incudo-stapedial joint; but fixation had not been achieved at all, due to a cushion of edematous tissue and fluid in the oval-window niche. Stripping the ossicle and its environment carefully of its mucoperiosteal cover, drying the bone thoroughly up to the very last moment before cement application, and tamping the liquid cement down by means of air pressure, produced a somewhat better seal, and, as Figure 13-1 (curve B) shows, a lesser BC loss. However, zinc oxide cements do not really combine with the bone, but adhere only by surface tension. The bone in the oval-window niche is fairly smooth and no undercuts had been attempted here. There-fore, this fixation could not be considered per-fect either; again a sizable, but slightly smaller lump of cement had been deposited around the stapes. It was not until a polymerizing cement ("Grip," manufactured by Caulk and Co.) was utilized that a satisfactory footplate fixation was achieved (Figure 13-1, curve C). The liquid primer supplied with this cement creeps deeply into all bone crevices, and after polymerization, forms a tight bond with the actual cement. (The author is obliged to L. Bernstein, M.D., D.D.S., for bringing his attention to these matters.)

It is interesting to note (Figure 13-1) that a mere impairment of stapedial mobility (Smith, 1943), without an addition of mass to the stapes, leads also to a minimal loss of BC responses.

It is seen from this series of experimental results that a combination of a large mass adhering to the stapes (e.g. a so-called "ice-berg" otosclerotic focus of the footplate) if associated with minimal fixation may produce a BC loss which clinically may be interpreted as being indicative of a diminished "cochlear reserve" and thus be considered a contra-indication to surgery.

Since the first publication of these findings

(28), the author has received a number of case reports (Drs. C. M. Kos, V. Goodhill, D. Meyers, and W. Kley) which appear to confirm the concept as presented here.

It should be mentioned that the maximal loss, which in the cat is centered around 500 c/s, will most likely be around 2000 c/s in man for reasons which will be discussed in section III. It seems to this author that differentiating stapes loading from a true sen-sorineural loss could be achieved by means of speech discrimination testing. A relatively good discrimination score would be expected in this condition (a point which may need further clinical confirmation) since stapes loading is really a conductive impairment. (The explanation given in the earlier report that this phenomenon might be due to a reverse loading of the ossicular chain in the sense of Bárány [2], could not be maintained on closer scrutiny.)

II. Simultaneous Occlusion of Both Cochlear Windows (28, 29)

This writer had originally supported W. House (13) in his belief that a simultaneous otosclerotic occlusion of both cochlear win-dows should severely reduce BC responses because it would completely immobilize the cochlear fluids. According to the classical hypothesis of Herzog (15), at least a com-pliant round window is mandatory for coch-lear BC responses. However, in none of his cases has House (13) been able to improve BC significantly or to obtain serviceable hear-ing by surgical restoration of compliant win-dows. J. Heermann's recent report on the same subject (14) was not very encouraging either.

These observations in human patients shed some doubt upon the above-mentioned con-cept. In subsequent experiments with cats it was found that a simultaneous occlusion of both windows did not produce a BC loss larger than that observed after occlusion of the oval window alone. (When the round window was occluded separately, the loss had been considerably less than that produced by occlusion of the oval window.) However, a prior closure of the cochlear aqueduct augmented the BC loss due to occlusion of the oval window. Thus it was shown that the cochlear aqueduct, being close to the round window, constituted an effective auxiliary outlet of the *scala tympani* with respect to compressional BC.

The extreme state of cochlear occlusion, a cochlea without *any* outlets whatsoever, cannot be realized in experimental animals for obvious reasons. A pertinent study was therefore conducted in cochlear models of the Békésy type (*29*). A displacement of the cochlear partition (the "basilar membrane") under vibratory ("BC") stimulation was indeed observed in such models, but only under one condition, namely, when the perilymphatic scalae were of unequal size. A subsequent analysis indicated that the shell of the model when put to vibration did not remain rigid but executed so-called *distortional* vibrations. That is to say, it altered its shape synchronously with the applied signal in the three dimensions of space. Figure 13-2 illustrates this point by means of schematic cross-sections and explains the origin of the displacement of the cochlear partition.

The distortional vibrations executed by a coiled cochlea are very likely more complex than those shown in Figure 13-2; but the point is that they are probably based upon the same principle. Thus it appears that the compressional mode of BC does not need any windows at all in order to produce a displacement of the basilar membrane as the classical theory had it (*15*), although its efficiency was found to increase with a compliant round window (*30*).

It must be concluded therefore that otosclerotic occlusion of both cochlear windows *per se*, even when involving the cochlear aqueduct, an occurrence which had been observed histologically by Ruedi (*25*), must not necessarily lead to severe depressions of BC responses. Whenever a combination of severe BC losses and occlusion of both windows is found, a concomitant severe sensorineural hearing loss ought to be suspected.

III. Carhart's Notch (*30, 34*)

In 1951, Carhart (*8*) first drew attention to the following curious observation with regard to patients with an otosclerotic stapedial fixation: after successful fenestration surgery, the BC response level often recovered, maximally by about 15 db around 2000 c/s, and

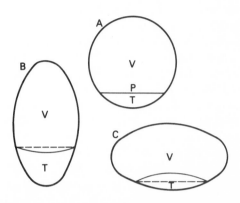

Figure 13-2. Distortional vibrations of the cochlear shell and their effect upon the instantaneous position of the basilar membrane (schematic after [*29*]).

The shell undergoes periodic changes in shape. The three instances shown are 90° apart in phase, the sequence being A-B-A-C-A-B-etc. If the cochlear partition (P) were dividing the entire space into two perilymphatic scalae of equal size, the ratio of their cross-sectional areas would remain unaltered at all times, and no displacement of the partition would ensue. However, when *scala tympani* (T) is smaller than *scala vestibuli* (V) the following is seen to happen. (The drawing overstates this case considerably.) At instant C, the area T becomes relatively smaller (it tends toward zero). At instant B it becomes relatively larger. Since the slice of fluid bounded within T cannot change its volume, the partition must be displaced in the manner indicated. Note the asymmetry of the positive and negative displacements (larger in *C* than in *B*). The resulting distortion (prominent 2nd harmonic) was actually observed in the model experiments in a correct phase relationship re the displacement of the partition.

somewhat less at adjacent test frequencies. Carhart pointed out correctly that in such cases the measurement of BC cannot be a perfect indication of the "cochlear reserve" in the affected frequency range, and suggested therefore that allowances be made for this

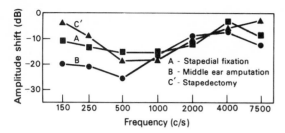

Figure 13-3. Shift of the CM response in cats after A) stapedial fixation; B) amputation of the middle ear (stapes retained); and C) stapedectomy. Average of five animals each. (Data from [*30*].)

phenomenon in assessing patients for surgery.

Various explanations have been offered for this phenomenon. The simplest, *viz.* that the notch might be due to the missing middle-ear BC contribution, was rejected by many "because (in the words of Carhart [*9*]) stapes fixation should cause reduced BC efficiency at low frequencies." Ranke (*23*) suggested that a fenestra made in the horizontal canal, i.e. beyond the fixed oval window, would in essence extend the length and volume of *scala vestibuli* and thus augment the fluid imbalance between the two perilymphatic scalae. Consequently, fenestration, by increasing the effectiveness of the *fluid inertial* component of BC, should improve the total BC response. Groen (*12*) submitted another interesting proposition. Based upon mathematical calculation, he showed that the air volume enclosed in the middle ear has its resonance point around 2500 c/s. He then reasoned that stapedial fixation should eliminate that portion of the effect which acts upon the inner ear *via* the tympanic membrane while retaining the lesser one acting directly upon the round window. Groen attributed the variability of Carhart's notch to the variation in frequency and in magnitude of the sub-component acting upon the round window. Carhart (*9*) in a recent summary cited various other attempts of explanation without actually taking sides in the argument.

The fact that the notch, to some extent, is also alleviated by stapedial surgery (mobilization and other function-restoring procedures) indicates that there are really two problems: 1) Carhart's notch as caused by stapedial fixation and 2) its alleviation by fenestration surgery.

The present author considers it fortuitous that his own animal experiments were originally started in cats. It turned out (Figure 13-3) a) that the notch produced by stapedial fixation in cats was very pronounced; b) that its maximum occurred between 500 c/s and 1000 c/s; c) that there was an even larger loss in the low-to-middle frequency range, after amputation of the middle ear, but with the stapes left in place. The degree of the loss and its place of maximum varied from species to species (cat, dog, guinea pig, and rat). The animal species coming closest to man in these respects was the rat. Stapedectomy, which was performed in cats only, improved the BC responses in the low frequency range with respect to those observed after stapedial fixation (Figure 13-3).

This complex set of events can only be understood on the basis of an analysis of BC into its various components. There is no need here to go into all of its details. (Reference is made to the appropriate papers [*30, 34*].) The following statements may suffice with respect to the problem at hand:

1. The contribution of the middle ear to the total BC response is made up of two components:

   a) the ossicular inertia (as originally defined by Bárány [*2*]);
   b) the compliance of the air enclosed in the middle ear spaces ("middle ear cavity effect" as postulated by Groen [*12*]).

2. The latter effect is largely responsible for the compliance of the tympanic membrane and is aided in this respect by the air column in the external ear canal.

3. The oval window acts as a leak with

respect to the inner-ear compressional component. Although not very effective in comparison with some other BC components, as long as the middle ear is intact, this oval-window release becomes important when the middle ear is absent.

4. There is a fluid inertial component of the inner ear which is diminished by stapedial fixation and augmented by stapedectomy.

From all these considerations, the following explanation evolves for the phenomenon at hand: The *magnitude* of Carhart's notch is determined by the relative importance of the middle ear contribution. Among the animals tested, it was found highest in guinea pigs and least in dogs, with man occupying an intermediate position. The *place* of the maximal loss along the frequency scale is determined by the resonant point of the ossicular chain for BC stimulation. The latter was lowest in cats and highest in rats (man being found at the high end of the scale). The middle ear cavity effect and the air column in the external ear canal play a subordinate role in this respect. Thus, Carhart's notch due to stapedial fixation is caused by the elimination of the middle ear BC contribution, and there is really no contradiction in the fact that in man it occurs at 2000 c/s, i.e. at a relatively high frequency. Structural restoration of the middle ear will restore normal BC response levels. On removal of the middle ear, with the stapes footplate remaining mobile, the loss is more pronounced because of the concomitant oval window leak.

Fenestration surgery increases the effectiveness of the fluid-inertial component and thus improves the BC response. In the cat, the only animal so studied, the fluid inertial component was most effective between 2000 and 4000 c/s, but the improvement never reached the response level of the intact ear. However, raising or lowering the fluid level in the oval window niche by about 1-1.5 mm did not produce measurable changes in the BC response level. Thus, the present experiments failed to verify the above-mentioned notion of Ranke (*23*), concerning the effect of a change in the perilymphatic mass balance upon fluid inertia.

IV. *The Occlusion Effect of the External Ear Canal (33)*

This effect has a long history (*16, 22*). Clinically, it is made use of in the form of the so-called Bing test: In normal-hearing persons, occlusion of one ear canal produces lateralization of BC sounds into the involved ear. A host of explanations has been offered over the years which cannot possibly be enumerated here. Suffice it to cite three which the present author considers most important.

1. Rinne (*24*), in 1855, suggested that the effect might be explained as a resonance phenomenon of the external ear canal. This concept has recently (1960) been revived by Huizing (*17*).

2. Mach (*19*), in 1863, formulated his well-known "outflow" theory which assumes that under BC stimulation the inner ear radiates sound *via* the middle-ear transformer (then acting in a reversed direction), through the external canal, into the surrounding air. This normal outflow, Mach postulated, would be impaired by an occlusion anywhere along this pathway. Allen and Fernandez (*1*) (1960) might be considered modern proponents of Mach's theory.

3. There is Békésy's explanation (*4*) of 1941. He found that under BC stimulation of the head the lower jaw moves in an out-of-phase relationship with respect to the skull itself. Since the mandibular capitulum borders anterior-inferiorly onto the osseous and also onto the cartilaginous ear canal, Békésy postulated that the relative motion of the lower jaw should set up periodic compressions and decompressions of the occluded canal which would subsequently be received as an AC signal. Békésy supported his concept by the finding that a plug inserted deeply into the bony canal, i.e. beyond its compressible soft portion, failed to produce the effect. Franke *et al.* (*10*) actually measured the out-of-phase motion of the lower jaw. However, there is some counter-evidence by Allen and Fernandez (*1*). They observed two patients in whom they were able to demonstrate the occlusion effect in both ears, although the

lower jaw, including the capitulum, was missing on one side. The effect appeared to be of the same magnitude as in the other normal ear. Reger (pers. comm.) observed another such case.

It is the consensus of opinion (*1, 3, 17, 20*) that occlusion of the external ear canal produces an improvement mainly in the low-frequency range, in gross proportion to inverse frequency. This was confirmed in the present experiments (cf. later Figure 13-7).

In the cat, the structural relation between the ear canal and the head of the mandible is rather remote. Nevertheless, occlusion tests were done before and after resection of the ascending mandibular ramus, including the capitulum. There were insignificant and non-systematic changes within the high-frequencies (3000 c/s and higher), presumably due to a thinning of the anterior wall of the soft part of the external canal by the surgical procedure. This finding shows that the role of the lower jaw as postulated by Békésy is probably a subordinate one.

The next question which needs to be answered is whether or not occlusion produces actual pressure changes in the external ear canal. Figure 13-4 gives CM and probe microphone readings with the canal open and occluded (the probe microphone being placed in the osseous portion of the external canal). The figure not only answers the above question in the affirmative (compare the db readings for both test situations!), but it also shows that the frequency response curves as given by the CM and those read by the probe microphone parallel each other fairly accurately in both test situations.

The use of the probe microphone permitted a unique test of Mach's outflow theory. (As far as this writer is concerned, all other arguments against Mach's theory given so far must be considered *indirect* evidence.) If Mach were correct, one would expect that removal of the tympanic membrane, the transducer acting upon the microphone, should produce a sizeable attenuation of the probe microphone response. As shown by the three examples of Figure 13-5 there was practically no alteration, neither in amplitude nor in phase, up to approximately 1000 c/s. At higher frequencies there were some changes, to be sure, both in amplitude and in phase, but they varied between animals in a non-systematic manner. (By contrast the cochlear response is much reduced by this procedure, predominantly for low frequencies.) This observation, especially the absence of attenuation in the low-frequency range, in which the occlusion effect manifests itself most prominently, constitutes clear-cut evidence against Mach. The slight alterations of maximally ±10 db,

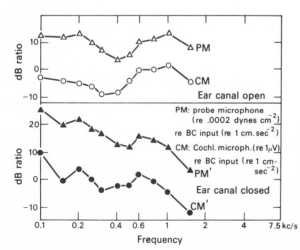

Figure 13-4. CM responses and probe microphone readings in the external ear canal re BC input (cat). Top: ear canal open; bottom: ear canal occluded. The frequency range was limited at 1500 c/s, since at higher frequencies the microphone required too high input values. The CM response within the frequency range shown had to be corrected for the BC resonant properties of the middle ear, in order to make them compatible with the probe microphone readings. (From [*34*].)

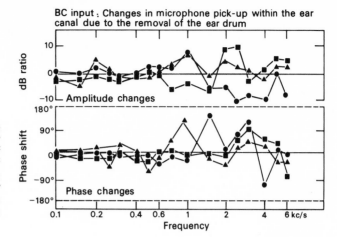

BC input : Changes in microphone pick-up within the ear canal due to the removal of the ear drum

Figure 13-5. Shift in probe microphone readings (amplitude and phase) for uniform BC inputs after removal of the tympanic membrane. The tip of the probe microphone was located in the osseous portion of the external ear canal (cf. procedure). Results from three individual cats are shown. (From [34].)

in the high-frequency range are, of course, due to the fact that after the removal of the tympanic membrane the microphone is looking into a different cavity with altered acoustic properties.

Next, the potential role of resonances in the external canal needs to be examined. Preliminary inspection of the raw data (CM responses *re* a given BC input for ear canals of various length) appeared to partially support this notion.

The results for each frequency were then plotted against the varying length of the ear canal, normalized for wavelength. That is to say, each individual result was expressed in terms of that fraction of wavelength a given

length of the ear canal had for each particular frequency. Figure 13-6 shows the results for a number of frequencies both with the ear canals open and occluded. Theory predicts that responses should be minimal for the open and maximal for the occluded ear canal at $\frac{1}{2}$ wavelength in the middle to high frequency range. Although, for obvious reasons, not all curves reach high enough, it is seen that this is probably a fair statement concerning the curve sections shown. There is only one low-frequency example included in the graph, 250 c/s. This frequency should form a maximum at $\frac{1}{4}$ wavelength with the ear canal open and at $\frac{1}{2}$ wavelength with the ear canal occluded. There is at least no contradiction to this

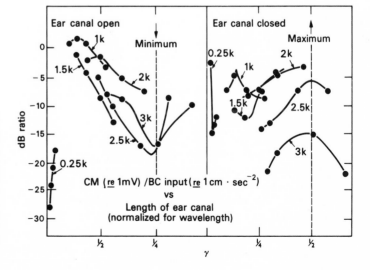

Figure 13-6. CM responses *re* BC input *vs* length of the ear canal, normalized for the wave length of each test frequency. Left: ear canal open; right: ear canal occluded. The "ear canals" of various length had been fashioned from thick-walled polyethylene tubing fitted tightly into the stump of the ear canal, after amputation of the pinna. Data from one individual cat (34).

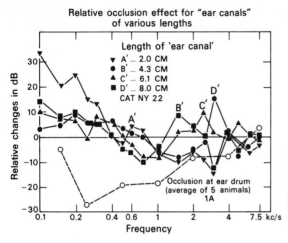

Figure 13-7. The relative occlusion effect for ear canals of various length in terms of the CM response shift for one individual cat (*34*). The data on the occlusion affected directly at the tympanic membrane are from a different series of experiments (*30*) and represent the average of five animals.

statement apparent in the short section of the curve on the left (canal open). However, with the canal occluded, the observational facts do not appear to support the prediction at all. (It must be noted that this observation was found for *all* low frequencies.)

It appears therefore that Rinne (*24*) and Huizing (*17*) were at least partially correct: the occlusion effect can indeed be explained on the basis of ear canal resonances with respect to middle and high frequencies. (Huizing based his entire conclusion upon similar considerations, but examined his results only for middle frequencies.)

Figure 13-7 gives the *relative* occlusion effect, i.e. the change in CM responses induced by occluding ear canals of various length, for one individual animal. In this and in the preceding figures, the results from one individual animal were presented, since averaging the results obtained from several animals tended to even out the sharp individual spikes in the middle and high frequency region, which varied slightly in position and magnitude from animal to animal. The spikes of course, are due to resonance phenomena in the ear canal. However, it is seen that the improvement of BC responses after occlusion of the ear canal was largest in the *low*-frequency region, increasing in approximate proportion to inverse frequency so that the resonance effects were largely obscured. Furthermore, as partly suggested already by Figure 13-6, the

effectiveness of the occlusion with respect to improving BC responses for varying sizes of the ear canal was given by a function having apparently *two* sharp discontinuities: as frequency went higher, it first decreased, then suddenly (between B' and A') it became much larger, eventually to revert to a steep loss. as the space was reduced to zero. Occlusion A', the most effective, was fairly close to the outer end of the osseous ear canal which in cats is very short. In other words, the occlusion was most effective when there was the least acoustic leak from the osseous canal.

These observations permit the following conclusion (Figure 13-8). Under the effect of BC stimulation, the osseous walls of the ear canal radiate sound into its lumen, part of which is taken up by the tympanic membrane and then transmitted to the inner ear *via* the ossicular chain. The head of the mandible may well play a small role in this process as Békésy (*5*) had postulated. As long as the ear canal is open, this system must act as a high-pass filter, i.e. low-frequencies must be attenuated. With the ear canal closed, the filter is eliminated (or at least partially eliminated, depending upon where the plug is situated) and transmission of low frequencies is improved accordingly. If the plug is inserted very deeply into the ear canal, the air cushion in front of the tympanic membrane becomes so small that the mobility of the tympanic membrane is impaired and ultimately eliminated altogether.

Figure 13-8. Left: Ear canal open; right: ear canal occluded. From top to bottom, 1st row: schematic cross-section of the ear canal; the mandibular capitulum is only shown in outline, since it lies in front of the cross-sectional plane. 2nd row: mechanical equivalent of the two situations; the piston (B - bone) produces an *ac* pressure within the cavity of the external canal which is terminated by the drum membrane (dm) and has a capacity (C_{ec}) and a mass (L_{ec}). There is an auxiliary pressure source (M = mandible). 3rd row: electrical equivalent; the inductance shunt to ground (L_{ec}) constitutes a high-pass filter. The two condensers represent the capacity of the air within the ear canal (C_{ec}) and that of the drum membrane (C_{dm}) respectively.

Note. In reality, the networks are more complicated; the present drawings attempt to show only the features essential to the discussion at hand.

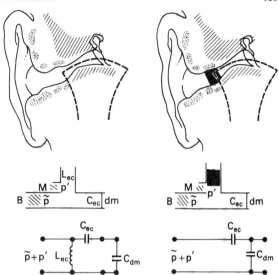

This has three consequences: a) it decreases the area of the osseous canal radiating sound into its lumen, b) it impairs the transmission through and also the contribution of the middle-ear to BC (it is for the latter reason that there is finally a BC loss); and c) the tuning of the external canal is shifted toward such high frequencies, that resonances for all lower frequencies are eliminated.

If this writer correctly understands a casual remark of Onchi (*20*), he may already have expressed a similar concept. Unfortunately, the translation of that particular article was rather poor so that one cannot be quite sure of Onchi's real notions.

The concept presented in the foregoing recognizes the existence of the often postulated *osseotympanic component* of BC. (The term was apparently first used by Bezold in 1885 [*6*]). Subsequently, this component was isolated quantitatively from older experimental data (*30*). In the cat, it turned out to be a sizeable component.

Finally, a few remarks are in order with respect to the clinical BC tests of Bing, Runge, Weber, and Gelle.

The results of the Bing (*7*) test in normal-hearing persons, i.e. lateralization into the occluded ear, is thus explained as a *combination of two factors*: a) *elimination of a high-pass filter effect* and b) *alteration of canal resonances*. Norm-

ally, both of these factors act upon the osseo-tympanic component of BC.

In the Runge (*26*) test, the ear canal is filled with water, which improves BC responses in the low-frequency range in normal-hearing subjects. This represents a *mass load of the tympanic membrane*. A detailed explanation of this phenomenon is given elsewhere (*31*).

With respect to the Weber (*35*) test, at least two different situations must be distinguished.

In *middle-ear effusions*, BC responses at frequencies below the resonant point of the middle ear (600 c/s in cats) were found to be slightly elevated (*34*). (This agrees with observations in human patients [*9*].) The phenomenon appears to be due to a combination of *mass loading of the tympanic membrane* and *increased friction* and must account for the lateralization into the involved ear.

In *stapedial fixation* and *ossicular discontinuity*, the mechanism is different. Considerable phase advances were found to occur, again at frequencies around and below the resonance point of the middle ear (*30*). These phase shifts, in spite of some amplitude losses taking place at the same time, appear to be responsible for the lateralization commonly observed in such cases. Sedee (*27*) has shown that, with regard to lateralization, phase advances in one ear may overcome relative amplitude deficiencies of up to 6 db. (Legouix and Tarab [*18*] and also Groen [*12*] had come to similar conclusions with respect to the Weber test.)

In the Gelle (*11*) test, air pressure is applied to the closed ear canal thereby diminishing BC responses in normal-hearing subjects. The air pressure displaces the drum membrane and thus, by decreasing its compliance, a) *attenuates the transmission of the osseotympanic component through the middle ear* and b) *reduces the middle-ear contribution to the total BC response.*

It is thus seen that in all these tests, in which BC sounds are lateralized into the involved ear (except in the Gelle test in which lateralization is toward the opposite ear), the explanations differ slightly but significantly from one another.

SUMMARY

A comprehensive study on bone conduction (BC), conducted mainly in experimental animals, yielded results some of which have direct bearings on clinical BC problems.

1. A combination of a large otosclerotic focus on the footplate with minimal fixation may produce appreciable BC losses which may simulate a concomitant sensorineural impairment.

2. Experiments in cochlear models have indicated that the compressional mode of BC stimulation can function even in the absence of any cochlear pressure outlets. Animal experiments showed that, although a compliant round window improves the response to compressional BC, occlusion of both cochlear windows does not have a very pronounced detrimental effect. The cochlear aqueduct was found to be an auxiliary pressure outlet of *scala tympani*, but only for BC stimulation.

3. Carhart's notch was shown to be due to the elimination of the middle ear. In particular, the magnitude of the loss is given by the relative contribution of the middle ear to the total BC response, and the place along the frequency scale by the resonant point of the ossicular chain in response to BC stimulation.

The alleviation of the notch observed after fenestration surgery is due to an improvement of the fluid inertial BC component of the inner ear.

4. The occlusion effect of the external ear canal (Bing test) is caused by a combination of a) elimination of the high-pass filter effect of the open ear canal and b) alteration of the resonant properties of the external ear canal. The first factor is responsible for the low-frequency emphasis, the latter for the sharply defined changes in the middle to high frequencies. Both affect the so-called osseotympanic component of BC.

Explanations are also given for the clinical tests of Runge, Weber, and Gelle. It is to be noted that, although the phenomena incurred are quite similar in all four cases (including the Bing test), the explanations differ slightly, but significantly, from one another.

The results of the entire study, which include many additional findings, will be published elsewhere in a series of five separate papers.

REFERENCES

1. Allen, G. W., and Fernandez, C.: The Mechanism of Bone Conduction. Ann. Oto. Rhino. Laryng. 69: 5–29, 1960.

2. Bárány, E.: A Contribution to the Physiology of Bone Conduction. Acta Oto-laryng. Suppl. 26, 1938.

3. Békésy, G. von: Zur Theorie des Hoerens bei der Schallaufnahme durch Knochenleitung. Ann. Physik. 13: 111–136, 1932.

4. Békésy, G. von: Ueber die Schallausbreitung bei Knochenleitung. Zeits. f. Hals-usw. Heilk 47: 430–442, 1941.

5. Békésy, G. von: Note on the Definition of the Term: Hearing by Bone Conduction. J. Acoust. Soc. Am. 26: 106, 1954.

6. Bezold: cit. after Politzer (*22*).

7. Bing, A.: Geschichtlicher Ueberblick ueber die Entwicklung der Hoerpruefmethoden seit 1850. Pp. 76–86 in Politzer (*22*).

8. Carhart, R.: Clinical Application of Bone Conduction. Arch. Otolaryng. 51: 798–807, 1950.

9. Carhart, R.: Effect of Stapes Fixation on Bone Conduction Response. International Symposium on

Otosclerosis, ed. H. F. Schuknecht, pp. 175–198, Little, Brown, Boston, 1962.

10. Franke, E. K., von Gierke, H. E., Grossman, F. M., and von Wittern, W. W.: Jaw Motions Relative to the Skull, and Their Influence on Hearing by Bone Conduction. J. Acoust. Soc. Am. 24: 142–146, 1952.

11. Gelle: cit. after Politzer (22).

12. Groen, J. J.: The Value of the Weber Test. Internatl. Symposium on Otosclerosis, ed. H. F. Schuknecht, pp. 165–174, Little, Brown, Boston, 1962.

13. House, W. F.: Oval Window and Round Window Surgery in Extensive Otosclerosis. Laryngoscope 69: 693–701, 1959.

13a. House, W. F., and Glorig, A.: Criteria for Otosclerotic Surgery and Further Experiences with Round-Window Surgery. Laryngoscope 70: 616–630, May 1960.

14. Heermann, J., Jr.: Zur Chirurgie des runden Fensters bei Otosclerose. Z. Laryng. Rhinol. 42: 669–708, 1963.

15. Herzog, H., and Krainz, W.: Das Knochenleitungsproblem. Theoretische Erwägungen. Zeits. f. Hals-usw. Heilk. 15: 300–306, 1926.

16. Hood, J. D.: Bone Conduction: A Review of the Present Position with Especial Reference to the Contribution of Dr. Georg von Bekesy. J. Acoust. Soc. Am. 34: 1325–1332, 1962.

17. Huizing, E. H.: Bone Conduction, the Influence of the Middle Ear. Acta Otolaryng. Suppl. 155, 1950.

18. Legouix, J. P., and Tarab, S.: Experimental Study of Bone Conduction in Ears with Mechanical Impairment of the Ossicles. J. Acoust. Soc. Am. 31: 1453–1457, 1959.

19. Mach, E.: Zur Theorie des Gehoerorgans. Akad. d. Wissensch., Wien, Sitxungsber. Math. Naturwi. Cl., II, Abth. 48: 283–300, 1863.

20. Onchi, Y.: The Blocked Bone Conduction Test for Differential Diagnosis. Ann. Oto. Rhino. Laryng. 63: 81–96, 1954.

21. Pfalz, R. K. J.: Centrifugal Inhibition of Afferent Secondary Neurons in the Cochlear Nucleus by Sound. J. Acoust. Soc. Am. 34: 1472–1477, 1962.

22. Politzer, A.: Geschichte der Ohrenheiklunde, vols. 1 and 2, F. Enke, Stuttgart, 1913.

23. Ranke, O. F.: Physiologie des Gehoers, in Ranke and Lullies: Gehoer, Stimme und Sprache. Springer, Berlin, 1953.

24. Rinne: cit. after Politzer (22).

25. Ruedi, L.: Histopathology of Sensorineural Degeneration and Other Inner Ear Changes in Otosclerosis. Internatl. Symposium on Otosclerosis, ed. H. F. Schuknecht, pp. 79–96. Little, Brown, Boston, 1962.

26. Runge, H. G.: Ueber die Lehre von der Knochenleitung und ueber einen neuen Versuch zu ihrem weiteren Ausbau. Zeits. f. Hals usw. Heilk. 5: 289–403, 1923.

27. Sedee: cit. after Groen (12).

28. Tonndorf, J., and Tabor, J. R.: Closure of the Cochlear Windows: Its Effect upon Air- and Bone-Conduction. Ann. Oto. Rhino. Laryng. 71: 5–29, 1962.

29. Tonndorf, J.: Compressional Bone Conduction in Cochlear Models. J. Acoust. Soc. Am. 34: 1127–1131, 1962.

30. Tonndorf, J., Campbell, R. A., Bernstein, L., and Reneau, J. P.: Quantitative Evaluation of Bone Conduction Components in Cats. (In preparation.)

31. Tonndorf, J., and Duvall, A. J., III: The Effect of Loading the Tympanic Membrane upon Bone Conduction in Experimental Animals. (In preparation.)

32. Tonndorf, J., Duvall, A. J., III, and Voots, R. J.: Comparative Studies on Bone Conduction in Cats, Dogs, Guinea Pigs, and Rats. (In preparation.)

33. Tonndorf, J., Greenfield, E. C., and Kaufman, R. S.: The Occlusion of the External Ear Canal and Its Effect upon Bone Conduction. (In preparation.)

34. Tonndorf, J., Greenfield, E. C., and Kaufman, R. S.: Quantitative Comparison Between Air- and Bone-Conduction Stimulation. (In preparation.)

35. Weber, E. H.: cit. after Politzer (22).

14

Factors Related to Bone–Conduction Reliability

DONALD D. DIRKS

DONALD D. DIRKS, Ph.D., is Associate Professor of Surgery, Head and Neck Division, Center for Health Sciences, University of California, Los Angeles

The clinical testing of bone conduction has long been essential and important in the measurement of cochlear reserve. However, as investigators (5, 8) have pointed out, the reliability of measuring bone conduction thresholds has been widely mistrusted. Several variables have been singled out in the literature (1, 10, 11, 13, 15) as having special influence on the reliability of bone-conduction measurements, such as the type of bone vibrator employed, the force exerted by the vibrator, the presence or absence of a masking stimulus in the nontest ear, and the location of the vibrator on the skull. If the assessment of bone-conduction thresholds is to enjoy full usefulness in the diagnosis of auditory disorders, the effects of the aforementioned variables on reliability must be defined and explained in more thorough terms. The present study was directed toward this end. Its primary purpose was to resolve some of the conflicts which now exist and to clarify the influence of the variables described on the bone-conduction measurement.[1]

GENERAL PROCEDURE

The present investigation was designed to

Reprinted by permission of the author from *Arch. Otolaryngol.*, **79,** pp. 551–558 (1964).

[1] This article is based on a PhD dissertation (1963) completed under the direction of Dr. Raymond Carhart at Northwestern University while the author was the recipient of a Predoctoral Fellowship from the National Institute of Mental Health, MF-13,341.

compare the reliability of bone-conduction measurements on a test-retest basis. A series of air-conduction thresholds and bone-conduction thresholds was obtained four times from each of 24 young adults with normal hearing. Normal hearers were useful in the present experiment since the basic problem studied was the effect of various experimental factors on the repeatability of bone measurements. All air and bone thresholds were measured with interrupted stimuli via the Békésy audiometer at the fixed frequencies of 250, 500, 1,000, 2,000, and 4,000 cps. The four sessions were divided into two test and retest sequences. In one of these pairs, the force of application of the vibrator on the skull was measured in the first meeting and replicated in the second. During the other pair of sessions only the usual precautions dictated by good clinical procedure were made to replicate the conditions of the first session during the second meeting.

Bone-conduction measurements were observed during the above test-retest sessions under all variations of the following experimental conditions: (1) with the vibrator positioned on the mastoid process or on the frontal bone; (2) with a hearing aid type vibrator or a grenade-shaped vibrator; (3) under conditions of no masking, of wide-band, or of narrow-band masking in the nontest ear. The thermal noises used in the present study were delivered to the nontest ear through an insert receiver. One wide-band noise and five narrow bands of noise, each of which surrounded one of the test frequencies, were employed in the above design. The various noise bands were administered at levels high enough to shift the bone conduction threshold on the nontest ear by 30 db at each test frequency.

EXPERIMENTAL APPARATUS

All subjects were seated in a double-walled industrial acoustics booth, Model 1202, at the Auditory Research Laboratory of Northwestern University. The Figure shows a block diagram of the experimental apparatus. All

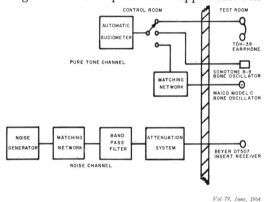

Vol 79, June, 1964

Block diagram of experimental apparatus.

pure tones were initiated by a General Radio oscillator, model 1304-B, which was part of a Grason-Stadler E800 Békésy automatic audiometer. To obtain air-conduction stimuli, the output of this audiometer was fed directly to an earphone, TDH-39-10Z, mounted on a rubber cushion, MX41/AR. The same automatic audiometer was employed as the source for bone-conduction stimuli. In this instance, the output of the audiometer terminated at one or the other of two bone vibrators, a hearing aid type receiver, Sonotone B-9, or a grenade type vibrator, Maico model C. The output signal was modified by a resistive matching network which was introduced between the source audiometer and the grenade-shaped bone vibrator.

The source of noise for the experiment was a thermal noise generator, Grason-Stadler E5539A. The output of this generator was led through a resistive matching network and into a custom-made band pass filter system. The noise signal, passed by the filter, was then fed to one channel of the speech audiometer, Grason-Stadler 162. This unit served here purely as an attenuation system. The output of the attenuation system was terminated by an insert receiver, Beyer DT507, which delivered the signal to the ear of the subject via one of five possible standard plastic earmolds.

Performance of Audiometer

Measurements of various kinds were conducted to determine the physical characteristics and stability of the automatic audiometer over the test period. Specifically, the magnitude and stability of its acoustic outputs, the linearity of its attenuation, and the travel rate of its pen and its table chart were observed.

Performance of Bone Vibrators

The output of each bone-conduction vibrator was determined by means of a Beltone artificial mastoid [2] and the necessary associated equipment. Measurements for stability, harmonic distortion, and linearity of the bone-conduction vibrators were performed during the experimental period.

The results of the measurements for harmonic distortion indicated that both vibrators were adequate for the present study. It should be noted that while the hearing aid vibrator was considered satisfactory for the experiment, the level of harmonic distortion at any test frequency was always smaller for the grenade-shaped bone vibrator. Likewise, the stability measurements also favored the larger grenade type vibrator.

Performance of Noise Channel

The performance of the noise channel was

[2] Appreciation is expressed to Dr. William Carver and Mr. Erwin Weiss of the Beltone Laboratories for their helpful suggestions concerning the artificial mastoid.

determined by describing the physical characteristics of the filter network and then by measuring the frequency response characteristics of the DT507 insert receiver. In addition, the acoustic output of the noise channel was measured before, during, and upon completion of the experiment.

On the basis of the measurements performed regarding band-width size and the output levels of the noise bands, the amount of threshold shift at a particular masking level was computed. It was then necessary to ascertain whether the shifts thus predicted actually occurred when bone-conduction stimuli were administered to a group of subjects with normal hearing. Five adults with complete unilateral sensorineural hearing loss, but with normal hearing in the other ear, were used as subjects. The shift in the bone-conduction thresholds from the mastoid process and frontal bone was observed on the good ear as the noise level was raised in 10 db steps.

The hypothesis that the bone threshold was shifted in a masking noise by an amount similar to the predicted air-conduction shift was found to be essentially upheld. From these results it was possible to tabulate the settings on the noise channel attenuator necessary to shift the threshold in the nontest ear by 30 db at each test frequency.

Measurement of Force

During the first experimental test and retest session, the force of application with which each bone vibrator was fixed to the skull was measured with a calibrated tension gauge immediately before testing. During the session designated as the retest run, the vibrator was readjusted until the force with which it had been affixed during the initial test session was replicated as closely as practical. During the final two test sessions, the force of application was not replicated, but it was measured.

A calibrated Pelonze tension testing gauge, model 57, was used to measure the force exerted by the vibrator on the subject's skull. By an adapter attached to the gauge, the vibrator was pulled away from the skull far enough to assure the passage of a 0.035 inch master gauge blade between the skull and vibrator. A detailed account of the calibration procedures and extensive physical measurements made throughout the study can be found elsewhere (7).

SUBJECTS

The 24 subjects employed in the present investigation were normal listeners whose ages ranged from 19 to 35 years. The mean age was 24.7 years. In order to be admitted to the experimental group, the subject was required to respond successfully to pure tone signals at each octave frequency from 250 cps to 4,000 cps at a hearing level of 10 db re USPHS norm. The better ear by air conduction was designated as the test ear if there were differences between ears.

RESULTS

Thresholds by Air Conduction

The mean and standard deviations by frequency for the air-conduction thresholds obtained by fixed frequency Békésy audiometry for both the test and nontest ears are reported in Table 14-1. The mean air-conduction thresholds obtained were superior at each frequency to the standard threshold

TABLE 14-1. MEANS AND STANDARD DEVIATIONS FOR AIR-CONDUCTION THRESHOLDS ON 24 EXPERIMENTAL SUBJECTS WITH NORMAL HEARING *

Frequency	Nontest Ear		Test Ear	
	Mean	SD	Mean	SD
250	23.4	3.4	22.3	2.9
500	11.0	4.7	10.2	4.0
1,000	7.5	5.1	7.0	3.8
2,000	7.6	6.1	6.7	6.1
4,000	10.6	7.0	10.9	7.9

* The computing center of Northwestern University was helpful in computing much of the data presented in this study.

All readings are reported in decibels re. 0.0002 dynes/sq cm.

as established by the US Public Health Survey (*2*). Actually, these thresholds were similar to the mean thresholds obtained in the 1955 Wisconsin State Survey (*9*) on a select group of young adults with normal hearing.

Bone-Conduction Test-Retest Variability

In order to evaluate the test-retest differences in the bone-conduction thresholds as a function of the experimental variables manipulated in the present study, an analysis of variance (*4*) was applied to the scores. Table 14-2 presents the results of this statistical

TABLE 14-2. SUMMARY OF ANALYSIS OF VARIANCE EVALUATING THE DIFFERENCES AMONG THE TEST-RETEST MEASUREMENTS AND THE EXPERIMENTAL CONDITIONS

Source	df	ms	F	P
Test-retest (TR)	1	47.31	0.83	ns
TR × force	4	15.15	0.96	ns
TR × position	1	105.43	0.37	ns
TR × masking	2	39.93	7.53	0.01
TR × vibrator	1	5.87	0.12	ns

procedure. The various experimental conditions are listed at the left of the table under "Source."

As evidenced in Table 14-2, the over-all main effect from test to retest did not reach a level of statistical significance. It appears that within the limits of the present experimental situation, initial bone-conduction thresholds were substantially repeatable during the retest sessions.

Interactions between test-retest and the conditions of force "controlled" and "uncontrolled," position of the vibrators on the skull, and type of vibrator were also found to be statistically nonsignificant. But, it was observed that the interaction between test-retest and the masking conditions did reach a level of statistical significance, in this case, the 0.01 level. Each of the above results is of particular interest since all have been suggested as possible sources of variation in the testing of bone conduction. Thus, the results

of the test-retest evaluation and the above variables should be discussed individually.

Some comment also seems to be necessary concerning the application of the above general findings on repeatability of bone measurements to groups of persons with hearing disorders. It does not appear unreasonable that repeatable bone thresholds similar to those observed in the present study could be obtained on cases with hearing loss if the techniques and precautions employed in this experiment were used and if the pathological process itself did not change from the test period to the time of the retest. In this regard, recall that Carhart and Hayes (*6*) and Jerger (*14*) concluded that the reliability of conventional bone-conduction audiometry was comparable to conventional air conduction audiometry. In the Carhart and Hayes investigation, conductive and sensorineural hearing losses were studied, and in the Jerger experiment persons with sensorineural loss were tested.

Relationship of Force to Test-Retest Bone-Conduction Variability

The rather important and somewhat surprising result was the lack of significance of test-retest bone-conduction thresholds between the conditions of controlled and uncontrolled force. The results of the analysis of variance procedure demonstrated that relatively the same repeatability of bone thresholds can be achieved when reasonable care is observed in replacing the vibrator for retests as when the vibrator force is meticulously replicated. This result is especially impressive since Konig (*15*), as well as Goodhill and Holcomb (*10*), have shown that changes in pressure can have definite effect on the measurement of bone thresholds.

The explanation for the aforementioned results is to be found in the data reported below. Recall that measurements of the force of application of each bone vibrator were made during every session of the present experiment, but it was only during the retest sessions of the force replicated series that any further adjustment of the vibrator was employed to achieve a duplication of an earlier state. Data were therefore available on the degree of consistency with which the force of application of the bone vibrator was reproduced during the retest, even though no special effort at replication of force had been made.

The results of these measurements on the forces which occurred during this study are summarized in Table 14-3. This table presents the means and standard deviations of the forces as measured during the pair of sessions wherein force of vibrator application was not replicated during the retest session. The *t*-ratio corresponding to each comparison between test and retest is also reported.

TABLE 14-3. MEANS AND STANDARD DEVIATIONS OF FORCE, IN GRAMS, EXERTED ON THE SKULL BY THE HEARING AID AND GRENADE-SHAPED VIBRATORS AT THE MASTOID PROCESS AND FRONTAL BONE DURING THE SESSIONS WITHOUT FORCE REPLICATED AND ALSO THE CORRESPONDING *t* RATIOS

Condition Vibrator/Placement	Means of Force Measurements		
	1st Session	2d Session	*t* Ratio
Hearing aid/mastoid	440.6	448.0	0.59
Hearing aid/frontal	576.7	597.4	1.43
Grenade/mastoid	689.8	650.4	1.81
Grenade/frontal	1,020.9	1,022.2	0.43

	Standard Deviations of Force Measurements		
	1st Session	2d Session	*t* Ratio
Hearing aid/mastoid	40.4	51.9	1.18
Hearing aid/frontal	66.1	78.6	1.40
Grenade/mastoid	118.6	125.9	0.71
Grenade/frontal	114.8	111.4	0.14

Four relationships stand out in Table 14-3. First, the two means and the two standard deviations for a given combination of vibrator and site of placement are numerically close to one another. Second, none of the *t*-ratios associated with them are high enough to achieve the 0.05 level of significance. Third, both the mean value of the force and its variability differ substantially from one combination of conditions to another. When using the grenade-shaped vibrator the force measurements were always larger than with the

hearing aid vibrator. The head band employed with the former vibrator allowed for a considerably tighter fit than did the band attached to the hearing aid receiver and accounts for a major portion of the increased force. Greater force was associated with frontal placement and with the use of the grenade vibrator than with placement on the mastoid process or use of the hearing aid type vibrator. Finally, means for forces of all conditions involved were greater than 400 gm.

It is the last fact which probably contributes significantly to the observation that performance was not more variable when force of application was not replicated. To explain, according to Harris (*12*), only small changes in bone-conduction thresholds occur after 400 gm of pressure is reached. Thus, the fairly large standard deviations of 50 or 60 gm which occurred from test to retest in the present study were probably tolerated without changing the bone thresholds appreciably because the forces involved were so high.

The practical implication of the foregoing observation is that the clinician may expect to achieve reasonable freedom from contamination of his bone-conduction audiometry by variations in force provided he uses a conventional bone vibrator and assures himself that it is applied to the patient's skull with substantial force. What the clinician must guard against is allowing the head band to become too loose or failing to fix the vibrator carefully and in a uniform position.

Effects of Vibrator Placement on Test-Retest Bone Variability

The interaction between test-retest and vibrator placement (mastoid process or frontal bone) as reported in Table 14-2 did not attain a level of statistical significance. This result is in agreement with the recent data on test to retest variability reported by Studebaker (*18*) on persons with normal hearing. In the same investigation, the author observed that intersubject variability favored the forehead as the site for the bone conduction vibrator. Earlier experiments by Pohlman and Kranz

(*17*), Békésy (*3*), Hart and Naunton (*13*), and Link and Zwislocki (*16*) also reported reductions in variability when measurements were made on the frontal bone rather than on the mastoid process.

In view of the number of earlier studies which are not in complete agreement with the picture observed in the present study when differences in means are compared by analysis of variance, it is advisable to report other measures of test-retest variability in the present instance. This is done in the form of the standard deviations of the difference scores between test and retest for the force uncontrolled conditions as a function of vibrator placement. The differences had been computed for the five test frequencies under each experimental condition. These difference scores were derived by subtracting each threshold obtained in the second session from its comparison threshold in the initial session. The results are reported in Table 14-4.

The standard deviations of the difference scores from the frontal bone measurements were found to be smaller in 27 out of 30 instances. Of the remaining three comparisons, the standard deviations were equal in two comparisons, and in one case the thresholds observed on the mastoid process were smaller. Purely on the bases of these data, the general conclusion which emerges is that the ability to reproduce bone thresholds from test to retest is less variable employing frontal placement than for comparable mastoid positioning. The observed superiority is not large in any particular instance, and, no doubt, individual exceptions may deviate substantially.

The very practical problem of which position to employ in clinical bone-conduction

TABLE 14-4. STANDARD DEVIATIONS OF THE DIFFERENCE, IN DECIBELS, BETWEEN TEST AND RETEST THRESHOLDS FOR BONE CONDUCTION WITH THE VIBRATORS POSITIONED ON THE MASTOID PROCESS AND FRONTAL BONE AND ALSO SIGNS INDICATING WHICH OF THE STANDARD DEVIATIONS IS GREATER

Condition	Frequency	Mastoid SD	Frontal SD	Sign
Hearing aid vibrator				
No masking	250	5.4	3.7	M > F
	500	5.6	3.8	M > F
	1,000	3.7	3.0	M > F
	2,000	2.8	3.0	M < F
	4,000	5.2	4.9	M > F
Wide band masking	250	4.6	2.6	M > F
	500	6.3	3.5	M > F
	1,000	5.1	3.9	M > F
	2,000	4.8	4.0	M > F
	4,000	5.5	4.7	M > F
Narrow band masking	250	4.7	3.9	M > F
	500	5.6	5.0	M > F
	1,000	4.9	4.2	M > F
	2,000	5.0	3.1	M > F
	4,000	5.3	4.5	M > F
Grenade shaped vibrator				
No masking	250	4.4	4.4	M = F
	500	4.5	4.3	M > F
	1,000	5.5	3.9	M > F
	2,000	5.9	3.1	M > F
	4,000	4.8	3.3	M > F
Wide band masking	250	7.9	4.9	M > F
	500	4.8	4.7	M > F
	1,000	4.9	3.3	M > F
	2,000	5.9	3.3	M > F
	4,000	6.0	5.1	M > F
Narrow band masking	250	7.0	4.8	M > F
	500	4.8	4.0	M > F
	1,000	4.8	3.1	M > F
	2,000	5.3	3.7	M > F
	4,000	5.3	5.3	M = F

testing has arisen. Advocates for the use of the forehead have based their argument on the increased reliability obtained from this site. In the present investigation, as in previous ones, certain variability measures have demonstrated consistently that frontal bone thresholds are somewhat less variable than those from the mastoid process. However, it is not always clear whether the superiority is large enough to be of clinical importance in routine tests. Further, there is also another problem which must be thoroughly considered. Reference here is made to the problem of loss in sensitivity when moving from the mastoid process to the frontal bone. Since approximately 10 to 15 db more energy is needed in the low frequencies to reach threshold when testing with the vibrator on the frontal bone, and, since the range in measuring bone thresholds is already restricted at 250 cps, even from the mastoid, there may be a loss in needed bone-conduction information from forehead tests when conductive and sensorineural components are present simultaneously in an ear. If the clinician is willing to accept the reduction in efficiency at the low frequencies and possibly minor losses of information in the low frequencies, then it would seem unreasonable not to measure bone conduction from the forehead and gain the vital extra dividend of added stability.

Effects of Masking on Test-Retest Variability

In Table 14-2, the F-ratio obtained from the interaction between test-retest and the three experimental masking conditions reached the 0.01 level of siginficance. Actually, this finding was probably the result of chance. It is a remarkable one when the means for each set of measurements were inspected. Under no experimental masking condition did the mean difference from test to retest exceed 2 db. The high F-ratio resulted rather from the direction of the difference of change between the test mean and the retest mean from one masking condition to another. However, these shifts were not consistent. In the narrow-band masking condition the retest

mean thresholds were larger than the test means, but in the other two masking conditions the means of test thresholds were smaller than the retest measurements. This result combined with a small variability obtained from the interaction between the test-retest masking conditions and subjects probably accounts for the statistically significant finding. Since 5 db steps are used ordinarily in measurements of bone conduction, the small mean differences from test to retest do not indicate that major changes will occur in the typical clinical test when masking is employed.

Effect of Type of Vibrator on Test-Retest Variability

In the performance of measurements on the artificial mastoid, somewhat smaller physical variations were observed with the grenade-shaped receiver than with the hearing aid vibrator. Results of the analysis of variance in Table 14-2 did not indicate statistically significant differences between the experimental test-retest scores when either vibrator was employed.

In relation to the present findings, it should be remembered that all the forces with which both vibrators were applied averaged more than 400 gm (Table 14-3). Therefore, the possible advantages of the grenade vibrator over the hearing aid vibrator at lower pressures as observed by Goodhill and Holcomb (10), may have been hidden in the present investigation by the greater force of application routinely employed.

SUMMARY

The present study was designed to compare the stability of bone-conduction measurements on a test-retest basis. The bone-conduction thresholds of 24 subjects were observed under various experimental conditions, including comparisons between (1) force of vibrator application, replicated and "uncontrolled"; (2) frontal and mastoid placements of the bone vibrator; (3) a hearing aid bone receiver and a grenade-shaped vibrator; and (4) conditions of no masking, wide-band, and narrow bands of masking in the nontest ear.

As a summary statement, the present study reaffirms that bone-conduction audiometry can have good inherent test-retest reliability. Moreover, it appears that more reliable information would be attained if bone-conduction tests were performed in clinical circumstances with the bone vibrator placed on the frontal bone and with either type of vibrator studied, as long as each exerts at least 400 gm of force on the skull.

REFERENCES

1. Bárány, E.: a Contribution to Physiology of Bone Conduction, Acta Otolaryng. (Stockholm), suppl. 26: 1–223, 1938.

2. Beasley, C. W.: Normal Hearing by Air and Bone Conduction, Hearing Study Series Bull., Washington, DC: US Public Health Service, 1935–1936, pp. 1–18.

3. Békésy, G. V.: Aur Theorie des Lorens bei der Schallaufnahme durch Knochenleitung, Ann. Physic., 13: 111–136, 1932.

4. Bennett, C. A., and Franklin, N. L.: Statistical Analysis in Chemistry and Chemical Industry, New York: John Wiley & Sons, Inc., 1954.

5. Carhart, R.: Clinical Application of Bone Conduction Audiometry, Arch. Otolaryng., 51: 798–808, 1950.

6. Carhart, R., and Hayes, C.: Clinical Reliability of Bone Conduction Audiometry, Laryngoscope, 59: 1084–1101, 1949.

7. Dirks, D. D.: Factors Related to Reliability of Bone Conduction, Doctoral dissertation, School of Speech, Northwestern University, 1963.

8. Feldman, A. S.: Problems in Measurement of Bone Conduction, J. Speech Hearing Dis., 26: 39–44, 1961.

9. Glorig, A., et al.: Determination of Normal Hearing Reference Zero, J. Acoust. Soc. Amer., 28: 1110–1113, 1956.

10. Goodhill, V., and Holcomb, A. L.: Cochlear Potentials in Evaluation of Bone Conduction, Ann. Otol., 64: 1213–1234, 1955.

11. Grossman, F., and Malloy, C.: Physical Characteristics of Some Bone Oscillators Used With Commercially Available Audiometers, Arch. Otolaryng., 40: 282–287, 1944.

12. Harris, J. D.; Haines, H. L.; and Myers, C. K.: A Helmet-Held Bone Conduction Vibrator, Laryngoscope, 63: 998–1007, 1953.

13. Hart, C. W., and Naunton, R. F.: Frontal Bone Conduction Tests in Clinical Audiometry, Laryngoscope, 71: 24–29, 1961.

14. Jerger, J. F.: Comparative Evaluation of Some Auditory Measures, J. Speech Hearing Res., 5: 3–17, 1962.

15. Konig, E.: Variations in Bone Conduction as Related to Force of Pressure Exerted on Vibrator, Trans. Beltone Inst. Hearing Res., 6: 1–12, 1957.

16. Link, R., and Zwislocki, J.: Audiometrische Knochenleitungsuntersuchungen, Arch. Ohr. Nas. Kehlkopfheilk., 160: 347–357, 1951.

17. Pohlman, A. G., and Kranz, F. W.: Monaural Tests on Bone Acuity Under Various Conditions, With Some General Comments on Bone Acuity, Ann. Otol., 35: 632–641, 1926.

18. Studebaker, G. A.: Placement of Vibrator in Bone Conduction Testing, J. Speech Hearing Res., 5: 321–331, 1962.

15

The Occlusion Effect in Bone-Conduction Hearing

DAVID P. GOLDSTEIN
CLAUDE S. HAYES

DAVID P. GOLDSTEIN, Ph.D., is Associate Professor of Audiology, Purdue University
CLAUDE S. HAYES, Ph.D., is Chairman, Department of Communicative Disorders, The University of Wisconsin

Wheatstone (1827) was the first to report an improvement in bone conduction hearing following occlusion of the ear. This phenomenon has come to be referred to as the occlusion effect and considerable clinical and experimental evidence has since been published in support of its existence.

Depending upon the type of occlusion, a threshold improvement of about 15 to 25 dB will be noted in the lower frequencies of 250 and 500 cps with a smaller shift occurring at 1 000 cps and little or no shift appearing above 1 000 cps (Pohlman and Kranz, 1925, 1926; Kelly and Reger, 1937; Watson and Gales, 1943; Sullivan, Gotlieb, and Hodges, 1947; Onchi, 1954; Rytzner, 1954). The occlusion effect can be demonstrated with the sound source located either on the mastoid or on the midline of the forehead (Pohlman and Kranz, 1925, 1926; Kelly and Reger, 1937; Keys and Milburn, 1961; Studebaker, 1962).

Bekesy (1960, p. 143) has attributed the occlusion effect to an increase in sound pressure level in the chamber formed in the ear canal by the occluding device. This sound pressure is supposed to arise from the walls of the meati which vibrate from the bone conduction signal and also, more importantly,

Reprinted by permission of the authors from *J. Speech Hearing Res.*, **8**, pp. 137–148 (1965).

from vibrations which are transmitted by the condyloid process of the mandible, adjacent to the exterior portion of the ear canal. The jaw, because of inertia, vibrates out of phase relative to the movements of the skull and therefore sets up the sound pressure in the ear canal. This sound dissipates into the larger volume of the surrounding air, when the ear is unoccluded but becomes an effective supplement to audition when the ear is occluded.

This investigation sought to test the hypothesis that there is, in fact, sound pressure generated in the external auditory meatus during presentation of a bone conduction signal and that following occlusion of the ear, there is an increase in this sound pressure. The hypothesis was tested for two locations of the bone conduction receiver on the head.

METHOD

The experiment was designed to obtain data on two variables; (a) the difference in decibels between a bone conduction threshold obtained with the ear unoccluded and the threshold obtained with the ear occluded (that is, the occlusion effect); and (b) the difference in decibels between a sound pressure level (SPL) measured in the medial third of the external auditory meatus when the ear is unoccluded and an SPL measured in the external auditory meatus when the ear is occluded. To test the role of position, data were obtained with the receiver located respectively on the forehead and on the mastoid.

Apparatus

Figure 15-1 shows a block diagram of the instrumentation used in this experiment. A pure-tone generator signal was fed to 2-dB step attenuators. A VTVM was connected across a Radioear B90 bone conduction receiver so that the experimenter could duplicate the bone conduction output level used for making SPL measurements with the ear open when making SPL measurements with the ear closed.

The pure tone pick-up system consisted of a probe tube which led to a B&K type 4132 condensor microphone. The microphone signal was amplified by a cathode follower and matched amplifier and was then led to a Hewlett Packard model 301A harmonic wave analyzer. All SPL measurements were made with this analyzer by tuning it to the particular frequency being measured. Bone conduction thresholds were determined according to the Carhart-Jerger ascending method (1959).

By adjustment of a microphone stand and laboratory clamp, the probe tube microphone could be positioned next to the lateral surface of the face on a line running through the intertragic notch and the corner of the mouth for insertion into the ear. The probe was a 5.25 inch length of polyethylene tubing with an inner diameter of .047 inches and an outer diameter of .067 inches. A small diameter probe tube was deliberately chosen so as to avoid any occlusion effect arising from the presence of the tube in the ear. A 45° bend was set into the probe tube so that after running through the intertragic notch, it curved into the auditory meatus. In this way, it was possible to occlude the ear using an

inoperative TDH-39 earphone with an MX41/AR cushion without disturbing the probe tube. Only the test ear was occluded.

Headrest

This experiment required that bone conduction threshold measurements be made from the mastoid and forehead position of the head and that movement of the bone conduction receiver from one position to the other be accomplished without disturbing an earphone placed over the test ear. A probe tube had to be placed in the external auditory meatus

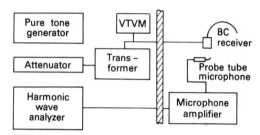

Figure 15-1. Block diagram of the pure-tone output and pick-up system.

to permit SPL measurements from bone conducted toens. A special headband was therefore constructed to: (a) hold a bone conduction receiver at either mastoid or the forehead and also to permit moving the bone conduction receiver from one position to the other without disturbing an earphone placed over the test ear; (b) prohibit head movement during the test period by tightening down on either temple with two end-padded screws; and (c) support the head on foam rubber pads in a comfortable position for the duration of a test.

Two bone conduction receiver holders were fabricated. One could be attached to the headband at either mastoid position while the other remained at the forehead position. One receiver could then be placed in either holder. Each holder was spring loaded and calibrated so that the receiver it held exerted a force of 800 gms against the head.

All measurements were performed in a sound-treated suite.

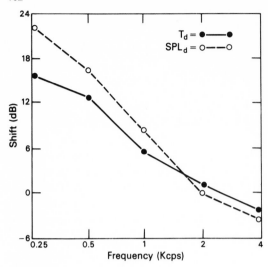

Figure 15-2. Mean shifts in threshold (T_d) and sound pressure level (SPL_d) with positions pooled.

position 1, frequency 1. This was followed by an SPL measurement at the same frequency with the input signal to the head, being just great enough to permit a reading on the harmonic wave analyzer when tuned to that frequency but no greater than the basic level needed for the reading. E recorded the input voltage level of the signal used when making the unoccluded SPL measurement. These two measures, threshold open and SPL open, were then repeated at the remaining four frequencies at that position. The ear was then covered by the occluding earphone and both measures were repeated at the five frequencies. Step 3 required moving the receiver to position 2, where both measures were repeated at the five frequencies with the ear occluded and finally the two measures were repeated for the last time in step 4 with the ear unoccluded.

Subjects and Procedures

Subjects consisted of 28 young adults. All were screened by pure-tone audiometry at a hearing level of 5 dB (ASA 1951) at the five test frequencies of 250, 500, 1 000, 2 000, and 4 000 cps. In addition the medical history in regard to auditory behavior had to be negative.

Following screening, the subject was instructed on the procedure for determining threshold. He was also told that at times he would be hearing tones but would be doing nothing, as indicated by E, and that at these times he was to remain especially still.

When it seemed clear that the instructions were understood, headrest and clamp were positioned over the subject's head. Next, the microphone was positioned at the side of the face, the probe was inserted into the ear and held in place by a strip of tape on the face.

Order of positions and of frequencies was randomly selected. Maintaining undisturbed occlusion while moving from one position to another permitted comparison of threshold shifts or SPL shifts across different positions. In the test sequence, unoccluded bone conduction threshold was first determined for

RESULTS

The mean shifts in threshold (T_d) and in sound pressure level (SPL_d), with positions pooled, are graphically plotted in Figure 15-2. Inspection of this figure revealed that both measures yielded the greatest shift at 250 cps with shifts decreasing steadily

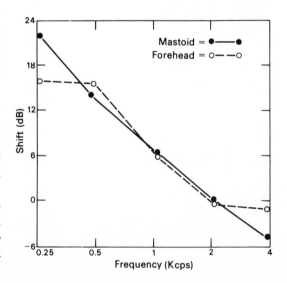

Figure 15-3. Mean shifts from mastoid and forehead position with measures pooled.

TABLE 15-1. SUMMARY OF MEANS AND STANDARD DEVIATIONS OF THE THRESHOLD SHIFTS (T$_d$) AND SOUND PRESSURE SHIFTS (SPL$_d$) AT THE MASTOID AND FOREHEAD POSITIONS FOR 28 NORMAL HEARING SUBJECTS

| Position | Frequency in cps | | | | | | | | | |
| | 250 | | 500 | | 1 000 | | 2 000 | | 4 000 | |
	T$_d$	SPL$_d$	T$_d$	SPL$_d$	T$_d$	SPL$_d$	T$_d$	SPL$_d$	T$_d$	SPL$_d$
Mastoid										
Mean	19.43	24.10	12.57	14.62	5.71	8.62	1.07	−.15	−4.14	−5.09
Standard Deviation	8.05	9.95	9.65	10.64	7.05	10.27	3.83	5.86	9.69	9.02
Forehead										
Mean	12.21	19.55	13.11	18.42	4.86	7.51	.43	−1.00	−.36	−1.58
Standard Deviation	6.51	9.89	6.58	7.08	3.52	6.82	2.99	6.10	4.04	5.67

in size as frequency increased up to 2 000 and 4 000 cps, where almost no shift occurred. Differences between measures can also be seen to follow the same frequency relationship. Figure 15-3 shows dB shift plotted on the ordinate and frequencies on the abscissa with pooled measures as the parameter. The same frequency relationship maintains, but a difference between positions can be seen at 250 cps.

Table 15-1 summarizes the means and standard deviations of the two measures at the forehead and mastoid positions. The reduced differences between the two measures at the higher frequencies can be attributed to the overall reduction of shift within either measure. Small negative shifts can be observed at the higher frequencies. This indicates that a threshold was poorer when an ear was covered and that the sound pressure was less under the same circumstances.

Table 15-2 summarizes the analysis of variance which considered the two measures, T$_d$ and SPL$_d$ at two positions and at five frequencies. Five significant results appeared. The significant main effect of frequencies reflects the difference between the large shifts at the low frequencies and the small shifts at the high frequencies. In view of the primary concern in this investigation with T$_d$ and SPL$_d$, the significant main effect of measures was examined by use of the Scheffe (1959) procedure for multiple comparisons. From this comparison, shown in Table 15-3, it is evident that the differences between the two

TABLE 15-2. SUMMARY OF THE ANALYSIS OF VARIANCE FOR THE EVALUATION OF MEASURES OF THRESHOLD SHIFT AND SOUND PRESSURE SHIFT

Source of Variation	df	Mean Square	F-ratio
Orders (O)	1	518.02	3.44
Subjects/O (S/O)	26	150.59	
Frequencies (F)	4	9556.94	11.53 *
F × O	4	144.81	1.75
F × S/O	104	82.85	
Measures (M)	1	566.42	13.53 *
M × O	1	24.28	< 1
M × S/O	26	41.87	
F × M	4	280.16	10.82 *
F × M × O	4	63.36	2.45
F × M × S/O	104	25.91	
Positions (P)	1	18.07	< 1
P × O	1	398.50	4.07
P × S/O	26	97.90	
F × P	4	374.73	6.15 *
F × P × O	4	139.77	2.29
F × P × S/O	104	60.97	
M × P	1	37.75	< 1
M × P × O	1	479.87	11.87 *
M × P × S/O	26	40.42	
F × M × P	4	21.96	< 1
F × M × P × O	4	6.00	< 1
F × M × P × S/O	104	26.54	

* P < .01 for given *df* or next lowest.

measures are statistically significant at the 1 percent level at 250, 500, and 1 000 cps but not at 2 000 and 4 000 cps. Figure 15-2 graphically describes the significant frequencies and measures effects. The third result, the frequencies-by-measures interaction, can be anticipated from examination of Figure 15-2 or Table 15-3. It can be seen from these that the differences between measures vary as a function of frequency. An examination of Figure 15-3 provides the explanation of the significant F ratio for the frequencies-by-positions interaction. This is seen in the change at different frequencies of the relationship between positions when the measures are pooled.

The measures-by-positions-by-orders interaction provided the fifth significant F ratio. This can be interpreted as meaning that the measures-by-positions interaction effect was not the same for the different orders. In view of the nonsignificant positions, positions-by-orders as well as measures-by-orders and measures-by-positions effects, this fifth result suggests that in interpreting these data, a cautious explanation of the role of position is warranted when one is comparing the occlusion effect to a sound pressure increase in the auditory canal.

It appears either that order had some confounding effect or that the higher order interactions involving order are attributable to chance which, under the null hypothesis, will occur some 1 percent of the time when multiple F ratios are calculated from samples taken from the same populations. The order effect was necessarily built into this experiment as a result of the desire to compare positions. To do this, the ear had to see the identical undisturbed occlusion for each position. The sequence of unoccluded, position 1; occluded, position 1; occluded, position 2 and unoccluded, position 2 was therefore followed, but for half of the subjects, the forehead was position 1 while for the other half of the subjects, the mastoid was position 1; hence the built in order effect, that is, forehead to mastoid versus mastoid to forehead.

Correlation

Table 15-4 summarizes correlation coefficients obtained between the two measures at each position. An examination of this table reveals that a low positive correlation exists between the occlusion effect and the sound pressure level alteration in the external auditory canal. The correlations tended to be a little higher when the bone conduction receiver was on the mastoid than when it was on the forehead. All coefficients at the mastoid

TABLE 15-3. SUMMARY OF THE S-METHOD OF MULTIPLE COMPARISONS WITH CONTRASTS ACROSS MEASURES

Measures	Frequencies in cps				
	250	500	1 000	2 000	4 000
T_d	15.82	12.84	5.29	.75	−2.25
SPL_d	21.82	16.52	8.07	−.57	−3.34
Differences across measures *		6.00 **	3.68 **	2.78 **	−1.32	−1.09

* The confidence limits at the 1 percent level were ±1.80.
** Significant at the 1 percent level of confidence.

position were significant when tested by a one tailed t-test procedure. The frequencies of 250, 500, and 1 000 cps, at the forehead, yielded significant correlation coefficients but the low values at 2 000 and 4 000 cps were not significant.

DISCUSSION

Huizing (1960) attempted to demonstrate experimentally that the occlusion effect is accompanied by an increase in sound pressure in the ear canal. He reported that the average sound pressure increase at the eardrum was greater than the accompanying occlusion effect, but he also stated that ". . . there seems to be no particular constant correlation between the increase in sound pressure measured and the accompanying threshold shift." He made all measurements with the bone conduction receiver on the mastoid. The differences between threshold shifts and the

TABLE 15-4. SUMMARY OF CORRELATION COEFFICIENTS OF THE THRESHOLD SHIFTS (T_d) AND SOUND PRESSURE SHIFTS (SPL_d) AND THE t SCORE OF THE CORRELATION COEFFICIENTS AT THE MASTOID AND FOREHEAD POSITIONS

Positions	Frequencies in cps				
	250	500	1 000	2 000	4 000
Mastoid					
Correlation coefficient	.42	.61	.50	.47	.66
† t score	2.40 **	3.97 *	2.94 *	2.68 *	4.51 *
Forehead					
Correlation coefficient	.36	.64	.41	.06	.18
† t score	1.94 **	4.24 *	2.29 **	0.29	0.90

† t = regression coefficient/standard error of the regression coefficient.
* $t_{.01}$ (df = 26) = 2.48.
** $t_{.05}$ (df = 26) = 1.71.

TABLE 15-5. A COMPARISON OF THE MEAN THRESHOLD SHIFTS (T_d) AND MEAN SOUND PRESSURE LEVEL SHIFTS (SPL_d) AND THE DIFFERENCES BETWEEN THESE TWO MEASURES OBTAINED IN THIS INVESTIGATION AND IN HUIZING'S STUDY

Investigation	Frequency in cps							
	250		500		1 000		2 000	
	T_d	SPL_d	T_d	SPL_d	T_d	SPL_d	T_d	SPL_d
Huizing	13.0	25.0	15.0	22.0	8.0	15.0	1.0	−10.0
Difference	12.00		7.00		7.00		11.00	
Goldstein	19.4	24.1	12.6	14.6	5.7	8.6	1.1	−.15
Difference	4.67		2.05		2.91		1.22	

sound pressure shifts had a similar trend to those obtained in this investigation, but were much larger. This can be seen in Table 15-5 which compares the differences obtained in the two studies.

It is not clear why the discrepancies between the Huizing study and the present study occurred. Two hypotheses present themselves: (a) Huizing placed his probe tube at a different depth in the ear canal than in the present study; and/or (b) the different methods of occlusion caused the discrepancies.

Huizing made sound pressure measurements "at the eardrum." In the present study the probe tube was always more than about 7 mm from the eardrum. If there were variations in pressure at different parts of this chamber, a greater or lesser SPL_d might be obtained, depending upon the location of the probe tube. Huizing made sound pressure measurements with the ear occluded, both at the eardrum and at $\frac{1}{4}$ wavelength (8.25 cm for 1 000 cps) back from the eardrum. He found distinct differences in sound pressure between the two positions with $\frac{1}{4}$ wavelength back position yielding a reduced pressure. This difference in pressure in the chamber formed by the occluding tube is quite reasonable, but does not help us since it took place a considerable distance outside of the ear canal. We are concerned with the possible differences in SPL within the chamber formed in the ear canal, the average length of which is 2.7 cm.

There appear to be no published references to variations in sound pressure in an occluded external auditory canal when the signal source is a bone conduction receiver. Weiner and Ross (1946) made sound pressure measure-

ments at different depths in the external auditory canal, but with unoccluded ears and with the signal emanating from a speaker in the field. They found little sound pressure variation in different parts of the canal at the low frequencies, in which we are interested. Variation did occur in the higher frequencies. This was attributed to resonance effects of the canal. In his report on calibration and use of probe tube microphones, Benson (1953) indicated that no variations in sound pressure greater than ±0.2 dB occurred in different parts of a 4.7 cc closed cavity that he used to calibrate microphones. Since the average volume of the ear canal is 1.04 cc, it is doubtful that the discrepancies between the excess SPL_d noted in the Huizing study over that noted in this study can be explained by differences in placement of the probe tube.

Huizing achieved occlusion with a soft-walled rubber tube in the ear which was closed off at different lengths. This produces a more secure closure than a MX-41/AR earphone cushion which was used in this study, since there is almost always some point around the phone cushion which does not come in perfect contact with the head. These points represent breaks in total occlusion. If faulty occlusion has the same effect upon sound pressure reading in the ear canal as upon the occlusion effect, then the hypothesis that differences in method of occlusion account for the differences between these studies would be rejected. If, however, these two measures are differently affected by changes in occlusion, the hypothesis might stand. Only a separate study relating the threshold change to the sound pressure change as a function of type of occlusion, would answer this question but in the discussion of impedance (see below) it will be seen that this may be a tenable hypothesis.

This discussion of the differences between the Huizing investigation and the present one is only about the mastoid position data since that is the only position employed by Huizing. The same comments undoubtedly hold true for the forehead data after one adjustment is made.

As can be seen in Table 15-1, the T_d, SPL_d differences were consistently greater for the forehead position than for the mastoid position. This probably stems from the fact that in the forehead position both ears were stimulated during the open condition more so than during the closed condition (since only one ear was occluded). This would result in a smaller T_d since, in effect, we were going from a binaural stimulation when the ear was open to a monaural stimulation when the ear was closed. Because it is not likely that this effect occurred as much, if at all, in the mastoid position, one can assume at least equivalent T_d, SPL_d discrepancies from the two positions and relate the discrepancies between positions to the aforementioned forehead situation. Dirks and Malmquist (1964) provided experimental evidence in a masking study which lends support to these assumptions.

Correlation

Regardless of any differences between the average magnitudes of the two measures, an estimate of their correlation is perhaps more meaningful. Contrary to Huizing's results, correlation coefficients derived from the present data suggest that these two measures are related. The coefficients were statistically significant at all positions and frequencies except 2 000 and 4 000 cps at the forehead. Furthermore, it is characteristic of a correlation coefficient to be attenuated by experimental error.[1] Thus, the obtained correlation

[1] For a complete discussion of this subject, the reader is referred to Walker, H. and Lev, J., *Statistical Inference*, Henry Holt and Company, New York, 1953, p. 300.

is likely to be somewhat less than the true correlation. Because of difficulties inherent in making some of the measurements involved in this investigation, it is likely that the correlations obtained in this study are somewhat attenuated over the true correlations. This would lend further support to the concept that the occlusion effect is related to increase in sound pressure in the external auditory canal.

Origin of SPL

Jaw vibrations relative to the skull are the most likely source of the SPL found in the external auditory canal. Franke, and others (1952), were able to measure the amplitude and phase of these vibrations relative to the skull (with a bone conduction receiver located on the vertex). They found that the lower jaw has a resonant frequency between 110 and 180 cps and vibrates relative to the skull less and less as the frequency of the driving signal is raised from resonance. This would account .for the frequency dependence of SPL_d.

Ayres and Morton (1951) suggest that the impedance which the eardrum sees probably plays a significant role in the occlusion effect. Covering the ear increases the impedance in the ear canal. This increase is greatest at low frequencies and least at high frequencies thus accounting for the frequency dependence of the occlusion effect.

If the sound pressure increase in the ear canal is the underlying cause of the occlusion effect, the degree to which the sensitivity of the ear is increased will likely be affected by the impedance of the ear canal. Since different occluding devices probably cause different changes of impedance, the particular mode of occlusion would, therefore, determine the relationship between T_d and SPL_d. For example, occlusion A may produce a greater relative SPL_d over T_d than does occlusion B, and this discrepancy may stem from differences in increase in impedance caused by the respective modes of occlusion. This may explain the discrepancies obtained between Huizing's data and the present.

SUMMARY

This experiment was designed to explore the relationship between a sound pressure generated in the external auditory canal from a bone conduction receiver and the improved bone conduction sensitivity which follows occlusion of the ear.

The method employed was to measure pure-tone, bone-conduction thresholds and the sound pressure in the external auditory canal with the ear open and with the ear occluded. These measures were obtained when the bone conduction receiver was located at the mastoid and when it was located at the forehead. The frequencies of 250, 500, 1 000, 2 000, and 4 000 cps were tested.

Analyses revealed differences between the threshold shifts and the sound pressure shifts which were significant at 250, 500, and 1 000 cps but not at 2 000 and 4 000 cps. Changes in sound pressure tended to be larger than concomitant changes in threshold. The results indicated that both measures yielded larger shifts in the low frequencies than in the high frequencies.

The two measures yielded positive correlation coefficients which were significant at all frequencies and positions except 2 000 and 4 000 cps at the forehead.

These data provided evidence that there is an increase in sound pressure level in the external auditory canal which accompanies occlusion of the ear during bone conduction testing but suggested that there was not a simple relationship between these two measures.[2]

[2] This investigation was supported by Public Health Service Fellowship No. MPM-18, 813 from the National Institute of Mental Health, and by a scholarship award from the American Speech and Hearing Foundation out of the Zenith Radio Corporation Fund.

REFERENCES

Ayres, E., and Morton, J., The subjective calibration of bone conduction receivers for hearing aids, *Acustica*, **1**, 109–113 (1951).

Bekesy, G., *Experiments in Hearing*. McGraw-Hill Book Co. N.Y. (1960).

Benson, R., The calibration and use of probe tube microphones. *J. acoust. Soc. Amer.*, **25**, 128–134 (1953).

Carhart, R., and Jerger, J., Preferred method of clinical determination of pure tone thresholds. *J. Speech Hearing Dis.*, **24**, 330–345 (1959).

Dirks, D., and Malmquist, C., Changes in bone-conduction thresholds produced by masking in the non-test ear. *J. Speech Hearing Res.*, **7**, 271–278 (1964).

Franke, E., Gierke, H., Grossman, F., and Wittern, W., The jaw motions relative to the skull and their influence on hearing by bone conduction. *J. acoust Soc. Amer.*, **24**, 142–146 (1952).

Huizing, E., Bone conduction, the influence of the middle ear. *Acta Otolaryng.*, Supplementum 155, 1–99 (1960).

Kelly, N., and Reger, S., Effect of binaural occlusion of the external auditory meati on the sensitivity of the normal ear for bone conducted sound. *J. Exp. Psychol.*, **21**, 211–217 (1937).

Keys, J., and Milburn, B., The sensorineural acuity level (SAL) technique. *Arch. Otolaryng.*, **73**, 710–716 (1961).

Onchi, Y., The blocked bone conduction test for differential diagnosis. *Ann. Oto. Rhino. Laryng.*, **63**, 81–96 (1954).

Pohlman, A., and Kranz, F., The problem of middle ear mechanics. Chapter III. Binaural acuity for air and bone transmitted sound under varying conditions in the external auditory canal. *Ann. Oto. Rhino. Laryng.*, **34**, 1224–1238 (1925).

Pohlman, A., and Kranz, F., The influence of partial and complete occlusion of the external auditory canal on air and bone transmitted sound. *Ann. Oto. Rhino. Laryng.*, **35**, 113–121 (1926).

Rytzner, C., Sound transmission in clinical otosclerosis. *Acta Otolaryng.*, Supplement 117, 1–137 (1954).

Scheffe, H., *The Analysis of Variance*, John Wiley & Sons, Inc., New York: p. 68 (1959).

Studebaker, G., On masking in bone conduction testing. *J. Speech Hearing Res.*, **5**, 215–227 (1962).

Sullivan, J., Gotlieb, C., and Hodges, W., Shift of bone conduction threshold on occlusion of the external ear canal. *Laryngoscope*, **57**, 690–703 (1947).

Watson, N., and Gales, R., Bone conduction threshold measurements: effects of occlusion, enclosures and masking devices. *J. acoust. Soc. Amer.*, **14**, 207–215 (1943).

Weiner, F., and Ross, D., The pressure distribution in the auditory canal in a progressive sound field. *J. acoust. Soc. Amer.*, **18**, 401–408 (1946).

Wheatstone, C., Experiments on audition. *Quart. J. Sci. Lit. Art*, **24**, 67–72 July–December (1827).

16

The Variability of Occluded
and Unoccluded Bone–Conduction Thresholds

DONALD D. DIRKS
JOHN G. SWINDEMAN

DONALD D. DIRKS, Ph.D., is Associate Professor of Surgery, Head and Neck Division, Center for Health Sciences, University of California, Los Angeles
JOHN G. SWINDEMAN is Director of Audiology, Casa Colina Hospital, Encino, California

It is well known that partial or complete closure of the external auditory meatus results in an increase in sensitivity for bone-conducted signals. Although the magnitude of the effect had been studied under various conditions of occlusion (Pohlman and Kranz, 1926; Kelly and Reger, 1937; Watson and Gales, 1943; Sullivan *et al.*, 1947; Naunton, 1957; Huizing, 1960), it was only recently that the stability and the intersubject variability of the effect was investigated by Elpern and Naunton (1963). These investigators, employing five occluding devices, obtained three estimates of the occlusion effect at each test frequency on normal hearing individuals. Two important conclusions emerged from their data. First, the occlusion effect was relatively unstable from test to retest; and second, the intersubject variability, as estimated by the standard error of estimate, was somewhat large. Since the standard deviations of the occlusion effect tended to vary inversely with frequency and the volume under the enclosure, the authors suggested that the occluding device itself was another source of variability—over and above that normally associated with bone conduction measurements. Thus, they reasoned that occluded thresholds might actually

Reprinted by permission of the authors from *J. Speech Hearing Res.*, **10**, pp. 232–249 (1967).

show a larger standard deviation than unoccluded thresholds.

More recent evidence, reported by Malmquist and Jerger (1966) indicated that the variability of occluded thresholds as exhibited by the intersubject standard deviations was smaller than the comparable variability of unoccluded thresholds. These investigators employed a TDH-39 earphone encased in a CZW-6 cushion as their occluding device, and covered the ears with Pederson earphones in the "unoccluded state." The latter condition was considered unoccluded, since the Pederson earphones cause no occlusion effect in the test frequency range from 500 to 4,000 Hz (Elpern and Naunton, 1963; Weston, 1965). The results of the Malmquist and Jerger (1966) data led to the conclusion that the variability associated with occluded thresholds is no larger and is possibly smaller than the variability observed during the unoccluded state. This conclusion somewhat contradicts the conclusions reached by Elpern and Naunton (1963). Thus, it was decided to investigate in further detail the test-retest and intersubject variability of the occlusion effect.

This investigation is a report of three experiments to determine the variability of the occlusion effect and of occluded and unoccluded thresholds on normal listeners, using both supra-aural and circumaural cushions as the occluding devices. Repeated measurements were made with a MX41/AR cushion employed as the occluder in the first investigation and a Grason-Stadler 001 cushion in the second. In the final experiment, an attempt was made to substantially reduce the error of measurement by replicating each threshold 12 times on a group of highly sophisticated subjects with normal hearing. The latter procedure allowed us to determine whether the variability of the occlusion effect was due mainly to differences between individuals or between trials and if the variability could be reduced by employing a more compactly fitting circumaural cushion rather than the customary supra-aural cushion.

EXPERIMENT I: METHOD

Subjects

Eleven young adults with normal hearing served as subjects for the experiment. Eight female and three male subjects were included in the group. For this investigation and in the remaining experiments, normal hearing was defined as 15 dB re ISO norms at 250, 500, 1,000, and 2,000 Hz. Each subject was screened at the 15 dB level prior to his inclusion in the investigation. The subjects were paid for their services.

Apparatus

Subjects were tested in a double-walled IAC booth, Model 1200A. The ambient noise level was 30 dB SPL in the frequency range from 60 to 120 Hz. In the range above these frequencies, the noise level dropped to 22 dB.

The pure-tone stimuli were generated from an audio oscillator (Hewlett Packard, Model 200AB) and then passed through an electronic switch (Grason-Stadler, Model 829D) and associated interval timer (Grason-Stadler, Model 471). The switch and timer were set to pass tones at the rate of 200 msec with a rise-decay time of 25 msec and a duty cycle of

50 percent. The signals were routed through a graphic attenuator of a Bekesy audiometer (Grason-Stadler, Type E800-4) at an attenuation rate of 2.5 dB per second. The signal was terminated in a TDH-39 earphone or in a Radioear B-70A bone-conduction vibrator. The TDH-39 earphones were encased in MX41/AR cushions.

Narrow bands of white noise, for conditions which required masking of the nontest ear, originated from a narrow-band masking unit (Beltone, Model NB 102). The noise was delivered to a second TDH-39 receiver mounted in an MX41/AR cushion. The masking noise was presented to the nontest ear at an effective level of 35 dB above the subject's air-conduction threshold at each test frequency.

The acoustic outputs of the pure-tone and noise channels were measured at intervals before, during, and after the experimental period. In the case of the pure-tone air conduction and noise stimuli, the signals were measured acoustically through a 6 cc coupler (Bruel and Kjaer, Type DB 0160) and associated Bruel and Kjaer microphone system. The output levels were read on the meter of an audio frequency spectrometer (Bruel and Kjaer, Type 2112).

The vibratory energy produced by the bone-conduction vibrator was measured on an artificial mastoid (Beltone, Model 5A). The output of the artificial mastoid was passed through an associated amplifier and the subsequent voltage was read on the audio frequency spectrometer (Bruel & Kjaer, Type 2112). The meter switch was set to read on the RMS scale. Appropriate corrections for the particular artificial mastoid, along with corrections for frontal bone measurements, were supplied by the manufacturer. These corrections were included in the computation of output levels in dB re 1 dyne RMS. The variations in output from both the air- and bone-conduction systems averaged less than 1.5 dB at any test frequency throughout the test period and, thus, were considered acceptable for the current investigations.

The bone-conduction vibrator was held in

place on the frontal bone by a metal holder attached to an adjustable rubber strap. The headband was adjusted on each subject to approximate a relative application force on the forehead of 750 grams, as measured with a calibrated tension testing force gauge (Pelonze, Model 57).

Procedure

Experimental subjects were tested under three basic conditions:

A. Air conduction
   1. Air-conduction thresholds on the test ear.
B. Bone conduction, Quiet
   1. Bone-conduction thresholds with both ears open.
   2. Bone-conduction thresholds with both ears occluded.
C. Bone conduction, Masked
   1. Bone-conduction thresholds with the test ear open and the nontest ear masked.
   2. Bone-conduction thresholds with the test ear occluded and the nontest ear masked.

Each subject was tested under all experimental conditions at 250, 500, 1,000, and 2,000 Hz. Three estimates of threshold were obtained at each condition for every test frequency. The frequency of the test tone was presented in random order, and the order of presentation for the conditions was counterbalanced for subjects and for test sessions. The right ear was used with five subjects and the left ear with the remaining six.

The testing period involved five one-hour sessions for each subject. At the start of each subject's first testing session, four one-minute practice tracings were obtained on each ear. Additional practice periods were included at the beginning of subsequent sessions. The subjects were instructed in a manner similar to that described in detail by Jerger (1960). Each subject traced an individual threshold for a one-minute period. The threshold was

determined by averaging the midpoints of the excursions at the 15-, 30-, and 45-second points during the tracing.

EXPERIMENT I: RESULTS

In the Elpern and Naunton (1963) study, the standard error of estimate and the correlation between trials of the occlusion effect were used primarily to determine the absolute and relative stability of the effect. For the present study, the results were analyzed not only in terms of the occlusion effect, but also from data of the occluded and unoccluded thresholds per se. The results of the average occluded and unoccluded thresholds from the Bekesy chart readings were converted into dB re 1 dyne RMS as determined on the Beltone artificial mastoid. All artificial mastoid outputs were read on the RMS volt meter of an audio spectrometer (Bruel & Kjaer, Type 2112).

TABLE 16-1. MEAN ABSOLUTE THRESHOLDS AND OCCLUSION EFFECTS IN DB AMONG THREE TRIALS FOR 11 SUBJECTS WITH MX41/AR CUSHIONS (EXPERIMENT I)

Condition	Hz			
	250	500	1 000	2 000
Air Conduction	24.0 *	7.2	1.2	4.5
Bone Conduction-Quiet				
Unoccluded	59.5 **	45.6	28.8	28.7
Occluded	35.8	26.3	21.3	29.3
Bone Conduction-Masked				
Unoccluded	63.2 **	49.6	34.0	34.4
Occluded	40.3	29.4	25.2	33.9
Occlusion Effect				
Quiet	23.7 ***	19.3	7.5	−0.6
Masked	22.9	20.2	8.8	0.5

* In dB re SPL.
** In dB re 1 dyne RMS (measured on Beltone, Model 5A, artificial mastoid).
*** In dB re occlusion effect (unoccluded thresholds—occluded thresholds).

Table 16-1 shows the average air-conduction and occluded and unoccluded bone-conduction thresholds for the 11 subjects, together with the average occlusion effect. The average results are based on three estimates of threshold for each subject in each condition. The occlusion effect was determined in the customary manner by subtracting the occluded bone-conduction threshold from the unoccluded bone-conduction threshold. The average occluded and unoccluded bone-conduction thresholds are reported graphically in Figure 16-1.

Table 16-1 and Figure 16-1 show that the occlusion effect decreased as a function of frequency. By 2,000 Hz, the occlusion effect was essentially negligible. Observe also that the bone-conduction thresholds obtained with noise in the contralateral ear mirror closely the threshold pattern found during the non-masking condition. The two curves are separated by approximately 5 dB, indicating that greater intensity was required to reach threshold when masking was present in the nontest ear than during comparable nonmasking conditions. Similar observations were reported and explained in a previous investigation by Dirks and Malmquist (1964). Finally, it should be noted that the mean occlusion effect was similar for both masking and nonmasking conditions.

were so small that these have not been reported in the current paper. The test-retest standard deviations were all between 1.5 to 2.0 dB.

Some general results can be readily observed from Table 16-2. First, and possibly most important in this study, is the relatively small difference in the standard deviations between the occluded and unoccluded thresholds at any frequency. The results are, of course, in general

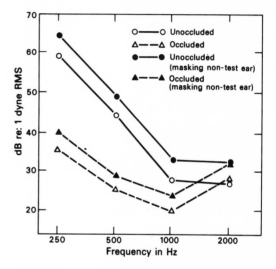

Figure 16-1. Mean absolute thresholds among three trials for 11 subjects with MX41/AR cushions (Experiment I).

TABLE 16-2. STANDARD DEVIATIONS IN DB FOR GROUPED THRESHOLDS AND OCCLUSION EFFECTS OBTAINED WITH MX41/AR CUSHIONS (EXPERIMENT I)

Condition	Hz			
	250	500	1,000	2,000
Air Conduction	3.6	3.5	3.9	5.9
Bone Conduction-Quiet				
Unoccluded	3.3	4.9	5.1	7.1
Occluded	3.5	5.4	5.4	6.6
Bone Conduction-Masked				
Unoccluded	3.0	6.5	6.4	7.9
Occluded	3.6	5.2	6.5	6.6
Occlusion Effect				
Quiet	4.1	3.7	4.0	2.7
Masked	4.4	5.1	4.5	2.9

Intersubject variability as estimated from the standard deviations of the group over three trials is reported in Table 16-2 for each experimental condition. Standard deviations for test-retest stability over the three trials

agreement with the findings of Malmquist and Jerger (1966), although no significant reduction in variability was observed during the occluded state of the present investigation. The results do not agree with those of Elpern and Naunton (1963), who suggested that the variability of occluded thresholds might be larger than those expected in the unoccluded state. Second, the standard deviations for the occlusion effect itself are similar to those observed for either occluded or unoccluded bone-conduction thresholds, and are only slightly larger than those found for air-conduction measurements. An exception should be observed at 2,000 Hz, where a relatively small standard deviation for the occlusion effect probably suggests the reduction in range in the occlusion effect itself at this frequency. In other words, the fact that there is practically no occlusion effect at 2,000 Hz no doubt accounts for the considerable reduction in variability at this particular frequency, even though the standard deviations for the occluded and unoccluded thresholds themselves are as large at 2,000 Hz as at any other test frequency.

than for bone-conduction thresholds themselves.

Pearson Product-Moment Correlations were also computed to determine the relative stability of air-conduction and occluded and unoccluded bone-conduction thresholds from trial to trial. These results are graphically displayed in Figures 16-2 and 16-3.

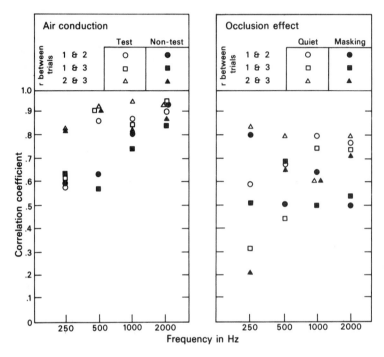

Figure 16-2. Correlations between trials for experimental conditions in Experiment I (air conduction and occlusion effect).

Analysis of variance was also applied to the data under all conditions and at each test frequency in order to determine whether the differences between individuals and/or between trials were the sources of variability. It would be much too lengthy to present the details of each analysis here, but the conclusions derived from the results patterned themselves in a clear-cut manner. As suggested from the data on standard deviations, the variability stems largely from variations between individuals rather than from test-retest variability, or from the trial factor. No greater test-retest variability was found for the occlusion effect

Observe that the test-retest air-conduction correlations are all high, ranging from 0.54 to 0.98. Correlations for bone-conduction thresholds (Figure 16-3) are generally high except for an occasional deviation. This result was found for the bone-conduction thresholds in both the occluded and unoccluded states. The test-retest correlations obtained for the occlusion effect itself are not quite as high as those for either air- or bone-conduction thresholds. The latter result indicates that there are slightly more changes in rank order from trial to trial for the occlusion effect than for air- or bone-conduction thresholds. However, the correlations from trial to trial in the present study are substantially higher than those reported by Elpern and Naunton (1963) and are in closer agreement with those obtained by Malmquist and Jerger (1966).

In summary, the correlation data indicate that air-conduction thresholds are highly reliable from test to retest. A similar result was observed for bone-conduction thresholds, whether occluded or unoccluded, although a few deviations from this pattern did occur. Considering the fact that all the subjects in these experiments are normal listeners, so that the range in thresholds is somewhat restricted, the correlations were surprisingly high.

bility was slightly smaller for occluded bone conduction thresholds than for unoccluded thresholds. In Experiment I of the present investigation, the standard deviations were essentially the same regardless of whether the test ear or ears were occluded or unoccluded. Malmquist and Jerger (1966) employed a TDH-39 earphone encased in a circumaural

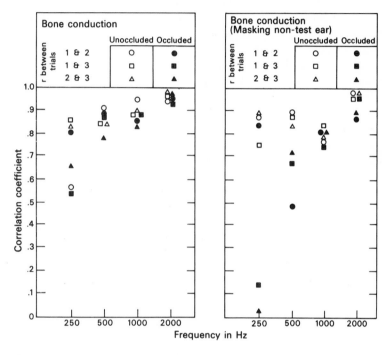

Figure 16-3. Correlations between trials for experimental conditions in Experiment I (bone conduction).

EXPERIMENT II

In the Malmquist and Jerger (1966) data, the investigators reported that intersubject varia-

cushion as the occluder, whereas in the first investigation of the present series, the occluding device was a supra-aural cushion. The results from both investigations suggested that the variability in the occluded condition might be reduced further if a cushion were employed which fitted more effectively over the entire external ear than was possible with the supra-aural cushion. Thus, a second experiment was designed, similar to the first, except that a Grason-Stadler 001 circumaural cushion replaced the MX41/AR cushion used in the first study.

METHOD

Procedure

The procedure for the second experiment was essentially the same as that employed in Experiment I. Eleven young adult subjects with normal hearing were tested under the same experimental conditions as used in Experiment I. The order of presentation of the conditions was counterbalanced for subjects and for test sessions. During the occluded conditions, both ears were covered with the Grason-Stadler 001 cushions. In the occluded masking conditions, the narrow bands of noise were presented at effective levels of 35 dB. Actually, the level of the noise could not be determined as precisely for this experiment as in Exepriment I, since there was no standard coupler available for the Grason-Stadler 001 cushions. The comparative dif-

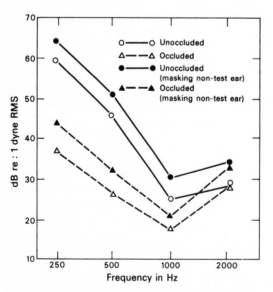

Figure 16-4. Mean absolute thresholds among three trials for 11 subjects with Grason-Stadler 001 cushions (Experiment II).

ference in subjective pure-tone threshold between the 001 and the MX41/AR cushions was determined for several normal-hearing subjects prior to the experimental sessions. The results indicated that it took more

intensity (approximately 1.5 dB at 250 Hz, 3.0 dB at 500 Hz, 6 dB at 1,000 Hz, and 3.0 dB at 2,000 Hz) to reach threshold with the Grason-Stadler 001 cushion than with the MX41/AR cushion. These results became our guideline in determining the noise levels necessary to obtain an effective level of 35 dB. Thus, when masking was to be introduced to the nontest ear, the tester merely added the above differences to the masker dial reading used with an MX41/AR cushion.

EXPERIMENT II: RESULTS

The results for Experiment II were analyzed in a manner similar to that in Experiment I. Table 16-3 shows the average thresholds for

TABLE 16-3. MEAN ABSOLUTE THRESHOLDS AND OCCLUSION EFFECTS IN DB AMONG THREE TRIALS FOR ELEVEN SUBJECTS WITH GRASON-STADLER 001 CUSHIONS (EXPERIMENT II)

Condition	Hz			
	250	500	1,000	2,000
Air Conduction	25.8 *	11.7	9.4	7.9
Bone Conduction-Quiet				
Unoccluded	59.8 **	46.2	24.8	28.6
Occluded	37.3	26.7	17.4	28.2
Bone Conduction-Masked				
Unoccluded	64.4 **	51.0	30.7	34.6
Occluded	44.6	32.5	21.1	32.8
Occlusion Effect				
Quiet	22.5 ***	19.5	7.4	0.4
Masked	19.8	18.5	9.6	1.8

* In dB re SPL.
** In dB re 1 dyne RMS (measured on Beltone, Model 5 artificial mastoid).
*** In dB re occlusion effect (unoccluded thresholds—occluded thresholds).

the various experimental conditions while Figure 16-4 contains a graphic description of the average results for bone-conduction thresholds. The bone-conduction thresholds are reported in dB re 1 dyne RMS as measured through the Beltone artificial mastoid, while the air-conduction thresholds are reported in dB re 0.0002 microbar as measured in a 6 cc coupler with the earphone encased in an MX41/AR cushion. Here the MX41/AR cushion was used only for calibration purposes, while the earphone was covered with the Grason-Stadler 001 cushion during the experimental sessions.

The mean occluded and unoccluded bone-conduction thresholds are similar to those obtained in the first study. As in the first

states. It should be noted that the test-retest standard deviations were again very small and hence are not reported separately.

Analysis of variance was applied to the data for each condition at every test frequency. As in the first experiment, the variability stems mainly from differences between indi-

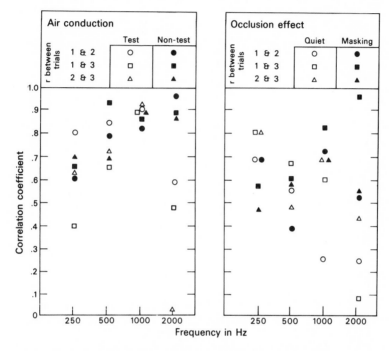

Figure 16-5. Correlations between trials for experimental conditions in Experiment II (air conduction and occlusion effect).

experiment, the bone-conduction thresholds obtained during the masking condition mirror those observed in the nonmasking condition, but again the curves are separated by approximately 5 dB. The occlusion effect is similar for both conditions.

The standard deviations for the group at each condition are reported in Table 16-4. Observe the small reduction in intersubject variability during the occluded state as compared to the standard deviations obtained with the test ear open. This result was obtained in both the nonmasking and masking conditions. The only exception was found at 250 Hz where the variability is substantially the same in both the occluded and unoccluded

TABLE 16-4. STANDARD DEVIATIONS IN DB FOR GROUPED THRESHOLDS AND OCCLUSION EFFECTS OBTAINED WITH GRASON-STADLER 001 CUSHIONS (EXPERIMENT II)

	Hz			
Condition	250	500	1,000	2,000
Air Conduction	3.8	2.9	4.8	2.8
Bone Conduction-Quiet				
Unoccluded	3.9	6.4	6.3	5.8
Occluded	4.2	4.7	5.7	5.4
Bone Conduction-Masked				
Unoccluded	3.4	6.8	7.3	8.1
Occluded	3.6	5.9	4.7	6.5
Occlusion Effect				
Quiet	6.0	4.2	3.1	1.9
Masked	5.2	4.8	4.8	4.4

viduals while the difference from test to
retest is statistically insignificant.

The results of correlations on test-retest data
are shown graphically in Figures 16-5 and 16-6
for all experimental conditions and for the
occlusion effect. The results lead to substantially the same conclusion as in Experiment I.

occluded thresholds, whereas in Experiment
II, in which a circumaural cushion was used,
standard deviations tended to be smaller for
the occluded condition. Since the variability
due to differences among persons was generally
large in both sets of data, it was decided to
reduce this source of variability as far as

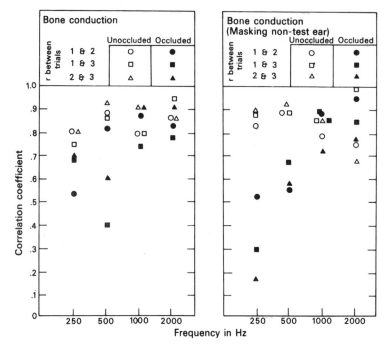

Figure 16-6. Correlations between trials for experimental conditions
in Experiment II (bone conduction).

The test-retest correlations were high for air-
conduction measurements and slightly reduced for bone-conduction thresholds, both
occluded and unoccluded. The test-retest
correlations for the occlusion effect were not
as high as for comparable air- and bone-
conduction measurements.

possible by using a more highly sophisticated
group of subjects than in the previous investigations. Further attempts to obtain the best
estimate of a subject's threshold were accomplished by testing each individual a total of
12 times at each test frequency.

EXPERIMENT III

The results of Experiments I and II suggested
that the variability of occluded bone-conduction thresholds might be related to the type of
occluder. In Experiment I, standard deviations were similar for both occluded and un-

METHOD

Procedure

Nine subjects with previous experience in the
Bekesy tracing task served as the experimental
group in Experiment III. They were tested 12
times at each of 5 conditions with individual

thresholds obtained at 500 and 1,000 Hz for each condition. These two frequencies were considered most desirable, since the occlusion effect is almost absent in the higher frequencies and since the lower frequencies present other problems, namely, harmonic distortion in the bone vibrator (Wilber and Goodhill, 1966) and difficulties in achieving appropriate masking levels which could interfere with the testing procedures.

The experimental conditions were as follows:

A. Air Conduction
   1. With an MX41/AR cushion
   2. With a Grason-Stadler 001 cushion
B. Bone Conduction (with masking in the nontest ear)
   1. Unoccluded
   2. Occluded with MX41/AR cushion
   3. Occluded with Grason-Stadler 001 cushion

Each of the above conditions was presented twice during a one-hour test session. Six one-hour test sessions per subject were necessary to trace 12 one-minute thresholds at both frequencies in each of the five conditions.

The conditions were presented in random order within each of the six sessions. The order of the frequency presentation was alternated from condition to condition and over trials. The noise levels necessary for an effective masking level of 35 dB, the instructions to the subjects, the practice for the subjects, and the method of scoring the tracings were comparable to procedures used in Experiments I and II.

Apparatus

The equipment used in this experiment was similar to that employed in the previous two, with one principal exception. A special apparatus was developed in order to couple the bone vibrator to the subject's forehead at a controlled and known force. The bone vibrator assembly is shown in Figure 16-7. It incorporates some of the features of a similar vibrator assembly described earlier by Jerger

and Jerger (1965). The apparatus permits application of the vibrator to the forehead or the mastoid process without the use of headbands or other elastic straps. The relative tension of a calibrated spring was employed to control the amount of vibrator application force at each subject's head. The device was calibrated so that forces of 250, 500, 600, 750, and 1,000 grams could be used. The subject's head was fixed in place with the aid of a specially modified headrest. A gauge was located on an arm, parallel and in synchrony with the spring, which monitored any movements of the subject's head or changes in the desired force. Thus, if the subject's head moved slightly during the testing period, it could be immediately observed by the tester. If any movement took place, the force was readjusted and the test readministered.

RESULTS

The results of Experiment III are shown in Tables 16-5 and 16-6. Table 16-5 contains the mean thresholds at 500 and 1,000 Hz for the various experimental conditions, while

TABLE 16-5. MEAN ABSOLUTE THRESHOLDS IN DB AMONG 12 TRIALS FOR NINE SOPHISTICATED SUBJECTS WITH NORMAL HEARING (EXPERIMENT III)

Condition	Hz	
	500	1000
Air Conduction		
MX41/AR cushion	9.0 *	2.4
Grason-Stadler cushion 001	11.7	7.4
Bone Conduction		
Unoccluded	48.3 **	34.7
MX41/AR cushion	35.9	32.0
Grason-Stadler cushion 001	36.0	29.1

* In dB re SPL.
** In dB re 1 dyne RMS (measured on Beltone, Model 5A artificial mastoid).

the standard deviations for the corresponding conditions are presented in Table 16-6.

Several results are noteworthy in Table 16-5. First, the air-conduction and unoccluded bone-conduction thresholds are in close agreement with those observed in the earlier studies. Second, the occluded bone-conduction thresholds are all slightly higher than those obtained during the first and second experiments. Thus, the occlusion effects are somewhat reduced from comparable results in the other studies. Whether the reduction in the magnitude of the occlusion effect is due to the sophistication of the subjects, together with the large number of threshold estimates obtained, is difficult to evaluate.

The standard deviations reported in Table 16-6 lead us to two major conclusions. First, the intersubject variability as estimated by the standard deviation is essentially the same for occluded and unoccluded bone-conduction

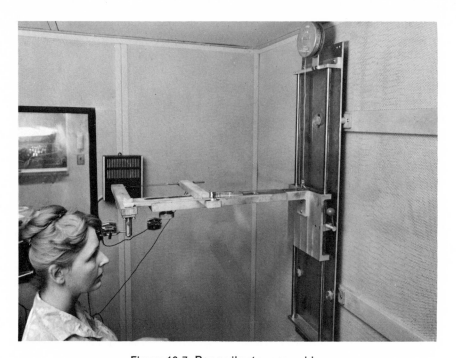

Figure 16-7. Bone vibrator assembly.

TABLE 16-6. STANDARD DEVIATIONS IN DB FOR GROUPED THRESHOLDS AND OCCLUSION EFFECTS OBTAINED FOR NINE SOPHISTICATED SUBJECTS WITH NORMAL HEARING (EXPERIMENT III)

Condition	Hz	
	500	1000
Air Conduction		
MX41/AR cushion	2.2	2.8
Grason-Stadler cushion 001	3.2	4.1
Bone Conduction		
Unoccluded	4.9	4.5
Occluded with MX41/AR cushion	4.8	5.6
Occluded with Grason-Stadler 001 cushion	4.7	4.9
Occlusion Effect		
MX41/AR cushion	5.8	2.3
Grason-Stadler 001 cushion	5.9	3.7

thresholds. Second, the variability of the occlusion effect itself is similar or smaller than the variability estimates observed for occluded and unoccluded bone-conduction thresholds. Since the standard deviations at 1,000 Hz decrease substantially from those observed at 500 Hz, it appears that the restricted range of the occlusion effect in the higher frequencies probably accounts for the decreased standard deviations of the occlusion effect as frequency rises.

The results from Experiment III essentially supported the conclusions reached in Experiments I and II. Thus, no further statistical analysis was performed on the data than is reported in Tables 16-5 and 16-6.

DISCUSSION

In the present experiments, data were obtained on the comparative variability between unoccluded and occluded bone-conduction thresholds. One conclusion emerged consistently from the results, namely, that the variability associated with occluded bone-conduction thresholds was no greater than the variability observed for unoccluded bone conduction measurements. In general, these results lend support to similar conclusions reached by Malmquist and Jerger (1966). However, in the present studies, it was not possible to substantiate their conclusion that occluded thresholds resulted in smaller intersubject variability than unoccluded thresholds, although there is a definite tendency toward this result in Experiment II. Thus, under controlled conditions, one should not anticipate greater variability from occluded than from unoccluded bone-conduction thresholds.

The source of the variability in all bone-conduction measurements, whether occluded or unoccluded, appears to stem primarily from differences between individuals rather than from variations from test to retest. This result might have been anticipated since numerous investigators (Carhart and Hayes, 1949; Dirks, 1964; Wilber and Goodhill, 1966) have suggested that the stability of bone-conduction measurements from trial to trial may be acceptable under controlled conditions. Fortunately, the intersubject variability for air conduction is substantially smaller than that for comparable occluded or unoccluded bone-conduction measurements and, therefore, does not constitute as great a problem for the clinician.

The variability of the occlusion effect itself was generally no larger than the associated variability for the occluded or unoccluded thresholds. As frequency increased, the standard deviations for the occlusion effect tended to decrease. Elpern and Naunton (1963) have reported a similar result. It seems reasonable to assume that the decrease in the variability of the occlusion effect at higher frequencies is related directly to the decreased range in the occlusion effect as frequency increases.[1]

[1] This investigation was supported by Public Health Service Research Grant No. NB 05883 from the National Institute of Neurological Diseases and Blindness and by the Hope for Hearing Research Foundation. The authors are indebted to the Health Sciences Computing Facility, UCLA, for statistical assistance.

REFERENCES

Carhart, R., and Hayes, C., The clinical reliability of bone conduction audiometry. *Laryngoscope*, **59,** 1084–1101 (1949).

Dirks, D., Factors related to bone conduction reliability. *Arch. Otolaryng.*, **79,** 551–558 (1964).

Dirks, D., and Malmquist, C., Changes in bone-conduction thresholds produced by masking in the non-test ear. *J. Speech Hearing Res.*, **7,** 271–278 (1964).

Elpern, B. S., and Naunton, R. F., The stability of the occlusion effect. *Arch. Otolaryng.*, **77,** 376–384 (1963).

Huizing, E. H., Bone conduction—the influence of the middle ear. *Arch. Otolaryng.*, Suppl. 155 (1960).

Jerger, J., Bekesy audiometry in analysis of auditory disorders. *J. Speech Hearing Res.*, **3,** 275–287 (1960).

Jerger, J., and Jerger, S., Critical evaluation of SAL audiometry. *J. Speech Hearing Res.*, **8,** 103–128 (1965).

Kelley, N. H., and Reger, S. N., The effect of binaural occlusion of the external auditory meati on the sensitivity of the normal ear for bone conducted sound. *J. Exp. Psychol.*, **21,** 211–217 (1937).

Malmquist, C. W., and Jerger, J. F., Some aspects of the normal occlusion effect. Paper presented at the Annual Convention of the American Speech and Hearing Association, Washington, D.C. (1966).

Naunton, R. F., Clinical bone-conduction audiometry: The use of a frontally applied bone-conduction receiver and the importance of the occlusion effect in clinical bone-conduction audiometry. *Arch. Otolaryng.*, **66,** 281–298 (1957).

Pohlman, A. G., and Kranz, F. W., The influence of partial and complete occlusion of the external auditory canals on air and bone transmitted sound. *Ann. Oto. Rhino. Laryng.*, **35,** 113–121 (1926).

Sullivan, J. A., Gotleib, C. C., and Hodges, W. E., Shift of bone conduction thresholds on occlusion of the external ear canal. *Laryngoscope*, **57,** 690–703 (1947).

Watson, N. A., and Gales, R. S., Bone conduction threshold measurements: effects of occlusion, enclosures, and masking devices. *J. Acoust. Soc. Amer.*, **14,** 207–215 (1943).

Wilber, L. A., and Goodhill, V., Real ear versus artificial mastoid methods of calibration. *J. Speech Hearing Res.* (in press).

Weston, P., Bone conduction and noise masking. *Acta Otolaryng.*, Suppl. 204 (1965).

17

Intertest Variability and the Air–Bone Gap

GERALD A. STUDEBAKER

GERALD A. STUDEBAKER, Ph.D., is Associate Professor, University of Oklahoma Medical Center

Among those concerned with the measurement of hearing loss there is a widespread belief that bone-conduction thresholds cannot be worse than air-conduction thresholds. Although an unqualified statement to this effect is rarely seen in the literature it is often heard in beginning audiology classes and is very often heard in lectures on audiogram interpretation given by "experts" to various medical and paramedical groups.

The reasoning usually is as follows: the air-conduction threshold is a measure of the sensitivity of the entire auditory system while the bone-conduction threshold is a measure of the sensitivity of only that part of the system excluding the outer and middle ear. Since a loss of sensitivity in part of a system cannot exceed the loss in the whole system, bone-conduction thresholds cannot be worse than air-conduction thresholds.

This argument is accurate as far as it goes, but it does not go far enough. Concluding the discussion at this point fails to take into consideration the very real subject of measurement variability and implies an exactitude of measurement which cannot be achieved in practice. This failure to discuss the effect of measurement variability on the air-bone relationship may be an effort to simplify the presentation or it may represent a lack of basic understanding on the part of the lecturer. In either case, it does create an idea about the air-conduction, bone-conduction

Reprinted by permission of the author from *J. Speech Hearing Dis.*, **32**, pp. 82–86 (1967).

threshold relationship which is misleading and which can result in several unfortunate consequences.

For example, the failure of test results in actual practice always to conform to "the way it is supposed to turn out" may make the inexperienced and insecure clinician anxious about his test findings. The tendency is to tamper with the test results or, at least, to be biased as to what is accepted as threshold. Even experienced clinicians modify bone-conduction calibration values if bone-conduction thresholds are as much as 10 dB worse than air-conduction thresholds in more than a very rare instance. Those who view these "modified" audiograms become even more convinced that "bone cannot be worse than air" and the circle is thus completed. Finally, those who hold this belief may reach the conclusion, when viewing audiograms based on accurate calibration, that the results are invalid or that the audiologist is incompetent.

The following discussion attempts to demonstrate that not only can bone-conduction thresholds be worse than air-conduction thresholds, but that, in a group of persons with normal middle ears, the bone-conduction thresholds should exceed air-conduction thresholds in a predictable percentage of cases as a result of the variability associated with procedures for finding the threshold.

The variability of pure tone air- and bone-conduction thresholds is a result of the influence of a number of factors. Some of these factors, such as sensory-neural sensitivity, subject fatigue, attention, and experience, affect both air- and bone-conduction thresholds in a similar way. Other factors such as the normal variability in the efficiency of the middle ear, length and shape of the external meatus, thickness of skin and subcutaneous tissue, and pressure of the vibrator on the head may affect the threshold obtained by either air or bone conduction without influencing the threshold by the other. These latter factors together with the changes which occur in the patient, equipment, or examiner between one test and another, affect air- and bone-conduction thresholds differentially even in the absence of middle ear malfunction. Either a positive or a negative air-bone relationship may result because of the way in which the bone conduction system is calibrated which is in turn dictated by the fact that both air- and bone-conduction hearing loss is expressed relative to a normal reference.

The most commonly used method of calibrating the bone-conduction apparatus is that proposed by Roach and Carhart (1956). In this procedure air- and bone-conduction thresholds are obtained on a number of subjects with normal middle ears. Calibration is achieved by calculating the means of the air- and bone-conduction threshold distributions at each frequency and correcting the bone-conduction thresholds by the amount of the difference between the means. This can be done by applying mathematical corrections to the obtained bone-conduction thresholds or by modifying the output of the audiometer. The use of an "artificial mastoid" for calibration of the bone-conduction system does not change this basic procedure. In either case the means of two distributions are made equal, that is, the mean difference is made to equal 0. With "artificial ears" and "artificial mastoids" the data were simply collected at a more remote place and/or time.

When both air- and bone-conduction thresholds are obtained on the same individuals, the difference between air- and bone-conduction thresholds for each subject may be plotted as a single distribution at each frequency. When each individual difference value is corrected by the amount of the difference between the means of the two distributions, as above, the mean of the distribution of differences is 0. Approximately one-half of the differences then are positive and one-half negative. The distribution of differences approximates the normal curve. This is true whether the group has completely normal hearing or consists of those with purely sensory-neural hearing losses. The distribution, in practice, may be slightly skewed in the direction of "bone better than air" because of the inadvertent inclusion of some people with slight conductive losses which resulted from a disease process too insignificant or too long ago to be remembered by the subject or detected on physical examination. The degree of skewness depends on the stringency of the selection standards set up for the group.

Assuming that the sample is truly representative of patients with no middle ear disease, the air-bone relationship obtained on patients should be distributed in approximately the same way as in the sample. In other words, approximately one-half of the air-bone relationships obtained on patients without middle ear disease should have bone-conduction thresholds worse than air-conduction thresholds. To the extent that the sample is representative of the population, the measures of dispersion calculated for the sample should also predict the dispersion in the population.

Table 17-1 shows the frequency with which various relationships between air- and bone-conduction thresholds can be expected, assuming a normal distribution of differences between air- and bone-conduction thresholds. The percentages are given for a standard deviation of the distribution of differences of 5 dB. This value seems a good estimate on the basis of unpublished data obtained on several separate samples collected at this Center. Interestingly, this is about the same as the variability associated with speech reception threshold-pure tone average comparisons as reported by Graham (1960).

TABLE 17-1. EXPECTED DISTRIBUTION OF THE AIR-CONDUCTION, BONE-CONDUCTION THRESHOLD RELATIONSHIP IN SUBJECTS WITH NORMAL MIDDLE EAR FUNCTION ASSUMING A STANDARD DEVIATION OF THE DISTRIBUTION OF DIFFERENCES OF 5 DB

Measured AC-BC Relationship	Actual AC-BC Relationship	Percentage in Interval
−20 or more	−20 or greater	0.02
−15	−17.5 to −12.5	0.60
−10	−12.5 to −7.5	6.06
−5	−7.5 to −2.5	24.17
0	−2.5 to +2.5	38.29
+5	+2.5 to +7.5	24.17
+10	+7.5 to +12.5	6.06
+15	+12.5 to +17.5	0.60
+20 or more	+20 or greater	0.02

Table 17-1 was developed by listing in the first column the measured air-conduction threshold, bone-conduction threshold differences which can be reasonably expected when testing a group of people without middle ear malfunction. The assumptions are that 5 dB steps are used and that the equipment has been calibrated to make the mean bone-conduction threshold equal to the mean air-conduction threshold. The second column shows the range of actual air-conduction and bone-conduction threshold relationships for each of the nominal relationships shown in the first column.

The intervals in the second column are set up as −2.5 to +2.5 dB and +2.5 to +7.5 dB, and so forth, on the assumption that the actual average threshold of a group of persons assigned a given nominal threshold is approximately 2.5 dB below the nominal value. Therefore, the bone-conduction threshold, in order to have the same nominal value as obtained by air-conduction (i.e., 0 dB "air-bone gap"), must fall within ±2.5 dB of the actual average air-conduction threshold.

The percentages in the ±2.5 dB interval were obtained by noting that ±2.5 dB is equal to ±0.5 standard deviations assuming a standard deviation of 5 dB. The area under a normal curve between ±0.5 standard deviation is equal to 38.29 percent of the total area under the curve. In other words, about 38 percent of all air-bone comparisons obtained on a group of persons with normal mid-

dle ears will have a nominal "air-bone gap" of 0 dB. Using the same reasoning, it is noted that about 24 percent of all comparisons would show bone-conduction thresholds 5 dB worse than air-conduction thresholds ($z = 0.5$ to 1.5) and another 24 percent with bone-conduction thresholds better than air-conduction thresholds by 5 dB etc. A total of about 87 percent of the measures would be expected to fall within the nominal limits of ±5 dB. However, fully 13 percent of all comparisons fall outside the ±5 dB limits. Of particular interest is the number of instances in which bone-conduction thresholds are worse than air-conduction thresholds by 10 dB or more. Between 6 and 7 percent fall in this category.

In actual clinical testing, the percentage of instances in which bone-conduction thresholds are worse than air-conduction thresholds will be somewhat smaller since the total patient load of any clinic includes large numbers of patients with conductive hearing losses. Nevertheless, the appearance of bone-conduction thresholds worse than air-conduction thresholds by 10 to 15 dB at any given frequency should be expected with some regularity. Their appearance should be considered cause for a change in the bone-conduction calibration only when the number of instances in which bone-conduction thresholds are worse than air-conduction thresholds by any given amount exceeds the expected percentage of measurements for that relationship.

The purpose of this presentation has been to show that bone-conduction thresholds can be worse than air-conduction thresholds on the basis of intertest variability. This, however, should not be construed to mean that bone-conduction thresholds worse than air-conduction thresholds by 15 or 20 dB can be simply ignored. It is possible that bone-conduction thresholds can be worse than air-conduction thresholds by 20 dB on the basis of normal variability. However, a statement to the effect that this difference is due to expected intertest variability will be correct only once out of every 5,000 times the statement is made. An observation of this type in any individual instance should be viewed with great skepticism and cannot be accepted until all controllable sources of error have been eliminated.

One other aspect of this discussion concerns the situation when the bone-conduction threshold is better than the air-conduction threshold by 5 to 15 dB. Although probability favors that a difference of this size represents a pathologic loss of middle ear efficiency, it must not be forgotten that on a number of occasions such a difference may represent only intertest variability.

ACKNOWLEDGMENT

This discussion is, in part, based on research supported by Vocational Rehabilitation Administration Project No. RD-1717-S.

REFERENCES

Graham, J. T., Evaluation of methods for predicting speech reception threshold. *Arch. Otolaryng.*, **72,** 347–350 (1960).

Roach, R. E., and Carhart, R., A clinical method for calibrating the bone-conduction audiometer. *Arch. Otolaryng.*, **63,** 270–278 (1956).

18

Clinical Applicability of the SAL Test [1]

TOM W. TILLMAN

TOM W. TILLMAN, Ph.D., is Professor of Audiology and Associate Director, Auditory Research Laboratories, Northwestern University

Through the years, dissatisfaction with the technique of conventional bone conduction audiometry has resulted in efforts to develop alternate methods for obtaining the information which bone conduction audiometry can yield. As early as 1953, Jerger suggested the use of the DL Difference Test as a means ". . . to predict bone conduction acuity without recourse to bone conduction audiometry in those cases in which the perceptive loss is due to cochlear lesion" (6: p 499). For a number of reasons, this method was never used extensively. In 1955, Rainville (13) described a new procedure for assessing cochlear function indirectly. In this technique, evaluation of the differential effect of air conduction and bone conduction masking of pure tones delivered by air conduction was used as a means of arriving at an estimate of bone conduction hearing level.

Rainville's method proved to be a somewhat cumbersome clinical tool, and in 1959, a variation of his test was suggested by Jerger and Tillman (7). This latter procedure was designated the Sensori-Neural Acuity Level (SAL) Test. In this test, the amount by which a bone-conducted thermal noise shifts the air conduction threshold of a subject with impaired hearing at a given frequency is compared to the shift produced at that frequency in normal ears by the same noise. Presumably, the subject who exhibits a shift of normal magnitude possesses a normal sensorineural mechnaism, while one whose threshold is shifted less than the normal amount has a sensorineural deficit equal to the difference between the mangitudes of his shift and that of the normal hearing subject.

Jerger and Tillman initially compared the results of the SAL test with those obtained by conventional bone conduction audiometry in a group of subjects with pure sensorineural type hearing losses. The close agreement between the two sets of data which they obtained led them to conclude that the new method was a valid tool for the assessment of sensorineural hearing acuity. The test therefore appeared to be an ideal substitute for conventional bone conduction audiometry because it, SAL, avoided the more serious limitations inherent in the latter method.

In spite of the apparent advantages of the new test, it was met with almost immediate criticism. Those who showed a reluctance to accept the SAL test appeared to be concerned chiefly with the effect which covering the ears of the subject with air conduction earphones might have on the magnitudes of the threshold shifts produced by the bone-conducted thermal noise signal. It was con-

Reprinted by permission of the author from *Arch. Otolaryngol.*, **78,** pp. 20–32 (1963).

[1] This research was supported by Contract AF 41 (657)-418 with the School of Aerospace Medicine, United States Air Force, Brooks Air Force Base, Texas.

tended that the methodology required by SAL would build into the norm an occlusion index [2] which would result in a spurious estimate of the sensorineural acuity level in cases of conductive hearing loss (2, 9, 12).

To be more specific, these workers felt that occluding the ears of the normal hearing criterion group with air conduction earphones would increase the bone conduction sensitivity of the group for the low frequency components in the noise. This occlusion index would then result in larger threshold shifts for the normal hearing criterion group in the low frequency range than would have occurred otherwise. It is well known that the individual with a conductive hearing loss does not yield a bone conduction occlusion index. Therefore, such an individual, even if his cochlear reserve were normal, might be expected to experience less than the "normal" threshold shift in the low frequency range and therefore spuriously high (poor) SAL levels in this range. Goldstein, Hayes, and Peterson (4) using the Rainville method have confirmed these expectations empirically. That is, in the low frequency region, the Rainville method yielded thresholds which were higher (poorer) than conventional bone conduction thresholds in the two conductive hearing loss groups which these investigators studied.

In addition to this observation, it can be reported that the SAL test has been routinely employed in the Hearing Clinics of Northwestern University for the past three years and the results which it has yielded have not always coincided with those of conventional bone conduction audiometry. The discrepancy between the results of the two methodologies has been particularly evident in patients with conductive impairments due to otosclerosis, and it has been in the direction reported by Goldstein, Hayes, and Peterson (4).

As a result of these observations, a critical evaluation of the SAL test was undertaken.

The experiment was designed with three purposes in mind. These were as follows:

A. To specify the magnitude of the discrepancy between the results of SAL and those of conventional bone conduction audiometry in subjects with conductive type hearing loss.

B. To explore methods of reducing the discrepancy between SAL and conventional bone conduction results in subjects with conductive impairments.

C. To reevaluate the validity of the SAL test in subjects with pure sensorineural type hearing loss.

SUBJECTS

To fulfill the aims of this experiment, four groups of ten subjects each were utilized. One of these groups contained subjects with normal hearing bilaterally. It served essentially as a "criterion population" against which to compare the performance of the other three groups.

The second group studied in this experiment contained subjects with bilaterally symmetrical conductive type hearing losses due to clinical otosclerosis. None of these individuals had undergone middle ear surgery of any type at the time of the experiment. This group was included in order to fulfill the first two aims of the experiment: namely, to determine the size of the discrepancy between the results of SAL and those of conventional bone conduction audiometry in subjects of this type and to investigate ways of reducing this discrepancy. Persons with otosclerosis were chosen exclusively for two reasons. First, we wished to have as homogeneous a group as possible. Second, our clinical experience with the SAL test had revealed that in the category of conductive impairment, the largest discrepancies between the results of SAL and those of conventional bone conduction tended to occur in individuals with clinical otosclerosis.

The last two groups comprised individuals with bilateral sensorineural type hearing losses. One of these groups contained individuals selected in such a way as to rule out

---

[2] The term "occlusion index" as it is used in this paper refers to the increase in bone conduction sensitivity produced by occluding the test ear of subjects with normal middle ear mechanisms.

presbycusis as a major etiological factor in the hearing loss. While no upper age limit was imposed on potential subjects for this group, none was selected whose hearing loss had not been first noted prior to age 50. This group is hereafter referred to as the sensorineural group. The second group of subjects with sensorineural type impairments was formed by selecting individuals whose losses were presumed to have resulted from the aging process. This group is hereafter referred to as the presbycusis group. These two groups were included in this experiment in order to extend the previously reported observations relating to the validity of the SAL test as a means of estimating sensorineural acuity level. The presbycusis group was specifically included because it was felt that such subjects represented one of the more difficult types of cases with whom the test would be used clinically.

Experimnetal data were gathered for only one ear of each subject. In the normal hearing group, the test ear was selected randomly. In the three pathological groups, the better ear was chosen as the test ear in those subjects where a difference in the degree of hearing loss for the two ears existed. In all other instances the test ear was selected randomly.

APPARATUS

Equipment

All experimental data were collected using a commercially available Békésy audiometer (Grason-Stadler, Model E800). At any given time, the periodically interrupted output of this pure tone signal source fed one of three possible transducers: (1) a TDH-39-10Z earphone mounted in an MX41/AR cushion; (2) a Sharpe Circumaural Earphone (Type B, Model HA10); (3) a hearing-aid-type bone conduction vibrator (Sonotone, 10 ohms).

Each of the two types of earphone was utilized to obtain audiometric tracings in quiet as well as those in the presence of the SAL noise. The bone vibrator was used to obtain conventional bone conduction data.

An integral part of the E800 Békésy audiometer is a white noise masking source. The signal from this source was fed to a hearing-aid-type air conduction receiver (Radioear, M-75). This insert type receiver was fitted with a universal earmold which had been altered so as to allow it to be terminated by a soft rubber tip. This device was used to deliver masking noise to the nontest ear in all conventional bone conduction tests.

A commercially available thermal noise generator (Grason-Stadler, Model E5539A) feeding another hearing-aid-type bone conduction vibrator (Radioear, B-70A) supplied the bone conduction masking signal necessary for the SAL test.

Rationale for Choice of Earphones

As stated earlier, one of the aims of the experiment was to explore methods of reducing the discrepancy between the results of the SAL test and those of conventional bone conduction audiometry in cases with conductive type hearing impairments. As previously pointed out, it has been postulated that the observed discrepancy in these cases is probably largely due to the effect on bone conduction hearing acuity produced by covering the ears of the subjects in the normal hearing criterion population with the air conduction earphones. The magnitude of the occlusion effect may be expected to vary inversely with the volume of air enclosed; i.e. the larger the volume enclosed, the smaller the occlusion effect (16). Since the TDH-39-10Z earphone housed in an MX41/AR cushion is the type generally employed in the clinical setting, this combination was one of the two utilized in this experiment for the collection of SAL data. It was felt that this would allow the specification of the magnitude of the discrepancy between the results of SAL and conventional bone conduction in conductive cases as this discrepancy is encountered clinically.

Sensorineural acuity level (SAL) test data were also obtained utilizing the Sharpe Circumaural type earphone. This earphone was chosen because it was felt that, by virtue of the larger volume of air which it encloses when placed over the ear of the subject, the bone conduction occlusion index which it produced in the normal hearing reference group would be smaller in magnitude than that produced by an earphone housed in an MX41/AR cushion. Therefore any discrepancy between the results of SAL and conventional bone conduction tests which is due to the occlusion index built into the norm should be reduced by employing the Sharpe earphone in the collection of SAL data.

Performance of Apparatus

The acoustic output of the pure tone section of the Békésy audiometer feeding the TDH-39-10Z earphone was calibrated before the experiment, at weekly intervals during the collection of data, and again at the end of the experiment. No systematic variation in acoustic output was noted over the course of this period. Since there is no accepted coupler designed for use with the Sharpe earphone, no attempt was made to specify the acoustic output of the system when this transducer was used.

Likewise, since no acceptable coupler for a bone conduction vibrator was available at the time data were being gathered, physical measurement of the vibrational output of the bone conduction apparatus was not made. However, the output of this system was monitored throughout the experiment in two different ways. First, the voltage produced by the electrical signal from the audiometer at a given attenuator setting was measured daily across the terminals of the bone vibrator at the five conventional bone conduction test frequencies. No systematic variation in these voltages was noted over time. Secondly, a psychoacoustic monitoring method was employed. Specifically, a bone conduction threshold tracing covering the frequency range from 200 through 5,000 cps was obtained prior to the experiment for my right ear, since I have normal hearing acuity bilaterally. This procedure was repeated at approximately three-day intervals throughout the course of the investigation. No systematic variation either in the bone conduction tracings thus obtained or in their companion air conduction tracings was observed.

The stability of the output of the SAL noise apparatus was also monitored psychoacoustically. The procedure was the same as just described except that in this latter instance two air conduction threshold tracings covering the frequency range from 200 to 5,000 cps were obtained each time. The first of these was accomplished in quiet and the second in the presence of the SAL noise produced by an electrical signal of 2.0 volts RMS across the terminals of the SAL vibrator. The threshold shifts resulting during the second run were computed at 50 cycle intervals from 250 through 500 cps, at 100 cycle intervals from 500 through 1,000 cps and at 1,500, 2,000, 3,000, and 4,000 cps. This procedure revealed a slight but systematic decrease in the magnitudes of the threshold shifts produced at 250, 300, 350, 400, and 450 cps as the experiment progressed. This finding suggests that a change in the frequency response characteristics of the SAL bone vibrator occurred with time. This change was taken into account in the interpretation of the data. (The method for doing so is discussed in one of the following sections.)

Acoustic Environment

All data for this experiment were obtained with the subject seated in an acoustic environment provided by a commercially available audiometric room (IAC Model 1202). The test equipment was housed outside this room. Measurement of the ambient noise level in the room itself indicated that the test environment was adequate to allow the valid measurement of bone conduction acuity in normal hearing subjects.

PROCEDURES FOR GATHERING DATA

Each of the ten normal hearing subjects was seen in two sessions separated by an interval of about three weeks. Procedures were counter-balanced from one subject to another, but a given subject followed exactly the same sequence of test runs during his two sessions.

Sequence of Tests

After a practice run, each subject accomplished five more threshold tracings by Békésy audiometry. The stimulus in all cases was a periodically interrupted sinusoid whose frequency was varied continuously. Four of these tracings were done by air conduction. In two of these four, the test signal was transduced by a TDH-39-10Z earphone mounted in an MX41/AR cushion. In the other pair of air conduction tracings, the Sharpe earphone was employed. The first test with each of the two earphones was accomplished in quiet and covered the frequency range from 100 cps through 8,000 cps. Immediately thereafter, a second tracing was accomplished covering the frequency range from 200 cps through 5,000 cps. This latter test was administered in the presence of the bone-conducted SAL noise. The intensity of the SAL noise was specified in terms of the RMS voltage produced across the terminals of the bone vibrator by the noise signal. In all cases, the gain control of the noise generator was adjusted to produce 2.0 volts RMS across the terminals.

The two air conduction audiograms for a given type of earphone were obtained consecutively, with the quiet tracing always preceding the one obtained in the presence of the SAL noise. However, half the subjects accomplished the two tracings under the TDH earphone first and the remaining half carried out the two tracings under the Sharpe earphone first.

In addition to the air conduction audiometry described above, a bone conduction threshold audiogram covering the frequency range from 200 through 5,000 cps was obtained for each subject on the Békésy audiometer. During this test the bone vibrator was positioned on the most prominent portion of the mastoid process of the test ear.

The order of the air conduction versus bone conduction tests was counterbalanced so that in half the subjects the bone conduction test was administered first and vice versa.

Except for the fact that they were seen for only one test session, the subjects in each of the three experimental groups were subjected to the same series of tests described above for the normal hearing criterion group.

Positioning of Transducers

In preparation for the two air conduction tracings for a given type of earphone, the bone vibrator employed for the SAL test was positioned in the center of the forehead in the manner described by Jerger and Tillman (7). The air conduction earphones were then placed in position. The two headbands were carefully isolated by interposing a sheet of sponge rubber between them. The air conduction tracings in quiet and in the presence of the SAL noise were then obtained. This procedure was followed in order to avoid moving the earphones between the two tests.

Masking

Whenever possible, during the conventional bone conduction test, the nontest ear was masked at an effective level of 25 db with a wide-band thermal noise signal delivered via an insert receiver. The frequency response of the insert receiver had been plotted prior to the experiment, and deviations from a flat response were taken into account in computing the intensity level of the noise necessary to produce the effective level of 25 db at each test frequency. Then, during each test run, the intensity level of the noise was continuously monitored so as to maintain a level sufficient to shift the air conduction threshold of the nontest ear by 25 db at each of the 15 frequencies for which bone conduction threshold data were to be abstracted. This rule was broken only in those cases where the severity of the subject's hearing loss at some frequencies made it impossible to achieve an effective level of 25 db. In these instances, the intensity level of the masking sound was increased to its maximum over-all level of approximately 102 db SPL re: 0.0002 microbar.

PROCEDURES FOR ANALYZING DATA

Designation of Threshold

Since the frequency of the stimulus for all air and bone conduction tests varied continuously from low to high, it was possible to abstract threshold at any frequency between the lower and upper limits of the range studied. However, only 15 frequencies were selected. These frequencies were chosen so as to cover the conventional bone conduction test range of 250 to 4,000 cps and at the same time to allow a relatively extensive evaluation of the low-frequency region where the occlusion effect exerts its influence. Specifically, thresholds were computed from the Békésy audiograms at 50 cycle intervals between 250 and 500 cps, at 100 cycle intervals between 500 and 1,000 cps, and at 1,500, 2,000, 3,000, and 4,000 cps. Each threshold was defined as the midpoint of the envelope of the tracing at the point of intersection with the marker on the audiogram chart for the frequency in question.

Drift of SAL Output

Since, as described earlier, monitoring of the SAL noise revealed a slight but systematic decrease in its effect on the thresholds at 250, 300, 350, 400, and 450 cps as time progressed, slight errors in the estimation of the sensorineural acuity levels at these frequencies in the pathological groups studied could have resulted. Fortunately, approximately half the pathological subjects in this experiment were tested in the three-week interval between the two tests on the normal group, and the remaining half were tested after the second test session on the normal group. It was, therefore, decided that any error introduced by the equipment artifact described could be minimized by combining the data from the two

test sessions on the normal group and using this composite performance as a reference against which to compare the performance of the pathological groups on the SAL test. It was further decided to utilize the performance of this "composite normal group" as the reference for the other tests included in this experiment.

Failure to Achieve Sufficient SAL Shift

The function relating masking (M) to effective level (Z) was originally defined by Fletcher and Munson (3). It was later confirmed in almost every detail by Hawkins and Stevens (5). Both investigations revealed that for values of Z exceeding approximately 10 to 12 db, Z and M were equal. Both also showed, however, that for values of Z below 10 to 12 db, the M-Z function was nonlinear. In this region the value of M associated with a given Z value always exceeded this latter value. For example, a Z of 0 db yielded an M of approximately 5 db.

In the clinical administration of the SAL test there will be instances in which the effective noise level during the SAL test will fall in this nonlinear region of the M-Z function. One instance in which this will occur is represented by the individual whose sensorineural impairment approaches the hearing level to which the normal hearing subject is shifted by the SAL noise. A second potential example is the individual with a conductive impairment. Since he does not experience the occlusion index in the low-frequency region which the normal hearing subject does, he will be less sensitive to the low-frequency components of the bone-conducted noise than is the normal subject. The point is that in any instance in which the effective noise level during the SAL test falls in this nonlinear region, a spurious estimate of the sensorineural acuity level will be obtained. This effect will result because the threshold shift recorded in such an instance will be too large.

On the basis of this reasoning, the decision was made to disregard SAL shifts in all instances in which the magnitude of the shift was less than 10 db. That is, in arriving at the mean SAL shift for a given group at a given frequency, all shifts of less than 10 db were arbitrarily assigned a value of o db. Of course, all cases in which the SAL noise failed to produce a threshold shift represent instances in which a valid measure of sensorineural acuity level is impossible. That is, all such instances are directly analogous to those in which no response can be obtained from tests such as air or bone conduction, because the individual's threshold hearing level exceeds the maximum output limit of the audiometer.

Failure to Reach Bone Conduction Threshold

Examination of the conventional bone conduction thresholds for the subjects in the sensorineural groups revealed that an occasional subject failed to respond at the maximum limit of the audiometer. Specifically, three subjects in the sensorineural group of nonpresbycusic origin failed to respond at the three lowest test frequencies, two gave no response at 400 cps, and one failed to respond at 450 cps. In the presbycusic group, only one subject failed to respond at 250 and 300 cps. Except for these instances, conventional bone conduction thresholds were recorded for all subjects at all test frequencies.

Reduction in Sample Size

In the instances noted above in which either bone conduction thresholds or SAL levels could not be recorded, air conduction test data were also discarded for that individual at the frequency in question. This procedure was followed because a legitimate comparison of the results of the air conduction, bone conduction, and SAL tests could be made only if data for all tests were available for each subject being considered. The total number of cases or ears in each experimental group for which data were available for all test conditions is listed in the Table. It should be noted that the sample size at any given frequency varies considerably from group to group. This circumstance was not considered

TOTAL NUMBER OF EARS AT EACH TEST FREQUENCY FOR WHICH DATA WERE OBTAINED UNDER ALL TEST CONDITIONS (AC, BC, AND SAL)

Frequency, cps	Group		
	Sensorineural	Presbycusis	Otosclerosis
250	2	4	5
300	3	5	6
350	4	5	9
400	5	6	9
450	5	6	9
500	5	6	9
600	5	5	9
700	5	5	9
800	6	5	10
900	6	5	10
1,000	6	7	10
1,500	8	8	10
2,000	7	8	10
3,000	7	7	10
4,000	6	7	10

to be a serious limitation, however, since the performance of a given experimental group was not to be compared with that of any other group. Only comparisons between results on specific measures, such as bone conduction and SAL, within a given group were important from the standpoint of this experiment.

RESULTS

Normal Group

Since most of the threshold measurements obtained in this study cannot properly be expressed in terms of absolute magnitudes, no detailed summary of the responses of normal hearers is presented here. Suffice it to reemphasize that the several sets of data for the ten normal hearing subjects became the reference levels against which the performances of the three groups of hearing impaired subjects were described.

Sensorineural Group

Figure 18-1 displays the mean air and conventional bone conduction threshold hearing levels obtained for this group. Note that the two configurations tend to interweave throughout

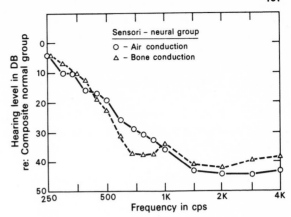

Figure 18-1. Mean hearing levels estimated by air conduction and bone conduction.

the frequency range tested and that at all test frequencies the bone conduction threshold is a fairly accurate estimate of the corresponding air conduction hearing level. The air conduction hearing levels reported in Figure 18-1 and in all subsequent figures were obtained using the TDH-39-10Z earphone housed in the traditional MX41/AR cushion.

Figure 18-2 displays the mean SAL estimates for this group obtained under the two types of earphones employed. In addition, the mean air conduction configuration is again displayed here. One striking feature of these data is the close agreement between the two sets of SAL data throughout the frequency spectrum. A second outstanding feature is the accuracy with which the SAL test results predict the mean air conduction hearing levels at frequencies below 1,000 cps. It is equally apparent, however, that at frequencies above 1,000 cps, results of the SAL test

tend to be systematically lower (better) than the corresponding air conduction hearing levels.

One may reason that this tendency for SAL to yield lower hearing levels than those estimated by air conduction in the high-frequency range is due to the "spread of masking phenomenon" described earlier by Jerger and his associates (8). These workers discovered that when exposed to an air-conducted narrow-band thermal noise masking signal, the ear with a sensorineural impairment experienced abnormally large threshold shifts at frequencies above that of the upper frequency limit of the noise band, ie, a "spread of masking" to regions devoid of energy from the noise band.

It should be noted here that as early as 1953, Lightfoot, Carhart, and Gaeth (10) published evidence that wide-band white noise at a fixed intensity level induces excess

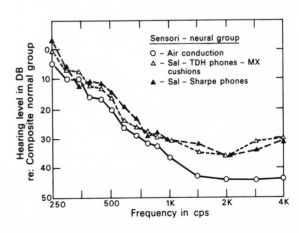

Figure 18-2. Mean hearing levels estimated by air conduction and by the SAL test applied under two different conditions.

threshold shifts at high frequencies in subjects with sensorineural losses whose air conduction audiometric configurations are similar to those displayed in Figure 18-1. Lightfoot, Carhart, and Gaeth did not attach a descriptive label to the excessive masking which they observed, but it seems certain to represent what Jerger and others later called the "spread of masking phenomenon."

In the present experiment, the mean hearing losses for the sensorineural group at frequencies above 1,000 cps were so great that, on the basis of conventional masking concepts, one would not have expected them to experience threshold shifts as a result of the SAL noise. However, mean shifts approaching 20 db were recorded for the sensorineural group at 800, 900, and 1,000 cps. The magnitudes of these latter shifts were not greatly different from those which would have been predicted on the basis of the noise level and hearing losses involved. It therefore seems safe to postulate that the audiometric configuration of the sensorineural group studied here functioned in the manner of a low-pass filter system and that the threshold shifts which yielded the SAL levels recorded in the frequency range above 1,000 cps resulted from a "spread of masking" from the components in the noise at 1,000 cps and below.

The validity of this hypothesis could easily be tested by employing narrow bands of noise centered around the specific test frequencies as the SAL noise stimulus. If the tendency for the SAL test to yield lower (better) hearing levels in the high-frequency range than those obtained via air conduction audiometry in sensorineural subjects of the type studied here should disappear when a narrow band of noise centered at the test frequency is used, then the hypothesis would seem tenable. Pending such an exploration, which will clarify underlying mechanisms, it must nonetheless be concluded that the SAL test, utilizing wide-band thermal noise, is inadequate as a means of predicting sensorineural acuity level in the high-frequency range for a significant portion of the sensorineural hearing loss population encountered clinically.

In view of the relative equivalence of the two sets of SAL data for the sensorineural group (Figure 18-2), it is sufficient to compare only the results of the SAL test, obtained under TDH earphones housed in MX41/AR cushions, with those of conventional bone conduction audiometry. This comparison is made in Figure 18-3. The relations are those one would expect from the foregoing discussion. First, below 1,000 cps, the results of the SAL test and those of conventional bone conduction, while not always in close agreement with one another, tend to be about equally good estimates of the air conduction hearing level. Second, above 1,000 cps, conventional bone conduction continues to esti-

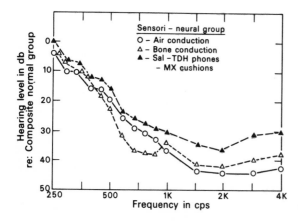

Figure 18-3. Mean hearing levels estimated by air conduction, bone conduction, and SAL.

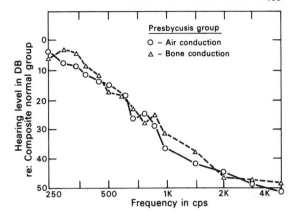

Figure 18-4. Mean hearing levels estimated by air conduction and bone conduction.

mate the air conduction hearing levels fairly accurately, while SAL tends to yield levels which are notably lower (better) than their companion air conduction hearing levels.

Presbycusis Group

The mean air and bone conduction configurations for the presbycusis group are shown in Figure 18-4. As with the first sensorineural group, the two sets of data are in relatively close agreement throughout the frequency range investigated. Similarly, as is apparent in Figure 18-5, the two sets of SAL test results obtained for the presbycusis group under the two earphones are almost identical. Finally, Figure 18-6 reproduces anew the air conduction, the conventional bone conduction, and the SAL hearing levels obtained with TDH-39 earphones for the presbycusis group. As one would expect from the parallelism between the first sensorineural group and the presby-

cusics, the results of the SAL test and conventional bone conduction are in close agreement at frequencies below 1,000 cps, while SAL thresholds are clearly lower (better) than bone thresholds above this frequency. In fact, the presbycusic group shows a greater discrepancy between the results of the two methods than that noted in the first sensorineural group.

Again, the "spread of masking phenomenon" is felt to account for the systematic tendency for SAL to yield lower (better) hearing levels than those yielded by either air or bone conduction audiometry in this region. Moreover, the fact that the discrepancy between SAL and conventional bone conduction is more pronounced for the presbycusic than for the sensorineural group seems to be explainable when one examines the air conduction hearing levels of the two groups. These levels for the presbycusis group are lower (better) in the frequency

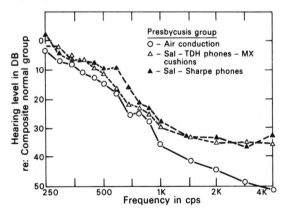

Figure 18-5. Mean hearing levels estimated by air conduction and by the SAL test applied under two different conditions.

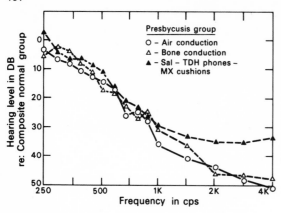

Figure 18-6. Mean hearing levels estimated by air conduction, bone conduction, and SAL.

range below 1,000 cps than the corresponding hearing levels for the sensorineural group. This factor acted to increase the relative effective level (Z) of the SAL noise in this frequency range for the presbycusis group, probably thereby enhancing the "spread of masking phenomenon."

Otosclerosis Group

The mean air and bone conduction audiometric configurations for this group are shown in Figure 18-7. It is apparent from the hearing levels involved and the magnitude and character of the air-bone gap that the otosclerosis group studied here was typical of a population without secondary sensorineural involve-

ment as described by previous investigators (1, 11).

As stated earlier, the thesis of those who have criticized the SAL test as an alternate method for assessing sensorineural acuity level has been that the occlusion index built into the SAL norms would result in erroneous estimates of the cochlear reserve in cases of conductive hearing loss. This point of view was perhaps most aptly stated by Naunton and Fernandez when they observed that any procedure which measures bone conduction with both ears of the subject occluded will yield results such that ". . . many of our otosclerotics and cases with other varieties of middle ear damage will appear to have mild low tone nerve deafness" (12: p. 318).

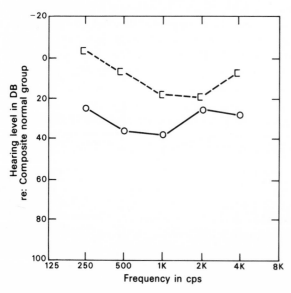

Figure 18-7. Mean audiometric configurations by air and bone conduction for otosclerosis group. Air conduction thresholds for 125 and 8,000 cps not shown.

The contention of Naunton and Fernandez is strongly supported by the data contained in Figure 18-8. This figure displays the configurations for conventional bone conduction and for SAL, measured under the two types of earphones employed. Evaluation of these data leads to two conclusions. First, in cases with otosclerosis, the SAL test yields sensorineural acuity levels which are markedly higher (poorer) at frequencies below 1,000 to 1,500 cps than the corresponding levels yielded by conventional bone conduction audiometry. Secondly, this discrepancy between the results of the two techniques is substantially reduced, but not by any means eliminated, when the SAL data are collected using the Sharpe earphone as opposed to the TDH earphone housed in an MX41/AR cushion.

In regard to the SAL curve for the Sharpe earphone shown in Figure 18-8, one note of explanation is in order. A small portion of the discrepancy between this curve and that for conventional bone conduction is artifactual. The arrows above many of the points on the SAL curve in Figure 18-8 indicate that the mean SAL responses at those points were at least as good as indicated and probably somewhat better. This was true because there were some instances at each of these points in which the individual subject's air conduction threshold was shifted by the SAL noise beyond the maximum output of the audiometer. The exact magnitude of the threshold shift could not be specified in these instances. That is, the shift was at least as great as the difference between the air conduction hearing level in quiet and the maximum output limit of the audiometer. However, the number of subjects for whom the exact threshold shift could not be specified at a given test frequency never exceeded two. Therefore, even taking this factor into account, a considerable discrepancy between the results of the two methods still exists in the low-frequency region. One must conclude that bone conduction audiometry and SAL do not yield the same estimates of sensorineural acuity level when otosclerotics are tested at low frequencies.

Undoubtedly the major reason for these discrepancies between results of the SAL test and those of conventional bone conduction audiometry is the occlusion index built into the SAL norms by virtue of occluding the ears of the normal criterion population with the earphones in question. It is true that the discrepancies between the curves displayed in Figure 18-8 are slightly larger than the occlusion indexes produced in normal listeners by each of these types of earphone (15). However, the discrepancies between the two SAL curves and the curve for conventional bone conduction essentially disappear at the point in the frequency range where the particular earphone ceases to produce a signi-

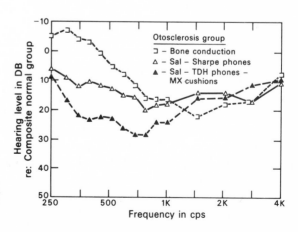

Figure 18-8. Mean hearing levels estimated by bone conduction and by the SAL test applied under two different conditions.

ficant occlusion effect in normal listeners. Specifically, no systematic changes due to occlusion were noted for these listeners above 500 cps with the Sharpe earphone or above 1,000 cps with the TDH earphone enclosed in an MX41/AR cushion (*15*). Reference to Figure 18-8 will reveal that above these frequencies, 500 cps for the Sharpe earphone and 1,000 cps for the TDH earphone, the SAL curves are essentially superimposed on the bone conduction curve. Thus, one must also conclude that the magnitude of the discrepancy in estimating sensorineural acuity levels of otosclerotics at low frequencies will vary with the ear cushion used to establish the norm for one's SAL test.

COMMENT

When the SAL test was originally proposed, it was argued that it enjoyed rather significant advantages over conventional bone conduction audiometry as a tool for estimating cochlear reserve. Certainly the SAL procedure makes it unnecessary for the clinician to decide when to mask the nontest ear and how much masking to apply, as he must decide when testing by conventional bone conduction audiometry. However, the results presented above for the otosclerosis group bear out the misgivings of those who have felt that the SAL test can yield spurious estimates of cochlear reserve in the low-frequency region for cases with conductive type hearing impairments. In addition, the data from the present experiment for the two groups with sensorineural losses raise the question as to whether the SAL test, administered using a wide-band thermal noise signal, represents a valid tool for the assessment of cochlear reserve even in cases of pure sensorineural hearing impairment. One has no alternative but to conclude that the SAL test as conventionally administered is not a suitable substitute for conventional bone conduction audiometry.

This statement is not meant to imply that the SAL test should be excluded from the armamentarium of the clinician. Because of

the unique results which SAL yields in conductive loss cases, it may in some cases provide useful diagnostic information of a qualitative nature which will supplement that gained through conventional bone conduction audiometry. Furthermore, Rintelmann and Harford (*14*) have recently reported using the SAL test in the detection of pseudohypoacusis in children. Therefore, it may prove to be of value to the clinician in manners which were not foreseen at the time of its development.

SUMMARY

The Sensori-Neural Acuity Level (SAL) test and conventional bone conduction tests were administered to normal hearers, two groups of subjects with sensorineural hearing losses, and to a group with conductive loss due to otosclerosis. SAL data were gathered under a conventional earphone and cushion as well as a circumaural-type earphone. The normal hearers served as a criterion group against which the performances of the other groups were evaluated.

Results of the two methods for the sensorineural groups agreed closely below 1,000 cps, but above this frequency SAL levels were lower (better) than bone conduction hearing levels. In the conductive loss group, the results of the two methods agreed closely above 1,000 cps, but at lower frequencies SAL yielded markedly higher (poorer) hearing levels than did conventional bone conduction tests. This discrepancy was reduced, but not eliminated, when SAL data were collected using the circumaural-type earphone.

In view of these findings, the SAL test cannot be considered an adequate substitute for conventional bone conduction audiometry. The threshold shift in the normal hearing criterion group required for the SAL test is modified at low frequencies by the ear cushion employed, and this appears to account for the discrepancies between the results of SAL and bone conduction audiometry in conductive cases. The "spread of masking phenomenon" appears to be responsible for the excessive threshold shifts which sensorineurals often show at high frequencies. Nonetheless, in certain cases, the SAL test may add qualitative information which supplements conventional bone conduction audiometry usefully.[3]

[3] Dr. Raymond Carhart, Professor of Audiology and Otolaryngology, Northwestern University, assisted in the preparation of this manuscript.

REFERENCES

1. Carhart, R.: Clinical Application of Bone Conduction Audiometry, Arch. Otolaryng. 51: 798–807, 1950.

2. Feldman, A. S.: Problems in the Measurement of Bone Conduction, J. Speech Hearing Dis. 26: 39–44, 1961.

3. Fletcher, H., and Munson, W. A.: Relation Between Loudness and Masking, J. Acoust. Soc. Amer. 9: 1–10, 1937.

4. Goldstein, D. P.; Hayes, C. S.; and Peterson, J. L.: A Comparison of Bone Conduction Thresholds by Conventional and Rainville Methods, J. Speech Hearing Res. 5: 244–255, 1962.

5. Hawkins, J. E., Jr., and Stevens, S. S.: The Masking of Pure Tones and of Speech by White Noise, J. Acoust. Soc. Amer. 22: 6–13, 1952.

6. Jerger, J. F.: DL Difference Test: Improved Method for Clinical Measurement of Recruitment, AMA Arch. Otolaryng. 57: 490–500, 1953.

7. Jerger, J. F., and Tillman, T. W.: A New Method for the Clinical Determination of Sensorineural Acuity Level (SAL), AMA Arch. Otolaryng. 71: 948–953, 1960.

8. Jerger, J. F.; Tillman, T. W.; and Peterson, J. L.: Masking by Octave Bands of Noise in Normal and Impaired Ears, J. Acoust. Soc. Amer. 32: 385–390, 1960.

9. Keys, J. W., and Milburn, B.: The Sensorineural Acuity Level (SAL) Technique: An Experiment with Some Observations, Arch. Otolaryng. 73: 710–716, 1961.

10. Lightfoot, C.; Carhart, R.; and Gaeth, J. H.: Efficiency of Impaired Ears in Noise: A. Thresholds for Pure Tones and for Speech, Project No. 21-1203-0001, Report No. 4, USAF School of Aviation Medicine, Randolph Field, Texas 1953.

11. McConnell, F., and Carhart, R.: Influence of Fenestration Surgery on Bone Conduction Measurements, Laryngoscope 62: 1267–1292, 1952.

12. Naunton, R. F., and Fernandez, C.: Prolonged Bone Conduction: Observation on Man and Animals, Laryngoscope 71: 306–318, 1961.

13. Rainville, M. J.: Nouvelle Methode d'assourdissement pour le releve des courves de conduction osseuse, J. Franc. Otorhinolaryng. 4: 851–858, 1955.

14. Rintelmann, W. F., and Harford, E. R.: The Detection and Assessment of Pseudohypoacusis Among School-Age Children, J. Speech Hearing Dis., to be published.

15. Tillman, T. W.: Some Comments on the Bone Conduction Occlusion Effect, unpublished manuscript, Evanston, Ill, Northwestern University.

16. Watson, N. A., and Gales, R. S.: Bone Conduction Threshold Measurements: Effects of Occlusion, Enclosures and Masking Devices, J. Acoust. Soc. Amer. 14: 207–215, 1943.

19

Critical Evaluation of SAL Audiometry

JAMES F. JERGER
SUSAN JERGER

JAMES F. JERGER, Ph.D., is Professor of Audiology, Baylor College of Medicine
SUSAN JERGER is Instructor, Department of Otolaryngology, Baylor College of Medicine

In spite of its undoubted clinical value, conventional bone-conduction audiometry suffers two serious limitations. One is the problem of calibrating clinical bone-conduction systems. Calibration on normal listeners requires an acoustic environment not generally available to the majority of clinicians. Calibration of the system on patients with pure sensori-neural loss (Carhart, 1950) minimizes the need for a superior acoustic environment but raises the equally disturbing problem of providing an external validating criterion of pure sensorineural loss independent of bone-conduction audiometry.

The second limitation of conventional bone-conduction audiometry is the problem of excluding the non-test ear from participation in the bone-conduction response (Naunton, 1960; Feldman, 1961). Essentially this is the problem of providing exactly enough masking noise to exclude the non-test ear without, at the same time, employing so much masking noise that the response of the test ear is affected (Jerger and Wertz, 1959). Such undesirable effects can result from either direct trans-cranial leakage or via the intermediary of central masking phenomena (Naunton, 1957; Dirks and Malmquist, 1964).

In 1955, M. Rainville described a procedure for assessing the status of the sensori-neural mechanism of hearing that circumvented

Reprinted by permission of the authors from *J. Speech Hearing Res.*, **8**, pp. 103–128 (1965).

these traditional problems of conventional bone-conduction audiometry. Instead of measuring the threshold for bone-conducted pure tones while masking the non-test ear with air-conducted noise, Rainville reversed the procedure and measured the masking effect on air-conducted tones produced by bone-conducted noise.

In 1960, Jerger and Tillman described a modification of the Rainville approach, called the SAL test. Although the SAL test is based on Rainville's principle, it represents a considerable simplification in procedure. The SAL test is carried out by measuring two thresholds, the threshold in quiet, and the threshold in the presence of a fixed level of bone-conducted noise. The difference, in dB, between these two thresholds is then compared with the difference produced by the same noise level in normal ears. Figure 19-1 illustrates this principle graphically. At any given frequency, N represents the normal pure-tone threshold in quiet. As the intensity of bone-conducted masking noise increases, masking begins and increases linearly. P represents the pure-tone threshold in quiet for an ear with hearing loss of L dB. If the entire loss is sensori-neural, then, as the bone-conducted masking-noise level is increased, masking will not begin until the normal function is reached (Palva, Goodman, and Hirsh, 1953). If, on the other hand, the hearing loss is entirely conductive, masking will begin at the same noise level as at the normal ear. The masking function will be linear but displaced to the left of the normal function by the distance ab, or θ, that is by the size of the conductive component.

If, now, we present bone-conducted noise at a single fixed intensity, W, then the threshold in noise for the pure sensori-neural will be at point a, and the threshold in noise for the pure conductive will be at point c. We are concerned, however, only with the difference between this threshold in noise and its counterpart in quiet.

In Figure 19-1, ND represents the normal difference, D_{sn} represents the difference for a pure sensori-neural loss, and D_c represents the difference for a pure conductive loss. The patient's sensori-neural level (SAL) is simply ND — D. In the general case ND — D = L — θ. In the case of pure sensori-neural loss, ND — D = L. In the case of pure conductive loss, ND — D = 0.

Note, however, that L may exceed ND. If this occurs in the case of pure sensori-neural loss, then $D_{sn} = 0$ and under this circumstance one can only say that SAL $\geq$ ND. In other words, the distance ND, the masking produced by the noise in normals, sets the upper limit of the test. By choosing a sufficiently high noise level, ND can be made to equal the upper limit of most conventional bone-conduction systems, that is, 50–60 dB at 1 000 cps and above.

Note, also, however, that point c may exceed the upper limit of the equipment used to measure the air-conduction threshold. This problem can be minimized by adjusting the noise level to produce a relatively small value for ND, that is, 20–30 dB. If, however, c does exceed the upper limit of the air-conduction systems, one can only say that SAL $\leq$ ND — D', where D' is the difference between the threshold in quiet and the upper limit of the instrument. This is a problem that, in our experience, seldom arises in practice.

By virtue of the procedure employed, the SAL test enjoys two distinct theoretical advantages over conventional bone-conduction

audiometry. First, the instrumentation can be readily calibrated on normal ears. Second, the interaural attenuation characterizing air-conduction audiometry greatly minimizes the problem of eliminating the non-test ear.

In spite of these theoretical advantages, the SAL test has found a varied reception among clinicians (Schröder, 1963). Michael (1963) reported that, in 31 consecutive cases, SAL was a better predictor of the post-operative

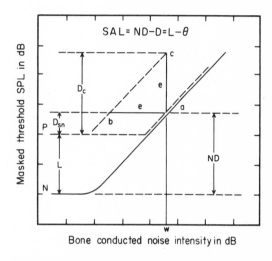

Figure 19-1. Diagram illustrating rationale for SAL audiometry (see text).

result of stapedectomy than conventional bone-conduction audiometry. Bailey and Martin (1963) reported similar success using spondees rather than pure tones as the SAL signal.

On the other hand serious doubts as to the validity of the SAL result have been raised by Naunton and Fernandez (1961), Goldstein, Hayes, and Peterson (1962), Tillman (1963), and Martin and Bailey (1964).

In view of these discrepant reports it seemed advisable to undertake a systematic evaluation of the SAL test. The present paper considers the effects of several relevant procedural variables on SAL audiometry, and the equivalence of SAL and bone-conduction thresholds.

APPARATUS

Air-conduction thresholds were obtained on a standard Bekesy audiometer (Grason-Stadler, Model E800). The pure-tone signal was interrupted at the rate of 2.5 ips and attenuated at the rate of 2.5 dB/sec. Unless otherwise noted, frequency changed at the rate of 1 octave/min. The output of the Bekesy audiometer passed through a speech audio-

illustrated in Figure 19-2, was built. One leg of a hospital-type table of adjustable height was pivoted so that the bone vibrator could be positioned on the subject's forehead. The force delivered to the bone vibrator by the tension of the spring on arm A could be varied by movement of arm B. The apparatus was calibrated for forces of 250, 500, 750, and 1 000 gram weight by substituting appropriate weights for the bone vibrator and determining

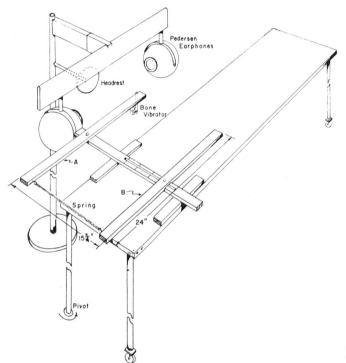

Figure 19-2. Apparatus used to couple bone vibrator to forehead with known, constant force.

meter (Grason-Stadler, Model 162) and terminated in a set of special earphones (Pedersen, type B-228A), consisting of loudspeakers mounted in approximately 7-inch spherical enclosures.

The bone-conducted noise source was a standard white-noise generator (Grason-Stadler, Model 901B). The output from this generator passed directly to a standard, commercially-available, bone vibrator (Radioear, type B-70-A). In order to couple the bone vibrator to the subject's head with a known and controllable force, a special device,

that position of arm B which oriented arm A in a plane parallel to arm B. In subsequent testing the bone vibrator was brought to a position in which it just touched the center of the subject's forehead with arm A held in this plane. Arm A was then freed so that the tension of the spring would apply the bone vibrator to the skull at the desired force.

For conventional bone-conduction audiometry the output from the Bekesy audiometer was connected directly to the bone vibrator. Bone thresholds were traced over the frequency range from 500 to 6 000 cps. The conventional frequency of 250 cps was omitted because of recent observations by Weiss (1961), on the Beltone Artificial Mastoid, that hearing-aid type bone vibrators transduce this frequency with considerable distortion.

PROCEDURAL VARIABLES

Occlusion Effect

It is well known that sensitivity to bone-conducted signals is affected by the condition of the external ear canal (Bárány, 1938). Covering the test ear with a standard earphone cushion, for example, increases sensitivity to bone-conducted signals in a systematic fashion (Naunton, 1957). This increase in sensitivity is called the "occlusion effect." Its magnitude, although variable among subjects, is, on the average, inversely proportional to the volume of air enclosed by the earphone cushion (Naunton, 1963). The term "relative" bone conduction is often applied to measurements obtained with the test ear open, and the term "absolute" bone conduction is applied to measurements obtained with the test ear occluded.

Conventional bone-conduction audiometry is typically carried out with the test ear unoccluded, that is, in the relative state. Either Rainville or SAL audiometry, on the other hand, must necessarily be carried out with the test ear occluded by an earphone cushion. Any attempt to compare SAL with conventional bone conduction must take this fact into account. If SAL is to be compared with BC, then both must be based on relative (that is, unoccluded) measures, or both must be based on absolute (that is, occluded) measures (Lightfoot, 1960).

One purpose of the present series of experiments was to determine whether SAL and conventional bone conduction (BC) results are equivalent when this factor is controlled. We elected to do this by studying only relative (that is, unoccluded) bone conduction. The effect of introducing occlusion will be con-

sidered in a subsequent section. In order to achieve the relative or unoccluded equivalent for SAL, we employed the Pedersen earphones which enclose a volume of air so large that the average occlusion effect is negligible (Naunton, 1963). Figure 19-3 compares the average BC threshold for six normal listeners under three test conditions; with both ears open, with both ears covered by MX41/AR cushions, and with both ears covered by the Pedersen

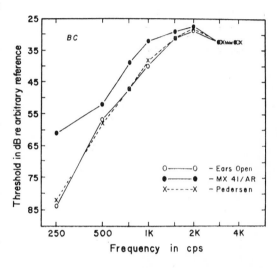

Figure 19-3. Average bone-conduction thresholds under three conditions, showing lack of occlusion effect for Pedersen earphones.

phones. In this and subsequent figures, the "arbitrary reference" to which ordinate values are referred is simply the zero line of the Bekesy audiogram with the compensating cam in the SPL or constant output position. For air-conducted tones this zero line corresponded to an SPL of approximately 10 dB as measured on a special coupler constructed to accommodate the Pedersen earphones. Note that, while the MX41/AR cushion produces the expected average occlusion effect, the Pedersen and the open-ear conditions are essentially equivalent. Through use of the Pedersen phones, therefore, it was possible to study both BC and SAL in the relative or unoccluded state and still keep both ears covered by earphone cushions at all times.

Force of Application

In order to determine the effect of varying the force of application of the bone vibrator, both BC thresholds and AC thresholds in the presence of BC noise were measured in three normal listeners. Figure 19-4a shows the result for AC thresholds in BC noise. For these measures the noise level voltage was −12 dB re 2 volts RMS measured across the terminals of the bone vibrator. Over the range from 250

Effect of Noise Duration

When the AC threshold in the presence of BC noise is measured by Bekesy audiometric technique, the subject is exposed to a constant, rather high, level of white noise for about 7 minutes. The question therefore arises, "does the length of time that the noise is on affect the SAL result?" In order to explore this possibility two subjects were tested in the following manner. First an AC threshold

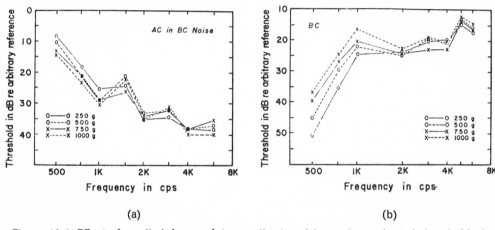

(a)   (b)

Figure 19-4. Effect of applied force of bone vibrator: (a) on air-conducted thresholds in bone-conducted noise; (b) on conventional bone-conduction thresholds.

to 1 000 grams we observe a slight effect in the region below 1 000 cps, in the expected direction. Threshold sensitivity for air-conducted tones decreases as the coupling force of the vibrator carrying the masking noise to the head increases.

Figure 19-4b shows that the effect is somewhat more pronounced for conventional BC thresholds. For these measures the non-test ear was masked by white noise at a sensation level of 50 dB. The present results for BC are in good agreement with the previous findings of König (1957) for a bone vibrator with a resonance peak at 2 200 cps.

On the basis of these results and recent recommendations of working group WG-1 of the International Standards Association (ISO/TC43), the applied force was held constant at 750 gram weight in all subsequent studies.

tracing was obtained in the usual fashion except that speeds were reduced to $\frac{1}{2}$ octave/min. for frequency change and 1.25 dB/sec. for attenuation change. Frequency moved in a "forward" direction (that is, from low to high) over the range from 300 to 6 000 cps. Again the bone-conducted noise voltage was −12 dB re 2 volts RMS. Upon completion of this standard tracing the direction of frequency change was abruptly reversed, and the subject continued to track thresholds as the frequency moved "backward" from 6 000 to 300 cps. After this tracing the noise level was raised 12 dB and the entire forward-backward procedure was repeated. Figure 19-5a shows the results for a subject with normal hearing. Figure 19-5b presents similar data for a subject with bilateral sensorineural hearing loss. Both figures suggest that, in spite of a total noise exposure of more than

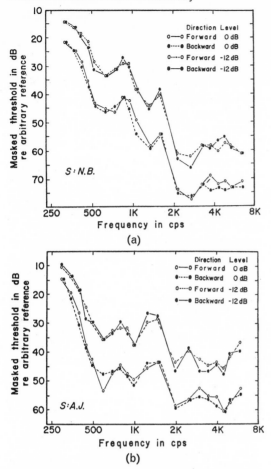

Figure 19-5. Effect of noise duration and direction of Bekesy frequency change on air-conducted thresholds in bone-conducted noise: (a) for a single subject with normal ears; (b) for a single subject with sensori-neural hearing loss.

56 minutes, there is no obvious noise duration effect. Furthermore, it is apparently immaterial whether the frequency changes from low to high or from high to low.

Linearity of Masking

Implicit in the rationale of the SAL test is the assumption that the masking produced by bone-conducted noise is a linear function of noise level. In order to test the validity of this assumption, air-conduction thresholds were measured in three normal subjects as bone-conducted noise voltage was decreased in 5 dB steps from a maximum of 2 volts RMS.

Two of the three subjects had normal hearing in both ears. In one of these the non-test ear was masked by white noise at a sensation level of 50 dB. This noise was supplied by a separate noise generator and was, therefore, uncorrelated with the bone-conducted noise. In the second bilateral normal, no air-conduction masking of the non-test ear was used. The third subject had normal hearing in the test ear but a severe sensori-neural loss in the non-test ear. Figure 19-6a shows results obtained on each subject at a typical frequency, in this case 1 000 cps. Note that the masking functions are reasonably linear with unit slope. No systematic differences among the three subjects were observed at this or other frequencies with the possible exception of 500 cps, the significance of which will be discussed in the next section. Figure 19-6b plots the mean masking function for all three subjects at each measured frequency from 500 to 6 000 cps. Masking functions for AC tones in BC noise do appear to be linear with unit slope across the frequency range of interest in SAL audiometry. The slope of the function for 500 cps is less than unit at low noise levels, but steepens to unity in the region of interest to

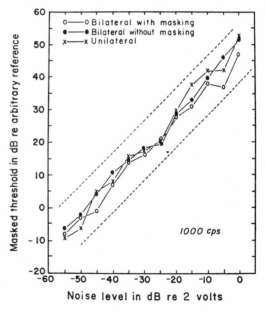

Figure 19-6a. Linearity of masking functions for air-conducted tone in bone-conducted noise: three normal ears at 1 000 cps.

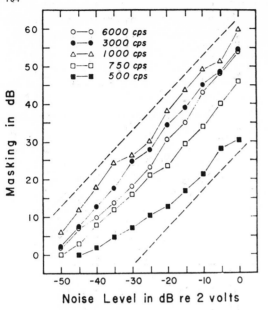

Figure 19-6b. Average functions at various frequencies in three normal ears.

SAL audiometry, from 0 to 20 dB below 2 volts RMS.

In order to test whether this linearity holds for subjects with hearing loss, AC, BC, and AC in the presence of two levels of BC noise were measured in one subject with conductive loss and in one subject with sensori-neural loss. The two noise voltages were 0 dB and −12 dB re 2 volts RMS. Figure 19-6c shows the result for the subject with conductive loss, and Figure 19-6d shows the result for the subject with sensori-neural loss. Results are plotted as hearing-threshold level relative to the norms for AC, BC, and SAL established for this equipment on 10 normal ears. SAL thresholds for a given noise voltage were computed by subtracting the subject's shift from the appropriate normal shift for that noise level. In both cases SAL results are equivalent for either noise level.

Effect of Correlated Noise in Non-Test Ear

In the SAL procedure we are interested only in the masking produced by the bone-conducted noise in the test ear. It is undeniable,

however, that the same noise also stimulates the non-test ear to a degre determined by the amount of sensori-neural hearing loss in that ear.

Recent studies of monaural versus binaural masking (Blodgett and others, 1962; Egan, 1964; Egan and Benson, 1964; Hirsh and Burgeat, 1958; Weston and Miller, 1964) have shown that the presence of such a correlated noise in the non-test ear has a measurable effect on the masking produced by the noise in the test ear. If the threshold first is determined in the presence of noise on the test ear only, and then uncorrelated noise is presented to the non-test ear, there is little or no effect. If, however, the added noise is correlated with that on the test ear, then the subject experiences a release from masking on the test ear, and the new threshold SPL may be several dB below the original level. This masking level difference (MLD) effect is quite

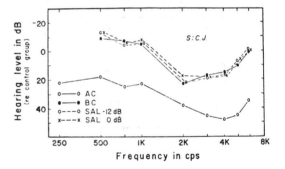

Figure 19-6c. Comparison of SAL thresholds at two noise levels in a single subject with conductive loss.

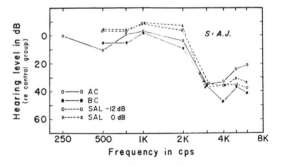

Figure 19-6d. Comparison of SAL thresholds at two noise levels in a single subject with sensori-neural loss.

clear-cut at frequencies below 1 000 cps, but fairly negligible above that point. An extremely thorough theoretical treatment of the entire phenomenon has been developed by Durlach (1963).

The magnitude of the MLD effect varies somewhat according to the method used to measure threshold. Egan (1964), using a two-alternative forced-choice technique, obtained an MLD of 9 dB at 500 cps, but Hirsh and Burgeat (1958) using a Bekesy-type threshold tracking technique obtained an MLD only slightly greater than 3 dB at this frequency.

Another interesting property of the MLD effect is its virtual independence of inter-aural noise intensity differences over an astonishing range (Egan, 1964; Weston and Miller, 1964).

The fact that the MLD effect exists should not, in and of itself, necessarily present any problem for SAL audiometry so long as the effect is common to both normals and patients with hearing loss. In this event it simply subtracts from the masked threshold, at frequencies below 1 000 cps, an amount which is constant for everyone. Furthermore the fact, noted above, that the effect is present over a rather wide range of inter-aural intensity differences in normals suggests that it should be present over an equally wide range of hearing loss asymmetry.

The possibility exists, however, that some kinds of hearing loss may have the effect of reducing the inter-aural noise correlation, even though the noise input signal itself is correlated at the two ears. It seems unlikely that any kind of conductive hearing loss could produce such an effect, but sensori-neural loss might very well disrupt the inter-aural correlation. In order to explore this possibility we measured MLD in four subjects with normal hearing and three subjects with bilateral sensori-neural hearing loss under the approximate conditions of SAL audiometry. After the monaural threshold in quiet had been determined, broad-band noise was introduced to the test ear by air conduction. Its level was then adjusted to produce the amount of masking typical of SAL audio-

metry at the test frequency. This condition of monaural signal and monaural noise is symbolized as Nm Sm (noise monaural, signal monaural). After threshold had been traced under this condition, correlated noise at the same intensity was added to the non-test ear and a new masked threshold was obtained. This condition is symbolized as NOSm (correlated noise to both ears, signal monaural). All thresholds were obtained by fixed-frequency Bekesy technique. Thresholds were tracked at 500, 750, 1 000, and 2 000 cps. Figure 19-7 shows the resultant MLD's, and,

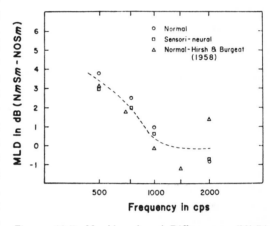

Figure 19-7. Masking Level Differences (MLD) as functions of frequency in normals and sensori-neurals.

for comparative purposes, data obtained by Hirsh and Burgeat (1958) on four normal listeners using a comparable threshold tracking procedure. We note the expected MLD effect at frequencies below 1 000 cps, but see no evidence that sensori-neurals are different from normals.

Certainly, however, this can be regarded as no more than a pilot investigation to be extended to a much larger sample of patients with sensori-neural loss. There may very well be varieties of sensori-neural loss not represented in this small sample which do have an important effect on inter-aural noise correlation. One thinks especially of the eighth-nerve disorders where timing relations may be quite aberrant.

Effect of Acoustic Reflex

The maximum bone-conducted noise used in this investigation, 2 volts RMS across the terminals of the BC vibrator, produces about 50 dB of masking in the range from 1 000 to 6 000 cps. This corresponds to an air-conducted noise at an overall SPL of about 80 dB. It is pertinent to ask, therefore, whether the SAL noise is sufficient to elicit the acoustic reflex in normal ears and, if so, whether the reflex contraction exerts a differential effect on air- and bone-conducted signals.

The answer to the first question is probably affirmative. Lilly (1964) has recently reported observation of the reflex in response to white noise at an average overall SPL of 69 dB. The occurrence of the acoustic reflex, per se, should not present any problem for SAL audiometry so long as it affects AC and BC signals equally. The possibility exists, however, that reflex contraction might attenuate the AC tone but not the BC noise. We reasoned that this possibility could be explored by comparing masking functions for AC tones in BC noise with masking functions for BC tones in AC noise. If the acoustic reflex exerts no differential effect, then both functions ought to remain linear. If, on the other hand, the acoustic reflex does, in fact, attenuate AC signals more than BC signals, then both functions should become non-linear and divergent. The function for AC tones in BC noise ought to accelerate, whereas the function for BC tones in AC noise ought to decelerate. We explored this possibility in one well-trained subject. Both types of masking were measured at 500 and 750 cps in the following manner. BC noise was introduced at the forehead at a maximum level of 2 volts and decreased in 5 dB steps as the subject tracked threshold for the tone by means of the Bekesy audiometer. Then noise was presented via AC and the threshold tracking tone was introduced to the bone vibrator on the forehead. In order to exclude the non-test ear from participation in the BC response, uncorrelated noise was presented to the non-test ear at a level 25 dB above the noise level in the test ear, an ingenious procedure recently recommended by Weston and Miller (1964).

Figure 19-8 shows the masking functions thus obtained. The abscissae for the two conditions have been adjusted so that the two functions for a given frequency approximately coincide. We note that the anticipated non-linearity does occur at 500 cps. The function for BC tone in AC noise does decelerate at high noise levels. Weston (1964) recently obtained a virtually identical result at both 250 and 500 cps when Pedersen earphones were used to deliver the AC noise. He attributes this non-linearity to the greater effect of the acoustic reflex on the AC noise than on the BC tone. We note, however, that the function for AC tone in BC noise remains within the linear portion of the curve. Apparently the acoustic reflex elicited by the SAL noise is not of sufficient strength to attenuate AC noise and BC signals differentially.

Finally, it should be noted that Weston (1964) observed this non-linearity when Pedersen phones were used to deliver the AC noise, but did not find it when conventional phones mounted in MX41/AR cushions were used. He attributed this difference to the fact that conventional receivers produce an occlusion effect which, according to Bárány (1938) and others, enhances bone conduction in the 500 cps region by generating an air-conducted component within the occluded external meatus. Weston reasons that, under this circumstance, the acoustic reflex will attenuate equally both the AC noise and the air-conducted component of the BC tone. Hence the shape of the masking function will not be altered by the reflex contraction.

RELATION TO CONVENTIONAL BONE-CONDUCTION AUDIOMETRY

Theoretically SAL and conventional bone-conduction audiometry ought to be measuring the same thing and should, therefore, yield identical results. In order to investigate this equivalence empirically, however, one must be aware and take account of two potential pitfalls. The first is the fact that the SAL result must necessarily be the equivalent of absolute bone conduction since it requires that the test ear be occluded by an earphone cushion. Rainville, himself, referred to this point in his original publication (1959, p. 7). It is not reasonable, therefore, to compare SAL thresholds with relative bone-conduction thresholds in patients with conductive hearing loss. A discrepancy at low frequencies will appear as a consequence of the occlusion effect. This discrepancy will necessarily arise from the fact that the normal standardization group is given the benefit of the occlusion effect in SAL audiometry, but denied it in relative bone-conduction audiometry. This is, of course, no problem as long as the same relationship holds for patients with hearing loss. But it is well known that one consequence of conductive hearing loss is to supply the patient with a "built-in" occlusion effect (Naunton, 1963). He, therefore, derives no additional benefit from the occlusion effect provided by the earphone cushion in the SAL procedure. Inevitably, then, at those frequencies where the occlusion effect is measurable, the SAL threshold will necessarily be poorer than the relative bone-conduction threshold by the amount of the occlusion effect provided by the particular earphone cushion being used.

Clearly, it is unreasonable to expect SAL and BC thresholds to agree in conductive loss unless the norms for both tests are derived in the same way, either in the relative or the absolute state.

The second pitfall is the very reason that thoughtful clinicians earnestly seek an alternative to conventional bone-conduction audiometry; namely, the problem of being sure that the non-test ear has, in fact, been excluded from the measured response. It is unreasonable to compare SAL and conventional BC results unless one can be absolutely sure that the BC threshold represents the test ear and the test ear only.

The purpose of the next series of experiments

was to determine empirically whether, in fact, SAL and BC results are equivalent in patients with conductive and sensori-neural hearing loss. The first pitfall was avoided by performing all measurements in the relative state. This was achieved for both SAL and BC by the use of the Pedersen earphones described in the previous section. The second pitfall was avoided by employing, as experimental sub-

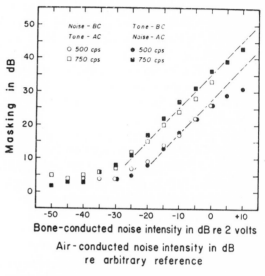

Figure 19-8. Comparison of masking functions for air-conducted tones in bone-conducted noise and bone-conducted tones in air-conducted noise.

jects, only patients whose non-test ear showed a severe or total sensori-neural loss. All subjects, even the normals on whom the SAL and BC systems were calibrated, were, in effect, "unilateral" hearers.

Standardization

The instrumentation described in the previous section was calibrated by measuring AC, BC, and AC-in-BC noise thresholds in 10 normal ears. Each of the 10 subjects used for this procedure had normal hearing in one ear and a severe or total sensori-neural loss in the other ear. On conventional manual audiometry no subject in this group responded to any bone-conducted signal on the poorer ear when the normal ear was masked. Four of the 10 subjects responded to no air-conducted signal at the limit of the equipment. The remaining six subjects gave some isolated responses in the hearing level range from 90 to 110 dB (ISO, 1964). Normal hearing on the good ear was defined by conventional audiometric thresholds not exceeding a hearing level of 20 dB (ISO, 1964) over the range from 250 to 6 000 cps. The average age of this normal group was 28.3 years, with a range from 12 to 54 years.

In the subsequent analysis of data, all results are referred to the average thresholds obtained on this normal group. Hearing loss by air conduction is defined as the difference, in dB, between the subject's threshold (midpoint of Bekesy tracing) and the average normal threshold (average mid-point of Bekesy tracings). Hearing loss by bone conduction is similarly defined. The SAL norm is defined as the difference, in dB, between the average threshold in quiet and the average threshold in BC noise. For purposes of standardization this latter threshold was determined for a BC noise of −12 dB re 2 volts RMS across the terminals of the bone vibrator. Hearing loss by SAL is defined as the difference between the subject's shift in threshold in the presence of BC noise and this normal shift in threshold. Table 19-1 shows the average shift in threshold

TABLE 19-1. AVERAGE DIFFERENCE BETWEEN AC THRESH-OLDS IN QUIET AND IN THE PRESENCE OF BC NOISE AT −12 DB RE 2 VOLTS IN 10 UNILATERAL NORMAL SUBJECTS

	Frequency in cps							
	500	750	1 000	2 000	3 000	4 000	5 000	6 000
Shift in Threshold	19.7	28.7	32.3	36.4	42.7	40.6	43.6	41.7

obtained on the normal group. These numbers constitute the SAL norm for this investigation.

In all conductive-loss cases the −12 dB level was used to define SAL. In the sensori-neural group, however, the severity of some subjects' losses, especially in the high frequencies, required that the BC noise be increased to 0 dB re 2 volts. In this circumstance 12 dB was added to the norms of Table

19-1 for the purpose of computing the hearing loss by SAL. This procedure seemed justified in view of the linearity of the masking functions shown in Figures 19-6a and 19-6b.

Conductive Loss

In order to compare SAL and BC in conductive loss, AC, BC, and SAL thresholds were measured in 10 subjects with asymmetrical conductive loss. All subjects in this group had a mild or moderate relatively pure conductive loss on one ear, and a severe or total sensori-neural loss on the other ear, in addition to any conductive component on this ear. Although the majority of these subjects gave no response to either AC or BC signals at the limit of conventional audiometric equipment on the poorer ear, some isolated responses to BC signals were noted at 500 and 1 000 cps. In all cases, however, the BC threshold of the non-test ear was at least 15 dB poorer than the threshold of the test ear, as measured by conventional manual audiometric technique. This configuration of loss made it possible to obtain reasonably valid BC thresholds on the better ear without the use of masking noise on the poorer ear.

Figure 19-9a shows results in a typical individual subject of this group. Note the close correspondence between SAL and BC, especially at 500 and 750 cps. Figure 19-9b shows the average result for the entire conductive loss group. Average SAL and BC thresholds are in relatively good agreement at all test frequencies.

Some previous investigators (Goldstein, Hayes, and Peterson, 1962; Tillman, 1963) have reported a discrepancy between SAL and BC at low frequencies in conductive loss. In the results of Goldstein and others, for example, the average Rainville threshold for their conductive group is 18 dB below the average BC threshold at 500 cps.

It must be emphasized that these investigators referred BC loss to "unoccluded" normals, but referred SAL loss to norms obtained in an "occluded" state. This procedure inevitably builds into the comparison a discrepancy equal to the amount of the occlusion effect produced by the earphone cushions used. Figure 19-9b shows that when this factor was eliminated by the use of earphones that did not produce an occlusion effect, there was no discrepancy between BC and SAL thresholds in this group of subjects with conductive loss.

subject in this group. Figure 19-9d shows the average result for the entire group. All three measures appear to be in reasonably good agreement.

Tillman (1963) has recently suggested that a systematic discrepancy may exist between SAL and AC thresholds in the high-frequency

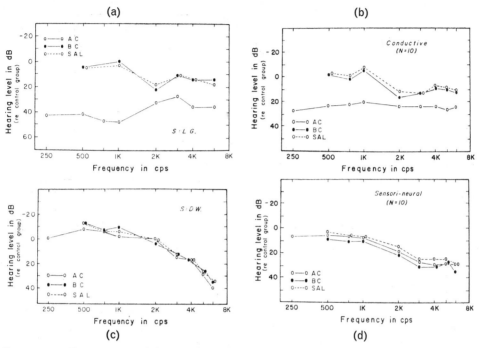

Figure 19-9. Equivalence of SAL and bone conduction. AC, BC, and SAL threshold hearing levels: (a) in a typical subject of the conductive group; (b) average of 10 "uni-lateral" conductives; (c) in a typical subject of the sensori-neural group; (d) average of 10 "unilateral" sensori-neurals.

Sensori-Neural Loss

AC, BC, and SAL thresholds were measured in 10 subjects with asymmetrical sensori-neural loss. All subjects in this group had a mild or moderate sensori-neural loss on one ear, and a severe or total sensori-neural loss on the other ear. Nine of the 10 subjects in this group gave no response to any BC signal on the poorer ear. In the remaining subject BC responses at a hearing level of 50 dB were noted at 500, 1 000, and 2 000 cps. Corresponding BC thresholds on the test ear of this subject were at the 40 dB level (ISO, 1964).

Figure 19-9c shows AC, BC, and SAL thresholds obtained on the better ear of a typical

region (1 000 to 4 000 cps) for pure sensori-neurals. Figure 19-10a compares his results with the present results for sensori-neurals and with the previous findings of Goldstein and others (1962) for sensori-neurals. Till-man's results above 1 000 cps show a much larger discrepancy between SAL and AC than either the present results, or those of Goldstein and others.

As a possible explanation for his finding, Tillman advanced the hypothesis that the abnormal masking effect previously observed by Jerger and others (1960) and by Rittmanic (1962) for frequencies above a noise band in sensorineurals might be operating in the SAL test. We find this explanation difficult to

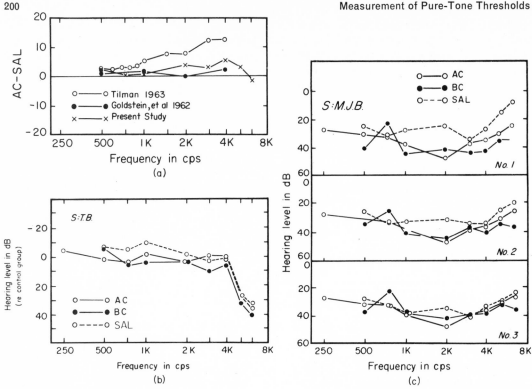

Figure 19-10. Analysis of Tillman phenomenon: (a) average difference between AC and SAL in three separate experiments involving sensori-neural hearing loss; (b) AC, BC, and SAL threshold hearing levels in a subject with sharply dropping high-frequency sensori-neural loss above 4 000 cps; (c) AC, BC, and SAL threshold hearing levels in a subject with sensori-neural loss obtained in three successive test sessions.

understand for two reasons. First, the effective pass band of most bone vibrators usually exceeds 4 000 cps, the highest frequency that Tillman measured. Second, the original observations of an abnormal masking effect above the noise band in sensori-neurals were made at effective noise levels in excess of those usually encountered in the SAL testing of sensori-neurals.

Nevertheless, we attempted to examine this hypothesis by testing a subject with a sharp loss in the region above 4 000 cps. Figure 19-10b shows the result. This kind of audiometric contour ought to be an optimal test of the abnormal-spread theory since it maximizes the effective level of the SAL noise. Yet we see nothing unusual at either 5 000 or 6 000 cps.

Certain observations made during our own experiments suggest an alternative explanation for Tillman's finding. After a considerable search we were successful in finding one subject who exhibited this behavior, that is, SAL above either AC or BC in the region above 1 000 cps. Figure 19-10c shows the result of three separate sessions with this subject. In session one we see the Tillman phenomenon. The second set of results was obtained after a short break during which the subject was admonished to listen more closely and try harder. The third set of results was obtained after another short break during which the subject was again instructed to listen more closely. The AC-threshold-in-noise condition was not singled out for any special instruction. The subject was simply told that the entire sequence of tests would be repeated and she must try harder. In other words, having found the Tillman phenomenon, we were able to make it disappear by careful instruction to the subject and repeated testing. The possibility that tester bias could have influenced these results is minimized by the fact that all thresholds were tracked by the Bekesy technique.

Effect of Occlusion

To this point we have compared SAL and BC only in the relative or unoccluded state. The question arises, therefore, "does the use of standard earphone cushions, which produce an occlusion effect, change the relationship between BC and SAL thresholds?" This possibility was investigated in two ways. First a group of 10 unilateral normals was tested with the good ear occluded by a standard SMR ear defender. We reasoned, here, that if direct occlusion of the external ear canal exerted a differential effect on BC and SAL responses, then the BC and SAL thresholds for this group, when referred to the norms for the unoccluded state, ought to differ in some systematic fashion. Figure 19-11a shows that this was not the case. Average BC and SAL thresholds for this group are quite similar.

It is well known, however, that the occlusion effect produced by an ear defender is both qualitatively and quantitatively different from the occlusion effect produced by an earphone-cushion combination, since, in the latter case, a much larger volume of air is enclosed. In order to explore this factor, three additional normal listeners were tested in the following fashion. First, BC and SAL thresholds were measured with the Pedersen earphones. Then the entire procedure was repeated with all conditions identical except that the Pedersen phones were replaced by Telephonic type TDH-39 phones mounted in MX41/AR cushions. We expected that both BC sensitivity and SAL shift would be changed in the latter condition, but reasoned that, if the occlusion effect produced by the MX41/AR cushions affected one measure more than the other, then the difference between the two BC curves ought to be different from the difference between the two SAL shifts. Figure 19-11b shows that this was not the case. In this figure the average difference is based on two separate threshold tracings by each of three subjects. The difference between the Pedersen and MX41/AR conditions (that is, the occlusion effect due to the MX41/AR cushions) is the same for BC and SAL.

We see, in these various findings, no evidence to suggest that the equivalence of BC and SAL thresholds demonstrated under Pedersen phones would be jeopardized by the use of MX41/AR cushions. To be sure the absolute values will differ, but the equivalence between BC and SAL in normal ears should

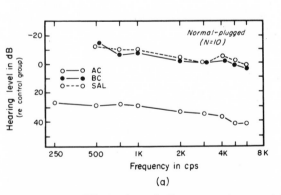
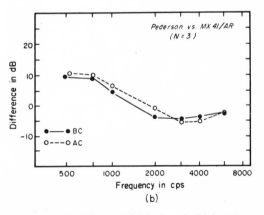

Figure 19-11. Effect of occluding normal ears: (a) average AC, BC, and SAL threshold hearing levels in 10 "unilateral" normals plugged by an ear defender; (b) average effect of occlusion by MX41/AR cushions on both BC and SAL thresholds in three normal ears.

hold for the occluded as well as the unoccluded state.

A recent paper by Burke, Creston, Marsh, and Shutts (1964), entitled "Variability of Threshold Shift in SAL Technique," con-

deviations of the distributions of AC, BC, and SAL in normal listeners. The standard deviations for AC are taken from Corso (1958) and are based on 60 normal ears. The standard deviations for BC are taken from the USPHS survey of 1935–36 (1938) and are based on 1 242 normal ears. The standard deviations for the SAL shift are taken from the paper

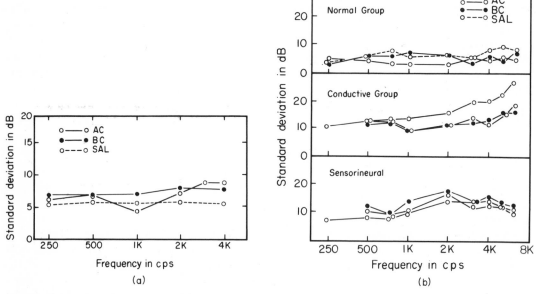

Figure 19-12. Variability of **AC, BC,** and **SAL:** (a) in normal ears (see text); (b) in normals, conductives, and sensori-neurals (present study).

tained a very curious piece of logic. The authors found that the threshold shifts obtained by the SAL technique in normal listeners were normally distributed with a standard deviation of about 6 dB. They concluded that ". . . this variability precludes the use of the SAL as a replacement for conventional bone-conduction audiometry and raises serious question as to its value as a diagnostic audiologic procedure." (1964, p. 159.)

These authors seem unaware that the norms for certain other audiometric procedures, notably conventional air-conduction and bone-conduction audiometry, are derived from data with a very similar distribution. Figure 19-12a, for example, compares the standard

of Burke, and others (1964) and are based on 30 normal ears. Note that variability among normals is, if anything, somewhat less for SAL than for conventional AC and BC.

The SAL norm, like the norms for AC and BC, is a statistical concept based on the central tendency of data reflecting both true individual differences and error of measurement. It is, in this respect, not different from the concepts of normal hearing by air-conduction and bone-conduction.

The fallacy in the argument of Burke and others, is the idea that their notion of "clinically acceptable error" (p. 156) applies to norms. If it did, we would have to reject air-conduction and bone-conduction audiometry for the same reason that they reject SAL.

Whenever one gathers data on normal thresholds, either by air-conduction or bone-conduction, either in quiet or in noise, one will inevitably observe that the data are normally distributed with a standard deviation of 6–8 dB. Now the SAL norm is simply the difference between air-conduction thresholds in quiet and in noise, and it is a well-known theorem in mathematical statistics (Cramér, 1951) that if A is a normally distributed random variable and B is an independent normally distributed random variable, then A-B is also a normally distributed random variable. Why the authors thought that SAL should be exempt from this very general probabilistic law is not made clear in their paper.

As their data very clearly show, the inherent variability of threshold shifts on which the SAL norm is based is neither more than nor less than the inherent variability on which other audiometric norms are based. If one concludes that this variability is sufficient to preclude the use of SAL for precise diagnostic audiometry, then clearly one must reject conventional air-conduction and bone-conduction audiometry on the same grounds.

Figure 19-12b compares the variability of AC, BC, and SAL in the three groups of 10 subjects each tested in the present series of experiments. In all groups the standard deviations for BC and SAL are reasonably comparable.

DISCUSSION

The present results encourage us to believe that the procedures underlying SAL audiometry are sound. Specifically, we have shown that: (1) the force with which the bone vibrator is applied to the head exerts no greater effect on the AC threshold in BC noise than on the conventional BC threshold; (2) neither the length of time the BC noise is on, nor the direction of frequency change of the Bekesy audiometer, exerts a significant

effect on the AC threshold in BC noise; (3) the linear masking functions characterizing air-conducted masking noise also hold for bone-conducted masking noise; (4) the acoustic reflex apparently does not confound the SAL test result; (5) SAL and BC threshold hearing levels are equivalent in both conductive and sensori-neural loss when both are measured in the relative state; and (6) occlusion of the ear canal with either ear defenders or MX41/AR cushion does not alter the equivalence of BC and SAL thresholds in normal ears.

Certain other procedural variables of hypothetical interest were not systematically explored in these experiments because of the earlier work of Keys and Milburn (1961). These investigators compared mastoid versus frontal placement of the bone vibrator and the use of narrow-band versus wide-band masking noise. Essentially, they found that neither refinement produced an appreciable effect on the SAL result.

We find, in these various results, no evidence inimical to the original recommended procedure for SAL audiometry, in which air-conduction thresholds are measured, either by standard manual or Bekesy audiometric technique, first in quiet, then in the presence of wide-band white noise delivered to the center of the forehead by a bone vibrator.

The meaningful clinical use of the SAL test requires, however, that the user understand the difference between absolute and relative bone conduction. In a typical clinical situation, where the earphones used to measure air-conduction thresholds are mounted in MX41/AR or similar earphone cushions, the SAL result must necessarily be the equivalent of absolute bone conduction. If the conventional bone-conduction system of the audiometer has been calibrated on open or unoccluded ears, then this system will measure relative bone conduction. SAL and BC will then differ in the low frequency region on conductive losses simply because the built-in occlusion effect of the patient with conductive loss gives him an artificial advantage relative to the normals on whom the BC system was calibrated, but does not influence the SAL result.

In this circumstance SAL and BC can be made to agree in conductive loss cases by simply calibrating the bone-conduction system on occluded normal ears. This can be accomplished by covering the test ear with the air-conduction receiver of the audiometer while testing the normal standardization group by bone conduction.

Finally, it must be observed that the masking level difference (MLD) phenomenon undoubtedly constitutes a source of slight error at frequencies below 1 000 cps, depending on the hearing level on the non-test ear. If the SAL system is calibrated on bilateral normals, then the maximum error would occur when a patient had normal hearing on the test ear and no hearing at all on the non-test ear. In such a patient the masked threshold on the test ear would presumably be unaffected by the correlated noise presented to the non-test ear and would, consequently, show a threshold shift greater than the norm by an amount equal to the maximum MLD effect (3 dB at 500 cps in the present experiment, but possibly ranging as high as 9 dB for a two-alternative forced-choice procedure). The potential error will be less than this maximum amount by the extent to which the difference between hearing levels on the two ears is less than maximal. According to the data of Weston and Miller (1964) the error should be fairly negligible when the difference between ears does not exceed 50–60 dB. The clinician must evaluate, for himself, the degree to which this potential error is likely to lead to a misleading result in the particular patient under study.

SUMMARY[1]

A series of experiments was conducted to evaluate SAL audiometry. Instrumentation was designed to assess both SAL and conventional bone-conduction (BC) audiometry in the relative (unoccluded) state. Results suggest the following conclusions.

(1) Varying the force of application of the bone vibrator from 250 to 1 000 gram weight has no greater effect on air-conduction (AC) thresholds in BC noise than on conventional BC thresholds.

(2) Neither the length of time the BC noise is on, nor the direction of frequency change of the Bekesy audiometer exert a significant effect on the AC threshold in BC noise, as measured by Bekesy audiometric technique.

(3) Masking functions for AC tones in BC noise are linear with unit slope, behaving, in this respect, like masking functions for AC tones in AC noise.

(4) The occurrence of the acoustic reflex apparently does not differentially affect the AC tone and the BC noise in the SAL procedure.

(5) SAL and BC threshold hearing levels are equivalent in both conductive and sensori-neural loss when both are measured in the relative state

(6) Occlusion of the ear canal with either ear defenders or an MX41/AR cushion does not alter the equivalence of BC and SAL thresholds.

[1] We are indebted to our colleagues at the Central Institute for the Deaf, especially James Miller, Ira Hirsh, and Peter Weston for their helpful suggestions throughout this research. This investigation was supported by Vocational Rehabilitation Administration Research Grant No. RD-1297S.

REFERENCES

Bailey, H. A. T., Jr., and Martin, F. N., A method for predicting post operative SRT. *Arch. Otolaryng.*, **77**, 177–180 (1963).

Bárány, E., A contribution to the physiology of bone conduction. *Acta Otolaryng.*, suppl. 26 (1938).

Blodgett, H. C., Jeffress, L. A., and Whitworth, R. H., Effect of noise at one ear on the masked threshold for tone at the other. *J. acoust. Soc. Amer.*, **34**, 979–981 (1962).

Burke, K. S., Creston, J. E., Marsh, A. J., and Shutts, R. E., Variability of threshold shift in SAL technique. *Arch. Otolaryng.*, **80**, 155–159 (1964).

Carhart, R., The clinical application of bone-conduction audiometry. *Trans. amer. Acad. Ophthal. Otolaryng.*, **54**, 699–707 (1950).

Corso, J., Proposed laboratory standard of normal hearing. *J. acoust. Soc. Amer.*, **30**, 14–23 (1958).

Cramér, H., *Mathematical Methods of Statistics*. Princeton University Press (1951).

Dirks, D., and Malmquist, Carolyn, Changes in bone-conduction thresholds produced by masking in the non-test ear. *J. Speech Hearing Res.*, **7**, 271–278 (1964).

Durlach, N. I., Equalization and cancellation theory of binaural masking level differences. *J. acoust. Soc. Amer.*, **35**, 1206–1218 (1963).

Egan, J. P., Masking-level differences as a function of interaural disparities in intensity of signal and of noise. *J. acoust. Soc. Amer.*, **36**, 1992 (1964).

Egan, J. P., and Benson, W., Masking-level difference for lateralization of a weak signal. *J. acoust. Soc. Amer.*, **36**, 1992 (1964).

Feldman, A. S., Problems in the measurement of bone-conduction. *J. Speech Hearing Dis.*, **26**, 39–44 (1961).

Goldstein, D. P., Hayes, C. S., and Peterson, J. L., A comparison of bone-conduction thresholds by conventional and Rainville methods. *J. Speech Hearing Res.*, **5**, 244–255 (1962).

Hart, C. W., and Naunton, R. F., Frontal bone conduction tests in clinical audiometry. *Laryngoscope*, **71**, 24–29 (1961).

Hirsh, I. J., and Burgeat, M., Binaural effects in remote masking. *J. acoust. Soc. Amer.*, **30**, 827–832 (1958).

Jerger, J., and Wertz, M., The indiscriminate use of masking in bone-conduction audiometry. *Arch. Otolaryng.*, **70**, 419–420 (1959).

Jerger, J., and Tillman, T., A new method for the clinical determination of sensori-neural acuity level (SAL). *Arch. Otolaryng.*, **71**, 948–955 (1960).

Jerger, J. F., Tillman, T. W., and Peterson, J. L., Masking by active bands of noise in normal and impaired ears. *J. acoust. Soc. Amer.*, **32**, 385–390 (1960).

Keys, J. W., and Milburn, B., The sensorineural acuity level (SAL) technique. *Arch. Otolaryng.*, **73**, 710–716 (1961).

König, E., Variations in bone-conduction as related to the force of pressure exerted on the vibrator. *Trans. Bel. Inst. Hearing Res.*, No. 6 (1957).

Lightfoot, C., The M-R test of bone-conduction hearing. *Laryngoscope*, **70**, 1552–1559 (1960).

Lilly, D. J., Some properties of the acoustic reflex in man. *J. acoust. Soc. Amer.*, **36**, 2007 (1964).

Martin, F. N., and Bailey, H. A. T., Jr., Clinical comment on the sensori-neural acuity level (SAL) test. *J. Speech Hearing Dis.*, **29**, 326–329 (1964).

Michael, L. A., The SAL test in the prediction of stapedectomy results. *Laryngoscope*, **73**, 1370–1376 (1963).

National Health Survey, 1935–1936. Normal hearing by air and bone conduction. *Hearing Stud. Ser. Bull.*, **4** (1938).

Naunton, R. F., Clinical bone conduction audiometry. *Arch. Otolaryng.*, **66**, 281–289 (1957).

Naunton, R. F., A masking dilemma in bilateral conduction deafness. *Arch. Otolaryng.*, **72**, 753–757 (1960).

Naunton, R. F., The measurement of hearing by bone-conduction, in *Modern Develpm. Aud.* (J. Jerger, Ed.), Academic Press, N.Y. (1963).

Naunton, R. F., and Fernandez, C., Prolonged bone-conduction: observations on man and animals. *Laryngoscope*, **71**, 306–318 (1961).

Palva, T., Goodman, A., and Hirsh, I., Critical evaluation of noise audiometry. *Laryngoscope*, **63**, 842–860 (1953).

Rainville, M. J., Nouvelle méthode d'assourdissement pour le relève des courbes de conduction osseuse. *J. Franc. Oto-Laryng.*, **4**, 851–858 (1955).

Rainville, M. J., New method of masking for the determination of bone conduction curves. *Transl. Bel. Inst. Hearing Res.*, No. 11 (1959).

Rittmanic, P. A., Pure-tone masking by narrow-noise bands in normal and impaired ears. *J. aud. Res.*, **2**, 287–304 (1962).

Schröder, K., Zur diagnostik der cochleareserve. *H. N. O. (Berl.)*, **11**, 33–38 (1963).

Tillman, T. W., Clinical applicability of the SAL test. *Arch. Otolaryng.*, **78**, 20–32 (1963).

Weiss, E., Personal communication (1961).

Weston, P. B., Bone-conducted tones masked by air-conducted noise. Unpublished masters thesis, Washington University (1964).

Weston, P. B., and Miller, J. D., Use of noise to eliminate one ear from masking experiments. *J. acoust. Soc. Amer.*, **36**, 2009 (1964).

part III

MEASUREMENT OF SPEECH THRESHOLDS

The audiometric assessment of hearing disorders frequently includes a speech threshold measurement and a suprathreshold measurement of speech discrimination function (see Part IV). A variety of speech thresholds have been defined, but only the spondee threshold (frequently called speech reception threshold or SRT)* is a standard part of speech audiometry.

Usually spondee threshold is defined as the lowest hearing level at which a subject repeats correctly 50 percent of the highly familiar spondaic words (two syllables, with approximately equal stress on each syllable) presented to him. The spondee threshold permits a rough estimate of the minimum stimulus intensity at which conversation will be understood. Measurement of spondee threshold also provides an independent check on the validity of pure-tone thresholds because there is well-documented agreement between spondee threshold and hearing sensitivity in the speech frequencies (500, 1000, and 2000 Hz). The articles in this section were selected to provide an understanding of spondaic stimuli, measurement methods, and interrelations with other measures.

Chaiklin's study of speech detection threshold, spondee threshold, and threshold of perceptibility for running speech, is included to show the effects of various threshold definitions on obtained results. The reader interested in further information on thresholds other than spondee threshold is referred to Egan's (1948) description of the various speech thresholds investigated at the Harvard Psychoacoustics Laboratory (PAL).

The lists of spondee stimuli developed at PAL were investigated at Central Institute for the Deaf (CID) by Hirsh *et al.* who sought to refine the criteria employed in the selection of the PAL spondaic stimuli (PAL Test No. 9). Their major goal was to produce a list of spondaic words that were more homogeneous in familiarity and intelligibility than the 84 stimuli of PAL Test No. 9. The 36 words they selected, largely drawn from the PAL words, are available in two

---

* We recognize that "speech reception threshold" is the more traditional usage, but chose to use the term "spondee threshold" because it is a more accurate description of the threshold being measured. Our usage is consistent with that of Tillman and Jerger, and Jerger, Carhart, Tillman, and Peterson (see Part I), among others.

recorded forms: CID Auditory Test W-1, which is a constant level recording, and CID Auditory Test W-2, which attenuates the words as the record progresses.

Hirsh *et al.* recognized that some of the CID spondaic words were more intelligible than others. To compensate for the intelligibility differences among the words in the final recordings, they raised the intensity of the least intelligible words and decreased the intensity of the most intelligible words. Subsequently, many clinicians observed that the CID recordings still resulted in obvious intelligibility differences among words. Curry and Cox present experimental data that substantiate this clinical impression, and they suggest shortening the CID spondaic word list to improve its homogeneity and, consequently, to improve the reliability of spondee threshold measurement. They also summarize Bowling and Elpern's (1961) data and suggestions for improving the homogeneity of the CID list.

Tillman and Jerger's study demonstrates the importance of familiarizing the patient with the stimulus words before spondee threshold measurement. They found that subjects not familiarized with the stimuli had spondee thresholds that were 4 to 5 db higher than thresholds obtained without familiarization. Hence, reliability of spondee thresholds in test and retest situations will probably suffer unless familiarization precedes the measurement process.

The article by Chaiklin and Ventry provides explicit procedures for spondee threshold measurement in 2-db or 5-db steps and presents data demonstrating that very little precision is lost by measuring spondee thresholds in 5-db steps rather than in the 2-db steps that most clinicians have favored in their clinical procedures.

The early work of Fletcher (1929), among others, established the relationship between the average of thresholds in the speech frequencies and spondee threshold. In a later publication Fletcher (1950) suggested that averaging the two lowest thresholds in the speech frequencies is the best method for predicting spondee threshold from pure-tone threshold data. A substantial number of studies have explored the 3-frequency and 2-frequency methods for predicting spondee threshold. We have selected the Siegenthaler and Strand article because it provides a critical summary of previous studies as well as original data on the same topic. They conclude that the 2-frequency method has slightly better predictive value than the 3-frequency method.

REFERENCES

1. Bowling, L. S., and Elpern, B. S. Relative intelligibility of items on CID auditory test W-1. *J. aud. Res.*, **1**, pp. 152–157 (1961).

2. Egan, J. P. Articulation testing methods. *Laryngoscope*, **58,** pp. 955–991 (1948).

3. Fletcher, H. *Speech and Hearing*. New York: Van Nostrand, 1929.

4. Fletcher, H. A method of calculating hearing loss for speech from an audiogram. *J. acoust. Soc. Amer.*, **22,** pp. 1–5 (1950).

20

The Relation Among
Three Selected Auditory Speech Thresholds [1]

JOSEPH B. CHAIKLIN

JOSEPH B. CHAIKLIN, Ph.D., is Professor of Audiology, University of Minnesota

Speech audiometry embraces the clinical procedures used in measuring auditory response to speech stimuli. Speech reception threshold (or threshold of intelligibility) and speech sound discrimination are the stimulus dimensions assessed most frequently in clinical practice. Speech reception threshold (SRT) is usually defined as the lowest hearing level at which a person repeats correctly 50 percent of the spondaic words heard by him. Speech sound discrimination (intelligibility function) is usually measured with lists of monosyllabic words phonetically balanced to include speech sounds in their approximate frequency of occurrence in daily conversation. The words are presented 30 to 40 db above SRT and the person under test says or writes the words as he hears them. The history of the development of SRT and intelligibility tests is well-documented elsewhere (2, 6, 8, 9, 10). The spondaic words of CID (Central Institute for the Deaf) Auditory Test W-1 and the phonetically balanced words of CID Auditory Test W-22 are the test materials in widest use at this time (9).

In some instances speech audiometry includes measures that employ running speech (or connected discourse) as a stimulus. The

Reprinted by permission of the author from *J. Speech Hearing Res.*, **2**, pp. 237–243 (1959).

[1] The research was supported by grants from the Speech Correction Fund, the Elks National Foundation, and the Veterans Administration.

thresholds of detectability, perceptibility, and intelligibility described by Egan (6) employ running speech as a stimulus. Thresholds of comfort and discomfort for speech are frequently included in speech audiometry as indexes of recruitment (11).

The published reports relating to speech thresholds provide rather incomplete data, particularly for the thresholds of detectability and perceptibility described by Egan. Thurlow and others (13) found threshold of detectability was 9 db lower than threshold for Psycho-Acoustics Laboratory (PAL) Auditory Test Number 9 (spondaic words) when they used 14 normal ears, but only 5.05 db lower for 237 hard-of-hearing ears. Hirsh (8) reported that the threshold of detectability for speech has a mean value of about 15 db and SRT for spondaic words (unspecified) is approximately 25 db (both *re* 0.0002 dyne/cm²). Preliminary work at the Central Institute for the Deaf (9) indicated an approximate threshold of 21 db (*re* 0.0002 dyne/cm²) for CID Auditory Test W-1 with inexperienced normal-hearing listeners. Corso (4) later established a threshold of 18.55 db (*re* 0.0002 dyne/cm²) for CID Auditory Test W-2 using 278 normal ears.

Falconer and Davis (7) studied the threshold of intelligibility for connected discourse (TICD) as a possible clinical tool for quick assessment of threshold for speech stimuli. They used a recording of Fulton Lewis, Jr., as a stimulus passage and for 50 normal ears found a mean TICD of 23.23 db (*re* 0.0002 dyne/cm²), in comparison with a mean threshold of 22.46 db (*re* 0.0002 dyne/cm²) for Auditory Test Number 9. They concluded that TICD, as administered in their study, is a reliable and valid threshold test.

The purpose of the present study was to investigate on an exploratory basis the relationships among speech reception threshold for CID W-1 spondaic words (SRT W-1), speech detection threshold (SDT), and threshold of perceptibility for running speech (TPRS).

PROCEDURE

Subjects

The subjects were 16 males and 14 females who ranged from 23 to 51 years of age with a mean age of 30 years, spoke American English as a first language, and had at least one ear with pure-tone thresholds at 500, 1000, and 2000 cps no higher than the 10-db hearing level.

Equipment

The basic test instrument was an Allison Laboratories diagnostic audiometer (Model 20A) equipped with Telephonics Corporation 10-ohm dynamic earphones (Model TDH 39). Speech stimuli were recorded and played back on an Ampex Corporation tape recorder (Model 350 P). The equipment has been described in greater detail in another article (*3*).

Calibration Checks

Calibration checks of the Allison audiometer speech circuit were performed periodically (*1*) with an Allison Laboratories Audiometer calibration unit (Model 300). The sound pressure output at the earphone was 24 db (*re* 0.0002 dyne/cm²) when a 1000-cps tone

was set at zero VU on the Allison audiometer VU meter and the hearing loss dial was set at 0 db. During all threshold measurements an additional 10 db of attenuation was inserted into the test earphone line by means of a nonreactive T-pad. This was necessary to provide an adequate range of attenuation below normal threshold for spondaic words.

Stimulus Materials

The same speaker (the experimenter) recorded all stimulus materials. The stimulus material for SDT and TPRS was a tape-recorded prose selection concerning ancient history. The running speech (connected discourse) script, which took five minutes to read, was read twice in succession providing 10 minutes of uninterrupted stimulus material. The script was read in such a fashion that most of the material peaked at zero VU. Lists A, B, and C of the 36 CID W-1 spondaic words (*9*) served as the stimulus materials for SRT W-1. They were recorded following the recording of the running speech section of the stimulus tape. The carrier phrase, "Say the word," peaked at zero VU, preceded each spondaic word. No special effort was made to peak the spondaic words at zero VU. A five-second interval elapsed between each spondaic word and the start of the succeeding carrier phrase. The sustained vowel [a] was recorded at zero VU at the start of the stimulus tape for use in adjusting input level at the start of each testing session. A single setting brought the carrier phrases and most of running speech to zero VU.

Threshold Assessment

The threshold tests used in this study were administered in the same fashion for all subjects. To control possible systematic order and fatigue effects a counterbalanced design was used. The counterbalancing procedure has been described previously (*3*). Three trials were made for each of the thresholds under study and the median of the trials was used as the final threshold estimate.* Written instructions were employed which the experimenter read to the subject after the subject had read them to himself. The right ear was tested unless the subject reported, during routine questioning, that his left ear was his better ear.

The following instructions were used for SDT:

Each time you hear something which sounds like speech, signal by raising your right index finger. Keep your finger raised as long as you hear something which sounds like speech. You do not have to understand the speech which you hear, but you should recognize the sounds as being speech—that is, the sound of someone talking. We will make several trials for this measurement. Be certain to put your finger down when you are not hearing something which sounds like speech.

At the start of each SDT trial the running speech stimulus was fully attenuated. The signal was increased in 2-db steps with five seconds of stimulation at each step. If the subject did not respond after five seconds the next higher step was tried. This procedure continued up to the level where the subject signalled properly for threshold determination. For each trial SDT was judged to be the lowest hearing level at which a subject indicated that he heard speech sounds continuously for five seconds. A five-second criterion for threshold estimate was used in an attempt to reduce the number of unreliable threshold estimates resulting from momentary reactions to stimulus intensity peaks not representative of the average intensity level of the speech stimulus.

The following instructions were used for TPRS:

[* For the purposes of this study, three trials were used to insure maximally reliable estimates, but I did not mean to imply that three trials are necessary for clinical threshold measurements. Apparently, the latter interpretation has occurred (see Newby, H. A. *Audiology*, 2nd ed. N.Y.: Appleton-Century-Crofts, 1964, p. 120). For most clinical purposes one trial is sufficient when the patient has been familiarized with the stimuli. JBC]

You are going to hear a recording of a man talking. The loudness of his voice will be decreased gradually. When his voice reaches a point where you can barely understand what he is talking about, *raise* your right index finger. It is a point where you may miss some of the words he is using, but where you still have a fair idea of what is being said. Keep your finger raised *as long as you can barely understand what is being said*. If I go below the point where you can barely understand what is being said, signal by lowering your right index finger. We will make several trials for this measurement. At the start of each trial I will make the speech loud enough to be understood easily. The only time your finger should be up is during the period when you are barely able to understand the speaker.

The test was started with the running speech signal set at 35 db above the normal reference level (24 db *re* 0.0002 dyne/cm²). The signal was attenuated at a slow rate (about 2 db per second) until the subject signalled that he could barely understand the recorded material. If, for five seconds, he continued to indicate that he barely understood the recording, the next lower 2-db step was tried. The same five-second criterion was applied for each succeeding 2-db decrease in signal strength. The signal was attenuated in this fashion until the subject lowered his finger to indicate that he no longer understood the stimulus passage. The lowest 2-db hearing level at which the subject barely understood the recording for five seconds represented TPRS.

The measurement of SRT W-1 was preceded by the following instructions:

You are going to hear a series of two-syllable words during the next few minutes. Your task will be to repeat the words as you hear them. At times the words will get very faint. When they get faint please try to guess at them. There will be no words longer than two syllables, and there will be no words shorter than two syllables. I am going to let you look at all the words which you will hear so that you can become familiar with them. There will be several trials for this measurement. At the start of each trial the words will be loud enough to be heard easily. After you have looked at the words, return them to me and the test will begin.

After the instructions were read, the subject was handed a stack of 36 cards. On each card there was typed one of the 36 CID W-1 spondaic words. After the subject had looked at each of the words the test was begun. At the start of each trial the spondaic words were set at 35 db above the normal reference level (24 db re 0.0002 dyne/cm²). The signal was attenuated in 5-db steps with one word being presented at each step until the subject failed to repeat a word correctly. The signal was then increased 5 or 6 db to an even step on the hearing-loss dial. At each succeeding 2-db decrement spondaic words were presented until (a) the subject repeated three words correctly without exceeding a maximum of six presentations, or (b) the subject missed four words without exceeding a maximum of six presentations. At each level, therefore, there were presented a minimum of three words (that is, three correct) or a maximum of six words (that is, three correct and three incorrect, or two correct and four incorrect). The threshold standard implicit in this method was that of 50 percent correct (three out of six). Thus at each level when the minimum limits described above were met, the experimenter moved to the next lower 2-db step. A tally of correct and incorrect responses was made as the test progressed. When four words were missed at each of three consecutive levels sampling was discontinued. This criterion for sampling discontinuance was used as a protection against premature acceptance of an early 50 percent-level as the lowest hearing level at which 50 percent of the spondaic words could be repeated correctly. For each of the three trials SRT W-1 was defined as the lowest hearing level at which the subject repeated three words correctly. It generally required about 15

minutes to complete the three trials for SRT W-1.

RESULTS

Table 20-1 summarizes the mean threshold values and standard deviatiosn for each test.

TABLE 20-1. MEANS AND STANDARD DEVIATIONS FOR SPEECH DETECTION THRESHOLD (SDT), SPEECH RECEPTION THRESHOLD (SRT W-1), AND THRESHOLD OF PERCEPTIBILITY FOR RUNNING SPEECH (TPRS), N = 30

Measure	Mean * (db)	Standard Deviation (db)
SDT	16.47	3.45
SRT W-1	25.47	3.85
TPRS	28.93	3.00

* Mean threshold values re 0.0002 dyne/cm².

The mean SDT was 16.47 (re 0.0002 dyne/cm²), the mean SRT W-1 was 25.47 db, and the mean TPRS was 28.93 db. Pearson product-moment correlations and t tests for related measures (4) were employed in statistical analyses which are summarized in Table 20-2. Values of t significant beyond the .001

TABLE 20-2. RESULTS OF THE t TEST FOR RELATED MEASURES AND PEARSON PRODUCT-MOMENT CORRELATION COEFFICIENTS FOR THE INTEREST COMPARISONS

Test	Mean (db)	Diff. (db)	S. E. Diff.	t	r
SRT W-1	25.47	3.46	.73	4.74 *	.27 †
TPRS	28.93				
SRT W-1	25.47	9.00	.66	13.64 *	.51 **
SDT	16.47				
SDT	16.47	12.46	.65	19.17 *	.35 †
TPRS	28.93				

* Significant beyond .001 level.
† Not significant at .05 level.
** Significant beyond .01 level.

level were found for each of the mean comparisons, indicating significant mean threshold differences among the tests. The correlational analyses produced low positive values of r for all three comparisons. The .51 correlation between SRT W-1 and SDT was significant (P = .01), but the SRT W-1-TPRS correlation ($r = .27$) and the TPRS-SDT correlation ($r = .35$) were not significant. The low correlations between thresholds raised the question of whether each of the three threshold tests might be unreliable enough to contribute to the low correlations between tests. To check on this possibility, average intercorrelations (*12*) were computed among the three trials that were made for each test. The average intercorrelations among trials yielded an r of .82 for trials of TPRS, an r of .87 for trials of SDT, and an r of .77 for trials of SRT W-1. These findings indicate that the separate tests were relatively reliable measures, hence the low correlations between tests may be presumed to have been primarily a function of differences between the tests rather than a function of their unreliability.

DISCUSSION

The results summarized above suggest that in the average case the instructions for each test served to produce significant differences among the thresholds. The relatively low correlations observed between tests are consistent with the variability in test relationships observed from subject to subject. For example, while the mean SDT was 9 db lower than the mean SRT W-1, several subjects had SDT and SRT W-1 determinations that were within 2 db of each other. Yet there were other instances in which these thresholds were 12 to 16 db apart. Sometimes SRT W-1 was within 2 db of TPRS but in several cases TPRS was 8 to 10 db higher than SRT W-1. Both SDT and TPRS evidenced little tendency to approximate each other. It was observed that TPRS was always higher than SDT, yet even here individual variation was apparent with differences between the two thresholds ranging from 6 to 20 db.

Comparison with Previous Findings

Egan (*6*) reported TPRS was 8 db above SDT as contrasted with the 12.47-db gap

betwen SDT and TPRS found in the present study. Hirsh's (*8*) reported mean SDT of 15 db (*re* 0.0002 dyne/cm²) agrees closely, however, with the mean SDT of 16.47 db reported above. The 9-db difference found between SDT and SRT W-1 agrees identically with the difference between SDT and threshold for spondaic words (Auditory Test No. 9) found by Thurlow and others (*13*) for normal ears. The mean SRT W-1 of 25.47 db reported in the present study agrees well with Hirsh's (*8*) general estimate of threshold for spondaic words (25 db *re* 0.0002 dyne/cm²) but it is higher than the tentative threshold of 21 db (*re* 0.0002 dyne/cm²) stated by Hirsh and others (*9*) for the CID recordings of CID Auditory Test W-1, and higher than the 18.55 db (*re* 0.0002 dyne/cm²) threshold Corso (*4*) found for CID Auditory Test W-2. Falconer and Davis' (*7*) finding that TICD agrees closely with the threshold for PAL Auditory Test No. 9 (spondaic words) is not consistent with the findings of the present study. Since TICD is the level at which a subject believes he understands all of the running speech material without perceptible effort, it is by definition a higher threshold than TPRS (where the subject is barely able to understand the stimulus passage). In the present study the mean TPRS was 3.46 db higher than SRT W-1 and while TICD was not measured, Egan's (*6*) estimate that it is about 4 db above TPRS appears reasonably accurate. One can estimate, thus, that if TICD had been measured in the present study it would have been approximately 7 db above SRT W-1.

Differences in stimulus materials, sample composition, or methodology may account for some of the differences noted above. For example, Corso tested 139 subjects, 18–24 years old, with W-2 recordings in an anechoic chamber, while in the present study 30 subjects, 18–51 years old,† were tested with dif-

[† Since the average age of subjects in this study was 30, it is probably not appropriate to view the SRT mean as a normative figure. The focus of the study was on relative values, hence it was feasible to use subjects older than the young adults used in most normative studies. JBC]

ferent recordings, in a room not having an-echoic properties. It appears that there is fairly good agreement that the normal threshold for spondaic words lies somewhere between 18–25 db (*re* 0.0002 dyne/cm^2), which is consistent with the 22 db (*re* 0.0002 dyne/cm^2) normal threshold specified for speech audiometers by the American Standards Association (*1*). The threshold relationships among SRT, TICD, and TPRS may be clarified by further research with larger populations.

SUMMARY

Sixteen male and 14 female subjects with normal hearing received the following threshold tests: (a) speech detection threshold (SDT), (b) speech reception threshold for CID W-1 spondaic words (SRT W-1), and (c) threshold of perceptibility for running speech. The stimulus materials, which were tape recorded by one speaker (the experimenter), consisted of a sample of running speech for SDT and TPRS measurements and lists A, B, and C of the CID Auditory W-1 spondaic words for SRT W-1.

The mean SDT was 16.47 db, the mean SRT W-1 was 25.47 db, and the mean TPRS was 28.93 db (all *re* 0.0002 dyne/cm^2). Statistical analyses revealed significant differences (values of *t* beyond the .001 level) and low positive correlations for all threshold comparisons. A discussion of threshold data from previous reports points out several areas of difference which might be resolved by further research.

REFERENCES

1. American Standards Association, *American standard specification for speech audiometers.* Report Z24.13-1953, Section 3.12.

2. Black, J. W., The origin and nature of the studies (in Studies in speech intelligibility, a program of wartime research). *Speech Monogr.*, 13, 2, 1946, 1–3.

3. Chaiklin, J. B., The conditioned GSR auditory speech threshold. *J. Speech Hearing Res.*, 2, 1959, 229–236.

4. Corso, J. F., Confirmation of the normal threshold for speech on C. I. D. Auditory Test W-2. *J. acoust. Soc. Amer.* 29, 1957, 368–370.

5. Edwards, A. L., *Statistical Analysis.* New York: Rinehart, 1946.

6. Egan, J. P., Articulation testing methods. *Laryngoscope*, 58, 1948, 955–991.

7. Falconer, G. A., and Davis, H., The intelligibility of connected discourse as a test for the "threshold for speech." *Laryngoscope*, 57, 1947, 581–595.

8. Hirsh, I. J., *The Measurement of Hearing.* New York: McGraw-Hill, 1952.

9. Hirsh, I. J., Davis, H., Silverman, S. R., Reynolds, Elizabeth G., Eldert, Elizabeth, and Benson, R. W., Development of materials for speech audiometry. *J. Speech Hearing Dis.*, 17, 1952, 321–337.

10. Hudgins, C. V., Hawkins, J. E., Karlin, J. E., and Stevens, S. S., The development of recorded auditory tests for measuring hearing loss for speech. *Laryngoscope*, 57, 1947, 57–89.

11. Newby, H. A., *Audiology; Principles and Practice.* New York: Appleton-Century-Crofts, 1958.

12. Peters, C. C., and Van Voorhis, W. R., *Statistical Procedures and their Mathematical Bases.* New York: McGraw-Hill, 1940.

13. Thurlow, W. R., Silverman, S. R., Davis, H., and Walsh, T. E., A statistical study of auditory tests in relation to the fenestration operation. *Laryngoscope*, 58, 1948, 43–66.

21

Development of Materials for Speech Audiometry[1]

IRA J. HIRSH
HALLOWELL DAVIS
S. RICHARD SILVERMAN
ELIZABETH G. REYNOLDS
ELIZABETH ELDERT
ROBERT W. BENSON

IRA J. HIRSH, Ph.D., is Dean of the Faculty of Arts and Sciences, Washington University and Director of Research, Central Institute for the Deaf

HALLOWELL DAVIS, M.D., is Research Associate, Central Institute for the Deaf

S. RICHARD SILVERMAN, Ph.D., is Director, Central Institute for the Deaf, and Professor of Audiology, Washington University

ELIZABETH G. REYNOLDS was a Research Assistant at Central Institute for the Deaf at the time this study was conducted

ELIZABETH ELDERT was an audiologist, Department of Otolaryngology, Washington University School of Medicine, at the time this study was conducted

ROBERT W. BENSON, Ph.D., is with R. W. Benson and Associates, Inc., Nashville, Tennessee

The sounds of speech have come to occupy an important place among the auditory stimuli that are used in clinical audiometry. By measuring a patient's ability to use his hearing in ways that are closer to everyday auditory experience, speech audiometry has not only added a kind of validity to pure-tone audiometry, but also certain speech tests have appeared to have diagnostic and prognostic value as well (10). The growth in the general acceptance and use of speech audiometry is accompanied by a need for standardization so that the test results in one clinic can be compared with those of another clinic. The present article deals with modifications of existing recorded auditory tests that yield new auditory tests, which appear to satisfy

Reprinted by permission of the authors from *J. Speech Hearing Dis.*, **17,** pp. 321–337 (1952).

[1] These materials were developed under contracts with the Veterans Administration (Contract V100lM-577) and the Office of Naval Research (Contract N6onr-272, Project No. NR142-170, Task Order III).

some clinical needs that were not fulfilled by older tests. In particular, tests will be described that permit the measurement of two clinical quantities: *hearing loss for speech* and *discrimination loss*.

BACKGROUND

During World War II, considerable effort was expended in the development of articulation testing methods for the evaluation of various types of military communications equipment. It turned out that certain of these tests, developed at the Psycho-Acoustic Laboratory, Harvard University, were applicable to the clinical evaluation of hearing.

Psycho-Acoustic Laboratory (PAL) Auditory Tests No. 9 and No. 12, for measuring the threshold of intelligibility for spondaic words and for sentences, respectively, were made available on phonograph records for clinical use—first for military rehabilitation centers and then for more general use. These two recorded tests permitted a quick and reliable measure of the threshold of intelligibility and its related clinical measure, the hearing loss for speech. They have been described by Hudgins *et al.* (*11*), by Hirsh (*9*), and others.

In a study of patients who were evaluated with respect to suitability for the fenestration operation, Davis (*2*) and his co-workers have formulated a general estimate of a patient's ability to hear speech by coupling the results on the threshold of intelligibility (or the hearing loss for speech) with a measure of the ability to discriminate among speech sounds at levels considerably above the threshold. This latter ability was measured by using the Psycho-Acoustic Laboratory's PB-50 lists, which are the phonetically balanced lists described by Egan (*5*). It appears that both types of tests are clinically useful and, indeed, that the latter measure of discrimination loss is the more useful clinical datum because the former, hearing loss for speech, can be predicted so reliably from the audiogram (*1, 6, 8*).

Several years have passed during which many audiometrists have had a chance to try out the spondee words and the PB-lists both by live-voice techniques and by way of phonograph records. During these years, reports have accumulated of several deficiencies in the Harvard tests, deficiencies mostly with respect to clinical use. Specifically, it has been reported informally that certain of the records of Auditory Test No. 9 yield slightly different thresholds from other of these records. Further, the large vocabulary that was assembled for the 20 PB-lists [published in Egan (*6*)] was too large for many clinical patients. The vocabulary appeared to need restriction in the dimension of familiarity. Finally, recorded versions of the PB-lists have not been available in suitably standard form.

This article does not purport to reveal any basically new concepts or techniques. It represents, rather, a report of modifications of these earlier tests in order to correct or eliminate some of these deficiencies that have been found as the tests have been used clinically.

Two basic improvements, from the clinical point of view, have been made. *First*, the vocabulary for the spondee lists and the PB-lists has been restricted so as to include only those words that meet certain criteria of familiarity. Furthermore, the vocabulary in each PB-list has been more rigidly phonetically balanced. The more rigid application of criteria of phonetic balance has resulted in a smaller test vocabulary, but one that appears to be sufficiently large for the small samples of lists that characterize clinical use. A *second* major improvement has been made possible by the use of recording on magnetic tape. With this recording technique it was possible to speak a given test word only once and then to copy it as many times as necessary to have it appear on different versions of a given test list. In the older tests, for example, the word *hothouse* appeared in each of six scramblings (word orders) of one spondee list. Since the test was made from original disc recordings, the word had to be spoken six times, once within each scrambling. With tape, one would have to speak the word only once, copy it six times, and cut and resplice the actual tapes in order to produce the word in its proper place in each of the six word orders.

An improved version of the Auditory Test No. 9 for clinical use is C.I.D. Auditory Test W-2 (spondees at descending levels). The comparable modification of Auditory Test No. 14 is C.I.D. Auditory Test W-1 (spondees at constant level). Finally, recorded versions of the modified PB-lists appear as C.I.D. Auditory Test W-22. A general description, method of construction, and preliminary test results for each of these three tests follows.

DESCRIPTION AND DEVELOPMENT

C.I.D. Auditory Test W-1

Test W-1 consists of six scramblings of a single list of 36 spondaic words. These are recorded at a constant level, each word at a level 10 db below the level of an introductory carrier phrase, "Say the word . . ." On the inside of each of the six record faces, a *1000 cps tone has been recorded at the level of the carrier phrases, that is, 10 db above the test words.* Since it was desirable that the carrier phrases be well above the level of the test words, especially for those playback levels at which the test words would be just barely intelligible, the tone could not be recorded at the level of the test words without endangering the monitoring meter of the test user. If, for example, the tone were recorded at the same level as the test words, and a playback were adjusted so that an ordinary VU meter read "0 VU," the carrier phrases would force the indicator to hit the pin at the right side of the scale.

Use of Test W-1. In general, Test W-1 permits the measurement of the threshold of intelligibility, the level at which a listener repeats correctly 50 percent of the words of a given list, by traditional methods of articulation testing. In clinical application, it may be used by the audiometrist who wishes to control manually (with an attenuator that is variable in decibel or some multiple of decibel steps) the intensity of the words presented to a listener.

Construction of Test W-1. The starting point for vocabulary was the group of 84 spondee words in PAL Test No. 9 (and No. 14). The most familiar spondees were obtained from ratings of judges who, working independently, rated the words in the Harvard tests on a three-point scale of familiarity. The words rated most familiar were spoken by an adult male and were recorded on a phonograph disc.

Two acetate discs were cut simultaneously, one for future rerecording and one for preliminary use. The talker monitored the carrier phrase "Say the word," carefully on a VU meter, and then spoke the following test word with "equal effort." When spoken in this manner the words varied from each other in intensity level by about ±2 db. Some words were spoken several times until

the talker felt that a satisfactory rendition had been obtained.

In a preliminary experiment, six listeners with normal pure-tone audiograms listened monaurally to the words through standard playback equipment (see Appendix A). The group included both experienced and inexperienced listeners. Instructions were as follows:

> You are going to hear a list of two-syllable words, like "baseball" and "armchair." A man's voice will say "Say the word" before each word. Listen for the word following. Some groups of words are louder, some are softer than others. Repeat through the microphone what you hear. If you hear only unintelligible sound after "Say the word," let me know by saying "Check."

Individual thresholds for speech (in db re 0.0002 microbar) were obtained for the spondaic word lists in the PAL Test 9. The method of scoring was that described in Hudgins *et al.* (*11*). Each listener then listened to the disc recording of the more familiar (CID) spondees at +4, +2, 0, −2, −4, and −6 db relative to the threshold that had been obtained for PAL Test 9. The order in which the lists were presented was the same for each listener. The order in which the different levels appeared, however, was varied for each listener and each list according to a random Latin Square design. In this design, dependent variables, such as learning and fatigue, are presumably weighted equally at each level in the averaged data for six listeners. All data for each listener were obtained in one listening session.

Raw data were recorded in terms of the number of errors per word for each listener. One word, relatively much easier than the others, might be repeated correctly even at levels 4 and 6 db below the threshold. Consequently, there would be very few errors for that word. And conversely, a difficult word might not be heard correctly, even at levels 2 and 4 db above the threshold, and would have many errors. In the analysis of this preliminary data an easy word was defined as one missed once or less by all six listeners. A difficult word was one missed five or more times by all six listeners. Words falling in both of these extreme categories were eliminated, and also the words that five of the six listeners found difficult or easy. In the 36 words left, a group of equally intelligible spondees was approximated.

The original disc reserve was then dubbed to tape. The 36 chosen words were cut out and spliced together with enough blank tape between words to facilitate the separate attenuation of individual words. This was called the *master tape* and all subsequent versions of the 36 words were recorded from this tape. One carrier phrase was recorded with good quality and even monitoring. This carrier was recorded separately from the words and therefore sounds qualitatively different from the words. This difference, however, in no way affects the results of the tests and is not very noticeable at levels around threshold where the test is given. This was called the *master carrier phrase*. It could be rerecorded any number of times by making a loop of it and running the tape around and around on the recording head of the tape recorder.

Six different word orders of the same 36 words were put together in the following manner. The master tape was dubbed to tape again six times. The order of the words in five dubbings was changed by cutting the words apart and resplicing them in different positions within each list. The master carrier phrase was then recorded once for each of the 216 words in the six lists at +10 db relative to the words. A carrier phrase was spliced in front of each word and the timing made such that one carrier phrase plus the word following plus the pause for a listener's response took six seconds. The six word orders were designated as Lists A, B, C, D, E, and F of W-1 and an appropriate recorded introduction was spliced in front of each. A copy of these lists as just described was made for experimental purposes and the original spliced version was held in reserve.

An experiment similar to the preliminary testing was then run. One Latin Square was done with inexperienced listeners, how-

ever, and another with experienced listeners. The six word orders were given to all listeners in the same sequence, although the levels at which different listeners heard different word orders were determined by a random Latin Square. Tentative speech thresholds were determined this time by using one of the experimental word lists. The words were presented at this threshold (0 db) and +4, +2, −2, −4, and −6 db. Raw data for each group of subjects were scored as errors for each word at each of the presentation levels.

Performance on the separate words varied little between the experienced and inexperienced listeners. For present purposes, therefore, their data were treated together. An inspection of the data showed that some words were still more difficult, some easier, than others in spite of the initial attempt to get a group of words homogeneous with respect to intelligibility. The degree of difficulty of a word was correlated with the intensity reading of the word on a VU meter. The easy words monitored at higher levels, the more difficult words at lower levels, relative to the average intensity reading for the 36 words. This correlation existed even though originally the words were spoken with "equal effort" and varied only ±2 db from an average intensity reading. It was therefore decided to push the more difficult words up 2 db and the easier words down 2 db.

A second set of the same six word orders was made from the master tape changing the levels of the more difficult or easier words by ±2 db in each rerecording of the master tape. The experiment described above was repeated. An analysis of the data showed that the words were now more homogeneous with respect to intelligibility and variations in the thresholds of individual words were, as adequately as could be measured by this method, chance variations. Since tape reproducers are not in general clinical use, and since there is no good way of copying large numbers of tape recordings, this last version of the six word lists was recorded on discs as Auditory Test W-1.

This final recording was done at the Technisonic Recording Studios. The word lists were recorded both at 78.26 rpm and 33⅓ rpm with the NARTB recording characteristic (*14*). A half-minute of a 1000 cps calibration tone, at the level of the carrier phrase, was put at the inner edge of each record so that individual operators can set their levels on a constant signal.

Preliminary Test Results for Test W-1. The articulation-vs.-gain function for Test W-1 as recorded on the final tapes is shown in Figure 21-1. The function represents the data of all listeners, six inexperienced and six experienced, and was drawn as the most representative curve for the series of individual curves superposed on each other at 0 db, or threshold. Therefore the function is to be interpreted as showing slope relative to threshold with no indication of the absolute levels involved.

The articulation score rises from 0 to 100 percent within a range of about 20 db. There is an increase from 20 to 80 percent within a range of 8 db and throughout this range the slope or rate of rise in score is about 8 percent per db. Since the threshold falls on the steepest part of the function, it is crossed very abruptly and, therefore, can be very sensitively determined with this test. There is a definite "tail" on the upper end of the curve. The rate of rise of the curve tapers off above 80 percent and does not reach the 100 percent point until about +14 db above threshold. Much of this tapering is due to the performance of the inexperienced listeners at levels above threshold. They were not familiar with the words or the listening situation and therefore continued to miss a few words even at levels above threshold where their scores should have been nearer 100 percent. Momentary inattention on the part of all listeners also contributed to the flattening of the function at the upper end. Below threshold the words drop out very quickly and there is little if any "tail" at this end of the curve.

The absolute thresholds for the experienced and inexperienced listeners were approximately the same, 20 db and 21 db re 0.0002 microbar, respectively. The difference between the two thresholds was not significant.

Preliminary checks were also made with the first disc recordings of Test W-1. Fourteen listeners (in groups of four or five) listened monaurally to all six scramblings at each of two levels, one below threshold and the other above. These levels were not the same for all listeners as each earphone used had a correction factor of its own which changed the output level. The two points obtained in each

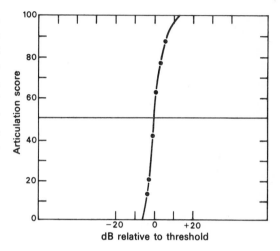

Figure 21-1. Articulation score as a function of level relative to individual threshold (Auditory Test W-1). Points represent average scores for 12 listeners.

case were connected by a straight line, the slope of which was close to 8 percent per db, and the approximate threshold was interpolated from this straight line function. The mean absolute threshold obtained in this way was 14.3 db re 0.0002 microbar and the standard deviation of the individual mean thresholds around this mean was 2.2 db.

It should be stressed here that the above results with the new W-1 disc recordings are tentative and await confirmation from those who use the test according to the instruction manual issued with the test.

C.I.D. Auditory Test W-2

Test W-2 employs the 36 words that were used in W-1 and also the same six word orders. Test W-2 differs from W-1, however, in that the intensity of the words is attenuated within each list at the rate of 3 db every three words. In the older PAL Test 9 the rate of attenuation was 4 db every six words. In the present test, it was attempted to employ a faster pace and also to avoid the necessity of a table for scoring by letting each word represent 1 db of attenuation on the average.

Use of Test W-2. This test is designed specifically for a rapid estimate of the threshold of intelligibility. The six word orders, labelled lists A through F, are the same as those of Test W-1. Instead of presenting a whole list or a portion of a list at a fixed intensity or several intensities, this test sweeps through an intensity range of 33 db by attenuating the level of the test words 3 db every three words. The rationale for this procedure consists of sampling three-word portions of the list at intensity levels that are 3 db apart. Ideally the intensity level at which a listener repeats 50 percent of a group (i.e., 1.5 words) would be the threshold. Actually, the threshold is approximated by assuming that the words are attenuated at an average rate of 1 db per word and that the threshold is the level at which the first group of three words is presented minus the number of words (or of decibels) that the listener repeats correctly.

Of course, a threshold calculated in this way will be in error because the 50 percent-criterion is not fully met unless 50 percent of the first group (i.e., the first 1.5 words) is first subtracted out of the total. The 1.5-db error involved is a constant of small magnitude relative to ordinary test results and may be neglected in clinical use. The absolute thresholds to be given below have taken this correction into account and represent, therefore, the best approximation to a 50 percent-response level. In general, the clinical norms, if established without this correction, should be 1.5 db lower.

Construction of Test W-2. When the master tape was dubbed again to tape for this test, the initial relative level of the same words was changed ±2 db in each rerecording as they

had been for the final version of Auditory Test W-1. In addition, in each rerecording every word was separately attenuated in such a way that when the words were spliced together in the same order as in W-1 the intensity within each list decreased 3 db every three words.

Two hundred sixteen copies of the master carrier phrase were made, one for each word in W-2. The first nine carriers for each list were recorded at the level of the first three words. The intensity of the rest of the carrier phrases for each list was decreased 3 db after every three carrier phrases. In the final spliced version of the test, therefore, the first nine carrier phrases are at the starting level of the test even though the intensity of the test words in these first three groups is already being attenuated. From the tenth item on, the carrier phrases are progressively attenuated, each carrier phrase remaining 6 db above the word that follows it.

A carrier phrase at the correct relative level was then spliced in front of each word. The lists were designated as lists A, B, C, D, E, and F of W-2, corresponding to the same lists in W-1. Appropriate introductions were then spliced in front of the lists. Finally, copies of this original spliced version were made for experimental purposes.

The experimental problem was to find out if there were any differences in difficulty among the lists. A group of six experienced listeners were given the six word orders of Auditory Test W-2. The tests were started at 40 db above 0.0002 microbar so that, assuming that the thresholds would be around 20 db, a listener would repeat approximately half the list before reaching threshold. Instructions to the listener were the same as for the experiments with Auditory Test W-1. The order in which each listener heard the W-2 lists was determined by a random Latin Square design.

An analysis of variance showed that different thresholds obtained by using different word orders varied no more than would be expected by random error. There were differences, however, in the average thresholds for six listeners as obtained with the different lists. Differences were of the order of ±1 db. It appears that the lists of words are not equal in difficulty unless each entire list is heard. When only part of the list is heard the difficulty of the list depends on which part is heard. For a given listener it cannot be said that all parts of the lists are equal in difficulty.

The six word lists were then recorded on discs at the Technisonic Recording Studios. These lists were also recorded at 78.26 rpm and at 33⅓ rpm with the NARTB recording characteristic (14). Again, as for W-1, a 1000 cps calibration tone was put at the inner edge of each record. This calibration tone is at the average level of the first nine carrier phrases and of the first three words.

Preliminary test results. The same 14 listeners who listened to the W-1 disc recordings also listened to the W-2 recordings. Each of the listeners heard all six scramblings of W-2 and individual thresholds were taken as the mean of the six scores for each listener. Lists were started at a level of 35 db re 0.0002 microbar and, as described, the level of each successive three words decreased 3 db. When the test is started at 35 db for normal ears half or more of the test is heard before threshold is reached.

The mean absolute threshold for 14 listeners was 17.7 db re 0.0002 microbar. (This includes the 1.5 db correction mentioned earlier.) The standard deviation of the individual thresholds was 2.6 db. The difference between the W-1 and the W-2 thresholds of about 3.5 db in favor of W-1 may result from presenting all 36 words at a given level instead of only three. In actual clinical practice Test W-1 should be administered, as described in the manual, by "bracketing" the threshold using small samples of four or five words at levels around threshold. Thresholds obtained in this manner will undoubtedly be closer to those obtained with W-2.

An analysis of variance showed that there were no significant differences in difficulty between the W-2 lists as they were recorded on disc. Again, however, as with the tape versions, there were differences of the order of ±1 db.

C.I.D. Auditory Test W-22

Test W-22 consists of a vocabulary of 200 monosyllabic words divided into four lists of 50 words each. Each list is phonetically balanced; that is, the speech sounds within the list occur with the same relative frequency as they do in a representative sample of English speech. Six scramblings of each list are available. The words have been spoken with the carrier phrase, "You will say," and the 1000 cps calibration tone on the inner face of every record is at the average level of the carrier phrases.

Use of Test W-22. This test is used to determine a patient's discrimination loss for speech. The discrimination loss for speech is the difference between 100 percent and the percentage of given speech material that a listener repeats correctly at a level that is sufficiently high so that a further increase in intensity is not accompanied by a further increase in the amount of speech material repeated correctly. Low discrimination scores, i.e., large discriminations losses, have been found to yield important diagnostic distinctions (2).

Construction of Test W-22. The most important task was the selection of the vocabulary to make up the phonetically balanced word lists. The following criteria for the vocabulary were set up. First, all the words must be one-syllable words with no repetition of words in the different lists. Second, any word chosen should be a familiar word. This second criterion is to minimize the effect of differences in the educational background of subjects. Third, the phonetic composition of each word list should correspond to that of English as a whole as closely as possible.

This third criterion was the most difficult one to satisfy because there are no satisfactory studies of spoken English in the literature. The sources used were Dewey's study (4) of the phonetic composition of newsprint and the Bell Telephone Laboratories' study (7) of business telephone calls in New York City. The two sources were given equal weight in the determination of the phonetic criteria for the word lists.

The sources were followed as closely as possible. First the distribution of syllable types (vowel-consonant, consonant-vowel-consonant, etc.) was determined. Then the distribution of vowels and consonants within each list was planned. Here the frequency of occurrence of consonants and consonant compounds in initial and final positions was considered. All distributions of phonetic elements were based on distributions of individual speech sounds rather than on groups of sounds.

The vocabulary of the 20 Psycho-Acoustic Laboratory PB-50 lists, a total of 1000 words, was used as a pool from which words were drawn for Auditory Test W-22. From this pool 120 words were used. The remainder of the vocabulary (80 words) was not drawn from any specific source.

Five people independently rated the entire PAL vocabulary for familiarity. They were instructed to rate about half the words in each PB-50 list as 1 (most familiar), about 25 percent as 2 (fairly familiar), and approximately 25 percent as 3 (very unfamiliar). Agreement among the five raters was good. A final rating in familiarity, based on the rating given by the majority of the raters, was then assigned to each word. Of the 120 words from the PAL lists used in Auditory Test W-22, 112 were rated as 1, 7 as 2, and only one, "isle," as 3.

The entire W-22 vocabulary, a total of 200 words, was checked with the Thorndike list (15). All words except "ace" appear on the Thorndike list. According to Thorndike, 190 are among the 4000 most common English words; 171 are among the 2000 most common words; and 144 are among the 1000 most common words. The W-22 vocabulary was also checked with the Dewey list (4). Of the 200 words, 128 appear on this list. All of these 128 words are among the first 2000 most common words on the Thorndike list.

The only words of doubtful familiarity are "ace," "ale," and "pew." These words received a rating of 2 by the board of judges and are relatively unfamiliar according to the Thorndike lists. "Isle," which was given a rating of 3 by the judges, is among the 3000 most common words according to Thorndike; as "aisle" it is in the first 5000; and as "I'll" it is in the first 2000. In general, the vocabulary consists of very common words.

The third criterion states that the phonetic composition of the lists shall correspond as closely as possible to that of English as it is generally spoken.

The first step in setting up a plan for phonetic balance was to decide on percentages for the various consonant-vowel arrangements found in monosyllabic words (Table 21-1).

TABLE 21-1. W-22 DISTRIBUTION OF SYLLABLE TYPES

Type	Percentage of words
VC	20
CV	22
CVC	36
VCC	4
CCV	2
CVCC	10
CCVC	4
CCVCC	2

This decision was based on the analysis of syllable types in the study by French, Carter and Koenig (7), with the following modifications. All vowel words were omitted. The high frequency of their occurrence depends on two words, "I" and "you." The percentage of consonant-vowel-consonant words was increased slightly and the percentage of words containing consonant compounds (two or more consonants in a row) was increased from 14.7 percent to 22 percent. The distribution of syllable types followed the French, Carter and Koenig study as closely as was practicable. In each W-22 list there were four initial consonant compounds and eight final compounds.

The next step was to decide on the distribution of vowels within each list (Table 21-2).

The mean of the percentages given by Dewey (*4*) and by French, Carter and Koenig (*7*) for the frequency of occurrence of each vowel was followed as closely as possible. The following modifications were made. The neutral vowel was omitted from the distribution, since this vowel does not ordinarily appear in monosyllabic words. The percentages for the other vowels were increased, therefore, by an appropriate amount to make up for the absence of the neutral vowel from the distribution. Percentages for long vowels were also increased in order to fulfill requirements for syllable distribution. In general, a plan for the distribution of vowel sounds was worked out which was practicable, and it was followed exactly in each list.

Finally, the distribution of consonants was determined (Table 21-3). As for the vowel sounds, the mean of the percentages given by Dewey and by French, Carter and Koenig for the frequency of occurrence of each consonant sound was followed. The percentage for each consonant was divided into a quota for appearance of that consonant in initial and final positions. This was done by referring to both Dewey and the French, Carter and Koenig study and following their divisions roughly. The number of words in each PB-list (50 words) is too small to permit precise division

TABLE 21-3. W-22 CONSONANT DISTRIBUTION

Sound	Number of occurrences in each PB list	
	Initial	Final
t	4	7
n	3	7
r	2	7
d	3	3
l	2	4
s	3	3
m	2	3
k	3	1
w	4	0
z	0	4
v	0	3
ð	2	1
h	3	0
f	1	1
p	1	1
b	2	0
j	2	0
ŋ	0	1
g	1	0
ʃ	1	0
θ	1	0
tʃ	1	0
dʒ	1	0
ʒ	0	0
	—	—
	42	46

TABLE 21-2. W-22 VOWEL DISTRIBUTION

Vowel Sound	Percent occurrence in each W-22 list
ɪ	12
æ	10
ɛ	10
ɑ	8
ʌ	8
i	10
e	10
o	6
u	6
ɑɪ	6
ɔ	4
ʊ	4
ɑʊ	2
ɪʊ	2
ɔɪ *	1
ɝ *	1

* The ɔɪ vowel occurs once in two lists and the ɝ sound in the other two lists.

of the consonants into quotas for initial and final positions.

Once the four PB-lists, each containing 50 different monosyllabic words, had been chosen they were recorded on magnetic tape. The talker used the carrier phrase "You will say." He monitored this phrase on a VU meter and then spoke the word as it would naturally follow in the phrase.

The four lists dubbed from live voice to magnetic tape were the master lists. Each list was then rerecorded six times and the words were cut and spliced in different orders to give six different word orders for each of the lists. There was no master carrier. Each phrase was kept intact as it had been spoken. The lists were designated Lists 1, 2, 3, and 4 and the word orders for each were lettered A through F. Appropriate introductions were then spliced into the recording. Copies on tape of the spliced version were made for experimental purposes and the original was kept for rerecording onto disc.

Trouble was encountered with signal transfer from one layer of tape to the layer directly underneath on the reel both on the original recording and on the copies. This phenomenon is recognized by the tape manufacturer but usually the level of the transfer signal is very low and is not noticeable in a continuous recording. The transfer signal on the recordings was 45 to 50 db below the signal and below threshold at lower playback levels. At the highest playback levels used in the experiment, however, particularly at 100 db, the "echo" was above threshold in the pauses between phrases. In the following experiments, the words were presented at a level 20 db above an intermixed white noise. The noise effectively masked the echo but did not interfere with the intelligibility of the words. When the lists were dubbed to disc the cutting head on the recording lathe was short-circuited between each phrase so that none of the echo was recorded.

An experimental check was made to determine whether the four lists were equal in difficulty. It was assumed that there would be no differences in difficulty among different word orders of the same list. Three groups of five listeners, a total of 15 in all, were used. They were screened at +10 db relative to normal threshold for all test frequencies on the Maico pure-tone audiometer. Each group of five came on eight consecutive evenings (Saturdays and Sundays excluded) and listened each evening for $2\frac{1}{2}$ hours including two or three rest periods.

Instructions were as follows:

You are going to hear lists of one-syllable words. All the words you will hear are on the printed sheet I have just given you. At the beginning of each session you will be given the chance to look at this list. Some lists will be very loud and others will be very soft. Listen carefully and write down as many words as you can.

Group I first listened monaurally to all 24 lists (six word orders of each of four lists) at 100 db re 0.0002 microbar. This procedure gave the listeners an indoctrination period in which the words were presented at a high level. Then they heard each of the 24 word lists at levels 10 db apart from 20 to 70 db re 0.0002 microbar. Lists and levels were randomized with the exception that no list was ever heard twice at the same level.

Group II listened under the same conditions. The lists and levels were in a different order, however, and an eighth level of 15 db re 0.0002 microbar was also used when it was found that not enough low scores at 20 db were being obtained to determine the bottom of the articulation curve. Group III first listened to all lists at 100 db. Then they listened to each word order at 50, 40, 30, 20 and 15 db re 0.0002 microbar. The scores from the first two groups were consistently near 100 percent correct above 50 db and it was felt that the shape of the upper part of the curve was well determined without running Group III at 60 and 70 db.

The articulation scores for each list are plotted as a function of sound pressure level in Figure 21-2. At higher levels there are no significant differences between the list scores. From 40 db down, however, there are greater differences. The gain function for List 1 was consistently lower than for the other lists. A second articulation curve (the broken curve) drawn through the scores for List 1 alone is shifted over on the scale approximately 2 db. A calculation of the average relative intensity of the words in each list as read from a VU meter showed that the words in List 1 were on the average 2.5 db lower than the words in any other list. Therefore, in the final recordings from magnetic tape to disc the intensity of List 1 was increased 2 db relative to the intensity at which the other three lists were recorded.

The threshold (50 percent-response) for these new PB-lists as determined from the experimental curve in Figure 21-2 is 24 db re 0.0002 microbar.

After inspection of the above data and the subsequent decision to raise the relative level of List 1 2-db, the six word orders of each list were recorded onto disc from tape. The lists were recorded at $33\frac{1}{3}$ rpm and 78.26 rpm. A calibration tone at the average level of the carrier phrase "You will say" was put on the inner band of every record.

Preliminary Test Results for Test W-22. The articulation function for Test W-22 has already been discussed under the construction of the test and is shown in Figure 21-2. This function was obtained using the experimental tapes. After the tapes were dubbed to disc for the final version of the test the articulation function was checked at two points using the disc recordings. The disc recordings were played to 15 listeners (in groups of 5) at 80 db re 0.0002 microbar to check the maximum articulation score and at 25 db to check scores close to threshold.

The average score at 80 db using the disc recordings was 98 percent as compared to a score of approximately 99 percent at 80 db read from the articulation function. At 25 db scores were higher with the 78 rpm recordings than with the $33\frac{1}{3}$ rpm recordings. The average score for the 78 rpm's was 63.4 percent, for the $33\frac{1}{3}$ rpm's, 56.3 percent. The $33\frac{1}{3}$ score agrees closely with the articulation score that would have been obtained at 25 db with the experimental tapes (see Figure 21-2).

Although the same word orders of a list monitor alike on both the 78 and the $33\frac{1}{3}$ rpm recordings, it is very possible that the high frequencies were given a boost of a few db on the 78 rpm recordings. This boost does not show up in the monitoring as the VU meter is responding primarily to the energy around 250 cps which is the peak energy of the speaker's voice. Since the high frequencies are important in the discrimination of many consonants a high frequency boost in the recording might be accompanied by an increased articulation score for the recordings affected.

These data showed no consistent differences between scores on the four different lists. All listeners were given ample opportunity to study alphabetical lists of the words, however, and heard scramblings of each list at least three times. In a shorter clinical procedure

where listeners may hear scramblings of two different lists once, some sort of differences between lists may appear from listener to listener. It can only be said that the averaged data of several listeners from several tests showed no consistent difference between lists.

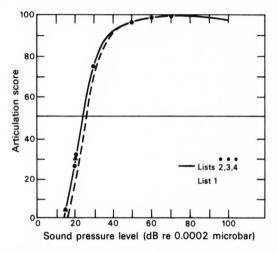

Figure 21-2. Articulation score (Auditory Test W-22) as a function of sound pressure level (experimental tape versions). Each point is the average of 15 listeners' scores on all six word orders of a list. The solid curve is drawn through points for Lists 2, 3, and 4. The broken curve is drawn through the points for List 1.

As with the W-1 and W-2 results these results await verification from several clinics using a large number of listeners.

DISCUSSION

Although this report is intended to be only a description of some new auditory tests, it seems appropriate to discuss the relations among these tests and their predecessors. This discussion is supported by experimental data on a relatively few listeners. Most of the conclusions must remain tentative until a larger amount of clinical information is available.

Relations Among The New Tests

There are two outstanding relations that have been established with groups of normal listeners: one concerns the relation between W-1 and W-2 and the other between W-1 and W-22.

Descending-Level vs. Constant-Level Spondees. It has already been shown that the threshold for W-2 is about 4 db above the threshold for W-1. That this difference is real is attested by some observations in which W-1 recordings were used as if they were W-2. Otherwise said, the W-1 recording was begun at a certain sound pressure level and the experimenter

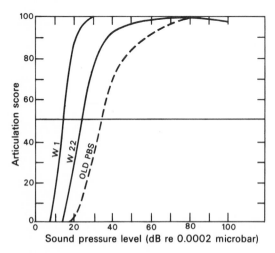

Figure 21-3. Relations between Auditory Test W-1, W-22, and the old PB-50 lists recorded at Technisonic Studios. The broken curve refers to the older version of the PB-lists. The solid curve labelled W-1 is the same curve found in Figure 21-1, but drawn relative to the average absolute threshold for 12 listeners. The curve labelled W-22 is the curve drawn for Lists 2, 3, and 4 in Figure 21-2.

attenuated the words by 3 db every three words. The results of this procedure yielded thresholds of the order of 18 db re 0.0002 microbar, the tentative standard threshold for W-2. It seems fair to conclude that the difference between the thresholds for W-1 and W-2 is attributable to the number of words that are presented at each level. From a restricted point of view, the W-1 threshold, at about 14 db,, represents the experimental ideal. When W-1 is put to clinical use, however, the tester ordinarily presents only four

or five words at each level. Thus, in clinical use, when all 36 words are not presented at each test level, the expected threshold will be more nearly 18 db, as for W-2.

Spondees vs. Monosyllables. Figure 21-3 shows the articulation-vs.-gain functions for all versions of W-1 and W-22. Two generalizations may be made: (1) The intelligibility of the spondee words (W-1) increases more rapidly with increase in intensity than does the intelligibility of the monosyllabic words of the PB-lists (W-22), and (2) the level at which a listener can repeat correctly 50 percent of a list of spondees is lower than for one of the PB-lists of monosyllables. The reasons for the lower spondee threshold have been treated adequately elsewhere (*5, 11, 12, 13*). It should be pointed out here, however, that the threshold for the present PB-lists (W-22) is much closer to the spondee threshold than have been the thresholds for previous PB-lists (see below).

Relations Between Present and Former Recorded Tests

It is clear that the results for normal listeners with these new recorded tests are not the same as the results for the older tests. Some of these differences need to be pointed out in detail.

Relation Between W-2 and PAL Auditory Test No. 9. The present W-2 threshold of 18 db is somewhat lower than the threshold for Test No. 9 (22 db). The reasons for this difference cannot be attributed entirely to the new recording procedure. First, the old threshold at 22 db is a clinical threshold, somewhat higher than experimental ones. Furthermore, the total spondee vocabulary in W-2 is only 36 words while the total vocabulary for Auditory Test No. 9 is 84 words, or 42 words on either version. In view of the relation between the intelligibility of a given list of words and the size of the vocabulary for the list, which has been pointed out by Miller, Heise and Lichten (*13*), it is not surprising that the threshold for the new tests with a smaller vocabulary should be lower. Again, it must be kept in mind that these thresholds are restricted to a psychophysical procedure in which only a few words are presented at each level. The low threshold that is obtained for W-1 indicates the order of difference that may be accounted for by these variations in the testing procedure.

Relation between W-22 and the older PB-lists. For some time a set of recordings of some of the PB-lists published by Egan has been available for distribution from the Technisonic Studios. These have enjoyed sufficient clinical use so that some tentative standards have become available. The articulation-vs.-gain function for these recordings is shown as a third curve in Figure 21-3. It is clear that the intelligibility of these older recordings at any given level is lower than for W-22 and that the function for the older recordings is not nearly so steep as that for W-22. Several reasons may be given for this difference. It has already been shown, in the above discussion of the development of Test W-1, that the intelligibility of a word is markedly dependent on its intensity relative to the other words in a list. The monitoring in W-22 is such that all of the words are much closer to each other in intensity than they were on the older recordings of the Egan lists. Furthermore, the vocabulary for W-22 consists of a total of 200 words while the total vocabulary in the Egan list was 1000 words. Again, noting the relation between intelligibility and vocabulary size (*13*), it is not surprising that the intelligibility of the smaller vocabulary should be higher at any given level than for the larger vocabulary*

There are certain clinical questions that arise concerning the usefulness of W-22 in measuring discrimination loss. The smaller vocabulary makes W-22 an "easier" test than

[* Comparison between the described speech-discrimination test and an older discrimination test based upon an earlier recording of the Harvard PB-Lists will be found in Silverman, S. R., and Hirsh, I. J., Problems related to the use of speech in clinical audiometry. *Ann. Otol. Rhinol. Laryngol.*, **64**, pp. 1234–1244 (1955): IJH, *et al.*]

the older PB-lists. Both the vocabulary and the greater internal homogeneity contribute to a steeper gain function for W-22 than for the older PB-lists (*12*) (see Figure 21-3). There is not available as yet sufficient clinical information to predict whether this higher intelligibility and steeper gain function will make the use of W-22 more limited in the measurement of discrimination loss than the use of the older PB-lists.

SUMMARY

Three new recorded tests for the hearing of speech have been described. Tests W-1, W-2, and W-22 have been constructed to take the place of recorded versions of PAL Auditory Tests 14 and 9 and the PB-lists published by Egan respectively. Two novel techniques have been introduced: (1) The use of magnetic tape recording has permitted the construction of several versions or word orders of a given test list in which all occurrences of a test item in the several versions are physically identical; (2) The criterion of phonetic balance in W-22 and the criterion of familiarity of test items in both tests have been more rigidly followed, resulting in easier, more homogeneous lists, but with a more limited vocabulary.

Preliminary results have been presented in which the intelligibility for these new tests is shown as a function of intensity. Furthermore, a relation between intelligibility for these new tests and their analogous predecessors has been established. The authors' recommendation for the clinical adoption of these tests is tentative, pending the accumulation of results on larger groups of listeners in both clinical and laboratory situations.[2]

[2] While this paper was in preparation clinical trials of W-2 and W-22 were conducted in the Hofheimer Audiology Laboratory (Washington University) and in the Hearing Clinic of Central Institute for the Deaf. Experience to date indicates (1) that W-2 is very satisfactory for determining the threshold for speech, but (2) that W-22 does *not* satisfactorily separate patients with mixed deafness from patients with pure conductive deafness. The older recordings of the Egan lists are more effective in this respect. The reasons for this difference are now being sought.

APPENDIX A

Equipment

The equipment necessary for reproducing the recordings of Auditory Tests W-1, W-2, and W-22 is represented by the American Standard Speech Audiometer [3] and includes the following elements:

1. A turntable and phonograph pickup with NARTB (National Association of Radio and Television Broadcasters) playback characteristic.

2. An amplifier.

3. A meter for monitoring the output of the amplifier.

4. An attenuator.

5. A calibrated earphone or loudspeaker.

The components are shown in the block diagram below:

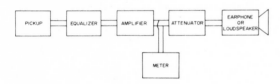

The turntable should be capable of playing recordings at a speed of $33\frac{1}{3}$ rpm or of 78.26 rpm. The pickup should exert a force not greater than 10 grams. The pickup should be equalized so that it reproduces the frequencies in accordance with the NARTB characteristic.

Appropriate amplifiers should be used in order to obtain the power level necessary to drive either the earphone or the loudspeaker. The output noise of the amplifier should be at least 50 db below the signal under all conditions. The meter should be provided to indicate the rms value of a 1000 cps tone. A VU meter is very convenient but it is not essential.

An attenuator should be provided with a maximum insertion loss of at least 110 db with indicated steps of 5 db or less. If the indicated steps are 5 db, an accessory vernier

attenuator with steps of 2 db or 1 db is very desirable.

The earphone or loudspeaker should be of good quality in order to meet the following requirements. The over-all response characteristic including the pickup and equalizer, amplifier, attenuator and earphone or loudspeaker should not deviate more than plus or minus 5 db from the NARTB characteristic over the frequency range from 200 to 5000 cps. Furthermore, at no frequency from 50 cps to 10,000 cps should the pressure exceed the pressure at 1000 cps by more than plus 5 db.

APPENDIX B

The following lists of words constitute the vocabulary of the three Auditory Tests described in this report. Only an alphabetical order is given here. The ideal test lists used in the recorded versions are randomized orders of these words. The reader can make up equivalent test lists from these alphabetized orders by suitable scrambling.

ALPHABETICAL LIST OF THE SPONDAIC WORDS USED IN AUDITORY TESTS W-1 AND W-2

1. airplane	19. iceberg
2. armchair	20. inkwell
3. baseball	21. mousetrap
4. birthday	22. mushroom
5. cowboy	23. northwest
6. daybreak	24. oatmeal
7. doormat	25. padlock
8. drawbridge	26. pancake
9. duckpond	27. playground
10. eardrum	28. railroad
11. farewell	29. schoolboy
12. grandson	30. sidewalk
13. greyhound	31. stairway
14. hardware	32. sunset
15. headlight	33. toothbrush
16. horseshoe	34. whitewash
17. hotdog	35. woodwork
18. hothouse	36. workshop

[3] *American Standard Specification for Speech Audiometers.* New York: American Standards Association (in preparation).

ALPHABETICAL LISTS OF THE WORDS IN AUDITORY TEST
W-22

List 1	List 2	List 3	List 4
1. ace	1. ail	1. add	1. aid
2. ache	2. air	2. aim	2. all
3. an	3. and	3. are	3. am
4. as	4. been	4. ate	4. arm
5. bathe	5. by	5. bill	5. art
6. bells	6. cap	6. book	6. at
7. carve	7. cars	7. camp	7. bee
8. chew	8. chest	8. chair	8. bread
9. could	9. die	9. cute	9. can
10. dad	10. does	10. do	10. chin
11. day	11. dumb	11. done	11. clothes
12. deaf	12. ease	12. dull	12. cook
13. earn	13. eat	13. ears	13. darn
14. east	14. else	14. end	14. dolls
15. felt	15. flat	15. farm	15. dust
16. give	16. gave	16. glove	16. ear
17. high	17. ham	17. hand	17. eyes
18. him	18. hit	18. have	18. few
19. hunt	19. hurt	19. he	19. go
20. isle	20. ice	20. if	20. hang
21. it	21. ill	21. is	21. his
22. jam	22. jaw	22. jar	22. in
23. knees	23. key	23. king	23. jump
24. law	24. knee	24. knit	24. leave
25. low	25. live	25. lie	25. men
26. me	26. move	26. may	26. my
27. mew	27. new	27. nest	27. near
28. none	28. now	28. no	28. net
29. not	29. oak	29. oil	29. nuts
30. or	30. odd	30. on	30. of
31. owl	31. off	31. out	31. ought
32. poor	32. one	32. owes	32. our
33. ran	33. own	33. pie	33. pale
34. see	34. pew	34. raw	34. save
35. she	35. rooms	35. say	35. shoe
36. skin	36. send	36. shove	36. so
37. stove	37. show	37. smooth	37. stiff
38. them	38. smart	38. start	38. tea
39. there	39. star	29. tan	39. tin
40. thing	40. tear	40. ten	40. than
41. toe	41. that	41. this	41. they
42. true	42. then	42. three	42. through
43. twins	43. thin	43. though	43. toy
44. up	44. too	44. tie	44. where
45. us	45. tree	45. use	45. who
46. wet	46. way	46. we	46. why
47. what	47. well	47. west	47. will
48. wire	48. with	48. when	48. wood
49. yard	49. young	49. wool	49. yes
50. you	50. your	50. year	50. yet

REFERENCES

1. Carhart, R. Speech reception in relation to pattern of pure tone loss. *JSD*, 11, 1946, 97–108.

2. Davis, H. The articulation area and the social adequacy index for hearing. *Laryngoscope*, 58, 1948, 761–778.

3. Davis, H., Morrical, K. C. and Harrison, C. E. Memorandum on response characteristics and monitoring of word and sentence tests distributed by CID. *J. acoust. Soc. Amer.*, 21, 1949, 552–553.

4. Dewey, G. *Relative Frequency of English Speech Sounds.* Cambridge, Mass.: Harvard Univ. Press, 1923.

5. Egan, J. P. Articulation testing methods *Laryngoscope*, 58, 1948, 955–991.

6. Fletcher, H. A method of calculating hearing loss for speech from an audiogram. *J. acoust. Soc. Amer.*, 22, 1950, 1–5.

7. French, N. R., Carter, C. W. and Koenig, W. The words and sounds of telephone conversations. *Bell Syst. tech. J.*, 9, 1930, 290–324.

8. Harris, J. D. Free voice and pure-tone audiometry for testing of auditory acuity. *Arch. Otolaryng., Chicago*, 44, 1946, 452–467.

9. Hirsh, I. J. Clinical application of two Harvard auditory tests. *JSD*, 12, 1947, 151–158.

10. ———. *The Measurement of Hearing.* New York: McGraw-Hill, 1952.

11. Hudgins, C. V., Hawkins, J. E., Karlin, J. E. and Stevens, S. S. The development of recorded auditory tests for measuring hearing loss for speech. *Laryngoscope*, 57, 1947, 57–89.

12. Levin, R. The intelligibility of different kinds of test material used in speech audiometry. M.A. Thesis, Washington Univ., 1952.

13. Miller, G. A., Heise, G. A. and Lichten, W. The intelligibility of speech as a function of the context of the test materials. *J. exp. Psychol.*, 41, 1951, 329–335.

14. *Recording and Listening Test Standards.* Washington, D.C.: Nat. Ass. Radio Telev. Broadcast., 1950.

15. Thorndike, E. L. *A Teacher's Word Book Of The Twenty Thousand Words Found Most Frequently and Widely In General Reading For Children And Young People.* New York: Teachers Coll., Columbia Univ., 1932.

22

The Relative Intelligibility of Spondees

E. THAYER CURRY
B. PATRICK COX

E. THAYER CURRY, Ph.D., is Director of the Speech Science Laboratory, University of Alabama, Tuscaloosa, Alabama
B. PATRICK COX, Ph.D., is Assistant Professor of Audiology, Gallaudet College

INTRODUCTION

The role of speech audiometry techniques has been extended beyond the realm of a simple, routine test. The notable example is the increased use of speech audiometric procedures and materials in the assessment of central auditory disorders. However despite the prominence and growing dependence on speech audiometry since its inception, only meager research has been devoted to scrutinizing the methodology involved. Techniques and materials for discrimination testing have received the attention of considerable research, but threshold assessment has scarcely been investigated. Thus the clinical audiologist may rely on statements such as that of Harris (1963) that "a commendable effort has gone into standardizing the Speech Reception Threshold Test with spondee words, and a Discrimination Score with Phonetically Balanced monosyllables. Scores and hundreds of clinics can arrive at virtually the same SRT and DS for a particular ear." However, the more sophisticated clinician realizes, in his day-to-day testing activities, that the materials and procedures of speech audiometry do not always produce the results one might expect. The threshold of hearing for speech,

for example, often varies more than would be expected from acceptable clinical error.

A review of the matter shows that with one notable exception little has been done to refine SRT test methodology since the early 1950's. Bowling and Elpern (1961) estimate the range of intelligibility of items in C.I.D. Auditory Test W-1. They presented randomized versions of Lists A and B, at increasing intensity intervals of 4 db, to 24 normal-hearing Ss (mn = 36 yrs of age), all inexperienced with auditory tests in general. They concluded:

"The range computed from data produced by these subjects was found to be 10 dB, which is considered to be unduly wide and detrimental to the precision of the test. Present results have led to the conclusion that the precision of auditory speech threshold measurements may be enhanced through the use of an indicated group of 22 words exhibiting a range of only 3.5 dB."

The C.I.D. Auditory Test W-1 is reported to fulfill criteria for stimulus materials designed for SRT evaluation (see Silverman and Hirsh, 1955), and is in fact the most widely-used clinical tool for assessing an individual's SRT. However, the comments of Bowling and Elpern are often corroborated in actual clinical tests in that these 36 words differ

Reprinted by permission of the authors from *J. aud. Res.*, **6**, pp. 419–424 (1966).

widely in level of intelligibility. If this is the case one of the most important criterial attributes for satisfactory SRT test materials may not be realized.

This study investigated the range of relative intelligibility of the words in the C.I.D. Auditory Test W-1 on a normal-hearing population. Such an investigation was expected to answer these important questions: (1) What is the range of intelligibility of the spondee words used, and (2) Is there a group of stimulus words within this test which falls within a more acceptable range of intelligibility and should therefore provide a more reliable tool for assessing the SRT?

PROCEDURE

Apparatus

The Ss were tested with an audiometer and in workspace which met specifications of the U.S.A. Standards Institute. SPLs for both the pure tone and speech output systems were measured with the Bruel and Kjaer Type 2203 meter at the onset, the middle, and the conclusion of the testing period. The pure tone levels for the prescribed frequencies fell within the recommended specifications (ASA 1951). The constancy of the speech signal was checked by measuring the output SPL of the 1000 c/s tone recorded on the experimental tape. The levels in the subsequent medial and final readings did not deviate more than 0.5 db from the initial reading.

Test Materials

A $33\frac{1}{3}$ rpm disc recording of the W-1 Test, Lists A–D (4 randomizations of the same 36 words) was transferred to a magnetic tape using an Ampex Type 350 tape recorder and the disc playback of the Allison Type 22 audiometer. This tape was then played to S through the Viking tape recorder associated with the Allison audiometer for the appropriate output channel. Each spondee was preceded by the carrier phrase, "Say the

word." S spoke his response into the audiometer's intercom microphone, whereupon correct responses were noted on a response sheet by the experimenter (E).

Subjects

Fifty students served, 18 males and 32 females, aged 17–40 yrs (mn = 21.2). Each had at least one ear with a pure-tone threshold better than 10 db HL (re ASA, 1951) for each audiometer frequency from 250–4000 c/s. Each spoke English as his native language and was reported to be unfamiliar with auditory tests in general.

Test Procedure

Each S was first given a pure tone test, then the following written instructions were given and also read face-to-face:

Now you are going to have a test a little different from the test you have just taken. Instead of listening for tones I want you to listen for some words. Please read along with me now. These are the words I will be giving you: airplane, armchair, baseball, birthday, cowboy, daybreak, doormat, drawbridge, duckpond, eardrum, farewell, grandson, greyhound, hardware, headlight, horseshoe, hotdog, hothouse, iceberg, inkwell, mousetrap, mushroom, northwest, oatmeal, padlock, pancake, playground, railroad, schoolboy, sidewalk, stairway, sunset, toothbrush, whitewash, woodwork, workshop.
Notice that each of these words has two syllables. On the recording I will play for you these words will be preceded by the phrase, "Say the word." There is no penalty for guessing so repeat the word even if you only hear part of it or have to guess. Remember, repeat the word as soon as you barely hear it.

These instructions served two purposes. First, S became more aware of the nature and purpose of threshold tests. Second, in view of the findings of Tillman and Jerger (1959) and other investigators, it was presumed that thresholds of Ss who had been given prior knowledge of the test vocabulary would be more independent of the practice effect and therefore more reliable.

Following the instruction session, S was fitted with binaural TDH-39 earphones (although the test was administered monaurally). The test ear was determined in a random manner. At the onset of the test, the attenuator was set at −10 db HL and a complete list (chosen at random) of the words was given at this level. The stimulus materials were presented at a rate of one list at each ascending 2-db step until S achieved 100 percent identification. Each S served as his own baseline control: the level at which an S gave his first correct response was referred to as his 0 db sensation level (SL). Any of the other spondees correctly identified at this

TABLE 22-1. COMPARISON OF RELATIVE INTELLIGIBILITY OF THE 36 SPONDEE WORDS

| Spondee | Mean Sensation Level in db | | Difference | Range of Responses of Subjects in Present Study |
	Bowling & Elpern	Present Study		
WORKSHOP	2.7	2.8	0.1	0–12
BASEBALL	5.0	3.0	—	0–8
HOTDOG	3.0	3.8	1.2	0–12
ICEBERG	4.8	4.0	0.8	0–14
AIRPLANE	4.7	4.2	0.5	0–12
ARMCHAIR	7.5	4.4	3.1	0–10
PLAYGROUND	4.5	4.6	0.1	0–10
DRAWBRIDGE	8.2	4.8	3.4	0–14
WOODWORK	4.3	4.8	0.5	0–10
HARDWARE	3.5	4.9	1.4	2–10
COWBOY	4.3	5.0	0.7	0–24
BIRTHDAY	6.3	5.6	0.7	0–22
GREYHOUND	7.0	6.0	1.0	0–18
EARDRUM	6.9	6.1	0.8	0–16
SUNSET	6.2	6.2	—	0–18
NORTHWEST	5.2	6.2	1.0	0–14
SIDEWALK	6.0	6.5	0.5	0–18
RAILROAD	4.8	6.5	1.7	2–16
DAYBREAK	8.3	6.6	1.7	0–14
DOORMAT	8.3	6.8	1.5	0–26
SCHOOLBOY	8.5	6.9	1.6	0–16
INKWELL	8.8	7.0	1.8	0–16
OATMEAL	7.0	7.6	0.6	0–12
MUSHROOM	10.3	7.7	2.6	2–18
MOUSETRAP	7.7	7.7	—	0–24
WHITEWASH	7.2	7.8	0.6	0–18
FAREWELL	6.3	8.0	1.7	0–24
PADLOCK	8.3	8.0	0.3	0–26
STAIRWAY	6.3	8.0	1.7	0–28
TOOTHBRUSH	7.5	8.0	0.5	2–14
PANCAKE	7.7	8.0	0.3	2–28
GRANDSON	12.2	8.4	3.8	0–16
HEADLIGHT	8.3	8.6	0.3	2–16
HORSESHOE	7.8	8.6	0.8	0–26
DUCKPOND	8.3	10.1	1.8	2–30
HOTHOUSE	12.7	10.9	1.8	0–44

Items ranked according to results of present study.

Items listed according to mean sensation level at which first correct identification occurred.

The range of mean sensation levels of the words within the brackets indicates a more homogeneous group of stimulus materials.

level were also scored as 0 db SL. Each additional list presented was then recorded as 2 db SL, 4 db SL and so on.

RESULTS

Columns 1 and 2 of Table 22-1 present comparable measures from Bowling and Elpern (1961) and from this study. In the present study, the over-all range of the mean SL values extended from 2.8 db (WORKSHOP) to 10.9 db (HOTHOUSE). Thus the average S first correctly identified the word WORK-SHOP at a level 8.1 db less intense than that at which he was first able to identify the test word HOTHOUSE. This range exceeds the 6 db criterion which is sometimes accepted clinically as the usual range of intelligibility.

In general, the findings of this experiment are in agreement with those of Bowling and Elpern, although the earlier study reported a greater range of 10 db. This discrepancy is probably due to differences in the experimental designs of the studies. Differences included the size interval used for stimulus presentation (2 vs 4 db), the number of Ss used, and the familiarity procedures used in this experiment. Column 3 indicates the differences for the individual words between the two studies.

Column 4 presents the range of responses. It is seen that the range of response increases as the mean SL (this is the well-known "ceiling" or "floor" effect). For example, the db range for BASEBALL is 0–12, whereas for HOTHOUSE it is 0–44. Thus even for normal-hearing individuals there is a wide range of responses for many of the items. This suggests that perhaps some of the items, particularly those with large ranges, are detrimental to the homogeneity of the test as a whole. For example, the brackets in Table 22-1 contain 27 of the spondee words which fell within a 4-db range. Therefore, by excluding only 9 of the original 36 test items, the homogeneity of the test would be enhanced, at perhaps negligible loss in reliability from other sources.

SUMMARY

Lists A–D of C.I.D. Auditory Test W-1 were presented monaurally to 50 normal-hearing subjects at increasing 2-db intensity levels. The range of individual spondee intelligibility was 8 db, considered unduly large. The least intelligible spondees tended to have greater range of response. The homogeneity of the recorded test could be enhanced by using 27 words which fell within a ±2-db range. The exclusive use of these 27 test items would improve the general efficiency of this speech audiometric procedure.

REFERENCES

1. Bowling. L. S. and Elpern, B. S. Relative intelligibility of items on CID Auditory Test W-1. *J. Aud. Res.*, 1961, 1, 152–157.

2. Harris, J. D. Research Frontiers in Audiology. Chapter 11 in: *Modern Developments in Audiology*, J. Jerger, Ed. New York: Academic Press, 1963.

3. Silverman, S. R. and Hirsh, I. J. Problems related to the use of speech in clinical audiometry. *Ann. Otol., Rhinol., Laryngol.*, 1955, 64, 1234–1245.

4. Tillman, T. W. and Jerger, J. F. Some factors affecting the spondee threshold in normal-hearing subjects. *J. Speech Hear. Res.*, 1959, 2, 141–146.

23

Some Factors Affecting the Spondee Threshold in Normal–Hearing Subjects[1]

TOM W. TILLMAN
JAMES F. JERGER

TOM W. TILLMAN, Ph.D., is Professor of Audiology and Associate Director, Auditory Research Laboratories, Northwestern University
JAMES F. JERGER, Ph.D., is Professor of Audiology, Baylor College of Medicine

The effects of subject sophistication on auditory test results vary with the particular stimulus being employed to assess auditory acuity. For example, Jerger and others (2) found that essentially equivalent pure-tone thresholds are obtained for highly sophisticated, highly practiced listeners and for listeners who have had no previous experience in pure-tone audiometric examinations. However, the same experiment suggested that the spondee threshold SPL for sophisticated subjects, who were relatively familiar with the spondee vocabulary, was some 5 to 7 db lower than that yielded by inexperienced subjects who were not familiar with the test vocabulary as such. It was found, moreover, that if spondee threshold measurements were repeated in these two groups, the second threshold SPL for the inexperienced subjects was approximately 3 db lower than the initial threshold SPL, while there was essentially no difference in the two thresholds for the sophisticated group.

The above findings led these same investigators (2) to formulate a more extensive experiment utilizing 96 unsophisticated normal-hearing subjects between the ages of 18 and 24 years. The design of the experiment allowed the assessment of the effect of prior knowledge of the test vocabulary on the spondee threshold. Prior knowledge of test vocabulary was imparted to half of the subjects by reading the entire list of spondee words to them immediately preceding the measurement of the spondee threshold. The mean spondee threshold SPL for the group given previous knowledge of the test vocabulary was approximately 3 db better than that for the group not given such knowledge.

Since the 3-db improvement observed in the preliminary experiment could have been due, in part, to knowledge of test vocabulary and, in part, to practice in the task of responding to words at threshold intensities, the present study was designed to isolate the effects of these two variables: (a) knowledge of spondee test vocabulary, and (b) practice in the task of responding to faint spondee words.

APPARATUS

The core of the apparatus used to measure spondee and 1000-cps thresholds consisted of a commercially available speech audiometer (Grason-Stadler, type 162) feeding a PDR-10

Reprinted by permission of the authors from *J. Speech Hearing Res.*, **2**, 141–146 (1959).

[1] This study was supported by funds provided under Contract AF41(657)-185 with the USAF School of Aviation Medicine, Randolph Field, Texas.

earphone mounted in an MX41/AR cushion. All spondee thresholds were obtained by playing portions of recorded List E of CID Auditory Test W-1 through this speech audiometer.

A separate pure-tone source, consisting of a commercially available clinical audiometer (Beltone, model 15-A), was fed through the speech audiometer to the same PDR-10 earphone. This portion of the apparatus was utilized in obtaining thresholds for a pure tone of 1000 cps.

The electrical signal across the earphone was measured periodically with a vacuum-tube voltmeter (Hewlett-Packard, model 400A). The acoustic output of the apparatus was calibrated by means of an ASA Type-1 coupler, calibrated condenser microphone (Western Electric, type 640AA), cathode follower (ADC, D5153), and vacuum-tube voltmeter (Hewlett-Packard, model 400A). All speech and pure-tone thresholds reported below are, therefore, expressed as the sound pressure level, reference 0.0002 microbar, developed in an ASA Type-1 coupler.

The sound pressure level developed by the earphone at octave frequencies from 125 to 8000 cps was measured before beginning the experimental testing and at three-day intervals throughout the course of the testing. The maximum variation in output over the testing period at the test frequency of 1000 cps was 0.5 db. This variation equalled or exceeded the maximum variation which occurred at any octave frequency from 250 to 4000 cps. However, maximum variations in output of 0.6 and 2.5 db occurred during the testing period at 125 and 8000 cps, respectively. Prior to the experiment, measurements demonstrated that the speech audiometer equalled or exceeded all specifications listed in the American Standard Specifications for Speech Audiometers (1).

SUBJECTS AND PROCEDURE

Three groups of 10 subjects each were selected from the female student body at Northwestern University. The age range of each group was restricted to 18 to 24 years, and no subject was

accepted who reported any history of ear pathology, excessive noise exposure or previous experience as a listener in auditory tests involving speech stimuli. All prospective subjects were screened audiometrically at a hearing level (hearing loss dial setting) of 10 db, reference USPHS norm, at each octave interval from 125 to 8000 cps, as well as at 1500, 3000, and 6000 cps. No subject was accepted who failed to respond to any test frequency at the screening intensity in either ear. Only one ear of each subject was used in the collection of the data reported below. The right ear was tested in half of the subjects, the left ear in the remainder. Subjects accepted for the experiment were assigned to the three experimental groups in a haphazard and nonsystematic fashion.

Each subject was seen in a single experimental session during which three thresholds were measured, the threshold for 1000-cps pure tone and two separate thresholds for spondee words. The measurement of the threshold for the 1000-cps tone always followed the initial spondee threshold and preceded the second spondee threshold.

Group A (Practice Only)

One group of 10 subjects, hereafter referred to as Group A, was included to test for the effects of practice only. In this group the first spondee threshold was obtained by playing words 1 through 18 of recorded List E of CID Auditory Test W-1. The second spondee threshold was obtained by playing words 19 through 36 of the same recording. The effects of practice alone on the spondee threshold could then be evaluated by comparing the mean threshold obtained in the first test with the mean threshold obtained in the second test.

Group B (Practice and Possible Prior Knowledge)

A second group of 10 subjects, hereafter referred to as Group B, was included to assess the combined effects of practice and possible knowledge of test vocabulary, prior to the second threshold. In this group, the first spondee threshold was obtained by playing words 1 through 18 of recorded List E of CID Auditory Test W-1. The second spondee threshold was then obtained by playing the same 18 words again. The effects of practice plus possible knowledge of test vocabulary could then be evaluated by comparing the magnitude of the two mean thresholds thus obtained.

Group C (Practice and Definite Prior Knowledge)

A third group of 10 subjects, Group C, was formed to evaluate the combined effects of practice and definite prior knowledge of test vocabulary on the spondee threshold. In this group, both spondee thresholds were obtained by playing words 1 through 18 of recorded List E of CID Auditory Test W-1. In addition, each subject was given prior knowledge of the test vocabulary by hearing the first 18 words of this list, in the manner described below, immediately preceding the measurement of the first spondee threshold. The effects of definite prior knowledge of test vocabulary could then be evaluated by comparing the mean initial threshold for this group with the mean initial thresholds obtained for Groups A and B.

All spondee thresholds were obtained by the up-and-down method, described in detail by Jerger and others (2), utilizing 2-db steps of attenuation. This method was chosen in preference to a simpler and less time-consuming clinical procedure because it allowed each threshold to be defined using exactly the same number of stimulus presentations. In other words, each spondee threshold was defined by presenting a series of 18 spondee words using the up-and-down method of threshold measurement. As noted earlier, these 18 words were always either words 1 through 18 or words 19 through 36 of recorded List E of CID Auditory Test W-1.

A clinical procedure utilizing 2-db steps of attenuation was employed to measure each subject's threshold for a 1000-cps pure tone. The procedure employed was the ascending technique described in the 1951 revision of the "Manual for School Hearing Conservation Programs" (3) prepared by the Committee on Conservation of Hearing of the American Academy of Ophthalmology and Otolaryngology.

The instructions read to subjects in the present study preceding the experimental session were essentially identical to those used by Jerger and others (2). The only changes were necessitated by the fact that the latter study employed only two test runs, while the present study used three test runs.

In addition to the instructions noted above, which were read to all subjects, the following instructions were read to the prior knowledge group immediately before the initial spondee threshold was measured.

Before the initial word test, I will read a series of 18 two-syllable words at a level which is easy for you to hear. You are to repeat back each word. These words are the same ones that you will later hear in the two word tests; however, they will be in a different order. Since the purpose of this initial reading is to make you familiar with the words, please listen carefully.

The first 18 words of List E of CID Auditory Test W-1 were then pronounced in alphabetical order by monitored live voice at a level 50 db above the present American norm of 22 db SPL.

RESULTS

Table 23-1 summarizes the experimental data. Group A, in which the first spondee threshold was obtained using the first 18 words of recorded List E and the second threshold using the second 18 words of the same recorded list, showed an improvement in threshold acuity of 1.1 db from the first to the second test. This is a very slight difference, and it would seem hazardous to conclude that it resulted from practice in the task of responding to spondee words at threshold intensities. This seems particularly true in view of the essentially

TABLE 23-1. MEAN SPONDEE AND 1000-CPS THRESHOLD SOUND PRESSURE LEVELS (DB *re:* 0.0002 MICROBAR IN ASA TYPE-I COUPLER) AND THEIR STANDARD ERRORS FOR THREE GROUPS OF 10 NORMAL HEARING SUBJECTS EACH: GROUP A, PRACTICE ALONE; GROUP B, PRACTICE AND POSSIBLE PRIOR KNOWLEDGE; GROUP C, PRACTICE AND DEFINITE PRIOR KNOWLEDGE

	First Spondee Threshold	Second Spondee Threshold	1000 cps
Group A			
Mean Threshold SPL	25.9	24.8	9.3
Standard Error of Mean	1.0	1.3	1.3
Group B			
Mean Threshold SPL	27.0	24.6	10.9
Standard Error of Mean	1.2	1.1	1.6
Group C			
Mean Threshold SPL	20.9	20.6	10.7
Standard Error of Mean	1.0	0.6	1.2

equivalent thresholds for the two spondee threshold tests in Group C. In this latter group, the two thresholds were obtained using the first 18 words of recorded list E after the subjects had been given previous experience with the test words. The 0.3-db improvement in this group from the first to the second test could hardly indicate an important practice effect.

In Group B an improvement of 2.4 db occurred from the first to the second spondee threshold test. The two thresholds in this group were obtained using the first 18 words of recorded List E. This group, it will be recalled, was included to assess the effect of possible knowledge of test vocabulary imparted to the subjects during the first spondee test as well as the effects of practice. In view of the relatively small change which occurred from the first to the second thresholds in Group A and the essentially equivalent thresholds obtained in Group C, it seems reasonable to conclude that the improvement noted in Group B was due to the knowledge of test vocabulary gained by the subjects as a result of the initial test.

Comparison of both the first and second spondee thresholds obtained in Group C (definite prior knowledge of the test vocabulary) with those for Group A (no prior knowledge) reveals that Group C yielded threshold SPLs 4 to 5 db lower than Group A. It seems reasonable to attribute this relatively large

difference solely to the fact that Group C had been given prior knowledge of the test vocabulary.

The above findings suggest that, at least insofar as short-term effects are concerned, practice in the task of responding to spondee words at near-threshold intensities exerts no important influence on the spondee threshold in normal hearing subjects. Conversely, it would appear that previous knowledge of the spondee test vocabulary has an important effect. Specifically, threshold SPLs as much as 4 to 5 db lower will be obtained from subjects who are given previous knowledge of the test vocabulary than from subjects who are not given this prior knowledge.

These findings have practical implications for the clinician as well as for those concerned with establishing a normative standard for the hearing of speech stimuli. In the routine clinical procedures requiring successive measurements of the speech threshold using spondee words, the initial threshold SPL established may be 4 to 5 db higher than succeeding ones unless time is taken to familiarize the subject with the test vocabulary preceding the initial threshold test.

In establishing an audiometric norm for speech, where spondee words are specified as the stimulus, one must apparently be concerned with the extent to which the criterion population is familiar with the test vocabulary. Such concern is necessary because the absolute value of the standard, as well as the relationship between hearing for pure tones and for speech, will be influenced rather importantly by the degree to which the criterion population has prior familiarity with the test vocabulary.

SUMMARY

The purpose of this experiment was to isolate the effects on the spondee threshold in normal-hearing subjects of (a) knowledge of spondee test vocabulary and (b) practice in the task of responding to spondee words at threshold intensities.

Two spondee thresholds were obtained for each of 30 subjects under varying experimental conditions utilizing recorded List E of CID Auditory Test W-1.

Results suggest two conclusions: (a) short-term practice in the task of responding to spondee words at threshold intensities exerts no important influence on the spondee threshold SPL in normal-hearing subjects; and (b) normal-hearing subjects given prior knowledge of the test vocabulary yield spondee threshold SPLs which are 4 to 5 db lower than those yielded by subjects not given such knowledge.

REFERENCES

1. *American Standard Sound Measurement Package, American Standard Specification for Audiometers for General Diagnostic Purposes*, approved March 21, 1951. American Standards Association, Inc., 70 East 45th St., New York 17, N.Y.

2. Jerger, J. F., Carhart, R., Tillman, T. W., and Peterson, J. L., Some relations between normal hearing for pure tones and for speech. *J. Speech Hearing Res.*, 2, 1959, 126–140.

3. Newhart, H., and Reger, S. N. (Eds.), *Manual for School Hearing Conservation Program* (rev. 1951, for Comm. on Conservation of Hearing, C. E. Kinney, G. D. Hoople, S. R. Guild, S. N. Reger, Eds., suppl., trans. Amer. Acad. Ophth., Otolaryng., 100 First Ave. Bldg., Rochester). Omaha: Douglas Printing Co.

24

Spondee Threshold Measurement:
A Comparison of 2- and 5-db Methods[1]

JOSEPH B. CHAIKLIN
IRA M. VENTRY

JOSEPH B. CHAIKLIN, Ph.D., is Professor of Audiology, University of Minnesota
IRA M. VENTRY, Ph.D., is Professor of Audiology, Teachers College, Columbia University

The general impression one gains from recent literature (Chaiklin, 1959; Jerger et al., 1959; Newby, 1958; Ruhm and Carhart, 1958; Tillman and Jerger, 1959) is that a 2-db measurement interval is typically used in measuring spondee threshold.[2] Probably many clinicians use a 2-db (or 1-db) measurement interval because they believe a small interval provides spondee threshold estimates that are more precise and more reliable than could be obtained with a larger measurement interval. On theoretical grounds this rationale seems weak. If a variable is continuously distributed, a relatively small increase (2- or 3-db) in size of measurement interval should have a negligible effect on precision, and no effect on reliability. A practical consideration that makes the use of small intervals questionable is that the intensity variations among currently used spondaic stimuli are larger than the small measurement intervals used by most clinicians. Finally, there is no apparent reason why spondee thresholds should be measured in steps smaller than the 5-db step ordinarily used to measure pure-tone thresholds.

It should be noted that small measurement intervals have not always been used for spondee threshold sampling. Some of the early spondee threshold methodologies (Fletcher, 1950; Watson, 1949; Watson and Tolan, 1949, p. 449) employed a 5-db measurement interval probably on the basis of equipment limitations rather than on theoretical bases. As far as we can determine, the most recent report of the use of a 5-db spondee threshold measurement interval is contained in an article by Whipple and Kodman (1960). The primary purpose of this article is to report experimental evidence supporting the use of 5-db steps in the measurement of spondee thresholds.

A secondary focus of the article is measurement method. Most descriptions of spondee threshold measurement methods have been imprecise or lacking in detail. A major portion of the present article is devoted to detailed descriptions of measurement methods that we believe will meet current needs in this area.

This article has been revised from the original and is reprinted by permission of the authors from *J. Speech Hearing Dis.*, **29**, pp. 47–59 (1964).

[1] The study was supported by U.S. Public Health Grant B-2741(C2R1) and by the Veterans Administration.

[2] The term "spondee threshold" (Tillman and Jerger, 1959) is used here in place of the more traditional "speech reception threshold" (SRT). The term "spondee threshold" is a more direct statement of what is being measured.

PROCEDURE

Subjects

Subjects were 100 adult male veterans selected from the clinic population of the Veterans

Administration Audiology and Speech Pathology Clinic, San Francisco. They ranged in age from 23 to 62 years with a mean age of 42.2 years. The etiologies and types of hearing loss for the subjects are listed in Table 24-1.

TABLE 24-1. DISTRIBUTION OF ETIOLOGIES AND TYPES OF HEARING LOSS FOR TOTAL SAMPLE; N = 100

Category	N
Etiology	
Otosclerosis	49
Otitis Media (inactive)	19
Undetermined	15
Acoustic Trauma	13
Presbycusis	1
Normal *	3
Type	
Mixed	60
Sensory-neural	31
Conductive	6
Normal *	3

* Right ear was normal for three cases with unilateral loss.

Seventy-one of the subjects were being seen at the clinic for routine audiometric testing related to otologic treatment, hearing aid evaluations, and diagnostic testing for the otolaryngology department. The remaining 29 subjects were being evaluated for compensation purposes and were part of a control group in a study of functional hearing loss (News Note, *JSHR*, 1962; Ventry, 1962).*

Subjects were selected using the following criteria: (a) absence of ear, nose, or throat conditions that might cause abnormal threshold fluctuations; (b) speech discrimination score not lower than 60 percent for the ear used in the study; (c) not more than 62 years of age; and (d) absence of functional hearing loss (Chaiklin and Ventry, 1963; Ventry and Chaiklin, 1962).

General Design

The general plan of the study was simple. First, pure-tone air-conduction thresholds were obtained for one or both ears. Next, spondee thresholds were measured using the 2-db and 5-db methods. To control order effects, 50 subjects had the 2-db threshold measured first, followed by the 5-db threshold. This order was reversed for the other 50 subjects. Eighty-five subjects had spondee threshold measurements on the right ear, and the remaining 15 had spondee threshold measurements on the left ear. An important feature of the general design was the control of bias that might result from the tester's knowledge of the results of a previous threshold measurement. The control of bias was accomplished either by having the second test conducted by a different tester who had no knowledge of the results of the first test (N = 43), or by means of an accessory "Random Variable Attenuator" (N = 57). The Random Variable Attenuator (RVA) permitted the tester to introduce an unknown amount of attenuation into the earphone line so that he could repeat a threshold measurement relatively free from the biasing effect of his knowledge of the first threshold obtained.[3] After making a threshold measurement the tester needed only to determine the amount of added attenuation in the line and then correct the audiometer dial reading by that amount. Following the measurement of spondee thresholds, the clinician proceeded with the remainder of the audiologic evaluation. All tests were administered by the authors or by the clinic's audiologists working under the close supervision of the authors. All tests were administered during a single test session except for the reliability substudy which required two sessions.

The test-retest reliability of the 2-db and 5-db methods was evaluated by retesting the 29 subjects referred to earlier. All reliability retests were conducted by the authors with the use of the RVA. The order of the retests was varied systematically to control order effects.

[* For more complete details, see Chaiklin, J. B., and Ventry, I. M., Chapter I: Introduction and Research Plan. In I. M. Ventry and J. B. Chaiklin (Eds.), Multidiscipline study of functional hearing loss. *J. aud. Res.*, **5**, pp. 219–230 (1965). JBC, IMV]

[3] The auxiliary RVAs were designed and constructed by Mr. L. Glen Pew, Electro-Acoustic Company, Palo Alto, California. The prototype for the RVA was designed for use in a study of simulated hearing loss conducted by Barrett (1959).

Equipment

Data were gathered in three test suites, two of which contained Industrial Acoustics Company audiometric testing rooms (Models 402 and 1201). The third two-room suite was of permanent construction. Two of the suites had Allison 21 series audiometers equipped with Telephonics Corporation TDH-39 earphones set in MX-41/AR cushions and Ampex 351 tape recorders as input sources for taped spondee stimuli. The third suite had an Allison 20A audiometer with provision for delivering only disc-recorded stimuli; the input source was a Garrard 301 turntable with a Garrard TPA 12 transcription arm and a General Electric variable reluctance cartridge (Model 4G-053). The calibration of both the pure-tone and speech circuits was checked periodically with an Allison Laboratories Audiometer Calibration Unit (Model 300). The pure-tone circuits were calibrated to the ASA standard (1951), but the speech circuits were calibrated to a zero hearing level of 29 db re 0.0002 dyne/cm² rather than the 22-db zero hearing level recommended by ASA (1953).[4]

Pure-Tone Threshold Measurement

Pure-tone air-conduction thresholds were measured with an ascending "on-effect" procedure

[4] The ASA standard for pure-tone audiometers (1951) produces test results that underestimate loss of auditory sensitivity for pure tones (Davis, 1959; Jerger et al., 1959). The 22-db (re 0.0002 dyne/cm²) sound pressure output recommended by ASA (1953) for calibrating zero hearing level in speech audiometers is a good estimate of the SPL required to reach average normal threshold for spondaic words (Chaiklin, 1959; Hirsh et al., 1952; Jerger et al., 1959). Therefore, the ASA standard for speech audiometers produces spondee thresholds that tend to be higher than pure-tone averages (Jerger et al., 1959). Several years ago, the VA adopted a 29-db (re 0.0002 dyne/cm²) calibration level for speech audiometers. This was done to bring the results of pure-tone and speech audiometry into better agreement with each other. The result is that the VA calibration for speech audiometers yields results that underestimate spondee thresholds in the same way that the ASA standard for pure-tone audiometers results in underestimates of loss of acuity for pure tones. It is important to recognize that some manufacturers of speech audiometers use the 22-db ASA standard and some use other calibration values.

similar to the procedure recommended by Carhart and Jerger (1959). Ascending series of short (approximately one sec.) tones were presented with successive stimuli separated by toneless intervals. The only important deviation from the procedure recommended by Carhart and Jerger was that each ascent was continued five db above the level at which a subject first responded. Threshold was usually defined as the lowest hearing level at which at least a 60 percent response criterion was met. Of course, the criterion percentage was dependent on the number of stimuli presented at each level. Occasionally a 50 percent response criterion was applied. However, the 5-db interval used in standard pure-tone audiometry is too large to allow routine application of the 50 percent response criterion frequently used with the classical psychophysical methods (Carhart and Jerger, 1959).

Spondee Threshold Measurement

The speech stimuli used in the measurement of thresholds were the 36 spondaic words of CID Auditory Test W-1 (Hirsh et al., 1952). All stimuli were presented either by means of the CID disc recordings of Auditory Test W-1 (lists A through F) or by taped dubs of the CID recordings with the identifying introduction to lists B through F omitted. Two further considerations should be noted: (a) the stimulus mode (tape or record) remained the same for a particular subject; that is, if the first spondee threshold was measured with taped stimuli, succeeding measurements employed taped stimuli; and (b) at no time was live-voice testing used in the measurement of spondee thresholds.

The procedure for instructing subjects before spondee threshold measurement was the same regardless of which of the two threshold measurement techniques was employed first. The following instructions, appropriate for both methods, were read to the subject before the first threshold measurement.

1. You're going to hear a recording of· a man reading a list of two-syllable words such as "blackboard" and "earthquake." Before each word the man will say, "Say the word.

. . ." For example, "Say the word 'earthquake.' "

2. Your job is to repeat each two-syllable word after you hear it, no matter how faint the word may be. You don't have to say, "Say the word." For example, if you hear "Say the word 'blackboard,' " you should say "blackboard." The words may become very faint, but please continue repeating them as well as you can until I tell you the test is over. It's important that you guess if you are uncertain of a word. Are there any questions?

3. The words you will hear are typed on cards lying on the table beside you. Please pick up the cards and read the words to me so that you can become familiar with them.

The subject then read aloud the 36 W-1 spondees which were typed on 3" × 5" cards. If a subject could not read the words the tester read them to him and asked him to repeat them aloud. The familiarization process served to reduce learning effects (Tillman and Jerger, 1959) and was consistent with the instructions provided with CID Auditory Test W-1 (undated). After the subject had been familiarized with the stimuli, he was told, "Remember, it's very important that you guess, no matter how faint the word may be, or if you only hear part of a word." Then the measurement of spondee threshold began.

Procedure for 2-db Method Spondee Threshold

A descending approach to threshold was used for both the 2-db and 5-db methods. The initial descending approach to threshold for the 2-db method was in 5-db steps with one spondee per step presented at succeedingly lower levels until the subject failed to repeat a word correctly. The intensity of the signal was increased five or six db to an even number on the hearing level dial. Sampling then proceeded in descending 2-db steps with a minimum of three or a maximum of six stimuli presented at each step. The intensity was decreased by 2 db each time it became apparent that a subject met or could not meet a 50 percent correct response criterion. It is obvious that six stimuli were not needed at each level. When a subject had made four errors

(before getting three correct) it was impossible for him to meet the 50 percent criterion. Similarly, when three correct responses had been obtained, nothing would have been gained by presenting the maximum of six stimuli.

Sampling was discontinued when (a) four words were responded to incorrectly at each of three consecutive levels, or (b) four words were missed at each of two consecutive levels with no correct response at either level, that is, eight consecutive errors with none correct. Threshold was defined as the lowest hearing level at which three words were repeated correctly out of a theoretical maximum of six stimulus presentations. It should be noted that the criteria for determining the sampling end-point were designed to prevent premature designation of threshold when three correct responses were obtained at several levels.

Procedure for 5-db Method Spondee Threshold

For the 5-db method the initial descending approach to threshold was accomplished in 5-db steps for 71 subjects and in 10-db steps for the 29 reliability subjects. The remaining procedure was the same for all subjects. One word per step was presented until the subject failed to respond correctly. The signal was then raised five db above the last level at which there was a correct response. Stimuli were presented in descending 5-db steps, following at each level the same criteria for minimum and maximum sampling described above for the 2-db method. The criterion for completion of threshold sampling with the 5-db method was four incorrect responses at two consecutive levels (a total of eight errors). As with the 2-db method, spondee threshold was defined as the lowest hearing level at which three words were repeated correctly out of a theoretical maximum of six stimulus presentations.

RESULTS

Order Effects

The first question considered was whether order of presentation resulted in a difference between spondee thresholds measured in 2-db and 5-db steps. Fifty subjects had the 2-db threshold measured first; the order was reversed for the remaining 50 subjects. There was no significant difference $(t = .43)$ between the mean difference scores for the 2-db and 5-db spondee thresholds as a function of order of presentation. All subjects, therefore, were considered as one group regardless of the order in which thresholds were measured.

Comparison of Measurement Methods

The mean spondee threshold obtained using the 2-db method was 25.72 db and the mean threshold for the 5-db method was 27.55 db. The difference (1.83 db) between the means was significant $(t = 6.54,\ P < .001)$.† The standard deviations were very similar for the two spondee thresholds $(SD_{2dB} = 20.26$ db; $SD_{5dB} = 20.54$ db); and there was little difference (.03 db) between the standard errors of the means. As would be expected, there was a high correlation[5] $(r = .99)$ between the results of the 2-db and 5-db measurement methods. These results are summarized in Table 24-2.

[† The journal version of this article reported an incorrect nonsignificant t ratio. In a letter to the editor (*J. Speech Hearing Dis.*, **30**, pp. 99-100, 1965), Gaeth called attention to the error. Our reply to Gaeth (*J. Speech Hearing Dis.*, **30**, pp. 100-101, 1965) acknowledged the mistake, which was caused by an arithmetical error, and presented supplementary data comparing the two methods. The following excerpt from our letter provides data that allow a fuller comparison of the two methods: "Of the 100 subjects used in the study, 49 had 5-db method STs that were within ±2 db of their 2-db method STs, 32 differed by ±3 to ±5 db, and the remaining 19 had STs from ±6 db to ±9 db of each other (one subject was +9 db). Twenty-three of the 5-db method STs were lower than the 2-db STs, 59 were higher and 18 were identical. The larger differences constituted less than 20 percent of the cases and were often associated with sloping pure-tone configurations which seem to produce slightly more ST measurement error. In this connection, it should be noted that 20 percent of the test-retest differences for the 2-db method were from +5 to +8 db, which suggests that size of interval is not the sole factor operating in extreme cases. It is possible that some of these differences are related to stimulus differences rather than to measurement method." JBC, IMV]

[5] All correlations reported are Pearson product-moment correlation coefficients.

TABLE 24-2. COMPARISON OF 2-DB AND 5-DB SPONDEE THRESHOLDS; N = 100

Method	Mean	SD	t	r
2-db	25.72	20.26		
			6.54 *	.99
5-db	27.55	20.54		

* Significant at < .001 level.

Measurement Method versus Pure-Tone Average (PTA)

Table 24-3 shows the correlations between spondee thresholds obtained with the two mea-

TABLE 24-3. MEAN PTAS (IN DB), CORRELATIONS BETWEEN SPONDEE THRESHOLDS AND PTAS, AND STANDARD ERROR OF ESTIMATES FOR PREDICTING SPONDEE THRESHOLDS FROM PTAS; N = 100

Method	2-freq. PTA			3-freq. PTA		
	Mean	r	$SE_{est.}$	Mean	r	$SE_{est.}$
2-db		.98	4.03		.97	4.90
	26.59			29.99		
5-db		.97	4.97		.96	5.78

surement methods and the two- and three-frequency PTAs. The table also shows mean PTAs as well as the standard errors of estimate for predicting either the 2-db or 5-db spondee threshold from either the two- or three-frequency PTA. It is readily apparent that a 5-db spondee threshold measurement method produces essentially the same degree of correlation with PTA as does the more commonly used 2-db measurement interval. It is also apparent from the standard errors of estimate reported in Table 24-3 that little predictive power (approximately one db) is lost when estimating a 5-db threshold from the two- or three-frequency PTA. It is important to note that the correlation coefficients and standard errors of estimate reported in Table 24-3 are very similar to results reported by other investigators (Fletcher, 1950; Graham, 1960; Quiggle et al., 1957). The similarities are even more striking when one considers the important differences among these studies in terms of samples, measurement intervals, stimulus materials, and measurement methods.

One qualification should be made concerning the high spondee threshold-PTA correlations reported above. They are, in part, a function of our sample. No subject in our study had a sharply sloping pure-tone configuration, at least through the speech frequencies; and, further, no subject had a speech discrimination score less than 60 percent. It can be assumed that the presence of either of these problems might reduce the correlations between PTAs and spondee thresholds obtained with either a 2-db or 5-db method. This assumption is partially supported by Graham's (1960) data, at least for the 2-db method. Nearly half of Graham's sample consisted of subjects with sensory-neural hearing loss, while only 31 percent of our sample had a similar loss. This difference could account for our finding a slightly higher correlation between spondee threshold and the three-frequency PTA than was found by Graham.

Measurement Method versus Pure-Tone Thresholds

Table 24-4 shows correlations between the spondee threshold measurement methods and

TABLE 24-4. MEANS AND STANDARD DEVIATIONS (IN DB) FOR PURE-TONE THRESHOLDS FROM 500 CPS TO 2000 CPS AND CORRELATION COEFFICIENTS BETWEEN THE 2-DB AND THE 5-DB METHOD SPONDEE THRESHOLDS AND PURE-TONE THRESHOLDS; N = 100

Frequencies	Mean	SD	$r_{2\text{-db}}$	$r_{5\text{-db}}$
500	26.30	21.80	.96	.95
750 *	30.48	22.24	.96	.95
1000	31.10	21.63	.96	.95
1500 †	33.52	21.16	.88	.87
2000	33.60	21.05	.79	.79

* N = 52.
† N = 61.

each of the pure-tone thresholds from 500 cps through 2000 cps including the interoctave frequencies of 750 cps and 1500 cps. Also shown in Table 24-4 are the mean thresholds and standard deviations for each frequency tested. Once again the 5-db method threshold compares favorably with the 2-db method threshold. Both methods show similar high positive correlations (ranging from .79 to

.96) with the speech-frequency pure-tone thresholds.

Test-Retest Reliability

Twenty-nine subjects were used for the evaluation of test-retest reliability. For the 2-db method 27 subjects (93 percent) had test-retest differences from 0 db to ±6 db; no subject had a test-retest difference greater than eight db. For the 5-db method all subjects had test-retest differences within ±5 db; 59 percent had identical thresholds on both measurements with the 5-db method. It is apparent that the small differences between the two methods are not significant.

DISCUSSION

The results of the data analyses indicate that spondee thresholds obtained with a 5-db measurement interval agree well with spondee thresholds measured in 2-db steps although the 5-db method thresholds are slightly higher.

The 5-db method is faster than the 2-db method, agrees well with pure-tone audiometry, and is highly reliable. For clinics that have speech audiometers graduated in 2-db steps, a 4-db measurement interval is recommended. Spondee thresholds measured with a 4-db measurement interval should have validity and reliability comparable to that demonstrated for a 5-db measurement interval. The validity and reliability of any measure is dependent, to a large extent, on measurement method. If, on the basis of the results of this study, a 5-db (or 4-db) measurement interval is adopted for routine clinical use, the general method employed should conform to that described below or in the *Procedure* section.

The literature on measurement of spondee threshold is marked by meager descriptions of test methods. Sometimes the entire description of methodology consists of the instruction to present several words at successive levels until the patient misses about half of the words. Frequently, methodology is not described at all. Jerger and others (1959) have also commented on the prevalence of cursory descriptions of spondee threshold test methods. They reported that it was necessary to devise their own methodology to achieve some degree of objectivity in their study of pure-tone and speech thresholds. Their procedure was based on the method described by Newby (1958, p. 112), a method which, in our opinion, is too general and unsystematic, Newby's instructions are:

> . . . start the record (or the delivery of the words by live voice) at a level [unspecified] above the patient's presumed threshold. As the patient repeats two or three words successfully, decrease the intensity by a few db. After two or three more words have been repeated correctly at this new level, decrease the intensity further. Continue in this way until the patient misses some words. By increasing or decreasing intensity in 1- or 2-db steps, try to find the point at which the patient is correct about half the time. This is his SRT by spondees.

Jerger and others (1959) used the following adaptation of Newby's method.

> Two or three words were initially presented at a level 20 to 30 db above the estimated threshold. Successive blocks of two or three words were then progressively attenuated in 10-db steps until a level was reached at which two consecutive words were repeated incorrectly. At this point the tester simply "jumped around" in no set order, from level to level in 2-db steps, presenting exactly four words per level. The spondee threshold was recorded as the lowest intensity at which a subject repeated two out of four words correctly.

This method is more explicitly described than Newby's method but still omits too many important procedural details.

The well-documented high correlation between spondee threshold and PTA may influence some clinicians to perform inappropriately casual spondee threshold measure-

ments. Indeed, the measurement process and the resulting thresholds may be biased by the clinician's tendency to estimate spondee threshold from the PTA. Well-defined methods can serve as a protection against this kind of tester bias. The more specific the method, the fewer unique decisions the tester must make; by having most decisions predetermined for the tester the obtained spondee thresholds gain a degree of independence that does not exist with "flexible" clinical methods. In addition, the relative freedom from bias gained through precise methods makes the spondee threshold a much more meaningful independent check on the validity of pure-tone audiometry. The problems discussed above illustrate the need for a well-defined system for spondee threshold measurement. The following methodological proposals, which are based on the present research and several years of cliuical trial, hopefully will meet this need.

The method we recommend for the measurement of spondee thresholds in 5-db steps is similar to that described in the *Procedure* section. The method involves three major steps: (a) instructions, (b) familiarization, and (c) measurement. We suggest that the following instructions be read to the patient immediately before the measurement of spondee threshold.

> The purpose of this test is to find the faintest level at which you hear words. You're going to hear some two-syllable words such as "baseball" and "mousetrap." Your job is to repeat each two-syllable word no matter how faint the word may be. For example, if you hear, "Say the word 'baseball,'" you should just repeat "baseball." The words may be very faint, but please continue repeating them as well as you can until I tell you the test is over. It's important that you guess at the word, even if you're not sure of it. Do you have any questions?
>
> Now, I want you to pick up the stack of cards on the table and read the words aloud to me. These are the words that you'll hear

during the test. I want you to become familiar with them. [The following final sentence of the instructions is to be read to the subject after he has been familiarized with the stimuli.] Remember, it's very important that you guess, no matter how faint a word may be or even if you only hear part of the word.

These instructions are similar to instructions used in previous research (Chaiklin, 1959; Jerger et al., 1959) and to the instructions provided with CID Auditory Test W-1. Deviations from the exact wording of the instructions may be far less critical than deviations involving essential ideas, such as the need for the patient to guess. We recognize that formal instructions may be inappropriate under certain circumstances, for example, in testing young children. However, we do believe it is important for clinics to adopt a specific set of instructions to be used whenever possible.

Familiarizing the patient with the spondee stimuli is the next important step. Familiarization serves to increase both the validity and reliability of spondee threshold results (Tillman and Jerger, 1959) and must, therefore, be incorporated into the measurement process. Familiarization can be accomplished by having the patient read the spondee words aloud, or by reading the words to the patient and having him repeat them back.

The 5-db measurement method is as follows: (a) assuming that pure-tone thresholds have been measured,[6] begin the initial descent 25 db above the two-frequency PTA (rounded to the nearest 5-db step); (b) descend in 5-

db steps, presenting one spondee per level, until the patient misses a spondee; (c) increase the intensity 10 db above the level arrived at in the previous step; (d) decrease the intensity in 5-db steps, presenting a minimum of three and a maximum of six spondees at each level; (e) continue to decrease the intensity in 5-db steps until the patient fails to repeat correctly three spondeees at two consecutive levels. Threshold is defined as the lowest level at which three spondees are repeated correctly out of a theoretical maximum of six stimuli. (See *Procedure* section for greater detail concerning sampling.) The entire measurement process for both ears, including instructions and familiarization, usually takes less than ten minutes.

We realize that some clinicians may be reluctant to change their measurement technique despite the evidence that a 5-db method compares favorably to a 2-db method and, in some respects, is superior. However, as was pointed out above, no detailed description of a 2-db measurement method is currently available to these clinicians. To meet this need we suggest the following 2-db measurement method (note that the instructions and familiarization process are the same for both the 2-db and 5-db methods): (a) begin initial descent 25 db above the two-frequency PTA (rounded to the nearest 5-db step); (b) descend in 5-db steps, presenting one spondee per level, until the patient misses a spondee; (c) increase the intensity five db or six db above the level found in the previous step, the object being to start at an even number on the hearing loss dial; (d) decrease the intensity in 2-db steps, presenting a minimum of two and a maximum of four spondees at each level;‡ (e) continue to decrease the intensity until three words are responded to incorrectly at each of three consecutive levels or until three words are missed at each of two consecutive levels with no correct responses at either level.

---

[6] At least two methods can be used to establish a starting point for the initial descent if pure-tone thresholds have not been measured prior to the measurement of spondee threshold. The first method is one recommended by Carhart and Jerger (1959) for pure-tone audiometry. They suggest starting ". . . at a hearing level of 30 to 40 db if the subject appears to have approximately normal acuity, and at a hearing [sic] of 70 db if only a moderate impairment seems to be present. Provided these levels are inadequate, subsequent presentations are increased in steps of 15 db until the subject's response is positive." The other method is to start at −10-db hearing level and ascend in 10-db steps until the patient repeats two spondees correctly at a given level.

[‡ We should have explained that we determined empirically that essentially the same results are obtained with either a 2 out of 4 or a 3 out of 6 criterion for the 2-db method. The 5-db method, however, suffers when a 2 out of 4 criterion is used. JBC, IMV]

SPONDEE RESPONSE DATA SHEET

Name: _N. K._____   Date: _12/21/62_   Tester: _1. JFW 2. JBC_

HEARING LEVEL	RIGHT	ERROR 1	ERROR 2	ERROR 3	ERROR 4
TEST NO. 1			CIRCLE EAR R L		
40	III				
38	III	shortstop			
36	II	baseball	NR	farewell	NR
(34)	III	N. R.	NR		
32	II	NR	sidewalk	NR	sandlot
30		NR	NR	sidewalk	NR
28		NR	NR	NR	NR
				SRT = 34	
TEST NO. 2			CIRCLE EAR R L		
40	III				
(35)	III	hotdog			
30	I	NR	NR	NR	NR
25		NR	NR	NR	NR
				SRT = 35	

Figure 24-1. Spondee threshold data sheet showing examples of the sampling process used with the 5-db and 2-db measurement methods. Correct responses are indicated by tally marks; errors are written out (NR = no response). Note: Test No. 1 shows a 3 out of 6 threshold criterion rather than the 2 out of 4 criterion advocated in the discussion section.

Threshold is defined as the lowest level at which two spondees are repeated correctly out of a theoretical maximum of four stimuli.

The data sheet shown in Figure 24-1 has proved to be a useful aid in the measurement process. It provides a permanent record and is simple to use. Correct responses are indicated by a tally mark, and incorrect responses are written to provide a means of examining error response patterns—some of which appear to have diagnostic significance.§ The use of the data sheet is illustrated in Figure 24-1.

Our experience during another study suggested that an ascending method may be an even more rapid method of measuring spondee threshold than a descending method. Unfortunately, we did not evaluate an ascending 5-db method and cannot, at this time, recommend such a procedure. It is not unreasonable to expect good agreement between thresholds obtained with either an ascending or descending measurement procedure.‖

There are several observations we would like to make concerning spondee stimuli. The intensity and intelligibility differences among currently used spondee stimuli suggest that there may be value in research designed to select spondee stimuli that are more comparable on these two dimensions, as well as being equated for familiarity. These stimuli would be easier to record and easier to monitor in clinical situations where live-voice testing is necessary. It would also seem advisable, in any new set of stimuli, to avoid pairs of stimuli with identical syllables. Combinations such as "hotdog"—"hothouse" and "inkwell"—"farewell" in the W-1 list introduce a discrimination task, particularly at weak signal levels, that is peripheral to the threshold being measured. A smaller population of stimuli would also seem desirable to produce greater homogeneity and to facilitate the related task of familiarizing the subject with the stimuli. Reducing the number of stimuli would also make it

easier to select spondees having equal intensity.

We have found it convenient to use tape recorded stimuli in the measurement of spondee threshold. The use of taped stimuli provides obvious advantages such as preservation of fidelity and ease of handling. In any event, live-voice testing is the least desirable method because it introduces an unnecessary source (the speaker) of intra- and inter-test variability.

SUMMARY

The monaural spondee thresholds of 100 hard-of-hearing adult males were measured with two different measurement intervals—a 5-db interval and a 2-db interval. Measurements with both methods were repeated for 29 of the 100 subjects. All tests were controlled for tester bias to insure independent measures. Recordings of CID Auditory Test W-1 served as test stimuli. Carefully specified methods were used for all threshold measurements. The 5-db measurement method resulted in spondee thresholds that (a) agreed well with 2-db method thresholds, (b) had high correlations with pure-tone thresholds, and (c) had high reliability.

On the basis of the results of this study it is recommended that spondee thresholds be measured in 5-db steps rather than in 2-db steps. The 5-db method is faster than the 2-db method and provides more than adequate accuracy for clinical needs. The change to a 5-db measurement interval should be accompanied by standard measurement techniques. Measurement techniques for both the 5-db and 2-db methods were described.

[§ See Chaiklin, J. B., and Ventry, I. M., Patient errors during spondee and pure-tone threshold measurement. In I. M. Ventry and J. B. Chaiklin (Eds.), Multidiscipline study of functional hearing loss. *J. aud. Res.*, **5**, pp. 219–230 (1965). JBC, IMV]

[‖ A study of the validity and reliability of spondee thresholds measured in ascending 5-db steps was reported by Chaiklin, J. B., Dixon, R. F., and Font, J., Spondee thresholds measured in ascending 5-db steps. *J. Speech Hearing Res.*, **10**, pp. 141–145 (1967). Validity and reliability for the ascending method were highly similar to results reported in the present study, but contrary to our earlier speculation, the ascending method was not significantly faster. JBC, IMV]

ACKNOWLEDGMENT

We wish to acknowledge the cooperation and assistance of the staff of the Audiology and Speech Pathology Clinic, Veterans Administration Hospital, San Francisco.

REFERENCES

American Standards Association, *American Standard Specification for Audiometers for General Diagnostic Purposes*, Z24.5-1951. New York: Amer. Standards Assoc., 1951.

American Standards Association, *American Standard Specification for Speech Audiometers*, Z24.13-1953. New York: Amer. Standards Assoc., 1953.

Barrett, L. S., Threshold relationships in simulated hearing loss. Ph.D. dissertation, Stanford Univ., 1959.

Carhart, R., and Jerger, J. F., Preferred method for clinical determination of pure-tone thresholds. *J. Speech Hearing Dis.*, 24, 1959, 330–345.

Central Institute for the Deaf, *Auditory Tests W-1 and W-2, Spondaic Word Lists: Description and Instructions for Use*. St. Louis: Central Institute for the Deaf, undated.

Chaiklin, J. B., The relation among three selected auditory speech thresholds. *J. Speech Hearing Res.*, 2, 1959, 237–243.

Chaiklin, J. B., and Ventry, I. M., Functional hearing loss. In J. F. Jerger (Ed.), *Modern Developments in Audiology*. New York: Academic Press, 1963.

Chaiklin, J. B., and Ventry, I. M., Functional hearing loss: V. Patient errors during measurement of speech reception threshold and the spondee error index (SERI), (in preparation). [See footnote § for reference. JBC,IMV]

Davis, H., For an international audiometric zero. *Asha*, 1, 1959, 47–49.

Fletcher, H., A method for calculating hearing for speech from an audiogram. *Acta otolaryng.*, Suppl. 90, 1950, 26–37.

Graham, J. T., Evaluation of methods for predicting speech reception threshold. *Arch. Otolaryng.*, 72, 1960, 347–350.

Hirsh, I. J., Davis, H., Silverman, S. R., Reynolds, Elizabeth G., Eldert, Elizabeth, and Benson, R. W., Development of materials for speech audiometry. *J. Speech Hearing Dis.*, 17, 1952, 321–337.

Jerger, J. F., Carhart, R., Tillman, T. W., and Peterson, J. L., Some relations between normal hearing for pure tones and for speech. *J. Speech Hearing Res.*, 2, 1959, 126–140.

Newby, H. A., *Audiology: Principles and Practice*. New York: Appleton-Century-Crofts, 1958.

Quiggle, R. R., Glorig, A., Delk, J. H., and Summerfield, Anne B., Predicting hearing loss for speech from pure tone audiograms. *Laryngoscope*, 67, 1957, 1–15.

Research News Note. Multidisciplinary Investigation of Functional Hearing Loss Enters Fourth (Final) Year. *J. Speech Hearing Res.*, 5, 1962, 291.

Ruhm, H. B., and Carhart, R., Objective speech audiometry: a new method based on electrodermal response. *J. Speech Hearing Res.*, 1, 1958, 169–178.

Tillman, T. W., and Jerger, J. F., Some factors affecting the spondee threshold in normal hearing subjects. *J. Speech Hearing Res.*, 2, 1959, 141–146.

Ventry, I. M., Relative efficiency of tests used to detect functional hearing loss. *International Audiol.*, 1, 1962, 145–150.

Ventry, I. M., and Chaiklin, J. B., Functional hearing loss: a problem in terminology. *Asha*, 4, 1962, 251–254.

Watson, L. A., *A Manual for Advanced Audiometry*. Minneapolis: Maico Company, 1949.

Watson, L. A., and Tolan, T., *Hearing Tests and Hearing Instruments*. Baltimore: Williams and Wilkins, 1949.

Whipple, C. I., and Kodman, F., Jr., The validity of objective speech audiometry. *J. Laryng. Oto.*, 74, 1960, 84–89.

25

Audiogram–Average Methods and SRT Scores

BRUCE M. SIEGENTHALER
RICHARD STRAND

BRUCE M. SIEGENTHALER, Ph.D., is Director, Speech and Hearing Clinic, Pennsylvania State University
RICHARD STRAND is at the Marshfield Clinic, Marshfield, Wisconsin

In this paper, the term *average method* does not necessarily indicate a statistical mean. Rather, it refers to any of several methods for arriving at a single value that indicates the general hearing level derived from the pure-tone audiogram. The averaging methods described in the literature are intended to yield either percent hearing loss or an estimate of the hearing loss for speech.

An individual's hearing loss for medicolegal purposes traditionally has been expressed by converting pure-tone audiogram thresholds into a single percent value.[1] However, the audiologist usually prefers a hearing-impairment score in decibels, and he usually prefers speech-reception tests for measuring functional level of hearing. Because in his clinical practice he must on occasion deal with percent hearing loss, he is interested in its relationship to the usual speech-reception-threshold test score.

The audiologist also is interested in audiogram-average methods in order to validate test results. For example, Hirsh[2] indicated that inconsistency between SRT and average threshold for pure tones should make the clinician suspicious of one or the other of the measurements. In addition, audiologists interested in primary auditory abilities desire to know whether pure-tone and speech-reception tests measure the same or different auditory abilities; describing the relationships between speech reception and pure-tone thresholds may help to clarify the meaning of hearing loss for speech as well as for pure tones.[3]

For these reasons, the audiological literature contains a number of studies of the relationships between acuity for pure tones and for speech. Carhart[4] found a product-moment correlation of 0.59 between the 1947 AMA percent method and speech-hearing thresholds, and a correlation of 0.69 between the three frequency-average and speech-hearing thresholds. In another study,[5] he found correlations between spondee threshold and AMA percent of between 0.49 and 0.82, depending on audiogram shape; the correlations between spondee threshold and three-frequency average were 0.80 for all types of audiograms, 0.79

Reprinted by permission of the authors from *J. acoust. Soc. Amer.*, **36**, pp. 589–595 (1964).

[1] "Tentative Standard Procedure for Evaluating the Percentage Loss of Hearing in Medico-Legal Cases," J. Am. Med. Assoc. **133**, 396–397 (1947).

[2] I. J. Hirsh, *The Measurement of Hearing* (McGraw-Hill Book Co., Inc., New York, 1952).

[3] J. D. Harris, H. L. Haines, and C. K. Myers. "A New Formula for Using the Audiogram to Predict Hearing Loss for Speech," Med. Res. Lab. Rept. No. 273 (Bur. Med. & Surgery, U.S. Navy Dept., Proj. NM 003 041.56.07, 24 Feb. 1956).

[4] R. Carhart, "Monitored Live Voice as a Test of Auditory Acuity," J. Acoust. Soc. Am. **17**, 339–349 (1946).

[5] R. Carhart, "Speech Reception in Relation to Pattern of Pure Tone Loss," J. Speech Disorders **11**, 97–108 (1946).

for flat, 0.75 for gradually descending, and 0.29 for markedly descending audiograms. Fletcher [6] reported that the mean of the two thresholds among the three frequencies 500, 1000, and 2000 cps gives a better approximation of speech-reception threshold than the three-frequency average. Harris, Haines, and Myers [3] used a multiple-regression technique to derive a formula to predict threshold for phonetically balanced word lists from the pure-tone audiogram. They found between-test correlations of 0.90, and a standard error for estimating SRT of 3.2 dB. Quiggle, Glorig, Delk, and Summerfield [7] independently derived a multiple-regression equation for the same purpose, using test W-1 as the criterion. Using their formula, standard errors of estimate are between 5.0 and 10.3 dB. In a study done by Graham,[8] correlations on the order of 0.90 were found between SRT measurements and four audiogram methods (three-frequency, two-frequency, Quiggle, and the Zarcoff method using bands of noise). His findings supported use of either the two-frequency or the three-frequency method in preference to the other methods.

Much of the research of the type mentioned above has been done on a single heterogeneous group of audiograms rather than on subcategories of audiograms, as was done by Carhart. Often, a given audiogram-average method has been tested against only one speech-reception test or against tests not in common clinical use, or a comparative evaluation of more than one averaging method has not been done. Because several methods are available for obtaining audiogram average, the audiologist is faced with the problem of which he should use in his clinical practice. The research available at this time has not indicated the best method for relating speech-hearing loss and pure-tone audiogram.

The purpose of the present study was to do

a comparison of several methods commonly known to audiologists for relating pure-tone audiograms and speech-reception thresholds, using several speech-reception-threshold tests and subcategories of audiograms. The intent was not to give a critique or discussion of each of the several available methods. Rather, given the methods, the intent was to do an empirical comparison among them.

I. PROCEDURE

The hearing-evaluation records on 535 patients in the Speech and Hearing Clinic audiology files at The Pennsylvania State University were used. Clinic folders were examined serially. A folder was utilized if valid test scores had been obtained and if an organic, binaural, peripheral hearing loss was present in at least one frequency in both ears according to notations made by the examining audiologist. Also, test scores had to be present for pure-tone air conduction in both ears at 250, 500, 1000, 2000, 4000, and 8000 cps, and for at least one of the following speech-reception-threshold tests: No. 9, W-2, picture-identification threshold [9] or nonstandard tests used in the clinic for determining speech-reception threshold when other procedures were not appropriate. The nonstandard tests, given by speech audiometer, were pointing to parts of the body, repeating numbers, and so forth. All of the testing was done by experienced clinicians in the sound-isolated room at The Pennsylvania State University Speech and Hearing Clinic. The binaural speech-reception-threshold testing was done in a sound field. A few test scores were obtained with recordings; the majority were obtained using live voice. The subjects on whom data were used were from 4 to 87 years of age, included 275 males and 260 females, and had a wide range of etiological and diagnostic categories. Hearing losses ranged from very mild to profound. Subjects given the picture-identification test (PIT) were in the age range four to fifteen

[6] H. Fletcher, "A Method of Calculating Hearing Loss for Speech from an Audiogram," J. Acoust. Soc. Am. **22**, 1–5 (1950).

[7] R. Quiggle, A. Glorig, J. Delk, and A. Summerfield, "Predicting Hearing Loss for Speech from Pure Tone Audiograms," Laryngoscope **67**, 1–15 (1957).

[8] J. T. Graham, "Evaluation of Methods for Predicting Speech Reception Threshold," AMA Arch. Otolaryngol. **72,** 347–350 (1960).

[9] B. Siegenthaler, J. Pearson, and R. Lezak, "A Speech Reception Threshold Test for Children," J. Speech & Hearing Disorders **19**, 360–366 (1954).

years. Subjects given tests No. 9 and W-2 were above twelve years. Subjects given nonstandardized tests covered the entire age range and tended toward severe hearing losses, lack of language, mental retardation, and uncooperativeness.

The clinic audiograms often did not have thresholds for frequencies 1500 and 6000 cps as needed for some of the audiogram-average methods. Frequently, lines on the audiogram between 1000 and 2000 and between 4000 and 8000 cps, accounting for the logarithmic progression in frequency, were established. Threshold for 1500 cps, to 5 dB, was obtained from a line connecting thresholds for 1000 and 2000 cps. The threshold for 6000 cps was estimated in a similar manner, but the thresholds at 4000 and 8000 cps were used as reference points.

The *better-ear* concept was employed to obtain an estimate of over-all binaural-hearing loss from the audiogram. That is, the lesser pure-tone loss was used to indicate hearing acuity at each frequency. (However, for the AMA method, each ear was considered separately prior to the binaural percent-loss computation.) Each better-ear audiogram was classified in the manner described by Carhart,[10] using the categories flat (F), gradual (G), marked (M), rising (R), and trough (T). All audiograms were grouped into an unselected (U) category, regardless of SRT test given, and subdivided by audiogram shape. The audiograms also were subdivided according to SRT test given and further according to audiometric category within SRT test.

An IBM-650 computer was programmed to assist in the following calculations. A single value from each pure-tone audiogram was obtained according to each of the following methods:

(a) 0.83 times mean decibel loss for frequencies 250 to 4000 cps inclusive;
(b) Fowler-revised method;[11]
(c) three-frequency average;[4]

(d) Harris *et al.* regression equation;[3]
(e) two-frequency average;[6]
(f) Quiggle *et al.* regression equation;[7]
(g) AMA method, 1947 revision.[1]

Product-moment correlations were computed between each audiogram-average method and subject SRT scores for each type of test given and for each audiogram class.

II. RESULTS AND ANALYSIS

Table 25-1 shows the product-moment correlation between audiogram-average method and speech-reception thresholds for each audiogram group. Generally, moderate and high correlations were found; i.e., most r's are 0.70 and up, and many are in the 0.80 and 0.90 range. The correlations for the F- and G-shaped audiograms appear to be consistently higher than those for the M, R, and T audiograms. Generally, the correlations for tests W-2 and No. 9 are higher than for the PIT and nonstandardized tests. The r values were tested for significance using the t method.[12] Only those values in italics in Table 25-1 are not significant at the 0.05 level. It is evident that the large majority of the correlations reached statistical significance and that many reached the 0.01 level (for a sample of fifteen, 0.64 is required for significance at the 0.01 level).

Although the correlations for nonstandardized tests, and R- and T-shaped audiograms for each type of test are shown in Table 25-1, in the main they are not treated further because of the very small numbers of subjects in these columns. The correlations in the U columns and for the "All SRT Tests" also are not considered further because the data in these areas are contained in F, G, and M columns of the Table.

One way of determining the best method for relating audiogram to SRT or of predicting SRT from the audiogram for a given audiology patient would be to note the patient's audiogram shape and the speech-reception test

[10] R. Carhart, "An Improved Method for Classifying Audiograms," Laryngoscope **55,** 640–662 (1945).

[11] E. P. Fowler, "A Simple Method of Measuring Percentage of Capacity to Hear Speech," AMA Arch. Otolaryngol. **36,** 874–890 (1942).

[12] E. Lindquist, *Statistical Analysis in Educational Research* (Houghton Mifflin Co., Boston, 1940), p. 212.

TABLE 25-1. PRODUCT-MOMENT CORRELATIONS BETWEEN EACH METHOD OF AUDIOGRAM AVERAGE AND SRT SCORES BY AUDIOGRAM TYPE

	All SRT tests						Test W-2						Test No. 9						PIT						Nonstandardized tests					
	U	F	G	M	R	T	U	F	G	M	R	T	U	F	G	M	R	T	U	F	G	M	R	T	U	F	G	M	R	T
	535	221	188	91	17	18	284	93	111	59	9	12	77	30	31	10	5	1	161	93	43	18	3	4	13	5	3	4	0	1
AMA	78	84	90	69	64	73	80	87	91	69	*60*	65	82	87	90	*61*	62	...	74	74	91	87	84	99	76	94	100	13	...	...
0.83	87	89	92	74	78	81	87	91	92	73	76	77	91	93	94	66	52	...	85	82	92	91	96	91	85	93	97	43	...	...
Fowler	80	87	90	71	71	73	82	89	91	71	*53*	65	84	90	90	65	61	...	75	77	90	88	89	94	78	96	99	07	...	...
3-freq.	87	88	92	75	75	80	87	89	92	75	*61*	75	91	92	95	*69*	57	...	85	81	93	90	81	95	87	90	97	00	...	...
Harris	84	90	92	73	72	79	85	90	92	73	*59*	76	89	93	95	*61*	52	...	82	82	92	90	84	93	79	96	98	25	...	...
2-freq.	87	88	92	79	77	84	87	89	91	79	*60*	79	90	92	95	70	61	...	88	81	93	92	84	84	95	91	98	41	...	...
Quiggle	87	87	92	76	70	79	86	89	92	76	*55*	77	91	92	95	69	40	...	85	80	93	91	76	94	91	97	97	00	...	...

NOTES: U indicates all audiograms for subjects having a given SRT test grouped together. F, G, M, R, and T indicate audiograms in the category flat-, gradual-, marked-, rising-, and trough-shaped, respectively. At the top of each column is the number of subjects contributing to that column. Decimal points preceding each r value have been omitted to conserve space. Correlation values italicized are *not* significantly different from zero at the 0.05 level. Columns with fewer than nine subjects were not evaluated for significance.

given, and referring to Table 25-1. The audiogram-average method, according to Table 25-1, having the highest correlation for the patient's-test data would be preferred. For example, if the W-2 test were given and the patient had an F audiogram, the 0.83 method is preferred because it has the highest r in the appropriate column of Table 25-1. Following are the methods preferred according to SRT test and audiogram type:

For test W-2

F: 0.83 method

G: 0.83 method, three-frequency, Harris, and Quiggle methods

M: two-frequency method

For test No. 9

F: Harris method and 0.83 method

G: two-frequency, Quiggle, three-frequency, and Harris methods

M: two-frequency method

For the PIT test

F: Harris method and 0.83 method

G: two-frequency, three-frequency, and Quiggle methods

M: two-frequency method

According to this listing, the two-frequency method has the most frequent occurrence of preference.

For general purposes, it is desirable to have a single method for relating pure-tone audiograms to different SRT test materials and audiogram types. To select a single pre-

ferred method, among the nine columns of interest in Table 25-1 (F, G, and M for tests W-2, No. 9, and PIT), the seven audiogram-average methods were ranked according to product-moment-correlation value. Table 25-2

TABLE 25-2. RANKS FOR THE SEVEN AUDIOGRAM-AVERAGE METHODS FOR NINE COLUMNS OF TABLE 25-1

	Audiogram-average methods						
	AMA	0.83	Fowler	3-Freq.	Harris	2-Freq.	Quiggle
Test W-2							
F	7	1	4.5	4.5	2	4.5	4.5
G	6	2.5	6	2.5	2.5	6	2.5
M	7	4.5	6	3	4.5	1	2
Test No. 9							
F	7	1.5	6	4	1.5	4	4
G	6.5	5	6.5	2.5	2.5	2.5	2.5
M	6.5	4	5	2.5	6.5	1	2.5
PIT							
F	7	1.5	6	3.5	1.5	3.5	5
G	7	4.5	6	2	4.5	2	2
M	7	2.5	6	4.5	4.5	1	2.5
Sum of ranks	61.0	27.0	52.0	29.0	30.0	25.5	27.5

gives the ranks. The two-frequency method, having the lowest sum of ranks, has superiority over the other methods although, except for the AMA and the Fowler methods, the differences in sum of ranks are small. The Friedman analysis of variance[13] was used to test for differences among the rankings. The X_r^2 value was 245.27, significant at the 0.001 level. A series of sign tests[14] was done to compare the r levels among the audiogram-averaging methods. The associated probabi-

[13] S. Siegel, *Nonparametric Statistics for the Behavioral Sciences* (McGraw-Hill Book Co., Inc., New York, 1956).

[14] See Ref. 13, p. 68.

TABLE 25-3. SIGN-TEST PROBABILITIES FOR DIFFERENCES IN
r VALUES AMONG AUDIOGRAM-AVERAGE METHODS

| | Audiogram-average methods | | | | | |
	AMA	0.83	Fowler	3-Freq.	Harris	2-Freq.
Quiggle	0.002	0.500	0.004	0.188 [a]	0.500	0.188 [a]
2-Freq.	0.016	0.500	0.008	0.188 [a]	0.637	
Harris	0.016	0.188 [a]	0.020	0.656		
3-Freq.	0.002	0.637	0.004			
Fowler	0.008	0.002				
0.83	0.002					

[a] P values greater than 0.188; exact values were not available.

lity values are shown in Table 25-3, and indicate that, although there was a significant value when comparing the AMA and the Fowler methods, both consistently had significant values when compared with the other methods. The other methods, however, when compared with each other showed high probabilities of being similar in correlation with SRT scores.

III. DISCUSSION

According to the previous data and analysis, the two-frequency method has an advantage over the other methods as a general procedure for relating the audiogram to speech-reception threshold. This advantage can be seen in Tables 25-1 and 25-2, which show that the two-frequency method had the highest correlation or was tied with other methods for highest correlation more times than any other method, and which also show that it had the lowest sum of ranks of all methods across the various SRT procedures and audiogram shapes. This general superiority also is seen in the "All SRT Tests" section of Table 25-1. However, according to Tables 25-1 and 25-2 and the series of sign tests shown in Table 25-3, the differences among the several audiogram-average methods are relatively small. This is seen especially among the 0.83, the three-frequency, the Harris, the two-frequency, and the Quiggle methods. Thus, the following conclusions seem warranted:

1. The two-frequency method appears to be the best, single, general method for relating pure-tone audiograms of various shapes to SRT-test materials of various kinds.

2. The 0.83, the three-frequency, the Harris, and the Quiggle methods can be considered nearly as good as and possible alternates for the two-frequency method when relating pure-tone audiograms to SRT-test scores.

3. The 1947 revision of the AMA method and the Fowler method appear to be less closely related to speech-reception thresholds than the other audiogram-average methods included in this study.

The finding that the AMA and the Fowler methods are separate from the other methods in their relationship to SRT scores and are similar to each other in this respect is not surprising in view of their communality. Both were designed for obtaining percent hearing loss, not for predicting decibels of hearing loss for speech (although the presumed relative contributions of various frequencies to speech intelligibility were considered in their design). Also, they have a common basis through Fowler's contribution to development of both methods.

It might be supposed that pure-tone thresholds and speech-reception thresholds measure different aspects of auditory acuity and that different auditory factors influence each type of threshold measurement. Therefore, it may be unrealistic to expect any audiogram method to reach a perfect correlation with SRT. The present methods may be the best that can be expected in view of the careful work that had gone into their development. This study neither does nor does not support the viewpoint that a search for a better method of relating pure-tone audiograms to speech-reception-test scores should be continued. Rather, it demonstrates a general preference for the two-frequency average as the method of choice for relating pure-tone threshold and speech-reception thresholds.

part IV

MEASUREMENT OF SPEECH DISCRIMINATION

Any minimum test battery for assessing hearing usually includes, in addition to threshold tests, some measurement of the ear's ability to understand speech at a level well above threshold. Such tests are referred to as tests of intelligibility, of articulation, or, more commonly, of speech discrimination. Estimates of suprathreshold hearing for speech are helpful in determining the anatomical site of a lesion in the auditory system, in assessing ability to communicate in social situations, and in evaluating hearing-aid performance. Because of difficulties in the development, administration, and interpretation of discrimination tests, many questions remain as to how accurately present tests satisfy these needs. Any particular speech-discrimination score is meaningful only when one knows which test was used and under what conditions it was given.

In this section we have assembled a collection of papers that discuss theoretical and practical problems in the use of speech-discrimination tests. An impressive number of intelligibility tests have been devised and investigated in the past twenty years; most, however, have not found their way into general usage. The majority of the papers in this section are concerned with the two most widely-used tests: the PB-50 lists, developed at Harvard University and described by Egan (1948), and the W-22 lists, constructed at Central Institute for the Deaf and described by Hirsh *et al.* in Part III. The student is encouraged to consult both of the foregoing references since they contain much useful information concerning speech audiometry.

Some of the theoretical considerations in measurement of speech intelligibility are discussed by Miller, Heise, and Lichten in the first paper presented here. The authors describe the differences one can expect with differences in speech stimuli, differences in size of test vocabulary, and differences in stimulus context. They find that repetition of stimuli produces only slight improvements in intelligibility. This paper should serve to introduce to the student the concept of "articulation function," the understanding of which is basic to much of the material presented in this section.

As it became apparent that the Hirsh recordings of W-22 yielded higher discrimination scores than the Rush Hughes recordings of PB-50, Silverman and Hirsh (1955) published a paper examining the differences between the two tests. Their paper showed differences between speakers and presented theoretical implications of clinical importance. We have selected a related article by Carhart which reviews many problems, including differences between PB-50 lists and W-22 lists, in clinical measurement of speech intelligibility. He shows that the disparity in results obtained with these tests may increase when sensorineural hearing loss is present, a point also suggested by Silverman and Hirsh. Carhart includes discussions of live-voice vs. recorded presentations of test stimuli, 25- vs. 50-word lists, presentation level, and test reliability. Carhart's article should impress upon the beginning clinical audiologist the importance of choosing tests according to the purpose for which they are to be used. Not emphasized by him, but implied in his comments, is the need for the audiologist to state, for any particular patient, the test employed and the conditions under which it was administered.

The next paper, by Campbell, concerns an attempt to improve the homogeneity and average level of word difficulty of the four W-22 word lists. Working from an analysis of errors with a clinical population, Campbell constructed new lists, containing W-22 stimulus items, which appear to satisfy his aims. The new lists, however, still do not provide the desired distribution of scores which, according to Campbell, could be achieved by replacing some of the easier W-22 words for the more difficult ones.

Live-voice presentation of speech-discrimination tests has been investigated by Brandy. He has shown that the same speaker, on different days, will present stimuli which result in different discrimination scores for the listener. Brandy's paper is one of those which questions the advisability of discrimination tests administered by live voice.

Prediction of speech-discrimination ability from other audiometric data is poor, particularly when sensorineural hearing loss is present. Ross *et al.* (1965) and Elliot (1963) have attempted to predict discrimination scores from other audiometric parameters, but with only limited success. It appears that general shape of the pure-tone audiogram has little to do with intelligibility performance, although amount of sensorineural loss is important to some degree. To illustrate this point, we have presented a short paper by Thompson and Hoel who demonstrate that individuals with "flat" hearing losses can have very poor discrimination for speech, particularly if the loss is greater than 50 db.

Space considerations have prevented us from including a number of papers concerning discrimination tests that are used infrequently (see for example, Kreul *et al.*, 1968 and Owens and Schubert, 1968). We have, however, included an article by Jerger, Speaks, and Trammell who describe lists of stimuli composed of "synthetic sentences." The use of such sentences, say the authors, may help to eliminate some of the problems encountered in traditional speech audiometry, particularly the problems related to stimuli that consist of single-syllable words. When synthetic sentences are made more difficult to identify by the addition of a competing message, test performance often, though not always, approximates that for single-syllable words. Comparative performance is discussed for a group of patients who reveal representative auditory problems.

REFERENCES

1. Egan, J. P. Articulation testing methods. *Laryngoscope*, **58**, pp. 955–991 (1948).

2. Elliott, L. L. Prediction of speech discrimination scores from other test information. *J. aud. Res.*, **3**, pp. 35–45 (1963).

3. Kreul, E. J., Nixon, J. C., Kryter, K. D., Bell, D. W., Lang, J. S., and Schubert, E. D. A proposed clinical test of speech discrimination. *J. Speech Hearing Res.*, **11**, pp. 536–552 (1968).

4. Owens, E., and Schubert, E. D. The development of consonant items for speech discrimination testing. *J. Speech Hearing Res.*, **11**, pp. 656–667 (1968).

5. Ross, M., Huntington, D. A., Newby, H. A., and Dixon, R. F. Speech discrimination of hearing-impaired individuals in noise. *J. aud. Res.*, **5**, pp. 47–72 (1965).

6. Silverman, S. R., and Hirsh, I. J. Problems related to the use of speech in clinical audiometry. *Ann. Otol. Rhinol. Laryngol.*, **64**, pp. 1234–1244 (1955).

26

The Intelligibility of Speech
as a Function of the Context of the Test Materials

GEORGE A. MILLER
GEORGE A. HEISE
WILLIAM LICHTEN

GEORGE A. MILLER, Ph.D., is at The Rockefeller University, New York City
GEORGE A. HEISE, Ph.D., is at Indiana University
WILLIAM LICHTEN was an undergraduate student at Harvard University when this study was
    conducted

For many years communication engineers have used a psychophysical method called the "articulation test" (2, 3). An announcer reads lists of syllables, words, or sentences to a group of listeners who report what they hear. The articulation score is the percentage of discrete test units reported correctly by the listeners. This method gives a quantitative evaluation of the performance of a speech communication system.

There are three classes of variables involved in an articulation test: the *personnel*, talkers and listeners; the *test materials*, syllables, words, sentences, or continuous discourse; and the communication *equipment*, rooms, microphones, amplifiers, radios, earphones, etc. The present paper is directed toward the second of these three classes of variables, the test materials.[1] The central concern can be stated as follows: Why is a stimulus configuration, a word, heard correctly in one context and incorrectly in another?

Three kinds of contexts are explored: (*a*) context supplied by the knowledge that the test item is one of a small vocabulary of items, (*b*) context supplied by the items that precede or follow a given item in a word or sentence, and (*c*) context supplied by the knowledge that the item is a repetition of the immediately preceding item. All three kinds of context enable the listener to limit the range of alternatives from which he selects his response. A word selected from a small vocabulary must be one of the few words agreed upon in advance. A word in a sentence must be one of the relatively few words that make a reasonable continuation of the sentence according to grammatical rules agreed upon in advance. A repeated word must be one of the few words similar to the word just heard. Not anything can happen, and the listener can set himself to make the required discrimination. Context, in the sense the word assumes here, is the *S's* knowledge of the conditions of stimulation. The experimental problem is to vary the nature and amount of this contextual knowledge in order to study its influence upon perceptual accuracy.

Reprinted by permission of the authors from *J. exp. Psychol.*, **41,** pp. 329–335 (1951).
[1] This research was carried out under Contract N5ori-76 between Harvard University and the Office of Naval Research, U.S. Navy (Project NR147-201, Report PNR-74).

EQUIPMENT AND PROCEDURE

The apparatus consisted of components from military communication equipment used during the recent war. The output voltage of a carbon microphone was amplified and delivered to the listener's dynamic earphones. The talker monitored his speaking level with a volume indicator (VU meter) that responded to the voltage generated at the output of the amplifier. A random noise voltage, with a spectrum that was relatively uniform from 100 to 7,000 cps, was introduced at the listener's earphones. The signal-to-noise ratio (S/N) was varied by holding the average voice level constant and changing the level of the noise. The S/N was measured by a vacuum tube voltmeter across the terminals of the earphones, and the measurements reported in the following pages represent the ratio in decibels of the average peak deflection of the meter for the words (in the absence of noise) to the level of the noise in the 7,000-cycle band. A S/N of zero db means, therefore, that the electrical measurements indicated the two voltages, speech and noise, were equal in magnitude. Since the earphones transduce frequencies only up to about 4,500 cps, however, the acoustic level of the noise was about 2 db lower than these electrical measurements indicate. The over-all acoustic level of the voice at the listener's ears was approximately 90 db re .0002 dyne/cm².

The speech channel was not a high quality system. Only the speech frequencies between 200 and 3,000 cps were passed along to the listener.[2]

Only two Ss were used throughout the experiments. Both had normal auditory acuity, and both were familiar with the design and theory of the experiments. The Ss were located in different rooms, connected only by the communication channel described above, and they alternated as talker and listener. Some particular S/N was set up in the channel, and the talker proceeded to read a list of test items. These items were pronounced after a

carrier sentence, "You will write. . . ." During this carrier sentence the talker adjusted his voice level to give the proper deflection of the monitoring VU meter, and then the test item was delivered with the same degree of effort. This procedure preserves the inherent variability of English words—the word "peep" has much less acoustic energy than the word "raw" when both words are pronounced with equal emphasis by a normal talker. By monitoring the carrier sentence rather than the test item, the relative intensities of the speech sounds are preserved in a natural fashion. The listener then recorded the item on a test blank, and these test sheets were later graded and the scores converted to percentages.

IMPORTANCE OF TEST MATERIALS

The kind of speech materials used to test communication systems is an important variable determining the results of the tests. Figure 26-1 illustrates how much difference the test materials can make. These three functions were obtained for the communication channel and the personnel described above. The test materials used for these three functions were the following.

(a) The *digits* were pronounced *zero, wun, too, thuh-ree, four, f-i-i-v, six, seven, ate, niner*. (b) The *sentences* were those constructed at the Psycho-Acoustic Laboratory (*1*). A sentence consists of five major words connected by auxiliary "of's," "the's," etc. The score shown in Figure 26-2 represents the percentage of these major words heard correctly. (c) The *nonsense syllables* used were also those published by Egan (*1*). To standardize the pronunciation and recording of the nonsense syllables, an abbreviated phonetic symbolism was used.

The values of S/N necessary for 50 percent correct responses are approximately −14 db for digits, −4 db for the individual words in a sentence, and +3 db for nonsense syllables. At a S/N where practically no nonsense syllables were recorded correctly, nearly all the

[2] For the convenience of those who may wish to apply one of the several schemes for predicting articulation scores, the frequency response of the system may be obtained by ordering Document 3250 from American Documentation Institute, 1719 N Street, N.W., Washington 6, D.C., remitting $1.00 for microfilm (images 1 in. high on standard 35 mm. motion picture film) or $1.00 for photocopies (6 × 8 in.) readable without optical aid.

digits were correctly communicated. Differences of this magnitude require explanation. What differences among these spoken stimuli make some easy to hear and others quite difficult? A list of perceptual aspects—rhythm, accent, grouping, meaning, or phonetic composition—can be suggested. Our experiments indicate, however, that these various characteristics of the stimulus that *did* occur are less important than the characteristics of the stimuli that *could* have occurred but didn't. The most important variable producing the differences is the range of possible alternatives from which a test item is selected. A listener's expectation (or, more precisely, his freedom of choice) is determined by the context in which the particular phonetic pattern occurs. When digits are used, the listener can respond correctly with a marginal impression of the relatively intense vowel sound alone, because all the digits, with the exception of *five* and *nine*, have different vowels. Since the alternatives are thus limited, the digit is interpreted correctly, although the same acoustic stimulus is quite ambiguous when the alternatives are not so limited. With nonsense syllables, however, this limitation of possibilities is far less helpful; the listener feels that anything can happen. To record the nonsense syllable correctly, a listener must perceive each phoneme correctly, and the perception of one phoneme in a syllable does not give a clue to the other phonemes in the same syllable. Not only must the listener hear the vowels correctly, but the less intense consonant sounds must also be distinguished.

SIZE OF TEST VOCABULARY

An articulation test is a rather unusual combination of the familiar psychophysical procedures. The experiment requires the listener to select, not one out of two or three, but one out of several thousand alternative responses. Thus the number of alternatives involved becomes an interesting variable.

Suppose we try to adapt spoken stimuli as closely as possible to the traditional method of constant stimuli. To this end we might use a single speech sound or a single syllable as the stimulus, present this speech unit at various intensities, and ask *S* to report whether or not he heard each presentation. This procedure determines a threshold of audibility for the particular speech unit. The practical value of this isolated datum is negligible.

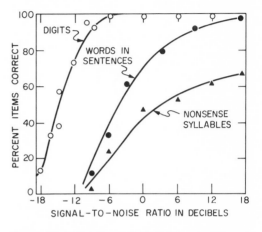

Figure 26-1. Relative intelligibility of different test materials.

The experiment must be repeated for all the forty or fifty different speech sounds or the thousands of different syllables of English. And then we know only about audibility, not intelligibility.

Consider this distinction between audible speech and intelligible speech. It is intuitively clear that the words *audible* and *intelligible* are not synonyms, and listeners give reliably higher thresholds when asked to make continuous discourse "just understandable" instead of "just audible" (2). The crux of the difference is that intelligibility involves a complex discrimination and identification, whereas audibility is simply a discrimination of presence or absence.

It seems reasonable, therefore, to call a speech unit intelligible when *it is possible for an average listener with normal hearing to distinguish it from a set of alternative units.* By a speech unit is meant any combination of vocal noises—phonemes, syllables, words, phrases, sentences. The act of distinguishing can take various forms—repeating the unit, writing it down, pointing to it, behaving in accordance with its content, etc. The critical part of this definition concerns the set of alternative speech units from which the particular unit is selected. This part of the definition reduces intelligibility to discriminability, and avoids the questions of semantic rules and meaning. Discriminability is a function of the number of alternatives and the similarities among them. The word "loot" is easily discriminated if all the alternatives are trisyllabic, but difficult to distinguish, other things being equal, in a set of alternatives that includes "boot," "loop," "jute," "lewd," "mute," "loose," etc.

An articulation test is analogous to a test of visual acuity where the percentage of correct judgments of a fixed set of test figures is plotted as a function of the level of illumination. A differential judgment is required under various favorable and unfavorable conditions. In such an experiment we determine the most unfavorable conditions under which the discrimination can be made, rather than the most unfavorable conditions under which the presence of the stimuli can be detected. These are clearly different thresholds and correspond to what we have called the thresholds of intelligibility and of audibility.

A difficult discrimination quickly becomes impossible as the conditions are made unfavorable, whereas an easy and obvious difference remains noticeable almost as long as the stimuli can be detected. The discrimination of a difference of 3 cycles in frequency, for example, is fairly accurate under favorable conditions—at 1,000 cps and 100 db. If the intensity is progressively reduced, however, such a small difference becomes imperceptible. For a simpler discrimination, say 30 cycles difference in frequency, the listener can respond accurately at all intensities down to 5 or 10 db above the threshold of audibility.

The situation is manageable so long as we have some index of the difficulty of the discrimination. Thus, in the tonal example, the difficulty can be gauged by the size of the difference in frequency. With the articulation test, however, such an index is not available. We could utilize known differences in the spectra of the sounds to construct an index of the distance between speech sounds, but this index is not yet available. For the present we must approach the problem in a simpler way.

Imagine a many-dimensional space with a separate coordinate for each one of the different frequencies involved in human speech sounds. Along each coordinate plot the relative amplitude of the component at that frequency. In this hyperspace each unique speech sound is represented by a single point. Each point in the hyperspace represents a single acoustic spectrum. The group of similar sounds comprising a phoneme is represented by a cluster of points in the hyperspace. If a language utilized only two different phonemes, the hyperspace could be split into two parts, one for each phoneme. The distance between the two phonemes could be made as large as the vocal mechanism permits, and discrimination would be relatively easy. But suppose the number of different phonemes in the language is increased from two to ten. With ten different phonemes the hyperspace must be divided into at least ten subspaces, and the average distance between phonemes must be smaller with ten phonemes than it is with two. The discriminations involved must be correspondingly more precise. If the number of alternative phonemes is increased to a thousand, then the listener is required to make even more precise discriminations.

In other words, the ease with which a discrimination of speech sounds can be made is limited according to the number of different speech sounds that must be discriminated. From this line of reasoning it follows that the number of alternatives can be used to gauge the difficulty of discrimination. This argument has been developed by Shannon (5) to give a measure of the amount of information in a message. The interesting aspect of this index of difficulty, or of amount of information, is that it does not depend upon the characteristics of the particular item, but upon the range of items that *could* occur.

The range of alternatives was used as the experimental variable in the following way. The listener was informed that each test word would be one of the items from a given restricted vocabulary. The size of the test vocabularly was alternatively 2, 4, 8, 16, 32, or 256 words. The talker always spoke one of the words from the prearranged list.

The words used in the restricted vocabularies were chosen at random from the list of phonetically balanced monosyllables published by Egan (*2*). For the two-alternative vocabulary, different pairs of words were chosen and typed on the listener's answer sheet. The talker read one of the pair, and the listener checked the item he heard. A similar procedure was used for the four- and eight-word vocabularies. For the 16-, 32-, and 256-word vocabularies the listeners had a list of all the words before them, and studied this list until they made their choice. The choice was recorded and a signal given to the talker to proceed to the next item. The *Ss* studied carefully the particular list used in any test and arranged the words according to the vowel sounds before the tests began.

The results are summarized in Table 26-1 and in Figure 26-2. Included with the data for restricted vocabularies are data for words from the original list of 1,000 monosyllables, obtained with no list of choices available to the listener. When these data are corrected for chance, the two-word vocabulary gives a threshold (50 percent of the words correct) at −14 db, the 256-word vocabulary gives a threshold at −4 db, and the unrestricted list of monosyllables gives a threshold at +4 db. With the same test words the threshold is changed 18 db by varying the number of alternatives. This result supports the argument that it is not so much the particular item as the context in which the item occurs that determines its intelligibility.

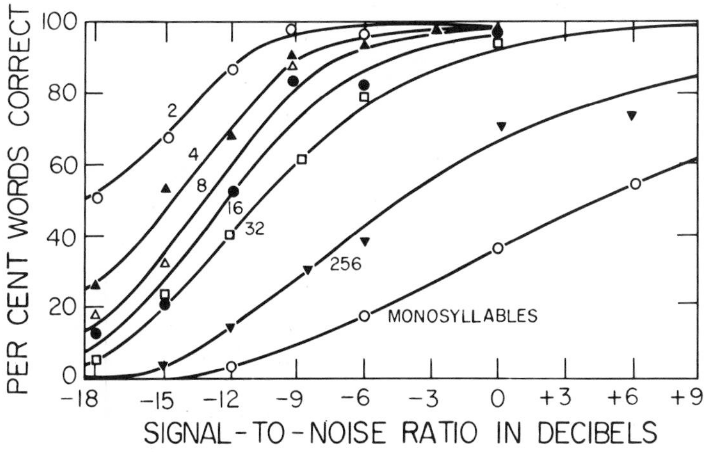

Figure 26-2. Intelligibility of monosyllables as a function of the size of the test vocabulary. (Data are not corrected for effects of chance.)

TABLE 26-1. PERCENT WORDS CORRECT IN ARTICULATION TESTS WITH VOCABULARIES OF VARIOUS SIZES

	Size of Vocabulary							
S/N in db	2	4	8	Digits	16	32	256	Monosyllables
− 21	49							
− 18	51	27	17	13	13	5		
− 15	67	52	32	38	19	20	2	
− 12	87	69	57	73	51	39	14	3
− 9	98	92	89	92	85	61	28	
− 6		94	95	99	82	81	39	17
− 3		96						
0				100	97	95	70	37
+ 6				100			76	53
+ 12				100			90	70
+ 18								82

CONTEXT OF THE SENTENCE

A word is harder to understand if it is heard in isolation than if it is heard in a sentence. This fact is illustrated by Figure 26-3. Sentences containing five key words were read, and the listener's responses were scored as the percentage of these key words that were heard correctly. These data are shown by the filled circles in Figures 26-1 and 26-3. For compari-

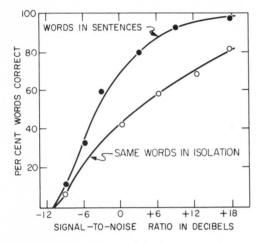

Figure 26-3. Effect of sentence context on the intelligibility of words.

son, the key words were extracted from the sentences, scrambled, and read in isolation. The scores obtained under these conditions are shown by the open circles of Figure 26-3. The removal of sentential context changes the threshold 6 db.

The effect of the sentence is comparable to the effect of a restricted vocabulary, although the degree of restriction is harder to estimate. When the talker begins a sentence, "Apples grow on ——," the range of possible continuations is sharply restricted. This restriction makes the discrimination easier and lowers the threshold of intelligibility. A detailed statistical discussion of the restrictions imposed by English sentence structure is given by Shannon (5), and is used in a simple recall experiment by Miller and Selfridge (4).

EFFECTS OF REPETITION

When an error occurs in vocal communication, the listener can ask for a repetition of the message. The repeated message is then heard in the context provided by the original message. If the original message enabled the listener to narrow the range of alternatives, his perception of the repeated message should be more accurate. A series of tests were run with various kinds of test materials to evaluate the importance of the context of repetition. These tests were run with automatic repetition of every item and, also, with repetitions only when the listener thought he had not received the test item correctly.

The improvement in the articulation scores obtained with automatic and with requested repetitions was found to be about the same. A slight but insignificant difference was found in favor of the requested repetition, and if we add to this the savings in time achieved by omitting the unnecessary repetitions, the requested repetition is clearly superior.

The advantage gained by repetition is small for all types of test materials. In Figure 26-4 data are given for the effects of repeating automatically the monosyllabic words. The difference in threshold between one presentation and three successive presentations is only

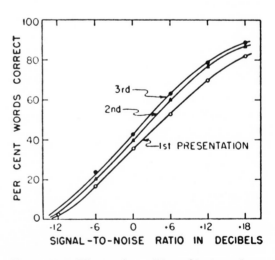

Figure 26-4. Effects of repetition of test words on the articulation score.

2.5 db. Similar data for words heard in sentences show a shift of 2 db, and for digits, 1.5 db.

These results indicate that the improvement that can be achieved by the simple repetition of a message is slight. The repeated message contains approximately the same information, and the same omissions, that the original message contained. If the listener thinks he heard the word correctly, he persists in his original response, whether it is right or wrong. If he thinks he heard the word incorrectly, he does not use this presumably incorrect impression to narrow the range of possibilities when the item recurs. In any case, no strong factor is at work to improve the accuracy on repeated presentations, and so we obtain only the slight improvement indicated in Figure 26-4.

The results indicate that far more improvement in communication is possible by standardizing procedures and vocabulary than by merely repeating all messages one to two times.

In general, therefore, the results are in qualitative agreement with the mathematical theory of communication presented by Shannon (5). A precise quantitative comparison of the data with the theory cannot be made in the absence of trustworthy information about the distributions of errors. Seemingly reasonable assumptions about the error distributions give results consistent with theoretical predictions, but a more thorough study would be rewarding. For a given signal-to-noise ratio the listener receives a given amount of information per second (according to Shannon's definition), and articulation scores can be predicted for different types of test materials on the basis of the average amount of information needed to receive each type of test item correctly.

SUMMARY

Articulation tests showed the effects of limiting the number of alternative test items upon the threshold of intelligibility for speech in noise. The number of alternative test items was limited by providing three kinds of context: (a) restricting the size of the test vocabulary, (b) using the words in sentences, and (c) repeating the test words. Differences among test materials with respect to their intelligibility are due principally to the fact that some materials require more information than others for their correct perception. The relative amount of information necessary for a given type of item is a function of the range of alternative possibilities. As the range of alternatives increases, the amount of information necessary per item also increases, and so the noise level must be decreased to permit more accurate discrimination.

REFERENCES

1. Egan, J. P. *Articulation testing methods, II.* OSRD Report No. 3802, February, 1942. (Available through Office of Technical Services, U.S. Department of Commerce, Washington, D.C., as PB 22848.)

2. Egan, J. P. Articulation testing methods. *Laryngoscope*, 1948, **58,** 955–991.

3. Fletcher, H., and Steinberg, J. C. Articulation testing methods. *Bell Syst. Tech. J.*, 1929, **8,** 806–854.

4. Miller, G. A., and Selfridge, J. Verbal context and the recall of meaningful material. *Amer. J. Psychol.*, 1950, **63,** 176–185.

5. Shannon, C. E. A mathematical theory of communication. *Bell Syst. Tech. J.*, 1948, **27,** 379–423, 623–656.

27

Problems in the Measurement of Speech Discrimination

RAYMOND CARHART

RAYMOND CARHART, Ph.D., is Professor of Audiology, Northwestern University

I. INTRODUCTION

Traditionally, a speech discrimination score is the percentage of test items a person can identify correctly by ear. Two decades ago lists of monosyllabic words, the PB-50 tests, were adapted to the measurement of the speech discrimination of the hearing impaired. These materials have since become thoroughly entrenched in otological and audiological practice. Unfortunately, a number of confusions regarding their use has persisted to the present. Our purpose is to review some of the factors that contribute to these confusions. The goal is to examine problems which, when kept in mind, can help otologists stabilize measurement of speech discrimination and unify their interpretation of its results.

II. TEST MATERIALS

The first problem is, "Which test materials shall one use?"

A test of discrimination for speech, as opposed to a threshold test, must consist of relatively nonredundant items. Otherwise, the multiplicity of clues available to the patient will obscure many of his inabilities to differentiate consonants and vowels accurately. It is for this reason that monosyllabic words have been chosen instead of conversa-

Reprinted by permission of the author from *Arch. Otolaryngol.*, **82**, pp. 253–260 (1965).

tional sentences or multisyllabic words, such as spondees. Monosyllabic words are sufficiently unpredictable for clinical subjects so that individual speech elements must be perceived relatively independently. On the other hand, they are not as confusing as nonsense syllables, which are so abstract that they baffle many subjects.

The traditional discrimination test in this country consists of 50 PB monosyllables. The original materials of this kind were the 20 PB-50-word lists developed at Harvard (6) during World War II. These lists are still used in some clinics and laboratories, but they contain enough unfamiliar words so that they can somewhat confound linguistically naive subjects. Consequently, several workers have since composed lists which are more familiar. For example, Haskins (9) developed four PB-50-word lists restricted to monosyllables taken from the speaking vocabularies of young children. Again, Hirsh et al (10) constructed the well-known W-22 test from words that (with one exception) appear in Thorndyke's tabulation of 20,000 familiar words.

The foregoing lists were all patterned so that they yielded only rough approximations of the phonetic balance found in everyday spoken English. Lehiste and Peterson (12), therefore, devised ten 50-word lists that conform very closely in balance to monosyllabic words as a class. These CNC lists, as they were called, were later improved by giving them more uniform distributions of word familiarity (*16*). Still more recently, Tillman et al (*20*) assembled other versions of the CNC test pattern, and other tests may be expected in the future.

Probably the most important consideration in choosing a particular discrimination test for clinical use is the linguistic background of the patient. Unfamiliar material tends to make the test more difficult (*15*). This fact does not mean that highly familiar words must always be used, since there are times when a relatively difficult test is preferable. However, the clinician must be on the lookout for instances where some words become nonsense items for his patient, as can occur particularly often with a young child.

Conversely, differences in phonetic balance among lists seem to be of only secondary influence as long as these are only moderate differences. This fact became apparent with the original PB-50-word lists. These 20 lists have proved to be reasonably equivalent forms, in spite of some deviation in phonetic balance. Likewise, we have found in our laboratory that discrimination scores are not changed importantly by shift from the PB-50 to the Lehiste-Peterson criterion of phonetic balance. In general as long as the test items are meaningful monosyllables for the patient and their phonetic distribution is appropriately diversified, one 50-word compilation is relatively equivalent to another.

III. TEST PRESENTATION

This generalization does not imply that major differences in discrimination scores do not occur. The contrary is true, but these large differences are brought about by other factors, such as changes in talker, in method of reproducing the test, in characteristics of the test equipment, and the like.

This circumstance brings us to the second problem facing the clinician: namely, the problem of determining the details of test presentation which he shall specify.

A major point of past controversy has been whether material should be administered by monitored live-voice, ie, spoken by the tester at the time of the test, or from a pre-recording. Critics of the live-voice procedure argue correctly that results obtained by different speakers cannot be compared unless the talkers have been demonstrated to be equivalent. Lacking this information, the best

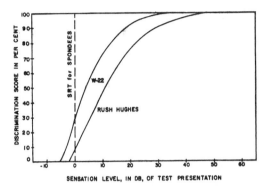

Figure 27-1. Articulation curves for normal hearers showing relation between two recorded tests.

one can do is to make comparisons only among the results obtained by a single talker and to remember that the significance of any particular score varies from one talker to the next.

A point often ignored in use of pre-recorded material is that each talker's unique characteristics are permanently built into the test he has recorded. There may be as much difference between one recording and another as between two live-voice talkers.

An excellent example of this fact is the well-known dissimilarity between the Rush-Hughes recordings and the W-22 recordings of PB-50 materials. The former, it will be recalled, constitute the version with which data were gathered in the late 1940's by Davis (*4*) and others. The latter are the later and widely used version prepared by Hirsh et al (*10*). The difference between the two versions is illustrated in Figure 27-1, which plots normal articulation functions for both versions. Notice that discrimination for W-22 improves

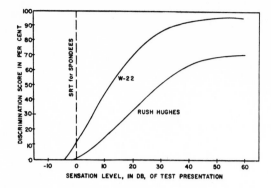

Figure 27-2. Articulation curves for an illustrative sensorineural loss showing relation between two recorded tests.

rapidly as the presentation level is raised, and that scores become nearly perfect relatively close to the speech reception threshold. The Rush-Hughes version is much more exacting, as evidenced by the more gradual improvement in discrimination as the presentation level is increased. It is not until extremely high levels are used that the Rush-Hughes scores are as good as the W-22 scores.

A somewhat comparable dissimilarity between these versions appears for clinical subjects, although the details of the relationship vary from person to person. Figure 27-2 presents an illustrative set of results. Notice first that performance on both tests is poorer than that obtained by normal listeners. This is apparent in two ways: namely each articulation function rises more gently, and it reaches a plateau before 100 percent scores are achieved. However, the most dramatic feature is that the deterioration in performance is proportionately much greater with Rush-Hughes than with W-22. For example, the plateau level is 94 percent for W-22 but it drops to 71 percent for Rush-Hughes.

As these examples emphasize, the clinician must remember that recorded tests are inflexible. Each version possesses a degree of difficulty which he must accept and to which he must adapt as best he can. Moreover, he has at his disposal only a very few recorded versions that are easily available. One or the

other of these may serve his clinical need, or neither may be very applicable.

Let us illustrate the clinician's dilemma by a further consideration of W-22. This version has become extremely popular for several reasons, one of which is that the Veterans Administration arbitrarily made it the basis for adjudicating service-connected hearing losses. Many clinicians now use the test without seriously questioning its appropriateness to their own needs. They do not ask whether it reveals the critical distinctions among their patients which it should. Among other things, they are not disturbed by relations such as Figure 27-3 illustrates. These are fairly typical of clinical findings. Here we see the cumulative frequency distribution for the scores of 170 hard of hearing veterans. Notice that no patient scored poorer than 26 percent, and that only 3.6 percent of these patients did not score at least 46 percent. These findings indicate that many of the test items were superfluous in this situation because they were so easy that almost no patient missed them. Notice also that only 39.4 percent of the patients yielded discrimination scores POORER than 90 percent. That is, 60

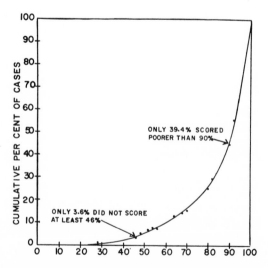

Figure 27-3. Cumulative distribution of discrimination scores obtained from 170 patients tested with W-22 recordings in a VA Audiology Center.

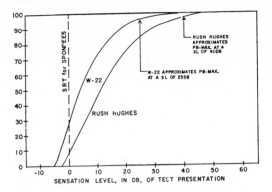

Figure 27-4. Articulation curves for normal hearers illustrating that the lowest presentation level yielding the maximum discrimination score varies with the test used.

percent of these patients obtained 90 percent or better. One may conclude that the test did very little to separate the performances of six out of every ten of these patients.

Please do not misunderstand the intent of these remarks. They are not a criticism of W-22 per se. They are a criticism of the clinician, be he audiologist or otolaryngologist, who uses a test without concern for its characteristics and for how these characteristics affect the test's usefulness to him. The Rush-Hughes version can be used just as uninsightfully, as can any other existing test. The simple fact is that no one has ever laid out the clinical criteria he felt a test should satisfy and then developed a set of recordings meeting those criteria.

Of course, variables other than the recording itself affect a test's characteristics.

One such variable is the equipment used. The American Standards Association (1) has decreed the specifications which a speech audiometer should meet. Since discrimination tests are particularly susceptible to variations in reproduction, one is not justified in comparing discrimination scores from two clinics where the same materials are presented in the same way unless the clinics also use comparable equipment.

Another variable that is critically important is the presentation level at which testing is done. Here we get into very complex problems even though the issue as it sometimes

is stated by clinicians appears very simple. To explain: clinicians often argue as to whether a discrimination test should be given 25 db above the patient's speech reception threshold, at 40 db above, or at some other level (such as the 110 db SPL advocated by Davis [4]). Here the underlying assumption has been that one should be measuring the best discriminations the patient can achieve on the test material. This maximum discrimination has sometimes been called the PB-Max score (3). The question is, "At what level is the PB-Max score achieved?"

The difficulties in selecting a presentation level which will guarantee measuring the PB-Max score can be illustrated by considering Figures 27-4 and 27-5.

Figure 27-4 compares normal articulation scores for W-22 and Rush-Hughes recordings when plotted against the sensation level of presentation. Note that W-22 yields scores good enough at a sensation level of 25 db to approximate maximum. It is necessary to rise to a 40 db sensation level before the same outcome is obtained with Rush-Hughes. Thus, one can be fairly certain of a score at 25 db approaching PB-Max if he is using W-22 on a patient with normal discrimination for speech, but he has no chance of this outcome if he is using Rush-Hughes. Incidentally, most talkers when using live voice obtain results close to those shown here for W-22.

Figure 27-5 expands the illustration by

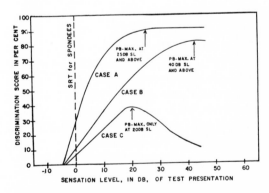

Figure 27-5. Three types of abnormal articulation curves illustrating that sensation levels at which maximum discrimination scores occur vary with the individual case.

showing three types of abnormal articulation function. These curves demonstrate that the presentation levels at which maximum discrimination scores are obtainable vary with individual clinical patients. Note that any level from 25 db up will yield PB-Max with patient A, but that this same situation is true for patient B only from 40 db up. Moreover, only a small range of levels around 20 db SL will allow patient C to achieve his best discrimination score. If, in these instances, the clinician were to test only at a sensation level of 25 db he would fail to obtain a reasonable estimate of the maximum discrimination score achievable by patient B, while using the 40 db SL would yield results far short of PB-Max for patient C.

The foregoing examples make eminently clear the fact that the clinician who tests only at one presentation level can be sure that he has a valid estimate of a person's maximum discrimination score only if the score approximates 100 percent. If the score is lower than this there is no way of knowing whether it represents the patient's best performance, ie, whether it is a score on the plateau of his articulation curve, or whether the test condition precludes his responding at his best capacity. The only way to resolve this dilemma is to administer enough lists at enough levels to allow the upper part of the patient's articulation function to be plotted. Admittedly, there are many circumstances wherein time limitations and other restrictions make it necessary to test discrimination for speech at only one level. Here the clinician has no choice but to use a level that is practical and likely to evoke maximum discrimination scores from most patients. But the clinician must recollect the uncertainty attending a single test score whenever he compares different patients or compares the same person under different circumstances of listening.

IV. MARGIN OF UNCERTAINTY

Another question of importance is, "What allowance must one make for the margin of uncertainty of the test he is using?"

Of course, precision of a patient's score depends on many factors. Some of these are related to the considerations which we have already mentioned. Obviously, failure to control key factors may increase the margin of error substantially. It is possible for a clinician to carry on such sloppy testing that his results have little meaning. We can discard such eventualities from further discussion with the comment that here we are discussing the uncertainty in test scores which remains after proper precautions are observed. The important point is that there is an irreducible minimum in the repeatability of test results. The problem before us is one of estimating this minimum so that allowance can be made for it.

Reliability varies from one test version to another, but an approximate picture of the precision possible with tests consisting of 50 monosyllables emerges from the following data obtained in our laboratory. Two versions of NU Auditory Test 4 were administered twice at each of five sensation levels to three groups of 16 subjects each. One group consisted of normal hearers, the second of patients with conductive losses, and the third of patients with sensorineural impairments.

A meaningful way to examine the results is to consider averages of the individual differences between test and retest scores, since these averages represent the means of the absolute discrepancies in scores. The Table presents these averages after the results have been corrected to compensate for the learning effect introduced by the experimental design.

The table highlights two relationships. As long as sensation levels were low, which meant that performance on the rising slope of the articulation function was being measured (notably at 0 and +8 db SL), averages of discrepancies tended to be a little less than 6 percent. Here, then, the margin of uncertainty as gauged by averages of discrepancies was about three test words. As soon as scores became high enough to evoke response on the plateau of the articulation function (at 32 db for sensorineurals but from 16 db up for conductives and normals) the averages of discrepancies dropped to 2

AVERAGES OF DIFFERENCES IN PERCENT BETWEEN DISCRIMINATION SCORES FOR TEST AND RETEST WITH NU
AUDITORY TEST 4 *

Sensation Level of Presentation	Normal Hearers †	Conductive Loss Group †	Sensorineural Loss Group †	All Groups Combined ‡
0 db	7.2	5.5	3.6	5.3
8 db	3.5	5.1	5.3	4.6
16 db	2.3	2.5	5.6	3.5
24 db	0.3	1.8	4.9	2.3
32 db	0.6	1.2	1.8	1.2

* Results shown are combined data for lists 1 and 2 after correction to compensate for the learning effect introduced by experimental design.
† 16 subjects, 32 test-retest comparisons.
‡ 48 subjects, 96 test-retest comparisons.

percent or less. This represents a margin of error of one test word.

To the degree that one may generalize from these data, two conclusions seem justified. First, precision varies with presentation level, being sharpest when the test is given so that the patient is able to do his best in discriminating speech. Second, the precision of a 50 monosyllable test, as gauged by the average discrepancy between test and retest scores, can be relatively good. There is little to be gained clinically by using a 100-item test so as to enhance the representativeness of the score.

Some authors, notably Elpern (7), have contended that the converse also is true: namely, that there is no point in using a 50-item test because adequate precision can be maintained with 25 words, ie, a so-called half-list. Elpern bases his argument on an analysis of W-22 scores. What he fails to remember is that about four tenths of the W-22 words are too easy to help differentiate among scores except very rarely. Consequently, when a half-list is used only about 15 of its 25 words function as effective test items under ordinary circumstances. This number cannot be considered adequate, at least when W-22 is used.

V. MEASUREMENT OF DISCRIMINATION

We come now to the question as to how measurement of discrimination for speech may serve the otologist in his diagnoses of auditory maladies.

First, we must recall Walsh's early emphasis on the idea that discrimination tests can help classify the amount of sensorineural involvement attending clinical otosclerosis. In an article that he wrote with Thurlow et al (21) we find the statement, "The maximum PB score varies with clinical diagnosis. It is highest in conductive deafness, slightly lower in conductive deafness with some nerve involvement causing high-tone hearing loss, and still lower if nerve involvement predominates." However, in accepting this conclusion, one must remember that discrimination must be measured with a difficult test like the Rush-Hughes version. The same degree of delineation will not occur with an easy test like W-22. Instead, as Walsh (22) has put it recently in speaking of responses of otosclerotic patients to W-22, ". . . everybody either gets 100 percent or 30 percent."

Second, we must remember that measurement of speech discrimination has in recent years become a helpful aid in differential diagnosis of relatively diverse conditions. For example, presbycusis may be classified in terms of whether patients have suffered a breakdown in clarity of speech perception which is out of proportion to the pattern of their pure tone loss. Schuknecht (17) has expressed the view that such a breakdown characterizes presbycusis due to neural rather than epithelial atrophy.

Another illustration is found when there is need to distinguish unilateral Meniere's disease from eighth nerve tumor. Moderate deterioration in speech discrimination is a frequent symptom in Meniere's disease. Thus Shambaugh (*18*), in describing the symptomatology of Meniere's, has said, ". . . impaired discrimination beyond the degree of pure tone loss is very characteristic. . . ." However, fair capacity in discrimination remains in this instance. By contrast, as is well known, acoustic neurinoma very often produces radical disruption of discrimination for speech. Here, the patient's score is likely to be near zero even with a very easy test. Hence, when the differentiation must be made between unilateral Meniere's disease and an eighth nerve tumor there are advantages in using an easy test, such as W-22 or NU Test 4, because scores on a harder test, like Rush-Hughes are likely also to be so poor for Meniere's disease that one malady will give results akin to the other.

Finally, we turn to use of speech discrimination in diagnosis of lesions within the central auditory system. Here the situation becomes very complex. Jerger (*11*) states, "Brain stem lesions may produce severe discrimination problems with no depression in the audiogram whatsoever." By contrast, lesions at higher levels in the auditory system do not disrupt speech discrimination to a noteworthy degree unless the material is distorted in some way to reduce its redundancies. Several kinds of material and various systems of distortion have been used. For example, Bocca (*2*) pioneered the use of filtered lists of phonetically balanced words. Such material can be presented via only one ear, in which event the score is appreciably poorer when hearing is done through the ear contralateral to a unilateral lesion of the higher auditory system. Or the same material can be administered binaurally with dissimilar distortions to the two ears, in which case the integrative mechanisms of the central auditory system are subjected to test. It is worth noting that the Rush-Hughes test is difficult enough so that it can serve as a distorted speech test when presented unilaterally (*8*), but it is of little value in binaural presentation because the same sound patterns are reaching both ears. It would appear that for the latter purpose one

must have differential stimulation such as Matzger's (*14*) system for filtering a single signal so that each ear gets a distinctive band of frequencies, although Linden (*13*) has failed to confirm Matzger's findings on the usefulness of this procedure.

One may epitomize the present situation by noting that, although speech audiometry has come to be recognized as an important tool in otoneurology, its present status in this area confuses the clinician. A plethora of special procedures has been suggested, but their significance and validity await confirmation. Already, however, the general principles are clear enough to suggest some of the ways that measurement with speech audiometry can assist in otoneurological diagnosis. Its contributions here are in addition to those it makes to differential diagnosis among more peripheral disorders.

VI. DIAGNOSING SOCIAL EFFICIENCY

An entirely different purpose for measuring speech discrimination is to evaluate a patient's everyday difficulties in hearing and to assess the practical significance of therapeutic and rehabilitative procedures for him. Here, the goal is to diagnose the social efficiency of his audition.

At present, one can perform such a diagnosis only in general and qualitative terms. We have very little positive information regarding the work-a-day meaning of discrimination scores. True, it is sometimes assumed that PB-word lists are representative of spoken English because of their parallelisms in phonetic composition. Every sophisticated person recognizes immediately that this cannot be the case. Monosyllables are more difficult to understand than are either longer words or connected utterances. Moreover, clinical measurement of discrimination for monosyllables is usually performed in quiet, whereas most everyday listening situations are characterized by fluctuating background noise of one degree or another. Finally, no one has done the extensive validational study that would be needed to estimate confidently a person's practical handicap from his discrimination score. Probably the closest approximation to such validation is the system for computing the Social Adequacy Index detailed by Davis (4), but this system merely ranks patients along a scale whose practical significance has not been clarified throughout its entire range. Consequently, every clinician must recognize that regardless of the monosyllabic word list he uses he is obtaining information which he cannot relate directly to everyday auditory efficiency.

Nonetheless, discrimination tests stand as the primary method by which we can ascertain whether or not a person has a multiple problem in receiving speech. That is, we can learn whether or not the patient combines loss of acuity, which is shown by pure tone audiometry and requires that signals be made more intense, with loss in precision of perceiving speech elements, which is shown by a discrimination test and is not improved by amplifying the signal. With this information at hand the insightful clinician can reach a qualitative judgment both about the circumstances in which his patient will have difficulty and about the magnitude of the trouble his patient will face. Of course, in reaching this judgment the clinician must consider both the life patterns of his patient and the characteristics of the test with which speech discrimination was measured.

As one example of how speech audiometry may be used in assessing therapeutic and rehabilitative procedures we have the question as to whether, after stapes surgery, a patient has maintained the clarity of perception he knew preoperatively. A good decibel gain can be at least partially nullified by a loss in discrimination. A relatively exacting test, like Rush-Hughes, is preferable in exploring such a question, because an easy test can fail to reveal moderate shifts which affect everyday efficiency.

Another important question is whether discrimination is affected adversely when a hearing aid is used. Again, a good decibel gain can be nullified by a loss in discrimination.

Two issues arisen in this instance. One is whether the patient suffers breakdown in discrimination with hearing aids as a class of amplifier. Many an elderly person, for example, is a poor hearing aid user because his phonemic regression interacts adversely with the limitations inherent in the good hearing aids of today. The second issue is whether the patient's discrimination changes importantly from one instrument to the next. We should assure ourselves that the particular hearing aid he procures is one with which he performs satisfactorily. Here a discrimination test serves as the basis for discarding undesirable instruments.

Today clinicians feel particularly frustrated when faced with the need to assess hearing aid performance. Negativistic attitudes have predominated ever since the Harvard research was reported in 1946 (5). It is often argued that differences in aided discrimination score are happenstance and are clinically meaningless.

Without attempting full consideration of the arguments involved, one comment must nonetheless be made. Almost without exception the tests used in the past to evaluate hearing aids have been inadequate in one of two ways. Sometimes, as in the study by Shore, Bilger, and Hirsh (19), tests have been too short to assure reliability. More often, as when W-22 is used, the test has been so easy that it lacks resolving power. This criticism applies to tests administered in noise as well as in quiet.

The present need, if we are to assess practical efficiency in speech discrimination relatively directly, is for new tests which pit their test items against backgrounds that simulate the competition encountered in everyday situations. Laboratory versions of such tests have been developed, but they are neither fully standardized nor available as yet to the clinician.

Meanwhile the clinician can recognize the limitations of contemporary tests and avoid attempting more precision of interpretation than they justify. Accepting this precaution, measurement of speech discrimination is useful in reaching the qualitative estimate of the outcome of surgery, of potential for hearing aid use, of relative efficiency with different instruments, and of phonemic perception in everyday life.

VII. SUMMARY AND CONCLUSIONS

A number of monosyllabic word tests designed to measure discrimination for speech are available today. The clinician must be clear as to the purpose for which he is measuring discrimination. He must choose both the test to use and the method for administering it so as to satisfy his purpose. Different criteria apply when a test is used in the diagnosis of auditory pathology and in determination of site of lesion than when it is used in estimating either the efficiency of hearing in everyday life or the potential value of a rehabilitative procedure such as a hearing aid. Finally, the clinician must remember that existing tests for speech discrimination are imperfectly standardized and lack validation. They have qualitative usefulness today, but with appropriate revision they can become much more definitive clinical tools.[1]

[1] This work was supported by grant K6 NB 16,244-02 from the National Institute of Neurological Diseases and Blindness, the Public Health Service, and by contract AF 41(657)-418, School of Aerospace Medicine, U.S. Air Force, Brooks Air Force Base, Tex.

REFERENCES

1. *American Standard Specifications for Speech Audiometers,* New York: American Standards Association, 1953.
2. Bocca, E.: Binaural Hearing: Another Approach, *Laryngoscope* **65**:1164–1171, 1965.
3. Carhart, R.: Speech Audiometry in Clinical Evaluation, *Acta Otolaryng* **41**:18–42, 1952.
4. Davis, H.: The Articulation Area and the Social Adequacy Index for Hearing, *Laryngoscope* **58**:761–778, 1948.
5. Davis, H., et al: The Selection of Hearing Aids, *Laryngoscope* **56**:85–115 and 135–163, 1946.
6. Egan, J. P.: Articulation Testing Methods, *Laryngoscope* **58**:955–991, 1948.
7. Elpern, B. S.: The Relative Stability of Half-List and Full-List Discrimination Tests, *Laryngoscope* **71**: 30–35, 1961.
8. Goldstein, R.; Goodman, A. C.; and King, R. B.: Hearing and Speech in Infantile Hemiplegia Before and After Left Hemispherectomy, *Neurology* **6**:869–875, 1956.
9. Haskins, H.: *A Phonetically Balanced Test of Speech Discrimination for Children*, thesis, Northwestern University, Chicago, 1949.
10. Hirsh, I. J., et al: Development of Materials for Speech Audiometry, *J Speech Hearing Dis* **17**:321–337, 1952.
11. Jerger, J.: Audiological Manifestations of Lesions in the Auditory Nervous System, *Laryngoscope* **70**: 417–425, 1960

12. Lehiste, I., and Peterson, G. E.: Linguistic Considerations in the Study of Speech Intelligibility, *J Acoust Soc Amer* **31**:280–286, 1959.
13. Linden, A.: Distorted Speech and Binaural Speech Resynthesis Tests, *Acta Otolaryng* **58**:32–48, 1964.
14. Matzker, J.: The Sound Localization Test, *Int Audiol* **1**:248–249, 1962.
15. Owens, E.: Intelligibility of Words Varying in Familiarity, *J Speech Hearing Res* **4**:113–129, 1961.
16. Peterson, G. E., and Lehiste, I.: Revised CNC Lists for Auditory Tests, *J Speech Hearing Dis* **27**:62–70, 1962.
17. Schuknecht, H. F.: Presbycusis, *Laryngoscope* **65**: 402–419, 1955.
18. Shambaugh, G. E., Jr.: *Surgery of the Ear*, Philadelphia: W. B. Saunders and Co., 1959.
19. Shore, I.; Bilger, R. C.; and Hirsh, I. J.: Hearing Aid Evaluation: Reliability of Repeated Measurements, *J Speech Hearing Dis* **25**:152–170, 1960.
20. Tillman, T. W.; Carhart, R.; and Wilber, L.: "A Test for Speech Discrimination Composed of CNC Monosyllabic Words," technical documentary report No. SAM-TDR-62-135, USAF School of Aerospace Medicine, Brooks Air Force Base, Tex, 1963.
21. Thurlow, W. R., et al: Further Statistical Study of Auditory Tests in Relation to the Fenestration Operation, *Laryngoscope* **59**:113–129, 1949.
22. Walsh, T.: Informal comment, *Trans Amer Otol Soc* **52**:79, 1964.

28

Discrimination Test Word Difficulty

RICHARD A. CAMPBELL

RICHARD A. CAMPBELL, Ph.D., is Research Audiologist, Veterans Administration Hospital, Miami, Florida

Several criteria for the construction of articulation testing materials were listed by Egan (1948). These criteria may be grouped into three different categories. The first category of criteria is that common, monosyllabic words be used; the second is that materials (lists) be of equal phonetic composition and representative of speech; the third is that the lists be equal in range and average level of difficulty.

The CID W-22 Auditory Test series developed by Hirsh and his associates (1952) has become a widely used clinical discrimination test. In the construction of this series considerable effort was made to meet the criteria within the first two categories above.

The criteria of the first category have been generally accepted without serious question.

The second category of criteria has been the source of considerable investigation (Lehiste and Peterson, 1959; Grubb, 1963) and some doubt. Whether this category of criteria is necessary for clinically useful audiometric discrimination tests, not whether it is necessary for articulation testing methods in general, would appear to be the issue. This issue has been recently discussed by Tobias (1964), who states that there is "overwhelming clinical and experimental evidence that indicates phonetic balance to be an interesting but unnecessary component of one of our current audiometric tests." The experimental evi-

Reprinted by permission of the author from *J. Speech Hearing Res.*, **8**, pp. 13–22 (1965).

dence that phonetic balance is not necessary may not be entirely overwhelming to all. However, experimental evidence that phonetic balance is necessary, in the interest of clinical validity, appears nonexistent. The validation studies called for by Silverman and Hirsh (1955), with the notable exception of Giolas and Epstein's (1963) study, are not to be found.

The third category of criteria are those common to the construction of any reliable and efficient set of equivalent tests and their use would appear unquestionable. The degree to which the W-22 discrimination tests meet these criteria has been of recent interest (Elpern, 1960, 1961) but attempts that have been made to evaluate the difficulty of the W-22 tests have not been completely adequate. These attempts were characterized by: use of populations consisting of many listeners with normal discrimination ability, inadequate descriptive statistics, lack of item analysis, and nonpertinent statistical inferences.

For example, Elpern reports on mean and standard deviations of many discrimination loss scores obtained on each of the four W-22 lists. The mean losses ranged from 13.6 percent to 18.3 percent (in order of list number). The standard deviations were from 13.9 percent to 18.5 percent (also in order of list number), all larger than their corresponding means. In this case it would be impossible to have a value which was one standard deviation less than the mean. This would require a discrimination loss of less than zero! The use of the standard deviation as a measure of dispersion under such conditions would appear questionable.

Do these lists differ significantly? Conventional statistical inference, or tests between lists, yield information on the probability of these lists having been drawn from the same parent population of lists. If the probability of these lists having come from the same population was too low to be reasonable, then one would say, at some level of confidence, that they were different.

Considering the uses to which these lists are being put one wonders if the question "could these lists have come from the same population?" is of interest. These lists are being used interchangeably as devices by which "discrimination loss" is described, thereby implying that all the lists measure the same thing in the same manner.

Thus, what differences are significant between lists is not a matter of statistical inference, but rather one of comparing existing differences with needed precision. The statistics used for descriptive purposes should be meaningful and appropriate. The lists should be compared on several measures, and these comparisons should be made within that listener population in which the need for precise evaluation of discrimination loss is greatest.

Clinical practice would make it apparent that only differences in discrimination scores in excess of about 5 percent are commonly thought to be meaningful. This reflects the general impression that test-retest variability is about 5 percent. To argue that differences of 5 percent (the test-retest variability) between lists are tolerable seems fallacious. For example, if a patient yielded a discrimination score of 80 percent on one list and a score of 70 percent on another list, a difference of 10 percent, this difference would probably be thought to be clinically important. However, if the second list were 5 percent more difficult at this score level, and his score were adjusted for inter-list differences, his adjusted score would be 75 percent, only 5 percent

different from that obtained on the first list. This 5 percent difference would probably not be considered clinically important. The effects of between-list variability should not be confused with the effects of test-retest variability.

For discrimination scores obtained on different lists to be "equivalent," there should be no measurable differences between lists. The smallest possible change between scores, or unit of measurement, is 2 percent (for whole lists), or 4 percent (for half-lists). Differences between tests should then be less than these units of measurement. Differences between lists which were less than one-half of the units of measurement would be of no concern.

The discrimination lists, then, ideally, should not differ in any of several measures, by more than 1 percent. Some measures which would seem appropriate are: (1) the extremes—least difficult and most difficult words; and (2) the quartiles—the 25th percentile, the 50th percentile (median), and the 75th percentile, in order of difficulty of words.

It is a basic tenet of test construction that the optimum range of item difficulty for a test is determined by the kind of differentiating that the test is called upon to do. If the test's purpose is to divide testees into only two categories, those above a certain proficiency level and those below, then the difficulty of items is best concentrated at the desired level of proficiency. In this way, if the testee's ability is even slightly above the desired level of proficiency, he tends to get all items correct. If his ability is slightly below this level he tends to get all items incorrect. In this manner, maximum differentiation is obtained.

If, however, the purpose of the test is to divide testees into several levels of proficiency, then the distribution of item difficulty should be essentially rectangular in form, with a range of difficulty similar to the levels of proficiency of interest. Having items whose difficulties are outside the range of interest reduces the efficiency of the test. Since these items are "always" either missed or answered correctly, they add to the length of the test without contributing to its ability to differentiate (Adkins, 1947; Guilford, 1954).

In the case of speech discrimination testing the general purpose is to determine on which of several levels of discrimination ability the patient should be placed. The range of clinically interesting discrimination loss scores would appear to be approximately from 10 percent to 70 percent. Any patient whose discrimination loss is less than about 10 percent would be classified as having "normal" discrimination and his discrimination ability would be of minimal clinical interest. On the other hand, any patient whose discrimination loss was greater than about 70 percent would probably be classified as having a "severe" discrimination problem, and clinical interest would become primarily rehabilitative rather than diagnostic.

Individuals who score in the 10 percent to 70 percent discrimination loss range are those for whom greatest reliability of measurement is needed. Small differences in scores within that range might affect surgical decisions, hearing aid recommendations, conclusions with regard to score consistency, the nature of an aural rehabilitation effort, or the amount of a monetary award.

The above comments pertain to a single general-purpose discrimination test. It may be helpful to have additional special-purpose discrimination tests available. In any case, a discrimination test should be developed and evaluated by analyzing the responses of individuals typical of the population for which the test was designed.

The following study was carried out to provide data on the difficulties of the items (words) of the W-22 test lists and to demonstrate the constructive steps to which such data can lead.

PROCEDURE

This study investigated the relative difficulty of words contained in the CID W-22 lists. The difficulty of words was assessed by means of the percentage of erroneous responses made to each word. The subjects were a relatively small but select group of veterans with discrimination losses, seen for audiological purposes at the Veterans Administration Out-patient Clinic, Atlanta, Georgia.

The lists were presented from recordings available from Technisonic Studios in St. Louis, and were played back monaurally through a Grason-Stadler #162 Speech Audiometer. The typical presentation level was +40 dB re the subject's speech reception threshold. No particular order of presentation of lists or orders was followed except that an attempt was made to utilize all lists and word orders an equal number of times.

A pool of 380 subjects was accumulated on whom detailed information was available regarding their behavior during audiological testing. From these 380 a group of 140 was selected in whom no behavior indicative of pseudo-hearing loss had been noted. From this group of 140 were selected those who (1) had sensori-neural or mixed type of losses, (2) had discrimination loss scores between 10 percent and 70 percent, (3) had been administered lists monaurally without masking or hearing aids, and (4) had been administered at least two different lists. The responses

TABLE 28-1. PARAMETERS OF DISTRIBUTIONS OF WORD DIFFICULTY OBTAINED ON THE FOUR LISTS OF THE CID W-22 AUDITORY TEST SERIES

W-22 List	Word Difficulty (% Errors)						
	Low	1st Quartile	2nd Quartile (Median)	3rd Quartile	High	Mean	Standard Deviation
1	0	7	17	40	83	25	32
2	2	10	19	36	86	25	29
3	2	10	15	32	71	22	24
4	0	12	22.5	35	71	26	26

of about 40 subjects per list were analyzed. If the same list had been administered twice to the same veteran, only the first presentation was tabulated.

RESULTS AND DISCUSSION

The distributions of word difficulty for the four lists are summarized in Table 28-1. (Further details of word difficulty are presented in the Appendix.)

It is obvious from Table 28-1 that the lists differ in word difficulty with regard to their means, medians, standard deviations, extremes, and quartiles. All difficulty distributions show positive (toward the more difficult) skew to various degrees. List 4 being least skewed, with list 2, list 1, and list 3 showing progressively increasing degrees of skewness.

The mean difficulties of the lists vary over a 4 percent range. The median word difficulties, however, vary over a 7.5 percent range. The standard deviations are, in all cases, equal to or greater than the means. In these lists 89 percent of the word difficulties lie within one standard deviation of the means rather than the 68 percent found in normal distributions.

A review of Table 28-1 and Table 28-2 shows that the whole lists and half lists consistently differ from one another by more than 1 percent, or 2 percent, with respect to nearly all of these characteristics. The word difficulties presented here are subject to sampling error, particularly with regard to intra-list (between subjects) comparisons. They represent, however, the best available estimates.

By using the pooled word difficulty data presented in Table 28-4 the 200 words were redistributed. Shown in the Appendix (Table 28-5) are eight half lists which were constructed. These half lists could be combined in pairs to make full 50-word lists. The words are listed in order of difficulty. Actual presentation could utilize scrambled orders, or an ascending or descending (in difficulty) method, or a procedure similar to the Block Up and Down method of Campbell (1963).

Table 28-3 lists the extremes and quartile

TABLE 28-2. COMPARISON OF PARAMETERS OF DISTRIBUTIONS OF WORD DIFFICULTY OBTAINED ON THE 48 CID W-22 DISCRIMINATION TEST HALF LISTS. ALL VALUES IN PERCENTAGE ERRORS

List	Low	Q_1	Median	Q_3	High
1A1	0	7	12	42	83
1A2	2	8.5	17	42.5	67
1B1	2	8.5	17	48	83
1B2	0	7	12	31	67
1C1	2	6	17	48	74
1C2	0	8.5	14	38	83
1D1	2	10	17	46.5	83
1D2	0	7	14	38	74
1E1	0	7	14	38	67
1E2	2	8.5	17	46.5	83
1F1	5	11	17	42	83
1F2	0	6	12	42.5	74
2A1	2	11	21	37	86
2A2	2	10	17	28.5	74
2B1	2	8.5	14	26	55
2B2	2	14	26	46.5	86
2C1	2	5	14	37	86
2C2	2	13	21	33	67
2D1	2	10	19	31	86
2D2	2	11	21	46.5	74
2E1	2	9.5	24	42.5	86
2E2	2	10	17	33	74
2F1	5	10	17	37	86
2F2	2	11	21	34.5	74
3A1	7	12	22	36.5	71
3A2	2	7	15	23	61
3B1	2	10	15	25.5	42
3B2	2	7	22	42	71
3C1	2	7	15	28	61
3C2	2	12	20	36.5	71
3D1	5	12	20	33	42
3D2	2	7	12	28	71
3E1	2	10	15	25.5	42
3E2	2	7	22	42	71
3F1	2	12	22	36.5	71
3F2	2	7	15	25.5	61
4A1	3	13.5	24	41	71
4A2	0	10.5	21	35	65
4B1	0	10.5	24	45.5	71
4B2	3	13.5	18	35	65
4C1	3	12	18	33.5	65
4C2	0	12	26	41	71
4D1	6	15	24	35	62
4D2	0	9	18	41	71
4E1	6	15	24	35	62
4E2	0	9	18	41	71
4F1	3	15	24	41	62
4F2	0	9	18	35	71

percentages of difficulty for each of these revised half lists. It is apparent that the quartiles of all lists do not differ by more than 1 percent. The easiest words of each half list do not differ by more than 2 percent in difficulty but the most difficult words of each

TABLE 28-3. COMPARISON OF PARAMETERS OF DISTRIBU-
TIONS OF WORD DIFFICULTY ON EIGHT MODIFIED DIS-
CRIMINATION TEST LISTS. ALL VALUES IN PERCENTAGE
ERRORS. BASED ON WORD DIFFICULTY DATA OF TABLE 28-4

List	Low	Q_1	Median	Q_3	High
M	0	10	18	36.5	67
N	0	10	18	37	67
O	2	10	18	37	71
P	2	9.5	18	37	71
Q	2	9.5	18	36.5	74
R	2	9.5	19	36.5	74
S	2	10.5	19	36	83
T	2	10.5	19	36	86

half list differ by 19 percent. Thus, utilizing the words contained in the W-22 lists as recorded by Technisonics and these data, eight half lists can easily be constructed which differ from one another enough to be of concern only with respect to the most difficult word of each.

The wide range of difficulty found in these words deserves further comment. With the range of clinical interest in mind it is apparent from these data that the W-22 lists fall short of the optimal distribution of word difficulty for a general-purpose discrimination test. About 25 percent of the words have difficulties of 10 percent or less and contribute little to the lists' ability to differentiate. At the other extreme, several words have difficulties greater than 70 percent and also contribute little to the lists' ability to differentiate. Furthermore, the distributions of word difficulties show definite skewness, instead of the more rectangular form desired. Thus, the efficiency of these lists would be greatly improved by replacing about 100 words, the easier and extremely difficult ones, by others which are of moderate difficulty.

SUMMARY

A review and discussion of criteria for the construction and evaluation of clinical speech discrimination tests has been presented. The need for such tests to be appropriate and homogeneous with respect to item (word) difficulty was emphasized. Word difficulty data obtained from a clinical population indicated that the CID W-22 word lists were inappropriate and nonhomogeneous in word difficulty. Reconstructed lists were presented which promise to be more homogeneous in difficulty.

REFERENCES

Adkins, D. C., *Construction and Analysis of Achievement Tests*. Washington: U.S. Government Printing Office (1947).

Campbell, R. A., Detection of a noise signal of varying duration. *J. acoust. Soc. Amer.*, **35**, 1732–1737 (1963).

Egan, J. P., Articulation testing methods. *Laryngoscope*, **58**, 955–991 (1948).

Elpern, B. S., Differences in difficulty among the CID W-22 auditory tests. *Laryngoscope*, **70**, 1560–1565 (1960).

Elpern, B. S., The relative stability of half-list and full-list discrimination tests. *Laryngoscope*, **71**, 30–36 (1961).

Giolas, T. G., and Epstein, A., Comparative intelligibility of word lists and continuous discourse. *J. Speech Hearing Res.*, **6**, 349–358 (1963).

Guilford, J. P., *Psychometric Methods*. New York: McGraw-Hill (1954).

Grubb, P., A phonemic analysis of half-list speech discrimination tests. *J. Speech Hearing Res.*, **6**, 271–275 (1963).

Hirsh, I. J., Davis, H., Silverman, S. R., Reynolds, Elizabeth G., Eldert, Elizabeth and Benson, R. W., Development of materials for speech audiometry. *J. Speech Hearing Dis.*, **17**, 321–337 (1952).

Lehiste, I,. and Peterson, G. E., Linguistic considerations in the study of speech intelligibility. *J. acoust. Soc. Amer.*, **13**, 280–286 (1959).

Silverman, S. R., and Hirsh, I. J., Problems related to the use of speech in clinical audiometry. *Ann. Oto. Rhino. Laryng.*, **64**, 1234–1245 (1955).

Tobias, J. V., On phonemic analysis of speech discrimination tests. *J. Speech Hearing Res.*, **7**, 102–104 (1964).

TABLE 28-4. PERCENTAGE OF ERRORS MADE FOR EACH WORD OF THE CID W-22 WORD LISTS
PRESENTED IN ORDER OF DIFFICULTY

CID W-22 Word List 1

yard	0	poor	7	him	12	stove	21	owl	48
it	2	ran	7	wire	12	skin	24	bells	52
none	2	there	7	toe	14	true	24	chew	55
you	2	hunt	10	wet	14	earn	26	east	60
me	5	or	10	as	17	she	26	ace	62
not	5	us	10	give	17	jam	36	ache	67
up	5	an	12	isle	17	twins	36	bathe	67
what	5	could	12	them	19	see	40	deaf	67
dad	7	day	12	law	21	thing	45	knees	74
felt	7	high	12	low	21	carve	48	mew	83

CID W-22 Word List 2

now	2	flat	10	too	14	new	26	cars	40
odd	2	live	10	does	17	thin	26	send	45
one	2	way	10	oak	17	with	29	ail	48
well	2	smart	12	buy	19	show	31	pew	52
die	5	then	12	move	19	chest	33	ill	55
star	5	tree	12	own	19	ease	33	tare	55
that	5	young	12	and	21	ice	33	gave	57
yore	5	ham	14	bin	21	cap	36	rooms	67
air	7	hurt	14	hit	21	jaw	36	key	74
eat	7	off	14	dumb	24	else	38	knee	86

CID W-22 Word List 3

book	2	raw	7	ate	15	ten	22	aim	39
no	2	have	10	glove	15	three	22	wool	39
do	5	may	10	jar	15	bill	24	chair	42
when	5	this	10	lie	15	hand	24	ears	42
are	7	add	12	pie	15	smooth	27	tan	42
done	7	end	12	shove	15	camp	29	owes	46
he	7	farm	12	tie	15	say	29	dull	61
if	7	is	12	though	20	cute	32	knit	61
on	7	oil	12	we	20	start	32	nest	61
out	7	use	12	year	20	king	34	west	71

CID W-22 Word List 4

who	0	why	9	leave	18	will	29	net	41
in	3	aid	12	of	18	arm	32	tea	41
jump	3	bread	12	shoe	18	than	32	ear	47
wood	6	bee	15	they	18	tin	32	chin	50
at	9	my	15	yes	21	am	35	nuts	56
clothes	9	ought	15	go	24	can	35	stiff	56
cook	9	toy	15	near	24	few	35	darn	62
men	9	where	15	yet	24	hang	35	save	62
our	9	art	18	pale	26	all	38	dust	65
through	9	his	18	so	26	eyes	41	dolls	71

TABLE 28-5. EIGHT MODIFIED DISCRIMINATION TEST HALF LISTS IN ORDER OF WORD DIFFICULTY. THESE HALF LISTS WERE DERIVED FROM DATA OF TABLE 28-4. THEY MAY BE PRESENTED IN VARIOUS ORDERS AND IN ANY COMBINATION OF TWO HALF LISTS FOR CONSTRUCTION OF FOUR WHOLE LISTS

M	N	O	P	Q	R	S	T
who	yard	no	book	odd	now	one	well
that	do	when	jump	in	none	it	you
star	die	yore	up	not	me	what	wood
eat	air	done	are	on	raw	out	if
there	ran	dad	poor	felt	he	our	at
this	have	may	cook	why	men	through	clothes
live	way	flat	or	hunt	us	add	oil
young	wire	bread	aid	use	farm	is	end
tree	smart	then	high	an	day	could	him
ate	shove	toe	hurt	too	off	ham	wet
glove	pie	tie	lie	jar	my	toy	where
of	as	isle	give	does	oak	bee	ought
his	they	shoe	art	leave	move	by	own
and	bin	hit	yes	though	year	we	them
low	stove	law	three	ten	hand	bill	yet
new	pale	so	skin	true	dumb	near	go
thin	she	earn	smooth	say	camp	will	with
ease	ice	tin	arm	than	start	cute	show
chest	king	few	am	can	hang	jaw	cap
see	cars	wool	aim	else	all	twins	jam
eyes	tea	net	chair	tan	ears	send	thing
bells	pew	chin	carve	owl	ail	ear	owes
ill	tare	chew	nuts	stiff	gave	east	knit
deaf	rooms	dust	ace	darn	save	nest	dull
ache	bathe	west	dolls	key	knees	mew	knee

29

Reliability of Voice Tests of Speech Discrimination

WILLIAM T. BRANDY

WILLIAM T. BRANDY, Ph.D., is Assistant Professor of Audiology, West Virginia University

PROBLEM

Hearing tests traditionally involve two kinds of auditory signals: relatively simple acoustic events such as pure tones and more complex acoustic events such as speech. Unlike the relatively uncomplicated pure tone, the variables in speech production are more difficult to control because there are more of them; these include vocal force or intensity, pitch, duration and consonant-vowel ratio, articulation, and voice quality (Hirsh et al., 1954; Fry, 1955; Fairbanks and Miron, 1957; Asher, 1958; Peterson and Lehiste, 1960).

No specifications exist regarding how the physical properties of the speech signal, as a complex waveform, should be controlled in routine tests of speech discrimination. When one examines attempts at speech discrimination test standardization, one observes that all tests have been equated in terms of printed symbols for words rather than in terms of the complex acoustic events that the words represent (Hudgins et al., 1947; Egan, 1948; Hirsh et al., 1952; Asher, 1958). When speech is considered in the acoustical sense (as a complex waveform), construction of equivalent lists must be thought of in terms of the standardization of signals and must, therefore, deal with acoustic events and not printed symbols.

Previous studies show that talker-by-list and talker-by-distortion interactions cause

Reprinted by permission of the author from *J. Speech Hearing Res.*, **9,** pp. 461–465 (1966).

significant variability in listener performance (Hirsh et al., 1954; Asher, 1958). From these studies one can conclude that acoustic waveforms of two or more talkers are sufficiently different to cause variability in listener performance even though the same word lists are used. This gives rise to the following question: Will a single talker's repetitions of a single word list vary acoustically and if so, will this variability influence listener performance significantly?

METHOD

It was felt that any twenty-five monosyllabic words would be adequate for this study because the words were intended only for internal comparisons among lists. The twenty-five words were chosen at random from List 3 of CID, Auditory Test W-22. These same words were randomized into three separate lists by using a table of random numbers. An adult male recorded each of the three lists on a separate day and under identical conditions. The talker received the same instructions (talk naturally; talk with equal effort; monitor the carrier phrase at zero on the VU meter) on each successive day of recording. The carrier phrase "write the word" preceded each test word. The talker stood in an IAC model 401 sound-treated room. An Altec model 633A microphone was located twelve inches from his mouth. The speech signals were recorded on an Ampex model 350 tape recorder.

There was a five second interval between presentations. Inasmuch as these three lists reflect, as closely as possible, the talker's original speech signals, they hereafter will be referred to as "live" presentations.

The live presentation made on the third day was rerecorded three times and spliced into three lists following the three original word orders. The interval between words on these spliced tapes was adjusted to five seconds. Variations in intensity for these rerecorded lists were approximated visually through the use of an Ampex VU meter and each word on these lists was corrected acoustically. This was done by dubbing the lists from the Ampex 350 tape recorder to an Ampex 601 tape recorder by way of an attenuator which was used to compensate for the intensive differences noted on the VU meter. The test word thereby were corrected on these new tapes in order for each individual test word to give approximately the same intensity when studied acoustically. These acoustically corrected lists hereafter will be referred to as "recorded" presentations.

The VU-level of each word in each of the six lists was observed visually. The mean VU-level of each of the six lists was calculated. A one-minute, 1,000 Hz tone generated from a Hewlett-Packard model 200AB audio oscillator was recorded at the mean VU level of the test words for each of the six lists and was spliced to the beginning of each appropriate list.

Twenty-four normal-hearing adults were used in this study. There were nineteen females and five males ranging in age from seventeen to fifty-five years; the median age was twenty-two years.

The speech signals were presented through a conventional Grason-Stadler model 162 speech audiometer by connecting the output of the Ampex model 601 tape recorder to the external jack of the speech audiometer. The 1,000 Hz tones at the beginning of each tape recording were used to calibrate the level of the speech signals of each list. All subjects were seated in a sound treated room and were instructed to write each test word on an answer sheet that was provided. The signals were presented monaurally through a TDH-39 dynamic earphone. Twelve subjects listened to the three live presentations and twelve listened to the three recorded presentations. All presentations were at 10 dB Sensation Level in order to maintain a condition of difficulty and to introduce variability into the data.

Statistically, the variable analyzed was twice the arcsin, in radians, of the square root of the proportion of correct responses (Walker and Lev, 1953). This transformed variable was analyzed with a two-way classification analysis of variance where observers and lists A, B, and C were the main effects. Data for recorded and live presentations were analyzed separately.

RESULTS

The means for each list and for each mode of presentation are shown in Table 29-1. Results

TABLE 29-1. MEAN SCORES FOR RECORDED AND LIVE PRESENTATIONS EXPRESSED IN PERCENTAGE SCORES OBTAINED BY ARCSIN TRANSFORMATION

Recorded			Live		
A	B	C	A	B	C
43.00	39.70	41.80	43.80	52.25	53.56

of the analyses of variance used to test for differences among the means are summarized in Table 29-2. Table 29-1 shows that the recorded mean scores varied by 3.30 percentage points while the live mean scores varied by 9.76 percentage points. Inspection of Table

TABLE 29-2. RESULTS OF ANALYSES OF VARIANCE USED TO TEST FOR DIFFERENCES AMONG MEANS OF LISTS FOR RECORDED AND LIVE PRESENTATIONS

Source	df	Recorded Mean Square	F	Live Mean Square	F
Subjects	11	0.6630		0.6394	
Lists	2	0.0020	0.010	0.0917	3.570 *
Error	22	0.0200		0.0257	

* Significant at 0.05 level.

29-2 shows no significant difference among lists for the recorded mode of presentation but shows a significant difference among lists for the live mode of presentation.

The three live presentations were studied further, following the procedure of Scheffé (1950). This revealed that list A varied significantly from lists B and C. In other words, for two of the three live presentations listener performance did not vary significantly, but listener performance for the third presentation did vary significantly from the other two.

When the among-lists variances for the two modes of presentation (Table 29-2) are compared directly, the resulting F ratio (0.0917/0.0020) is significant beyond the 0.05 level. Thus it can be stated that the variation among lists was significantly larger for live presentations than for recorded presentations.

DISCUSSION

The results of this study show that recorded presentations which are equivalent in acoustic output provide more reliable listener performance than do live presentations which are unequivalent in acoustic output. This supports the contention that the construction of equivalent speech discrimination tests must be thought of in terms of the standardization of acoustic signals and not printed symbols.

The assumption that one talker produces the same acoustic signal on successive readings of a given printed word is untenable when the results of this investigation are considered. The fact that listener performance for live list A was significantly different from listener performance for live lists B and C suggests that a given talker can present words in relatively the same acoustic fashion on some days but that his presentations on other days will vary. This variability in the acoustic output of a talker's live presentations can, in turn, cause variability in listener performance.

In routine live speech discrimination tests, the talker often does not attempt identical modes of presentation for each reading. Since equivalence cannot be assumed for successive readings of the same word lists when the talker attempts identical modes of presentation, it is assumed that even more variability will be introduced when he changes his mode of presentation on successive readings.

SUMMARY

Speech, as a complex acoustic event, has innumerable variations and deviations in waveform. It has been shown in previous studies that two or more speakers produce variation in observer performance because of talker-by-list and talker-by-distortion interaction. From these studies one can conclude that acoustic waveforms of two or more talkers is sufficiently different to cause variability in listener performance when these talkers present the same word lists.

The extent of one talker's time-to-time variation in live versus recorded presentations of monosyllabic words was studied at relatively low sensation levels. Twelve subjects with normal hearing listened to three recorded presentations and twelve subjects with normal hearing listened to three live presentations of these words under identical conditions.

Results of subjects' performance were evaluated by analysis of variance. For the live mode of presentation, there was a significant difference among lists, one list being significantly different from the other two. For the recorded presentations, the difference among lists failed to reach a significant level. This study shows that recorded presentations (equivalent in waveform) are more reliable than live presentations (unequivalent in waveform). Since one talker introduces significant variability on successive days of live testing when using identical modes of presentation, it is assumed that even more variability will be introduced when one speaker changes his mode of presentation on successive days.[1]

[1] This article is based upon a Master of Science thesis completed at the University of Pittsburgh in 1962 under the direction of Robert C. Bilger and is adapted from a paper presented at the 1963 convention of the American Speech and Hearing Association. The writer gratefully acknowledges Bilger's guidance and assistance throughout the planning, execution, analysis, and reporting of this investigation.

REFERENCES

Asher, W. J., Intelligibility tests: a review of their standardization, some experiments, and a new test. *Speech Monographs*, **25,** 14–28 (1958).

Egan, J., Articulation testing methods. *Laryngoscope*, **58,** 955–991 (1948).

Fairbanks, G., and Miron, M. S., Effects of vocal effort upon the consonant-vowel ratio within the syllable. *J. Acoust. Soc. Amer.*, **29,** 621–626 (1957).

Fry, D. B., Duration and intensity as physical correlates of lingusitic stress. *J. Acoust. Soc. Amer.*, **27,** 765–768 (1955).

Hirsh, I. J., Davis, H., Silverman, S. R., Reynolds, E. G., Eldert, E., and Benson, R. W., Development of materials for speech audiometry. *J. Speech Hearing Dis.*, **17,** 321–337 (1952).

Hirsh, I. J., Reynolds, E. G., and Joseph, M., Intelligibility of different speech materials. *J. Acoust. Soc. Amer.*, **26,** 530–538 (1954).

Hudgins, C. V., Hawkins, J. E., Karlin, J. E., and Stevens, S. S., The development of auditory tests for measuring hearing loss for speech. *Laryngoscope*, **57,** 57–89 (1947).

Peterson, G. E., and Lehiste, I., Duration of syllable nuclei in English. *J. Acoust. Soc. Amer.*, **32,** 693–703 (1960).

Scheffé, H., Statistical methods for evaluation of several sets of constants and several sources of variability. *Chem. Eng. Prog.*, **50,** 200–205 (1950).

Walker, H. M., and Lev, J., *Statistical Inference*. New York: Henry Holt & Co. (1953).

"Flat" Sensorineural Hearing Loss and PB Scores

GARY THOMPSON
RICHARD HOEL

GARY THOMPSON, Ph.D., is Assistant Professor, Speech Department, University of Washington
RICHARD HOEL is Instructor in Audiology, University of Minnesota

Many clinical workers in the field of speech and hearing hold the view that speech discrimination scores depend primarily on shape of the pure tone audiogram. Obviously, sharply falling audiograms frequently produce poor discrimination scores. For less obvious reasons, "flat" losses may produce poor discrimination scores, too, if they are sensorineural in type. We have investigated the relationship between "flat" sensorineural loss and speech discrimination scores in the following manner.

Subjects were adults seen at the Houston Speech and Hearing Center over a three-year period. The age range was limited to 16-65 years. All subjects had a "flat" sensorineural hearing loss in at least one ear. A "flat" loss was defined as one in which the hearing at one frequency varied by no more than 10 db from that at any other frequency. "Sensorineural" was defined as an air-bone gap no greater than 10 db. Speech discrimination scores were tabulated for all subjects and the results are shown in the following table.

Inspection of these data on "flat" sensori-

Reprinted by permission of the authors from *J. Speech Hearing Dis.*, **27**, pp. 284–287 (1962).

TABLE 30-I. SPEECH DISCRIMINATION SCORES IN FLAT SENSORINEURAL HEARING LOSSES OF VARYING SEVERITY. RECORDED W-22 PB WORD LISTS WERE USED

Average Pure Tone Loss in db re Audiometric Zero	Mean Discrim. Score	Number of Subjects
10–19	94%	10
20–29	94%	4
30–39	90%	5
40–49	67%	12
50–59	49%	26
60–69	38%	16
70–79	7%	9
80–	3%	21

neural hearing losses shows no significant speech discrimination impairment accompanying the mild hearing losses. However, for hearing levels of 40–49 db and greater a marked reduction in intelligibility is noted. Moreover, for losses greater than this, the discrimination scores become progressively worse.

There has been no attempt here to compare discrimination scores of "flat" vs. "sloping" losses. The purpose has been to discourage the practice of overgeneralization in regard to discrimination scores on the basis of pure-tone audiogram shape.

A New Approach to Speech Audiometry

JAMES JERGER
CHARLES SPEAKS
JANE L. TRAMMELL

JAMES JERGER, Ph.D., is Professor of Audiology, Baylor College of Medicine
CHARLES SPEAKS, Ph.D., is Associate Professor, Department of Communication Disorders and Director, Communication Sciences Laboratory, University of Minnesota
JANE L. TRAMMELL is an Audiologist, Methodist Hospital, Houston, Texas

In the short span of two decades speech audiometry has become a basic tool of audiologic evaluation. Speech signals are used to measure threshold, to assess suprathreshold intelligibility, to measure progress in lipreading and auditory training, to evaluate hearing aid performance, to predict the success of otologic surgery, and to aid in the diagnosis of both peripheral and central auditory disorders. They are useful, and often essential, in virtually every phase of modern audiology from research to rehabilitation.

Although the groundwork for the use of speech signals in auditory measurement derives from many sources, the genesis of what we now know as clinical speech audiometry is attributable in large measure to the pioneering work of Raymond Carhart. In a series of papers published in the late 1940s and early 1950s (Carhart, 1946a, b, c, 1953a, b, c; Carhart and Thompson, 1947) he established such basic concepts as the relation between pure-tone and spondee thresholds, the PB max, and the evaluation of hearing aids by aided PB scores; then outlined the several uses of these concepts in the total audiologic evaluation and rehabilitation of the hearing-impaired. Striking testimony to his contribution

Reprinted by permission of the authors from *J. Speech Hearing Dis.*, **33**, pp. 318–329 (1968).

is the fact that present-day clinical speech audiometry is still based on the concepts outlined by Carhart almost 20 years ago.

Traditionally the materials of speech audiometry have been lists of single words, either monosyllabic (the PB lists) or bisyllabic (the spondee lists). The testing paradigm has been repetition from an open message set. The tester presents a word and the subject repeats back what he heard. In choosing his response, the subject may draw from an open or undefined set of all the words in his response repertoire.

In the light of present knowledge we can, of course, see several disadvantages to this traditional methodology. First, the use of single words, and especially single-syllable words, imposes severe limitations on our capacity to manipulate a crucial parameter of ongoing speech, its changing pattern over time. In order to add this dimension to speech audiometry it is necessary to develop materials based on relatively longer samples of speech than single words.

Second, the traditional testing paradigm has at least two important disadvantages: (1) the open message set, and (2) the problem of scoring the subject's responses.

The open-set method leaves uncontrolled the subject's previous linguistic history and the extent to which this variable may affect his response. It is preferable to utilize a closed-set paradigm in which the population of all possible responses to a given test item is rigidly specified.

The scoring problems arising from the repetition method are well known to clinicians. Under conditions of less than ideal electronic communications systems it is sometimes ambiguous as to whose speech discrimination is being tested, the patient's or the audiologist's. This problem can be alleviated to some extent by the use of written responses, but this technique is not without its own problems. The "write-down" approach also is somewhat more tedious and time-consuming for the clinician, which perhaps accounts in part for its failure to achieve wide clinical application. A better solution is to structure the test procedure in such a way that the patient's response is a simple motor act, such as pushing a button, rather than the relatively more complex act of repetition and its attendant ambiguities.

These considerations led us to develop, during the past four years, both new speech materials and new test procedures and to evaluate their use in clinical speech audiometry.

NEW MATERIALS

The new speech materials (Speaks and Jerger, 1965) that we have developed are "artificial" or "synthetic" sentences; artificial in the sense that they are not "real" sentences, synthetic in the sense that the sequence of words that comprises the sentence follows specifiable rules of syntax. We decided against using real English sentences because the meaning of such a sentence is often conveyed by only one or two key words, which would have defeated our purpose at the outset.

Table 31-1 contains four examples of synthetic sentences. Each resembles the others in some respects. For example, all have seven words and nine syllables. A closer examination reveals, however, some important differ-

TABLE 31-1. TYPICAL EXAMPLES OF SEVEN-WORD SENTENCES CONSTRUCTED ON THE BASIS OF CONDITIONAL PROBABILITIES

Order of Approximation	Example Sentences
First	Due his fit along sick near nearly
Second	Three came home on any woman can
Third	Agree with him only to find out
Fourth	Only to find broken on the line

ences. Note that, although none is an actual sentence that occurs in English, each of the last three seems to read more like a sentence than the one that precedes it. Said differently, the sequence of words in each successive sentence is a closer approximation to the kind of sequence that we normally would expect with real English sentences.

The four sentences in Table 31-1 represent four degrees or levels of approximation to real sentences. All words for the sentences were chosen from the Thorndike and Lorge (1944) count of the 1000 most familiar words. Words for a "first-order" sentence were selected at random from this pool. No word in the sentence is dependent on the word that precedes it. This, of course, is extremely unlike the natural events in language. Thus, the first-order sentence does not approximate a real sentence at all well.

We can improve on this circumstance by allowing each word to be dependent on the single word preceding it. That is to say, we can construct a sentence using a sequence of word pairs that are linked together naturally in real speech. In such a sentence, the choice of the second word is not free or random, but is highly dependent on the first word, just as the third is on the second, the fourth on the third, and so on until we reach the last word in the sentence. When this procedure is followed the result is a "second-order" sentence: one that is characterized by a sequence of word pairs. Third- and fourth-order sentences are constructed similarly, except that sequences of word triplets and quadruplets are used respectively. Of course, if the procedure were extended far enough, the result would be a real sentence.

These rules can be applied uniformly, time after time, to build a series of alternative sentences that are relatively homogeneous. Table 31-2 contains 10 alternative third-order

TABLE 31-2. EXAMPLE MESSAGE SET CONSISTING OF 10 ALTERNATIVE SYNTHETIC SENTENCES CONSTRUCTED AS THIRD-ORDER APPROXIMATIONS TO REAL SENTENCES

Alternative Sentences

1. Small boat with a picture has become
2. Built the government with the force almost
3. Go change your car color is red
4. Forward march said the boy had a
5. March around without a care in your
6. That neighbor who said business is better
7. Battle cry and be better than ever
8. Down by the time is real enough
9. Agree with him only to find out
10. Women view men with green paper should

sentences. They are homogeneous in the sense that all have seven words and a controlled, but not necessarily equal, number of syllables. But the most important feature that determines the degree of homogeneity is that each is based on the word-triplet rule. Expressed differently, the amount of redundancy, related to the dependence of any one word on the other words in the surrounding context, is relatively similar among the 10 alternatives. Standard articulation tests carried out with the message set shown in Table 31-2 substantiate the notion of similarity among the alternatives (Speaks, Jerger, and Jerger, 1966).

The discussion to this point has been limited to sentence lengths of seven words. Of course, other lengths can be used, and in fact there may be circumstances in which a longer or shorter sentence might be preferable. For purposes of speech audiometry, we have found that seven words are optimal.

TESTING PROCEDURE

Our procedure contrasts with the traditional approaches used in speech audiometry in two important ways. First, the patient identifies the message instead of repeating aloud what he hears. Second, his response is drawn from a closed set of response alternatives.

The message set shown in Table 31-2 is placed on a console in front of the patient and is available to him throughout the entire session. His task is simply to push a button on the console corresponding to the sentence that he heard. A variety of systems can be devised to inform the tester of the patient's response. The simplest and least expensive method is to provide the tester with a panel containing 10 light bulbs that correspond to the 10 buttons on the patient console. It is a fairly simple matter to record the patient's performance on a response sheet.

If appropriate instrumentation is available, the entire procedure can be automated for ease of testing. Our preference has been to use a two-channel tape recorder. The sentences are recorded on one channel. On the second channel, coding pulses are recorded in synchrony with the sentence. The number of pulses corresponds to the sentence identification number, that is, one pulse for the first sentence, two pulses for the second sentence, etc. The pulses trigger a logic circuit (Grason-Stadler Modular Programming System, Series 1200) that provides an automatic data acquisition and storage system. This system informs the subject when to rest, attend, listen, and respond. The number of messages presented and the number of correct responses are accumulated automatically on separate mechanical counters.

CLINICAL FINDINGS

How do the synthetic sentence identification (SSI) materials compare with conventional PB word lists in the assessment of discrimination loss? Do the two methods yield equivalent results or lead to equivalent conclusions?

We learned, at a very early stage, that, if the sentences were presented in quiet, the task was much too easy to reflect fine shades of difficulty in speech understanding. No matter how poor a patient's PB max might be, his performance-intensity (PI) function for SSI always rose to 90–100 percent at sufficiently high intensities.

We tried various methods for making the task more difficult. The most successful approach was simply to add a competing speech message to the sentences. The same talker who had originally recorded the sentences read a long passage of continuous discourse concerned with events in the life of David Crockett, an early pioneer in the history of Texas. This served as the competing speech message. It was recorded on tape and mixed electrically with the sentences.

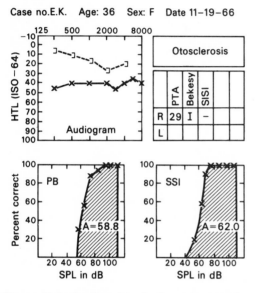

Figure 31-1. Audiometric findings in a patient with conductive loss due to otosclerosis. Comparison of the PI functions for PB and SSI shows that thresholds, maxima, and areas are all similar.

After some preliminary exploration we found that a message-competition ratio (MCR) of 0 dB was quite suitable for clinical evaluation. It seemed to produce a listening task at a level of difficulty roughly equivalent to a PB score.

Our next step was to test a series of hearing-impaired patients by both PB and SSI. For PB words, 25 words were presented at each intensity level tested and a different group of words was used at each level. For sentences, 10 messages were presented at each intensity. The same 10 messages were used throughout, but presented in different random orders.

Complete PI functions were constructed, for PB in quiet, and for SSI at MCR = 0 dB. By complete PI functions, we mean that the patient's performance was catalogued over a broad range, extending from the intensity at which he could perform at a rate of 0–30 percent through a maximum intensity of 110 dB SPL.

Basically we found that, with certain qualifications the two methods, PB and SSI, yielded equivalent results. The qualifications concern systematic differences between the two methods when the audiogram slopes, either gradually or markedly, from low to high frequencies.

The following cases typify results obtained in a consecutive series that now exceeds 150 patients.

Conductive and Cochlear Disorders

Figure 31-1 shows results obtained in the left ear of a patient with a conductive loss due to otosclerosis. Both the PB and the SSI functions rise to a maximum of 100 percent. In comparing these functions we found it useful to compute an area measure in order to reflect both sensitivity and maximum performance in a single number. This measure was calculated by placing the PI function over a grid and summing all squares (arbitrary units) enclosed by the curve to an upper boundary of 110 dB SPL. In general this area index shows closer correspondence between the two functions than either the initial slope or the maximum value. Note the close agreement in this patient. The PB area is 58.8, the SSI area 62.0. Note, also, that the "thresholds" or 50 percent levels of the two functions are in good agreement—61 dB for PB and 62 dB for SSI.

Figure 31-2 typifies results obtained in patients with relatively mild flat cochlear losses and good speech understanding. Both thresholds and areas are quite similar.

Figures 31-3 and 31-4 show results in patients with distinctly sloping audiometric contours. Here we note a sizeable discrepancy between the two functions. Although the maxima are

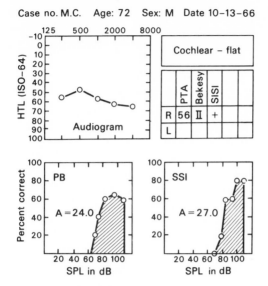

Case no. M.C.   Age: 72   Sex: M   Date 10-13-66

Figure 31-2. Audiometric findings in a patient with moderate cochlear loss and a flat audiometric contour. PB and SSI are similar.

similar, the SSI area is consistently larger than the PB area.

On the other hand, Figure 31-5 shows results on a patient whose audiometric slope is similar to the slope in Figure 31-4, yet whose PB and SSI functions are quite similar. The SSI function is, in fact, somewhat poorer than the PB function, but areas are similar.

These four cases illustrate important points of similarity and difference between PB and SSI. Except in the case of a relatively severe loss, there is a fairly systematic relation between audiometric slope and discrepancy between PB and SSI. When the contour is flat, the two functions agree. But as the slope becomes more severe, PB declines more rapidly than SSI. The discrepancy is greatest in patients with good hearing at low frequencies, but with a severe drop in the high frequencies.

Such a relation is quite understandable in terms of the frequency regions important for PB and SSI. Performance on PB materials is more critically dependent on frequencies above 1000 Hz than SSI. We have shown (Speaks, 1967), for example, that the point of intersection for high-pass and low-pass filtering is only 725 Hz for SSI, whereas French and

Steinberg (1947) found the value to be 1900 Hz for monosyllabic words. It follows, therefore, that if a patient has retained good hearing in the region below 1000 Hz he will encounter little difficulty with SSI, but mounting difficulty with PB words as high-frequency sensitivity diminishes. If however, low-frequency sensitivity is also impaired, then he will find SSI as difficult as PB, independent of audiometric contour (Figure 31-5).

In any event, patients with good hearing at low frequencies and poor hearing at high frequencies pose an interesting dilemma. Where the SSI area is vastly larger than the PB area we may reasonably ask which of the two provides a more accurate statement of the patients' hearing difficulty in everyday life. Does the SSI area underestimate it? Does the PB area overestimate it? The tentative answer seems to be that both statements are true. The best predictor of hearing handicap seems to be about midway between the two areas.

To illustrate this point we selected five pairs of subjects, matched according to hearing handicap scale (HHS) (High, Fairbanks, and

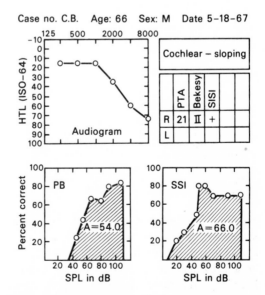

Case no. C.B.   Age: 66   Sex: M   Date 5-18-67

Figure 31-3. Audiometric findings in a patient with mild cochlear loss and a precipitously sloping audiometric contour above 1000 Hz. SSI area is somewhat larger than PB area.

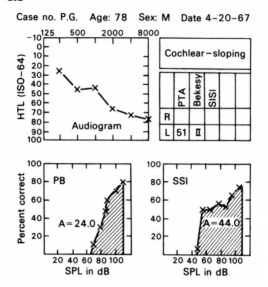

Figure 31-4. Audiometric findings in a patient with a moderate cochlear loss and a gradually sloping audiometric contour. SSI area is considerably larger than PB area.

Glorig, 1964). One member of each pair had a flat audiometric contour, the other a sloping contour. Table 31-3 summarizes PB area,

TABLE 31-3. PB, SSI, AND AVERAGE AREAS IN 10 SUBJECTS PAIRED ACCORDING TO AUDIOMETRIC CONTOUR AND HEARING HANDICAP SCORE

Subject	Audio-metric Contour	Hearing Handicap Score	PB Area	SSI Area	Average Area
1	flat	12%	70.2	73.8	72.0
2	sloping	12%	59.3	85.5	72.4
3	flat	20%	62.0	63.6	62.8
4	sloping	18%	54.4	65.9	60.2
5	flat	40%	52.5	54.0	53.8
6	sloping	41%	32.5	85.9	59.2
7	flat	48%	45.0	47.4	46.2
8	sloping	50%	27.0	55.5	41.3
9	flat	62%	32.3	40.1	36.2
10	sloping	69%	5.2	45.6	25.4

SSI area, and the average of these two areas for each of the five pairs. Note that, when the audiometric contour is flat, either SSI or PB area provides the same estimate of hearing handicap. Whenever the loss is sloping, however, the PB area overestimates and the SSI area underestimates the amount of handicap. The best predictor of actual hearing handicap

in the sloping cases (i.e., the predictor yielding an area in close correspondence with the analogous area for flat loss) seems to be a simple average of the two areas.

It is probably an oversimplification, however, to conclude that one area overestimates handicap and the other underestimates it. This conclusion is necessarily restricted to handicap as measured by the hearing-handicap scale devised by High et al., the only satisfactory tool presently at our disposal for this purpose. Although this scale is an excellent research instrument, our own interpretation of the various items leads us to conclude that it is heavily weighted with items primarily responsive to sensitivity loss, a situation which, again in our opinion, places the PB area at a possible disadvantage.

A more refined scale of hearing handicap might reveal that the SSI area tells us something about how the patient gets along in certain listening situations, while the PB area tells us about his extraordinary difficulty in certain other listening situations.

Presently, however, we can only conclude that the two sets of information seem to be complementary.

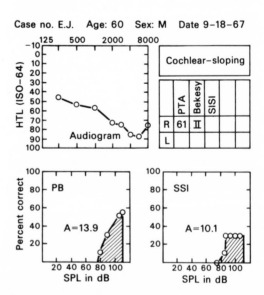

Figure 31-5. Audiometric findings in a patient with a severe cochlear loss and a gradually sloping audiometric contour. PB and SSI areas are similar.

Case no. I.W.   Age: 44   Sex: F   Date 2-6-67

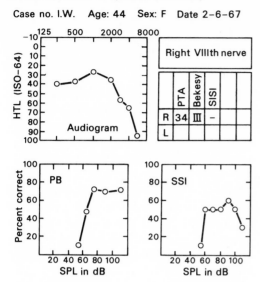

Figure 31-6. Audiometric findings in a patient with a right VIIIth nerve disorder. PI functions for PB and SSI are similar, although the SSI function shows "roll-over" at the higher speech levels.

Eighth Nerve and Central Disorders

Figure 31-6 summarizes findings in a patient with VIIIth nerve audiometric findings. SISI was negative, and the Bekesy audiogram was type III. Here PB and SSI functions are similar, although SSI shows a slightly lower maximum and a rollover at high speech levels.

Figure 31-7 summarizes findings in a patient with a surgically confirmed lesion of the left brain stem affecting the afferent auditory pathway. Note that speech scores are lower on the right, or contralateral, ear. Again, PB and SSI functions lead to the same conclusion. On the affected right ear, maxima are similar, but the SSI area is somewhat smaller than the PB area. Both functions show the rollover phenomenon at high speech levels.

DISCUSSION

Our clinical and research experience with the SSI procedure during the past four years encourages us to believe that it may represent a valuable addition to the body of materials and techniques presently available for speech audiometry. In comparison with conventional PB testing it has several advantages.

First, the message set is closed. There are only 10 possible answers to each test item, they are always the same, and they are exactly specified. This means that all patients, no matter what their backgrounds, familiarity with the various words of the language, etc., must choose responses from the same linguistic pool. This is a decided advantage over the open set repetition technique.

Second, the scoring system is unambiguous. The patient's response is a button push that can be scored as either correct or incorrect by machine without the need for human decision-making processes. This feature virtually eliminates a source of error that has always plagued conventional PB testing.

Third, each test item is a multiword sentence rather than a single word. This has both a theoretical and a practical advantage. Theoretically a sentence has greater face validity than an isolated word as a unit of speech understanding. At the practical level

Case No. R.H.   Age: 43   Sex: M   Date 2-10-67

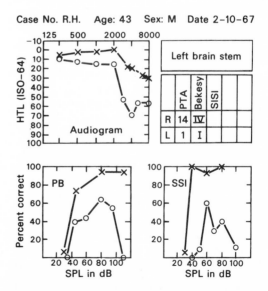

Figure 31-7. Audiometric findings in a patient with a left brain stem lesion. Both PB and SSI functions for the affected ear are similar in maxima and both demonstrate the "roll-over" phenomenon.

multiword sentences are of sufficient duration to permit the easy manipulation of various temporal parameters of the ongoing speech waveform such as temporal interruption, compression, etc. In contrast, the relatively short duration of even bisyllabic words imposes severe constraints on this very convenient method of speech degradation.

Fourth, the generation of equivalent forms is easily accomplished. More importantly, however, the same form of 10 sentences can be used over and over by reordering the 10 items in a new random order. In our experience three trials (i.e., 3 blocks of the same 10 sentences in different orders) are sufficient for most subjects to reach an asymptotic level of performance. Thereafter, these same 10 sentences can be used again and again under a variety of conditions without the intrusion of further learning or practice effects.

It should be noted, however, that the percent-correct score based on a single 10-item trial is not usually as stable as a PB score based on a 25-item trial. When great stability is required we usually base the score on responses to 3 trials or 30 items. In defining PI functions on hearing-impaired listeners, one 10-item trial per level yields data of quite acceptable stability. On the other hand, where a single score must represent a given condition, as, for example, in the comparison of different hearing aids, we typically use as many as 10 trials of 10 items each. Under these conditions extremely stable scores may be anticipated.

Although the SSI test procedure has many potential applications in the general area of speech perception, its use in the clinical evaluation of the hearing-impaired has been especially fruitful. In many patients, especially those with conductive, flat cochlear, VIIIth nerve, and CNS lesions, the SSI procedure led to the same result as the PB test. In other, especially sloping cochlear disorders, the two sets of information seemed to be complementary.

We believe that the clinician with an investigative turn of mind may find SSI an interesting, provocative, and possibly fruitful avenue to explore in evaluating the complex problems of speech understanding faced by the hearing-impaired listener.

ACKNOWLEDGMENT

This project was supported by Public Health Service Grant No. NB 05044 from the National Institute of Neurological Diseases and Blindness, by the Vocational Rehabilitation Administration under Research Grant No. RD 1904-S, and by the Veterans Administration, Prosthetics and Sensory Aids Service, under Research Contract V1005 M-1239. Since completion of this research, Charles Speaks has become an associate professor of communication disorders at the University of Minnesota.

REFERENCES

Carhart, R., A practical approach to the selection of hearing aids. *Trans. Amer. Acad. of Ophthal. Otolaryng.*, **50**, 3–11 (1946a).

Carhart, R., Individual differences in hearing for speech. *Ann. Otol. Rhinol. Laryng.*, **55**, 1–34 (1946b).

Carhart, R., Tests for selection of hearing aids. *Laryngoscope*, **56**, 1–15 (1946c).

Carhart, R., Hearing aid selection by university clinics. *J. Speech Hearing Dis.*, **15**, 106–113 (1950).

Carhart, R., Basic principles of speech audiometry. *Acta Otolaryng.*, **40**, 62–71 (1953a).

Carhart, R., Instruments and materials for speech audiometry. *Acta Otolaryng.*, **40**, 313–323 (1953b).

Carhart, R., Speech audiometry in clinical evaluation. *Acta Otolaryng.*, **41**, 18–42 (1953c).

Carhart, R., and Thompson, Eva. The fitting of hearing aids. *Trans. Amer. Acad. Ophthal. Otolaryng.*, **51**, 3–10 (1947).

French, N. R., and Steinberg, J. C., Factors governing the intelligibility of speech sounds. *J. Acoust. Soc. Amer.*, **19**, 90–119 (1947).

High, W. S., Fairbanks, G., and Glorig, A., Scale for

self-assessment of hearing handicap. *J. Speech Hearing Dis.*, **29,** 215–230 (1964).

Speaks, C., Intelligibility of filtered synthetic sentences. *J. Speech Hearing Res.*, **10,** 289–298 (1967).

Speaks, C., and Jerger, J., Method for measurement of speech identification. *J. Speech Hearing Res.*, **8,** 185–194 (1965).

Speaks, C., Jerger, J., and Jerger, Susan, Performance-intensity characteristics of synthetic sentences. *J. Speech Hearing Res.*, **9,** 305–312 (1966).

Thorndike, E. L., and Lorge, I., *The Teacher's Word Book of 30,000 Words.* New York: Columbia Univ. (1944).

part V

MASKING

Masking in both laboratory and clinic involves essentially the same process: the elevation of threshold for one signal by the presence of a second signal—that is, by a masker. The need for masking in clinical audiometry is based on two facts: (1) an intense stimulus delivered to an earphone placed over one ear may cross to the opposite ear via bone conduction, via air conduction, or via both routes; and (2) bone-conducted signals tend to stimulate both cochleas simultaneously and nearly equally, even at low-intensity levels. These two circumstances sometimes make it difficult to know which ear is actually being stimulated. A common approach to resolving this problem is to reduce or eliminate the participation of the ear not under test by using a masking noise to elevate its threshold.

Clinical masking is one of the most complex audiometric procedures to understand and to execute. It is complex because it involves so many variables that operate simultaneously, some of them under very tenuous control. Masker spectrum, minimum masking levels, interaural attenuation, central masking, and occlusion effects are only some of the variables that must be considered. Most audiometry texts do not provide sufficient information to permit the student to understand the bases and procedures for clinical masking. The seven articles in this section were chosen to provide a representative sample of current approaches to clinical masking. The fact that six of the seven articles were published after 1957 reflects the recency of the application of laboratory data and theory on masking to masking procedures in the clinic.

Sanders and Rintelmann's study compares the relative efficiency of narrow-band noise, white noise, and saw-tooth noise—three of the most commonly available clinical maskers. They found that narrow-band noise was generally superior to the other two. Their discussions of masking noises, of the critical-band concept, and of their data's clinical implications provide an excellent foundation for understanding the masking process.

Bilger and Hirsh's article on masking of tones by bands of noise is included to provide more detailed information about the critical-band concept. Having investigated the masking effects of narrow bands of noise at different frequencies and noise levels, Bilger and Hirsh found that the critical-band hypothesis predicts masking effects rather precisely under certain conditions but not under others (high-noise levels, in particular). They also describe the remote masking phenomenon that has received so much attention since the publication of their article. The interested student is referred to the works listed by the authors at the end of their article.

Dirks and Malmquist's study of the effects of central masking on bone- and air-conducted stimuli shows the average central-masking effects one can expect at various masker-sensation levels. The study also clarifies the reason why masking shifts are greater for frontal than for mastoid vibrator placements.

Chaiklin's paper on interaural attenuation could have been placed in any one of several sections. We included it here because it provides normative data on values of interaural attenuation. These data are essential in determining the need for masking in air-conduction audiometry and in estimating maximum permissible masking levels for both air- and bone-conduction testing. The article is also of interest because of Chaiklin's concise explanation of interaural attenuation and his discussion of the mechanism of cross-hearing.

Studebaker, in his article on clinical masking, shares our opinion concerning the deficiencies in textbook presentations of masking procedures. He reviews the major variables involved in masking, surveys the major research findings that bear on each variable, and proposes clinical masking procedures. In addition, he presents a 56-item bibliography that emphasizes the clinical aspects of masking.

The succeeding article by J. D. Hood presents similar information and recommendations but employs different methods for illustrating various masking principles and places greater emphasis on certain topics. For example, it provides a more comprehensive treatment of cross-hearing, masking noises, and the critical-band concept.

The establishment of minimum masking norms for each masker—an increasingly common clinical practice—is criticized by Veniar in this section's final article. She points out that individual subjects deviate considerably from normative standards and suggests that a more valid procedure is to establish minimum masking levels for each subject. The method she describes is a thought-provoking approach to masking that may prove especially valuable in difficult masking situations.

32

Masking in Audiometry

JAY W. SANDERS
WILLIAM F. RINTELMANN

JAY W. SANDERS, Ph.D., is Associate Professor of Audiology, Vanderbilt University, and the Bill Wilkerson Hearing and Speech Center
WILLIAM F. RINTELMANN, Ph.D., is Professor of Audiology and Associate Director Audiology Research Laboratory, Department of Audiology and Speech Sciences, Michigan State University

THE PROBLEM [1]

One of the major problems in audiometry is that of determining thresholds in monaural and asymmetrical binaural hearing losses. The clinician confronted with a patient whose two ears differ in acuity may have serious difficulty in obtaining accurate measures of hearing for the poorer ear. Under such circumstances, the clinician may arrive at estimates of hearing for the poorer ear that are better than the actual thresholds in that ear. Such erroneous results may even lead to attempted middle ear surgery on an ear having a profound sensorineural hearing loss.

When the two ears differ sufficiently in acuity, the intensity of the tone presented to the poorer ear may be raised to such a level that it is heard in the better ear, either across the head by air conduction or through the head by bone conduction. A number of investigators (*10, 12–14, 22*) have shown that pure tones may cross the head by air conduction when the air conduction thresholds differ by 50 to 60 db. On the other hand, in bone conduction testing the interaural attenuation is essentially zero (*10, 12, 13, 15, 16*). Indeed,

Reprinted by permission of the authors from *Arch. Otolaryngol.*, **80**, pp. 541–556 (1964).
[1] This study was supported by grant NB-01310, grant NB-5329, and grant NB-1048, all from the National Institutes of Health, Public Health Service.

false bone conduction thresholds for the poorer ear may be obtained at approximately the same hearing levels as the bone conduction thresholds in the better ear. Thus it is possible to obtain responses to a bone conduction stimulus at the 0 db hearing level in a dead ear if the opposite ear has normal sensorineural acuity.

The problem is complicated still further by the fact that false air conduction thresholds at the 50 to 60 db hearing level can be obtained in the poorer ear even when the better ear exhibits a 50 to 60 db air conduction loss if bone conduction thresholds in the better ear are at about the 0 db hearing level. In this instance, the test tone presented to the poorer ear by air conduction at a hearing level of 50 to 60 db has reached an intensity level sufficient to stimulate the nontest cochlea by bone conduction.

As a result of crossover of the test tone an audiogram may be obtained for the poorer ear showing an air-bone gap with both air and bone thresholds considerably better than actual acuity in that ear.

The answer to the problem, of course, is to eliminate responses from the better ear through the use of masking noise in that ear while attempting to obtain bona fide responses from the poorer ear. The presence of a masking noise in the good ear shifts the threshold in that ear to a higher hearing level, permitting test tones of greater intensities to be presented to the poorer ear without danger of crossover. The degree of threshold shift produced in the good ear varies with the intensity of the masking noise. However, as Carhart (2) and Naunton (15) have pointed out, certain cases, notably patients with a conductive impairment in the better ear, pose a special problem in masking. The effect on the cochlear sensitivity and thus on the bone conduction threshold of a masking noise applied to a conductively deafened ear is reduced by the amount of the air-bone gap present in that ear. A masking noise at a 50 db effective level for the normal ear[2] when put into an ear with a 40 db conductive loss will shift the air conduction threshold in that ear to a hearing level of 50 db but will only shift the bone conduction threshold to a hearing level of 10 db. Since many commercially available audiometers do not produce much more than 50 db of effective masking, false threshold measurements for a poorer ear may be obtained in conductive hearing losses even when the maximum amount of masking available is applied to the better ear. Thus it may be seen that the problem of obtaining true threshold responses from a poorer ear might not be overcome in many cases simply by putting a noise into the opposite ear. In order to avoid being misled by false audiometric results, the clinician needs to understand the relative effectiveness and the limitations of the various kinds of masking noise.

PURPOSE

The effectiveness or masking efficiency of a particular noise depends not only upon the intensity but also upon the nature of the noise. For example, previous studies (4, 21) have shown that a pure tone can be used to mask other pure tones but that over a range of test frequencies the masking efficiency of a

single frequency is low compared to the efficiency of a noise composed of many frequencies. Consequently, the masking noise produced by the commercially available audiometer is usually some form of noise composed of many frequencies.

The two types of masking noise that have been used most commonly in clinical audiometry are saw-tooth noise and white noise. Recently, a third type, narrow band noise, has become available.[3] The purpose of the present study was to compare these three types of masking noise and to determine their relative efficiencies in solving the problem of eliminating false threshold responses. First, the physical characteristics of the noises were compared in order to form a basis for understanding the masking effectiveness of each noise. Second, a comparison was made of the degree to which each type of noise shifted threshold in a normal ear. Finally, pure tone audiograms were obtained for a number of persons with impaired hearing who presented special problems in masking. In each case four audiograms were obtained, one with no masking and one with each of the three types of masking noise.

THE MASKING NOISES

Saw-Tooth Noise

Saw-tooth noise, one of the two most commonly used for masking in pure tone audiometry, is a noise in which the basic repetition rate (the fundamental frequency) is usually that of the line voltage (60 or 120 cps) and which contains only those frequencies that are multiples of the basic repetition rate. The intensities of these multiple frequencies decrease as their frequencies increase. The acoustic spectrum of the saw-tooth noise used

[2] A masking noise at a 50 db effective level for the normal ear would shift the pure tone threshold in the normal ear to a hearing level of 50 db.

[3] Actually, narrow band noise is not a third type of noise per se but is rather a restricted frequency band of white noise. Although white noise and narrow band noise are the same except for band width, in the present study the terms "white noise" and "narrow band noise" will be used to differentiate between white noise of unlimited spectrum and white noise in a limited band.

in this study is shown in Figure 32-1. As can be seen in the figure, the fundamental frequency for this particular noise was 78 cps, and the additional frequencies present are multiples of that fundamental (156 cps, 234 cps, etc). The figure also shows that the energy systematically decreases as the frequency increases.

Noises referred to as "complex" or "square wave" noise are similar to saw-tooth noise

Narrow Band Noise

Although narrow band noise has only recently become available on American audiometers, a number of investigators (3, 4, 11, 14, 20) have used narrow bands of noise for masking in experimental studies. Actually, the concept of masking with narrow bands of noise was suggested by Fletcher's work in the formulation of the critical band hypothesis (6, 7).

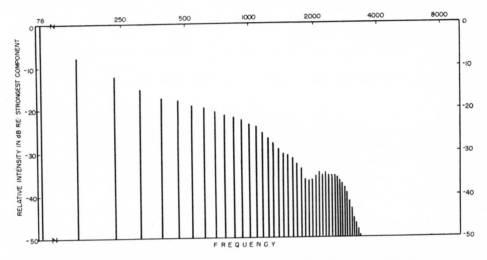

Figure 32-1. The acoustic spectrum of a saw-tooth noise through a PDR-8 earphone.

in that they are composed of a fundamental frequency plus the components that are multiples of the fundamental.

White Noise

White noise, sometimes referred to as thermal noise, and also frequently used as a masking noise in pure tone audiometry, is a noise containing all of the frequencies in the audible spectrum at approximately equal intensities. However, as with any other sound delivered by a transducer, the spectrum is limited at the ear by the frequency response of the earphone. As shown in Figure 32-2, the acoustic spectrum through the TDH-39 earphone is essentially flat out to 6,000 cps but drops rapidly beyond that point.

Fletcher pointed out that in masking with thermal noise, the only components of the noise that have any masking effect are those whose frequencies lie within a narrow band around the frequency of the test tone and that, when the tone is just audible against the noise background, the total acoustic power of the components within that narrow band is the same as that of the pure tone. Fletcher defined this restricted range of frequencies as the critical band. The results of further investigations (1, 4, 9) have supported the critical band hypothesis.

Narrow band noise is produced by selectively filtering white noise and may be defined as a cluster of frequencies encompassed in a restricted range. The frequency around which the cluster is grouped and the width of

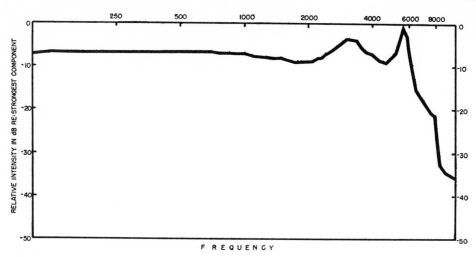

Figure 32-2. The acoustic spectrum of a broad band white noise through a TDH-39 earphone.

the frequency range are matters of choice. A given narrow band of noise may be described in terms of its band width and its rejection rates. The width of the band is defined as the span of frequencies whose energies are no more than 3 db below that of the peak component, and the rejection rate is defined as the decrease in intensity over a one-octave range on either side of the band.

For maximum masking efficiency, a narrow band must be at least as wide as the critical band defined by Fletcher. As the band width increases beyond the critical width, masking efficiency decreases in that the additional energy present does not contribute to masking. Although the overall level of the noise is raised by the energy present in frequencies beyond the critical band width, the level of masking produced by the noise remains the same. The band widths and rejection rates of the six narrow bands used in this study are shown in Figure 32-3. The band widths, determined at the level 3 db down from the peak intensity, are all greater than the critical band widths for the different frequencies.

Comment

A comparison of the acoustic spectra shown in Figures 32-1 and 32-2 leads to the theoretical expectation that white noise has greater masking efficiency than saw-tooth noise, at least in the highest frequencies. As shown in the figures, most of the energy in the saw-tooth noise is concentrated in the lower portion of the frequency range, whereas white noise has its energy spread uniformly throughout the range from 100 to 6,000 cps. A consideration of Figure 32-3 leads to the further theoretical expectation that, for equal energy delivered to the ear, narrow band noise is more efficient than either of the other two types when the narrow band is matched in frequency to the pure tone it masks. This occurs because the narrow band noise concentrates all of its energy into a limited range of frequencies clustered around the frequency of the pure tone to be masked. To illustrate, suppose we take the white noise shown in Figure 32-2 and the 1,000 cps narrow band shown in Figure 32-3 and produce each at an overall sound pressure level of 80 db. The energy of the white noise would be distributed over a range of approximately 6,000 cps, whereas the narrow band noise would be the same energy spread over essentially only 190 cps. According to the critical band hypothesis, the effective masking level of a noise depends upon the energy present in a restricted band of frequencies, the critical band, around the test tone, and not upon the total energy of the noise. Since the critical band width is the same for white noise and narrow band noise, the determining factor in masking is the level per cycle, that is, the intensity of each one-cycle band, rather than the overall intensity. Moreover, since the level per cycle is determined by dividing the overall intensity by the width of the noise band, it can be seen that for equal overall intensity a narrow band of noise will have a higher level per cycle than will a broad band white noise, because the same amount of energy is spread over a much smaller range of frequencies in the narrow band. Thus, for equal overall intensity, narrow band noise with a higher level per cycle might be expected to produce more masking than white noise.

APPARATUS

The apparatus used in the present study is shown schematically in Figure 32-4. The saw-tooth noise from a commercially available audiometer (Maico, model MA-8) was recorded on magnetic tape and fed from a tape reproducer (Magnecorder, type PT63AN, amplifier model PT63J) through the auxiliary circuit of a noise generator (Grason-Stadler, model E-5539A) which served as an amplifier. The noise level was controlled with an attenuator set (Hewlett-Packard, model 350A) with impedance matching networks. A mixing transformer was used to mix the signal from the tape with the test stimulus (pulsed pure tone) from a Békésy audiometer (Grason-Stadler, model E-800). The combined signal was then transduced by a PDR-8 earphone.

The white noise used in the study was produced by a noise generator (Grason-Stadler, model E-5539A) and controlled by an attenuator set (Hewlett-Packard, model 350A) with impedance matching networks. A mixing network was used to combine the white noise with the pulsed stimulus from the Békésy audiometer, and the composite

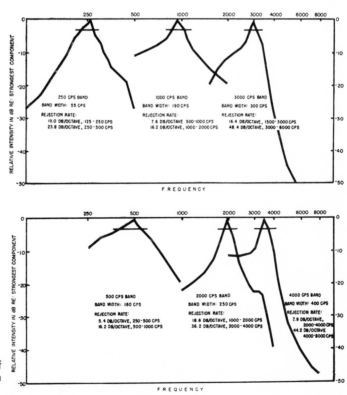

Figure 32-3. The acoustic spectra of six narrow bands of noise through a hearing aid type receiver.

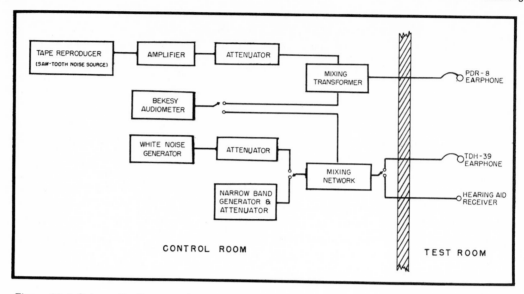

Figure 32-4. Schematic diagram of the apparatus used to obtain pure tone thresholds in quiet and in the presence of three different masking noises.

signal was then transduced by a TDH-39 earphone.

A narrow band noise generator (Amplivox prototype, not available commercially) was used to provide the narrow band noise. The noise was combined in the mixing network with the pulsed stimulus from the Békésy audiometer, and the combined signal was then transduced by a hearing aid type receiver fitted with a rubber tipped insert.

Acoustic measurements of the various masking noises and of the audiometer stimuli were made with an artificial ear assembly. The NBS-9A coupler (6 cc) was used with the PDR-8 and TDH-39 earphones, and the NBS-type 2 coupler (2 cc) was used with the insert receiver. Regular calibration checks were made throughout the period of analysis and testing to insure the stability of the equipment.

MASKING AUDIOGRAMS

To determine the relative efficiencies of the three types of noise employed in this study, masking audiograms were obtained at three

different intensity levels for each type of noise with ten young, normal hearing subjects. The apparatus shown in Figure 32-4 was used in this portion of the study. For each type of noise, the masking noise and the pulsed pure tone stimuli from a Békésy audiometer were mixed into the same receiver. The subject traced his threshold for fixed frequencies in quiet and at each of three intensity levels for each type of noise. The noise levels used were 50 db, 70 db, and 90 db sound pressure level. The mean shifts in threshold were expressed as threshold shifts re: the NBS norms.

The results are shown in Figure 32-5. The curves shown in the figure are the hearing levels to which the normal ears studied were shifted by each type of noise at three different intensity levels. For instance, when the overall intensity level for each type of noise was 50 db sound pressure level, subjects with normal hearing had their thresholds for pure tones shifted by each type of noise to the hearing levels shown in *audiogram 1* of Figure 32-5. Of course, a person with impaired hearing would have his air conduction thresholds shifted to the same hearing levels as those shown for the normal ear, providing his air conduction thresholds in quiet were better than the masked thresholds.

Saw-Tooth Noise

As can be seen in Figure 32-5, saw-tooth noise produced a much greater shift in the lower frequencies than in the highs. This is reasonable when one remembers the acoustic spectrum of the saw-tooth noise. As Figure 32-1 shows, most of the energy in the saw-tooth noise was concentrated in the lower frequencies. By 3,000 cps the noise level is 43 db below that of the peak intensity at the fundamental.

Also shown in Figure 32-5 is the non-linearity of obtained masking with saw-tooth noise. That is, a given increase in the intensity of the masking noise does not produce an equal increase in masking.

Since the frequency of the fundamental in a saw-tooth noise may vary from one noise generator to another, thus varying the spectrum, one might expect two different saw-tooth noises to give somewhat dissimilar masking results. To examine this possibility, the results obtained in the present study were compared with the masked thresholds for saw-tooth noise obtained by Liden (*12*) and with those obtained by Palva (*16*). The masking obtained with two levels of saw-tooth noise produced by four different audiometers is shown in Table 32-1. The table shows that audiometers A, B, and D produced quite similar results through 1,000 cps, whereas audiometer C produced lesser amounts of masking

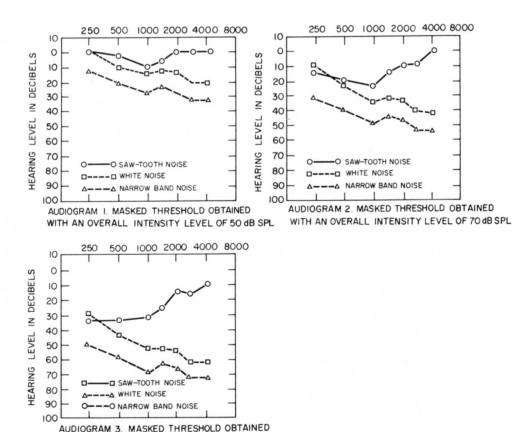

Figure 32-5. Masking audiograms obtained with three types of masking noise at three intensity levels.

TABLE 32-1. SAW-TOOTH NOISE MASKING* OBTAINED IN THE PRESENT STUDY (AUDIOMETER D) COMPARED WITH MASKING REPORTED BY LIDEN (*12*) (AUDIOMETER A) AND PALVA (*16*) (AUDIOMETERS B AND C)

	250	500	1,000	2,000	3,000	4,000
Masking noise at 70 db SPL						
Audiometer A	13.0	17.5	21.8	13.0	16.4	11.7
Audiometer B	11.3	20.0	22.2	6.0	†	5.6
Audiometer C	11.2	12.9	8.9	0.0	†	0.1
Audiometer D	13.7	20.3	23.8	10.1	9.9	0.6
Masking noise at 90 db SPL						
Audiometer A	24.0	30.0	32.6	25.0	28.9	24.0
Audiometer B	25.8	35.2	33.1	13.3	†	11.4
Audiometer C	24.8	23.6	23.6	9.0	†	0.0
Audiometer D	32.7	33.8	32.8	15.6	17.9	11.6

* Threshold shift in decibels in a normal ear.
† Measurement not made.

at these frequencies. For the higher frequencies, audiometer A produced the most masking, audiometers B and D were similar in results, and audiometer C produced the least masking.

The variability in the results obtained with four different noise generators suggests that it would be dangerous to generalize regarding masking effectiveness from one saw-tooth noise to another. However, the results of the comparison do indicate that the saw-tooth noise used in the present study (audiometer D) was not too unlike that produced by different audiometers.

White Noise

The masked audiograms obtained with white noise shown in Figure 32-5 demonstrate that white noise tends to be least effective in the lower frequencies. This occurs because the human ear is less acute in the lower frequencies.

A comparison of the masked thresholds for white noise shown in audiograms 1, 2, and 3 of Figure 32-5 suggests that, unlike saw-tooth noise masking, the masking obtained with white noise is linear. That is, beyond a certain minimum level, each addi-

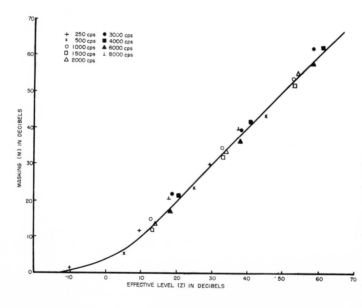

Figure 32-6. Relation between masking (M) and the effective level (Z) of a white noise used for masking. M is the change in the threshold of a pure tone in the presence of the noise. Z is the number of decibels that the total energy in a critical band is above the threshold energy for a pure tone whose frequency is at the center of the band. The solid line is the relation reported by Hawkins and Stevens (*9*).

tional decibel of masking noise produces an additional 1 db shift in threshold. This one-to-one linear relationship between noise intensity and threshold shift is not unexpected. According to Fletcher (6), when a pure tone is just audible against the noise background, the total acoustic power of the components within the critical band surrounding the tone is the same as that of the pure tone. The effective level of the noise is the total acoustic power within the band minus the pure tone threshold in quiet. Beyond a certain minimum level we would expect to find a one-to-one relation between the effective level of the noise and masking, the threshold shift produced by the noise.

Figure 32-6 shows the relation between the masking obtained with ten normal hearing subjects in the present study and the effective levels of the noise used. As can be seen in the figure, the data from the present study are in good agreement with those reported by Hawkins and Stevens (9) and give further support to the critical band hypothesis.

The relation between masking and effective level is shown in another way in Figure 32-7. In this figure one set of curves shows the masking actually obtained with normal

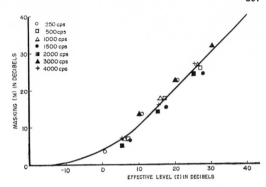

Figure 32-8. Relation between masking (M) and the effective level (Z) of six narrow bands of noise used for masking. M is the change in the threshold of a pure tone in the presence of the noise. Z is the number of decibels that the total energy in a critical band is above the threshold energy for a pure tone whose frequency is at the center of the band. The solid line is the masking-to-effective-level for white noise reported by Hawkins and Stevens (9).

hearing subjects, at three different noise intensity levels. The second set of curves shows the predicted masking for the same intensity levels determined by computation using the critical band data.[4] The mean differences averaged over all frequencies between obtained and predicted masking are 0.2 db at the 50 db level, 0.2 db at the 70 db level, and 0.8 db at the 90 db level. The close agreement between obtained and predicted masked thresholds indicates that high degree of accuracy with which masking by white noise can be predicted.

Narrow Band Noise

As shown in Figure 32-5, the masked audiograms for narrow bands of noise are similar to those for white noise in two respects. First, the greatest shifts in threshold were obtained at those frequencies where the ear is the most sensitive. Second, narrow band masking shows the same one-to-one linearity between masking and noise intensity as does white noise masking.

The relation between masking and the

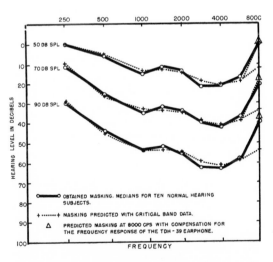

Figure 32-7. A comparison of the masking obtained with white noise at three different intensity levels for ten normal hearing subjects and the masking predicted with the critical band data of Fletcher (6).

[4] The predicted masking at a given noise level is equal to the total energy in the critical band minus the pure tone threshold in quiet.

effective level of narrow band noise is shown in Figure 32-8 with the data compared to the relation reported by Hawkins and Stevens (9) for white noise. The results of the present study suggest that the masking-to-effective-level relation is essentially the same for the two types of noise. This finding is in agreement with that reported by Bilger and Hirsh (1) for the 1,000–1,420 cps noise band.

Since narrow band noise appears to have the same masking-to-effective-level relation as white noise, the critical band data should be just as applicable in the prediction of masked thresholds with narrow band noise. Figure 32-9 compares masked thresholds

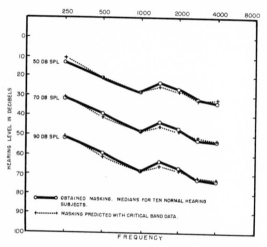

Figure 32-9. A comparison of the masking obtained with narrow bands of noise at three different intensity levels for ten normal hearing subjects and the masking predicted with the critical band data of Fletcher (6).

obtained with normal hearing subjects to the masked thresholds predicted through computation based upon the critical band data. As can be seen in the figure, the thresholds agree closely. The mean differences are 0.3 db at the 50 db level, 0.1 db at the 70 db level, and 0.1 db at the 90 db level. From these results it would appear that the critical band hypothesis is as valid for narrow bands of white noise as it is for a wide spectrum white noise, providing the narrow bands are at least as wide as the critical bands. This

finding does not seem unreasonable in light of Fletcher's (6) concept of equivalance of energy—namely, that when a pure tone is just audible in the presence of noise, the total acoustic power of the components within the critical band surrounding the tone is the same as that of the pure tone. Although the results of the present study are in agreement with those reported by Bilger and Hirsh, they are at variance with the findings of several other investigators. Egan and Hake (4), testing at 410 cps, found masking to be 3 db less than the effective level of a narrow band of noise. Schafer and others (19), testing at three frequencies, found masking to be 1 to 2 db less than the effective levels of narrow bands of noise. Palva (16, 17), commenting on these findings, repeated Garner's (8) explanation that when a single band of noise is used, some of the energy "spills over" onto the adjacent frequency areas of the basilar membrane. Actually, discrepancies of 3 db or less are not of great importance clinically, and the results of the present study suggest that the mean discrepancy averaged over six frequencies is less than 1 db.

Comment

As shown by the masking audiograms in Figure 32-5, when the noises are equated in terms of overall level, saw-tooth noise is the least efficient of the three types of masking noise, because of its dearth of energy in the higher frequencies; white noise is substantially more efficient than saw-tooth noise in the middle and higher frequencies; and narrow band noise is the most efficient of the three types at all of the frequencies tested.

Table 32-2 shows the advantage of narrow band noise over saw-tooth and white noise at each of the three masking noise levels used at each test frequency. As might be expected, the advantage over saw-tooth noise is greatest in the higher frequencies, whereas the advantage of narrow band noise over white noise is greatest in the lower frequencies. It may be noted in Table 32-2 that at 250 cps the advantage of narrow band

TABLE 32-2. THE MASKING ADVANTAGE IN DECIBELS OF NARROW BAND NOISE OVER SAW-TOOTH NOISE AND WHITE NOISE AT THREE MASKING NOISE LEVELS

	250	500	1,000	1,500	2,000	3,000	4,000
Advantage * of narrow band noise over saw-tooth noise							
At 50 db SPL of noise	12.7	18.7	18.1	18.4	26.7	32.5	33.8
At 70 db SPL of noise	18.0	18.7	24.6	28.9	36.6	42.6	53.2
At 90 db SPL of noise	19.0	25.2	24.1	37.9	51.1	54.6	62.2
Advantage † of narrow band noise over white noise							
At 50 db SPL of noise	12.7	14.7	13.6	11.9	13.2	11.1	12.5
At 70 db SPL of noise	20.2	15.7	14.1	11.9	13.2	13.1	12.0
At 90 db SPL of noise	21.7	15.7	14.6	11.9	11.7	10.1	11.5

* Obtained masking with narrow band noise minus obtained masking with saw-tooth noise.
† Obtained masking with narrow band noise minus obtained masking with white noise.

noise over white noise seems to increase at higher noise levels. Actually, the difference in advantage at different noise levels is an artifact. Because of the poorer sensitivity of the ear at 250 cps, no threshold shift was produced by white noise at 50 db sound pressure level. At those noise levels and frequencies where both noises produced threshold shifts, the masking advantage of narrow band over white noise reflects the linearity of the masking produced by each.

A greater advantage of narrow band over white noise in the lower frequencies results from the fact that, although both types of noise have less efficiency in the lows, narrow band noise wastes relatively less energy in components outside the critical bands. Although the critical bands at 250 and 500 cps are narrower than those in the middle frequencies, it is more feasible to produce narrow bands in the lows that are only slightly wider than the critical bands. The narrow bands used in the present study are much closer to the critical band widths in the lower frequencies than in the higher.

Previous studies (5, 10, 14, 20) have suggested a greater efficiency for narrow band noise as compared with broad band white noise. The masking audiograms in the present study, shown in Figure 32-5, support this finding and confirm the theoretical expectation stated earlier in this study; namely, that for equal energy delivered to the ear, narrow band masking is more efficient than saw-tooth

or white noise. Consequently, the clinician faced with a patient who presents a masking problem should expect to find that narrow band masking is considerably more effective than the other two types in eliminating the danger of obtaining false threshold responses in the poorer ear.

CLINICAL APPLICATION

The final step in the present study, after analysis of the physical characteristics of the three types of noise and measurement of the masking produced by each type in a normal ear, was a return to the original problem of eliminating false threshold responses resulting from crossover of the test stimulus in hearing-impaired subjects. Three cases were selected to illustrate serious masking problems, and each case was tested with no masking and with each of the three types of masking noise under consideration. Because narrow bands of noise were available only at 250, 500, 1,000, 2,000, 3,000, and 4,000 cps, thresholds for the poorer ear were obtained only at those frequencies. For each case, all audiometric results were obtained during a single testing session. The Hood technique (10) of masking was employed with each type of noise.

Case A.—The patient was a 66-year-old female. This patient had normal hearing in the right ear except for a moderate sensorineural loss in the higher frequencies. She had a complete loss of hearing in the left ear due to surgical intervention for labyrinthine hydrops.

Figure 32-10 shows the results of pure tone audiometry with this patient when no masking was used and when the better ear was masked with each of the three types of noise.

by air conduction with no masking or with saw-tooth noise in the right ear, the patient could not tell in which ear she heard the tone. When the tone was presented to the left ear by bone conduction with no masking or with saw-tooth noise in the right ear, the patient was convinced she heard the tone in the left ear—the dead ear. This confusion is

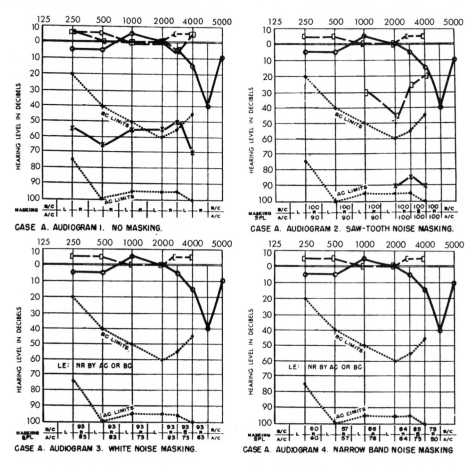

Figure 32-10 (case A). Audiograms obtained for a hearing impaired subject, with no masking and with each of three types of masking noise.

Audiogram 2 shows that saw-tooth noise did not prevent crossover of the test tone in the higher frequencies, even at the maximum masking intensity available, whereas *audiograms 3* and *4* show that responses from the nontest ear were eliminated at all frequencies by both white noise and narrow band noise.

It is worth noting that when the test tone was presented to the left ear (the dead ear)

not unusual and illustrates the fact that the clinician must not place too much reliance on a patient's report as to the ear in which the test tone is heard.

CASE B.—This patient was a 40-year-old female with a diagnosis of bilateral clinical otosclerosis. After middle ear surgery, the patient's left ear developed a complete loss of hearing. Surgery was not performed upon the right ear; thus this ear retained a conductive hearing loss with a sensorineural component in the higher frequencies.

The audiometric results obtained for this case with no masking and with each of the three types of masking noise are shown in Figure 32-11. *Audiograms 2 and 3* show that

frequencies than those used for saw-tooth and white noise.

CASE C.—This 58-year-old male also had a diagnosis of bilateral clinical otosclerosis. Postsurgical serous labyrinthitis had left this patient with a profound sensorineural hearing loss in the left ear. The unoperated right ear

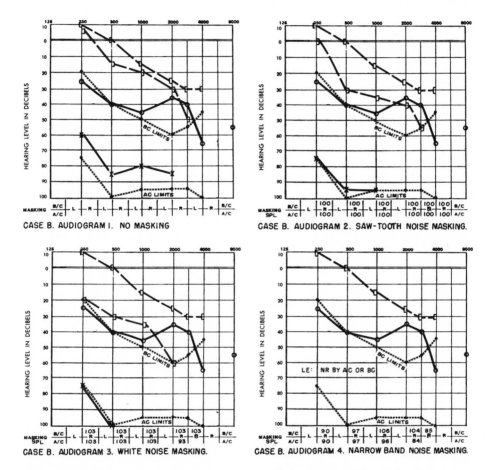

Figure 32-11 (case B). Audiograms obtained for a hearing impaired subject, with no masking and with each of three types of masking noise.

in this case neither saw-tooth nor white noise was successful in preventing crossover of the test tone by air conduction and by bone conduction from the poorer ear to the better ear even when the maximum masking intensities available were used. However, as *audiogram 4* shows, masking was successfully accomplished with narrow band noise even with lower intensity levels at all but two

had a conductive loss with a sensorineural component in the higher frequencies.

The audiometric results for this case are shown in Figure 32-12. In this case, too, although white noise again showed a greater efficiency in masking than did saw-tooth noise, neither was successful in eliminating false responses in the poorer ear due to crossover of the test tone to the better ear.

However, as in case B above, the better ear was successfully masked with narrow band noise. The presence of a response by air conduction at 3,000 cps with a narrow band masking noise of 105 db sound pressure level in the right ear suggests that this is actually a true left ear response rather than a false response due to crossover of the test tone.

The audiometric results for case A shown above illustrate that when air conduction acuity is good in the better ear, masking sounds are not reduced in their capacity to produce threshold shifts in that ear. Although saw-tooth noise did not prevent false responses

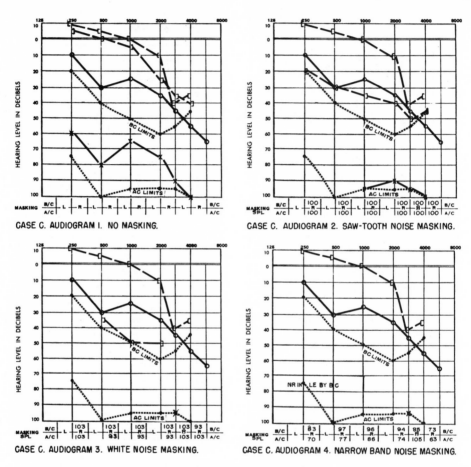

Figure 32-12 (case C). Audiograms obtained for a hearing impaired subject, with no masking and with each of three types of masking noise.

With no air-bone gap present in the right ear at that frequency, a narrow band noise of 105 db sound pressure level would have shifted the right ear threshold to a hearing level of approximately 90 db, thus effectively ruling out the possibility of a crossover response in the right ear at a hearing level of 95 db.

in this case, it was possible to achieve full protection with white noise. The results for cases B and C, however, illustrate that, as pointed out by Carhart (2) and Naunton (15), a conductive hearing loss in the better ear does increase the difficulty of obtaining true responses from the poorer ear. In these two cases, false responses could be eliminated only with narrow band noise.

A further consideration of the results shown for the three clinical cases might lead to the suggestion that successful masking could have been accomplished with white noise masking in all three cases if higher intensities of white noise had been available. This is possibly true and requires further comment.

One difficulty in the use of white noise at high intensity levels is the problem of patient discomfort. This would not have been a problem in cases B and C above, since the noise level would be substantially reduced by the conductive block, but it is a problem in certain other cases. It is of no use to the clinician to have a high level of white noise available if the patient will not tolerate it. In this respect, too, narrow band noise has an advantage. Studebaker (20), using a loudness balancing method with white noise and narrow band noise, has shown that when the two types of noise are equated by subject adjustment to the same loudness, narrow band noise at that level produces considerably more masking than does white noise. This means that for equal masking with the two kinds of noise, narrow band noise subjects the patient to less loudness, thereby reducing patient discomfort and fatigue. An even more important advantage is with the patient who will not tolerate sound at high loudness levels. With these cases it is often possible to mask successfully with narrow band noise when it would not be possible with white noise.

Also, while it is true that successful masking might have been accomplished with white noise in all three of the clinical cases reported here if higher levels of white noise had been available, it should be remembered that levels beyond approximately 105 db SPL are often not available on pure tone audiometers; and, regardless of the maximum intensities available, a given level of narrow band noise will produce more masking than the same overall level of white noise.

Although the problem of overmasking did not arise in the present study, it is always a danger when masking noise is used at high intensity. Just as the pure tone test stimulus might cross the head and be heard in the nontest ear, so might the masking noise cross the head and interfere with threshold determination in the test ear. Various studies (15, 17, 18) have shown that white noise transduced through an earphone in a standard cushion crosses over at a level of about 50 db above threshold in the test ear. The use of narrow band noise does not bring greater interaural attenuation (15), since the determining factor in overmasking is the level per cycle transmitted across the head, rather than the overall level. However, the danger of overmasking can be decreased by delivering the noise through an insert receiver—a small hearing aid type receiver with a rubber tipped insert that fits into the ear canal. A number of studies (5, 10, 15, 17, 18, 20, 21) have shown that use of such a receiver can bring about a substantial increase in interaural attenuation. Several investigators (5, 10, 22) have reported attenuation of 80 to 90 db, thereby practically eliminating the problem of overmasking.[5]

One further comment is necessary at this point. The results of this study should not be interpreted as implying that narrow band masking is a panacea that will end all problems in masking. Although false responses were eliminated with narrow band noise in the clinical cases shown, it is certainly possible to obtain false responses due to crossover of the test tone even when using high levels of narrow band noise. To illustrate, suppose we have a patient with a profound sensorineural loss in the left ear and a 50 db conductive loss in the right ear. At 500 cps, a narrow band noise of 120 db SPL will shift the air conduction threshold in the right ear to 90 db hearing level. However, the bone

[5] In the present study the narrow band noise was presented through an insert receiver, although danger of overmasking was not a problem. The results obtained with narrow band masking would have been essentially the same if a standard earphone had been used.

conduction threshold in the right ear would be shifted to a hearing level of only 40 db because of the 50 db conductive block in that ear. As a result of crossover of the test tone by bone conduction, it would be possible in this case to obtain false responses from the poorer ear to air conduction presentation at about the 95 db hearing level and to bone conduction presentation at about the 45 db hearing level. Thus, although narrow band noise will produce greater masking than either of the other two types, it will not completely eliminate the problem of false responses in all cases, at least with the maximum levels now available. In such cases the clinician's only recourse is to employ the Hood method of masking (*10*) to demonstrate that the thresholds obtained are actually false responses.

CONCLUSION

The results obtained in this study [6] indicate that of the three types of noise studied, narrow band noise is the most efficient as a masking noise in pure tone audiometry. The masking audiograms for normal hearing sub-

[6] Dr. George E. Shambaugh, Jr., Dr. Raymond Carhart, Dr. Tom W. Tillman, and Mr. Robert Johnson gave assistance.

jects and the clinical results for hearing-impaired subjects show that for equal intensity levels, narrow band noise produces greater threshold shifts than does either of the other two types and thereby affords the clinician greater protection from false responses due to crossover of the test tone. The advantage of narrow band noise over the other two types is great enough to make it distinctly preferable, at least for the special problem cases.

SUMMARY

Three types of masking noise (saw-tooth, broad band white, and narrow band noise) were compared to determine their relative efficiencies as masking noises in pure tone audiometry. The physical characteristics of each type of noise were examined and the noises were used to obtain masking audiograms for ten normal-hearing subjects. Three hearing-impaired subjects, considered critical cases for masking, were tested with each type of noise. The results show that at equal overall intensity levels, white noise has greater masking efficiency than does saw-tooth noise but narrow band noise is considerably more efficient than either of the other two types.

REFERENCES

1. Bilger, R. C., and Hirsh, I. J.: Masking of Tones by Bands of Noise, J. Acoust. Soc. Amer., 28:623–630, 1956.
2. Carhart, R.: Assessment of Sensorineural Response in Otosclerosis, Arch. Otolaryng., 71:141–149, 1960.
3. Dirks, D. D.: Factors Related to Reliability of Bone Conduction, PhD Dissertation, Northwestern University, 1963.
4. Egan, J. P., and Hake, H. W.: On Masking Pattern of Simple Auditory Stimulus, J. Acoust. Soc. Amer., 22:622–630, 1950.
5. Feldman, A. S.: Problems in Measurement of Bone Conduction, J. Speech Hearing Dis., 26:39–44, 1961.
6. Fletcher, H.: Auditory Patterns, Rev. Mod. Physics 12:47–65, 1940.
7. Fletcher, H., and Munson, W. A.: Relation Between Loudness and Masking, J. Acoust. Soc. Amer., 9:1–10, 1937.
8. Garner, W. R.: Hearing, Ann. Rev. Psychol. 3: 85–104, 1952.
9. Hawkins, J. E., Jr., and Stevens, S. S.: Masking of Pure Tones and of Speech by White Noise, J. Acoust. Soc. Amer., 22:6–13, 1950.
10. Hood, J. D.: Principles and Practice of Bone Conduction Audiometry, Laryngoscope 70:1211–1228, 1960.
11. Jerger, J. F.; Tillman, T. W.; and Peterson, J. L.: Masking by Octave Bands of Noise in Normal and Impaired Ears, J. Acoust. Soc. Amer., 32:385–390, 1960.
12. Liden, G.: Speech Audiometry, Acta Otolaryng (Stockholm), suppl. 114, pp 72–76, 1954.
13. Liden, G.; Nilsson, G.; and Anderson, H.:

Masking in Clinical Audiometry, Acta Otolaryng. (Stockholm), 50:125–136, 1959.

14. Liden, G.; Nilsson, G.; and Anderson, H.: Narrow Band Masking With White Noise, Acta Otolaryng. (Stockholm), 50:116–124, 1959.

15. Naunton, R. F.: Masking Dilemma in Bilateral Conduction Deafness, Arch. Otolaryng., 72:753–757, 1962.

16. Palva, T.: Masking in Audiometry, Acta Otolaryng (Stockholm), suppl. 118, pp 156–172, 1954.

17. Palva, T.: Masking in Audiometry: Further Studies, Acta Otolaryng. (Stockholm), 49:229–239, 1958.

18. Palva, T., and Palva, A.: Masking in Audiometry, Acta Otolaryng. (Stockholm), 54:521–531. 1962.

19. Schafer, T. H., et al: Frequency Selectivity of Ear as Determined by Masking Experiments, J. Acoust. Soc. Amer., 22:490–496, 1950.

20. Studebaker, C. F.: On Masking in Bone Conduction Testing, J. Speech Hearing Res., 5:215–227, 1962.

21. Wegel, R. L., and Lane, C. E.: Auditory Masking of One Pure Tone by Another and Its Probable Relation to Dynamics of Inner Ear, Physic Rev., 23:266–285, 1924.

22. Zwislocki, J.: Acoustic Attenuation Between Ears, J. Acoust. Soc. Amer., 25:752–759, 1953.

33

Masking of Tones by Bands of Noise

ROBERT C. BILGER
IRA J. HIRSH

ROBERT C. BILGER, Ph.D., is Associate Professor, School of Medicine, University of Pittsburgh

IRA J. HIRSH, Ph.D., is Dean of the Faculty of Arts and Sciences, Washington University, and Director of Research, Central Institute for the Deaf

INTRODUCTION [1]

There appear to be at least two widely accepted notions concerning auditory masking. The first, called the *critical band*, suggests that the masking of a pure tone by noise is mediated by only a narrow band of frequencies in the noise that are near the frequency of the tone being masked. The second has to do with the relation between the amount of masking (that is, the difference between the masked threshold and the threshold in the quiet) and the level of the masking noise. For wide-band masking noise, this relation appears to be linear; that is, an increase of x db in the level of the noise will be accompanied by an increase in masking of x db. These two notions provide the theoretical point of departure for the experiments to be reported here.

In 1940, Fletcher [2] postulated that of all the frequencies in a wide-band noise, only those lying within a certain band would produce masking of a pure tone whose frequency lay in the middle of that band. This critical band was quantified by Fletcher and Munson,[3] who measured the masking of pure tones by a wide-band noise, filtered so that it yielded equal masking for all frequencies. We must distinguish between the general notion and its quantification, for it will become one of our conclusions that the quantification is quite adequate but the applicability of the critical-band concept is not so general as has been supposed.

From the theory and experiments that followed Fletcher's paper,[2] there have emerged at least three ways of defining a critical band. First, and most directly connected with the original definition, the critical band is defined as that band of frequencies in a noise beyond which broadening the band will not further increase the masking of a pure tone in the center of the band. Second, a critical band may also be defined as that band width of noise whose over-all energy is equal to the energy of a pure tone in the center of the band when the tone is just barely masked by the noise. Third, and as a corollary of the second, a critical band of noise is that band width whose absolute threshold is equal to the threshold of a pure tone in the center of the band.

The first definition has not been directly tested except for some results published by Fletcher (reference 2, Figure 17) for which

Reprinted by permission of the authors from *J. acous. Soc. Amer.*, **28**, pp. 623–630 (1956).

[1] This research was carried out under Contract No. AF18(600)-131, between Central Institute for the Deaf and the U.S. Air Force. Reproduction for any purpose of the United States Government is permitted.

[2] H. Fletcher, Revs. Modern Phys. **12**, 47–65 (1940).

[3] H. Fletcher and W. A. Munson, J. Acoust. Soc. Am. **9**, 1–10 (1937).

the experimental details are not available. Tests of the critical-band values according to this definition are also provided by extrapolation in the results of Schafer et al.[4] and, although slight differences are shown for the three frequencies that they investigated, the values are clearly not out of line.

The second definition actually arose from the experiments of Fletcher and Munson.[3] According to this definition, values given by Fletcher[2] for the critical band as a function of frequency have been corroborated by Hawkins and Stevens.[5] (Fletcher's values for the critical band width as a function of frequency, as reproduced by Hawkins and Stevens will be used in this paper.)

The third definition has been tested and values found adequate, except at low frequencies, by Hirsh and Bowman.[6]

In general, then, it appears that the values for the critical band that have been published by Fletcher[2] and by Hawkins and Stevens[5] are correct and fairly repeatable in a variety of experimental arrangements. One of the most obvious limitations, however, has to do with the level of the masking noise. Intensity levels of the masking noise did not exceed 100 db in the experiments of Fletcher and Munson or of Hawkins and Stevens. Schafer et al.[4] measured masking by narrow bands of noise at only one moderate level. Hirsh and Bowman[6] tested critical-band values only at threshold. The critical-band concept implies, however, that masking should increase linearly with the level of the masking sound, particularly according to the second definition of the critical band given above; namely, that band whose total energy is equal to that of the pure tone masked. Actually this implication of linearity was verified by Hawkins and Stevens[5] when pure tones or speech were masked by wide-band, white noise. Hirsh and Bowman[6] also observed this linearity for the masking of speech by white noise.

If we look back to the classical paper of Wegel and Lane[7] on the masking of tones by tones, we do not always find a linear relation between the masking of the test tone and the level of the masking tone. They show, for example, that while a linear relation between masking and the level of an 800-cps masking tone is observed when the frequency of the test tone lies near 800 cps, sigmoidal functions are seen for higher frequencies of the test tone (reference 7, Figure 2). This curvilinearity has been interpreted as resulting from combination tones and other harmonic combinations that complicate studies with pure tones.

But bands of noise yield similar phenomena. Hirsh and Bowman[6] reported, for example, that the threshold of intelligibility (spondaic words) increases linearly with the level of masking noise when that noise has a broad band or is confined to frequencies between 400 and 1000 cps. The relation was positively accelerated when the masking noise was restricted to frequencies above 1000 cps and was sigmoidal in shape for bands of noise below 400 cps. Even more bizarre shapes for the masking functions when brief acoustic clicks are masked by white noise were reported by Hirsh, Rosenblith, and Ward.[8] These authors tentatively interpreted these results by regarding the noise as a band (160 to 6600 cps) and the click that was masked as having a broader spectrum. The audibility of a click, like the intelligiblity of speech, could be mediated by different parts of the audible spectrum, depending upon what was available in the unmasked portion. Changing level presumably shifted the responsibility, so to speak, from one region of frequencies to another.

Miller[9] also studied the masking of speech by 250-mel bands. In his case, however, masking effects were shown not as threshold shifts but as decreases in the articulation score for lists of monosyllabic words that were

[4] T. H. Schafer et al., J. Acoust. Soc. Am. 22, 490–496 (1950).

[5] J. E. Hawkins, Jr., and S. S. Stevens, J. Acoust. Soc. Am. 22, 6–13 (1950).

[6] I. J. Hirsh and W. D. Bowman, J. Acoust. Soc. Am. 25, 1175–1180 (1953).

[7] R. L. Wegel and C. E. Lane, Phys. Rev. 23, 266–285 (1924).

[8] Hirsh, Rosenblith, and Ward, J. Acoust. Soc. Am. 22, 631–637 (1950).

[9] G. A. Miller, Psychol. Bull. 44, 105–129 (1947).

presented at a constant level. It is difficult, of course, to trade decrements in intelligiblity for shifts in the speech threshold for comparative purposes, but we may note nonetheless a difference in relation between articulation score and the level of the band of noise, as the frequencies in the band are changed. For white noise and for bands of noise below 1000 cps, the intelligibility of the words continues to drop to zero as the noise level is increased. For bands of noise above 1000 cps, however, the articulation score drops to a minimum value (which value increases with the frequencies in the band), after which no further decrease in intelligibility is observed as the noise level is increased. Although Miller's explanation, stemming from conclusions of Wegel and Lane,[7] to the effect that low frequencies mask high frequencies better than high frequencies mask low frequencies, may satisfy his own observations, it is not at all applicable to the accelerating functions of Hirsh and Bowman [6] for threshold elevation due to increasing the level of high-frequency bands of noise.

These apparent exceptions to an admittedly more orderly relation of linearity between masking and the level of masking sound, led us to seek further explanation in the pattern of masking produced by different bands of noise. In particular, we were interested in knowing how well the masked threshold of a tone as a function of frequency would follow the frequency characteristic of a band of noise. Further, it was of importance to know how this behavior would change with the level of the band of noise.

It is surprising that, in spite of a fairly large experimental literature on masking, there has been relatively little reported on this matter. Fletcher and Munson [3] give some results for certain bands of noise but they did not examine masking as a function of the level of these bands nor did they report the cut-off characteristics of the filters used. Egan and Hake [10] studied the masking of pure tones by a single band of noise, 90 cps wide and centered around 410 cps. They varied the band

[10] J. P. Egan and H. W. Hake, J. Acoust. Soc. Am. **22,** 622-630 (1950).

level from 40 to 80 db. Their results are of direct concern here but we wished to know about other frequencies and higher levels as well. Schafer et al.[4] using mixtures of tones in lieu of bands of noise, have shown the response of the ear in terms of pure-tone thresholds at frequencies within and near these bands at three widely spaced frequencies, but their results may not yet be generalized with respect to masking level.

As an attempt to fill in some of these gaps, then, the present studies were designed to provide information on the masking patterns of different bands of noise at different noise levels. Seven of the 11 bands used by Hirsh and Bowman [6] were employed as masking sounds. These bands, each corresponding to a pitch interval of 250 mels, had the following limits of frequency: 394–670, 670–1000, 1000–1420, 1420–1900, 1900–2450, 2450–3120, and 4000–5100 cps. Our interest in the ability of the ear to follow the filter characteristics led us to use these bands with two rates of cutoff or slope beyond the band limits, namely 36 and 54 db per octave. Masked audiograms as a continuous function of frequency were obtained in the presence of these noises at over-all sound pressure levels of 40, 60, 80, and 100 db.

APPARATUS AND PROCEDURE

Filter Characteristics

Each section of our variable electronic filters (Spencer-Kennedy Laboratories, Model 302) rejects beyond the cut-off frequency at the rate of 18 db per octave. To obtain bands of noise with cut-off slopes of 54 db per octave three sections were used as high-pass and three as low-pass filters. Two sections of the filters were used on each side of the band to obtain the bands of noise with cut-off slopes of 36 db per octave. Each section was tuned separately by setting the variable frequency control so that the level of a pure-tone signal at the cut-off frequency was 1.75 db below the level of a tone in the pass-band of that section. After each section had been tuned separately, the sections for the low-pass side of the pass-band were checked to make sure that any two sections were down 3.50 db at cutoff (36 db per octave) and that all three sections were down 5.25 db at cutoff (54 db per octave). This procedure was repeated for the high-pass side of the pass-band.

The electrical response of the filters was further mapped out with pure tones. For each pass-band the response as a function of frequency was recorded on an automatic frequency-response recorder (Sound Apparatus Company, Model FR-1). The results of these measurements are presented in Figures 33-2–8, along with the results of these experiments. In these figures the solid curves represent the bands with a rejection rate beyond cutoff of 54 db per octave, while the dashed lines represent the bands with slopes of 36 db per octave.

Audiometer

Figure 33-1 is a block diagram showing the way in which the circuits that provided the filtered noise were mixed with the circuits that provided the pure-tone signal. The output of a pure-tone oscillator (General Radio, Model 1304-A) was fed to an internally timed electronic switch, so that a pulsed tone with a clickless onset, pulsing 3 times per second, was available as a signal. After suitable amplification and control attenuation, this signal was fed to a modified portion of a sound level recorder in such a way that its level was controlled by a motor-driven attenuator. The direction of attenuator change was controlled by the listener. Level was also recorded indirectly as a function of frequency, a mechanical link between the oscillator and the recorder affording the necessary synchronization. The apparatus thus described constitutes a modified Békésy audiometer.

Listening Tests

Each of five observers was instructed to push his attenuator-control button as soon as he heard the interrupted tone and to release the button as soon as he could no longer hear

the tone. At the beginning of each experimental session two audiograms were made in the quiet. The first of these runs was used only for practice and general "settling." The second was used as the observer's audiogram in quiet. After the two unmasked audiograms had been made, masked audiograms were made for each of the four levels of a particular band of noise. In all, each observer partici-

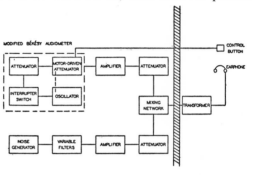

Figure 33-1. Block diagram of apparatus.

pated in fourteen such sessions, one each for each of the seven bands of noise, with two rejection rates for each band. Monaural thresholds were taken on the better ear of each listener. All audiograms were started at 100 cps and frequency always proceeded from low to high.

RESULTS

Main Experiment

A visually interpolated midline was drawn through the envelope of each Békésy audiogram. The point at which this midline intersected a frequency marker was taken as the threshold for that frequency. Thresholds were tabulated for 39 frequencies between 150 and 6000 cps. These threshold values were then converted to sound pressure level (db above 0.0002 microbar in an ASA Type-1 coupler [11]).

[11] American Standard Method for the Coupler Calibration of Earphones, Z24.9-1949, American Standards Association, New York.

The results for the 394–670 cps band of noise are presented in Figure 33-2. In this and in subsequent figures (Figures 33-3–10), the left-hand ordinate, to be used in reading pure-tone thresholds for the quiet and noise conditions, is in db above 0.0002 microbar. The threshold curve across the bottom of the figure is a smoothed curve based upon the mean thresholds for the five listeners over all trials in quiet. The right-hand ordinate (SPL per cycle of noise) is to be used in reading the noise level (electrical response of the filters) for each of the four levels.

Each masked threshold plotted represents

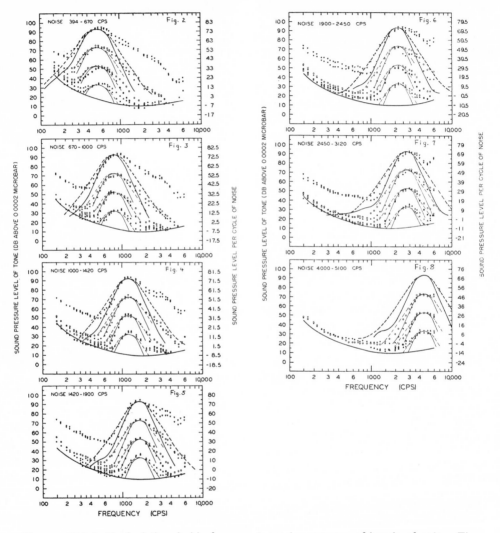

Figures 33-2–8. Masked thresholds for pure tones in presence of bands of noise. The right-hand ordinate gives the noise level per cycle in the band: solid curves show the noise spectrum when the filter rejects at the rate of 54 db/octave beyond the cut-off frequencies shown at the upper left, while the broken curves give the same spectrum for a cut-off rate of 36 db/octave. The four sets of curves show level per cycle corresponding to over-all band levels of 40, 60, 80, and 100 db above 0.0002 microbar. Open symbols show thresholds for 36-db-per-octave bands, while filled symbols show thresholds for 54-db-per-octave bands. Different symbols refer to the several over-all band levels: triangles for 40, squares for 60, circles for 80, and inverted triangles for 100 db. Thresholds are to be read from the left-hand ordinate. The right and left ordinates are displaced by the critical band width (in db) for the midfrequency of the band. Thus in or near the band, the left ordinate may also be used to read effective level for the noise.

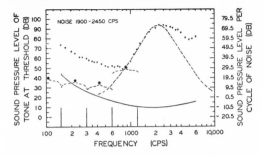

Figure 33-9. Octave-band analysis of noise from earphone compared with masked thresholds and with electrical filter characteristics for the band 1900-2450 cps.

the mean for the five listeners. Filled symbols represent the masked threshold data obtained with bands of noise having slopes beyond cutoff of 54 db per octave while open symbols represent masked threshold data obtained with the band set for a slope of 36 db per octave. Data for the over-all level of 40 db SPL are represented by triangles, for 60 db by squares, for 80 db by circles, and for 100 db by inverted triangles.

The points in Figures 33-2–10 constitute *masked audiograms* rather than the traditional masking audiogram in which the data reported are db of masking. The amount of masking can be determined from our figures by subtracting the quiet threshold from the masked threshold. We have chosen to report the masked threshold, rather than masking, in order to be able to include the response characteristics of the filters on the same figures.

Critical Bands and Linearity. To facilitate the comparison of the values of various critical band widths reported by Fletcher [2] and by Hawkins and Stevens [5] with our data, we have positioned the right-hand ordinate (db per cycle of noise) in such a manner that coincidence of the points with the filter-response curves indicates agreement between these measured masked thresholds and corresponding values that would be predicted by published values [5] of the critical band. This alignment was accomplished by placing o db per cycle of noise directly across from 17 db of the left-hand ordinate in Figure 33-2, 17 db being the critical band width reported

for 520 cps, the middle frequency of the 394–670 cps band of noise. Inspection of Figure 33-2 reveals that the coincidence of the masked thresholds (points) obtained for the frequencies at the center of the band of noise and the noise spectrum (curves) is obtained, at least within the limits of accuracy of Békésy-type audiometry. Further inspection also shows that masking, within the 394–670 cps band of noise, increases linearly with increases in the level of the band of noise.

In Figures 33-3–8 the two ordinates were positioned in the same manner relative to the critical band width of the center frequency of the particular band of noise. Inspection of these figures indicates the same agreement for previously reported critical band widths [2,5] and for the linearity of masking within the band.

Symmetry. The patterns of the masked thresholds shown in Figures 33-2–8 are highly consistent in the relation they bear to the filter characteristics. First, when we compare the pattern of the masked thresholds to the response characteristic of the band, we see that all of these patterns are dissymmetrical, even those for the 40-db sound pressure levels. This dissymmetry indicates an inability of the ear to follow the slope of the filtered noise above the high-frequency cutoff, in contradistinction to how well it follows the slope of the noise below the low-frequency cutoff. This dissymmetry at low levels is in dis-

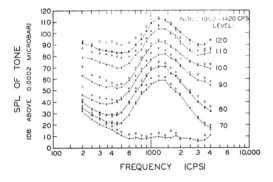

Figure 33-10. Masked thresholds for pure tones in the presence of six over-all band levels of noise (1000–1420 cps). Open symbols show monaural thresholds, while filled symbols show binaural thresholds.

agreement with the symmetrical patterns reported by other investigators.[10]

As the over-all sound pressure level in each band is increased from 40 to 80 db, the slope of the masked audiogram for frequencies above the band remains relatively constant, but as the level is increased further to 100 db the slope of the masked audiogram above the band changes radically.

Differences between the Two Slopes. The ear's ability to follow the filtered-noise spectrum is shown best by the effect of changing the cut-off slope of the filter. The results shown in Figures 33-2–8 indicate, first, that the slope has no effect on the masked thresholds for tones lying in or slightly below the band. On the low-frequency side of the filter, the points representing masked thresholds stay close to the respective curves for the two slope settings of 36 and 54 db per octave. Points converge again, indicating no effect of cut-off slope, at more remote frequencies, but this part of the results will be discussed below. Above the band, even though the masked thresholds diverge considerably from the filter characteristics, the differences between the masked thresholds for the two cut-off slopes are usually seen.

"Remote" Masking. We have already noted how, in Figures 33-2–8, the masked thresholds fall very closely on the filter response curves as we move downward in frequency from the center of the band. But as we approach low frequencies that are fairly remote from the band, a much more unusual phenomenon occurs. If the over-all noise level in the band is 80 or 100 db we observe, in addition to the "proper" masking in or near the band, a threshold elevation for these low frequencies that is very nearly constant as a function of frequency. Furthermore, this remote masking, after it appears, does not seem to be related linearly to the masking level. For example, we find approximately 10 db masking for the 80 db noise, but this masking increases by more than 20 db as the noise level is raised to 100 db.

The appearance of masking beyond the

limits included by the band of noise used plus its extrapolated effects according to the critical-band calculations, suggests the possibility of masking of a different kind from that covered by the critical-band hypothesis. Before considering this further, however, we had first to test whether some low-frequency noise might actually be present at the input to the ear.

Acoustical Measurements. The response curves shown in Figures 33-2–8 were obtained from electrical measurements alone. We have not attempted to introduce corrections for variations in the response of the earphone to a constant voltage as a function of frequency. (Such corrections do enter, however, in the pure-tone thresholds.) To investigate the acoustic spectrum of the noise produced by the earphone, we [12] fed the output of the earphone to a Western-Electric 640-AA microphone through a 6 cc coupler (ASA, Type-1 [11]). The microphone's output was connected to a General Radio (Type 1550-A) octave-band analyzer. This analysis was carried out for only one of our bands, 1900–2450 cps, with only one slope, 36 db/octave. The results are shown in Figure 33-9 along with the electrical response and the masked thresholds for this particular over all level (100 db). The heavy dots show the effective level (Z, to be read on the left ordinate) of the midfrequency in the octave-band, corrected for slope. Although the acoustic noise does not decrease as rapidly as does the electrical response of the filters, as the frequency is lowered, it does drop and furthermore is below those effective levels that would be sufficient to cause masking in these low frequencies. We conclude, therefore, that noise, either in our amplifying system or from other sources, was not sufficiently intense, in the earphone, to have produced the low-frequency masking shown in Figures 33-2–7.

Follow-up Experiments. Since acoustical measurements of the noise below the band indicated that the masking of frequencies well below the band of noise was not the result of noise

[12] We are indebted to Dr. J. R. Cox who supervised these tests.

at the earphone, we sought more detailed information about the relation between the masked audiogram and over-all level in the band. A follow-up experiment was planned, therefore, to determine the masked audiograms at band levels between 70 and 120 db SPL, in steps of 10 db, for the 1000–1420 cps band, with a single slope beyond cutoff of 36 db per octave. Five highly trained listeners who had not participated in the previous experiment were used. The experiment involved two sessions for each listener. In addition to the two quiet audiograms at the outset, each session consisted of listening in three levels of the noise, spaced at 20 db intervals. Only one session was conducted for a listener on any one day. In this first follow-up experiment, monaural audiograms were taken for the better ear. The same experiment was repeated binaurally.

The results of these follow-up experiments are presented in Figure 33-10. The monaural results are represented by open symbols and the binaural results by filled symbols. The binaural masked thresholds for each band level are connected by straight lines.

The sound pressure levels for binaural thresholds represent the response of the more sensitive phone at each frequency. For the range of frequencies reported (200–4000 cps) the phones differed by no more than 3 db, and differences occurred at only the highest frequencies.

Comparing the open symbols in Figure 33-10 to the open symbols in Figure 33-4, we see that the patterns of the masked thresholds for the same band are essentially the same for the two groups of listeners. Figure 33-10 indicates that the masking at the low-frequency end does not increase as a linear function of band level, but accelerates between noise levels of 80 and 110 db SPL. Considering the binaural thresholds (filled symbols) we see that the masking as a function of band level in the high-frequency end of the audiograms tends to accelerate for band levels below 100 db but is more or less linear with higher levels.

Cross-Hearing. The reader may be wondering why we have brought binaural hearing into this later study. The reason has to do with the fact that for certain levels and/or bands, the listener may report that the barely audible tone has moved to the opposite ear, even though both tone and noise were being delivered to the same ear. It was for this reason that the results for 100 db of the band 4000–5100 cps were not given in Figure 33-8. The shift in localization made the listening task extremely difficult to do, and even more difficult to interpret.

In order to eliminate possible distortions in the masking functions that would relate masking to noise level, the follow-up studies included binaural tests in which both the tone and the noise were presented to both ears, in phase. The effect of the cross-hearing can be seen in Figure 33-10. For example, monaural thresholds for high frequencies (open symbols) do not continue to increase as the noise level is increased from 100 to 120 db. But the increase in the binaural threshold shows that masking does continue to increase with level, even above 110 db.

In an attempt to determine whether this cross-hearing was due to air to to bone conduction, one of us (IH) listened for monaural masked thresholds under four different conditions of the opposite ear: (1) opposite ear open and unoccluded, (2) opposite ear covered by a dummy phone but unoccluded, (3) opposite ear open but occluded by an earplug, and (4) opposite ear covered by a dummy phone and occluded by an earplug. Since this cross-hearing was minimal for the first condition (opposite ear uncovered and unoccluded) and maximal for the fourth condition (opposite ear covered and occluded), we have assumed that the cross-hearing present in this situation can be attributed to bone conduction.

With respect to the differences between the monaural and binaural experiments, it is interesting to note that the average (mean for the five listeners) binaural thresholds in the quiet are consistently 3 db below the average monaural thresholds in quiet.[13] The differences between the masked monaural and

[13] Shaw, Newman, and Hirsh, J. Exptl. Psychol. **37,** 229–242 (1947).

binaural thresholds will require further research.

Masking Functions. The "remote" masking that was evidenced in the low frequencies in Figures 33-2–7 is shown in greater detail in Figure 33-10, for the one band, 1000–1420 cps. The low-frequency masking seems to appear when the over-all level reaches 80 db. Then it increases in an accelerating manner as the level is increased to 110 db, after which deceleration is observed. Cutting through these graphs at certain frequencies, we can

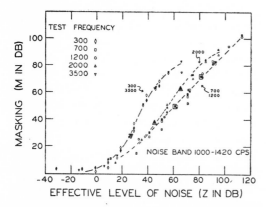

Figure 33-11. Masking for five selected frequencies as a function of the effective level (*Z*) obtaining at the particular frequency. Data from Figures 33-4 and 33-10.

obtain other graphs that show directly the relation between masking and the level of the band of noise. An example, taken from Figures 33-4 and 33-10, is shown in Figure 33-11.

The ubiquity of the critical band and its correlate *effective level* (*Z*) was shown most clearly by Hawkins and Stevens [5] when they plotted amount of masking as a function of effective level. On such a plot the results for all frequencies lay along the same straight line, whose slope was 1. We have used the same coordinates (*M vs Z*) in Figure 33-11, combining comparable data from Figures 33-4 and 33-10. Masking is the difference between the masked and the quiet thresholds.

Effective level was obtained by adding the critical band width for each frequency plotted to the noise level per cycle *at that frequency*, as read from the curve (noise spectrum) of Figure 33-4. Five frequencies were chosen for this display, representing a frequency in the center of the band (1200), one an octave below the upper cutoff (700), one an octave above the lower cutoff (2000), and the last two far below and above the band (300 and 3500 cps), but still showing reliable threshold measures. The different symbol shapes are associated with the different frequencies. Symbols that are half-filled are taken from Figure 33-4, representing monaural thresholds at 40, 60, 80, and 100 db SPL from the main experiment. Open symbols represent the binaural results, while filled symbols represent the monaural results of follow-up experiment (five different listeners) on this band in which the band level was increased in 10-db steps from 70 to 120 db.

Clearly, the results for 700 and 1200 cps show a linear relation and fit very well the straight line drawn. This line was not drawn to fit the points but is rather a theoretical line with a slope of 1, passing through a point at which the effective level equals the masked threshold. The critical-band theory of masking would predict this fit for 1200 cps, and it is interesting to note that it also fits 700 cps, a frequency slightly below the noise band.

It is apparently coincidental that the results for 300 and for 3500 cps can be fitted by the same curve. The important observation is that this curve lies well above the straight line and indicates, therefore, that masking can occur when the effective level of the noise (entering the ear) is well below the level of the tone being masked. We do not believe that this coincidence indicates similar processes above and below the band. It should be noted that the masking above the band continues to decrease as the test frequency is raised; but the "remote" masking remains constant throughout the range of frequencies tested below the band. Our knowledge of the results for 3500 cps led us to draw a separate curve for 2000 cps, rather than to consider these data as errors or random deviations from the straight line. The results for 2000 cps apparently represent an intermediate condition between the strict critical-band data that hold for 1200 cps and those that involve some kind of distortion, as in the case of 3500 cps.

DISCUSSION AND CONCLUSIONS

There appear to be at least three groups of phenomena to be discussed; those above, those below, and those within the band of frequencies that constitute a masking noise.

If we restrict our discussion to the masking of frequencies that lie within or very near the noise band, the critical-band notion seems verified with respect to actual values reported in the literature and the implied linear relation between masking and the level of the noise.

Wegel and Lane showed long ago that low frequencies could mask high frequencies and this effect is also shown here for frequencies that lie above the band. It seems difficult and unfruitful, however, to think of the cause of such masking as simple harmonic distortion, produced by a kind of built-in peak-clipper, for these effects are already clear at moderate levels and involve many frequencies between the "fundamentals" in the band itself and a group of second harmonics. It may be that such masking has a source similar to that for the low-frequency masking (see following).

The major experimental findings, so far as new knowledge is concerned, have to do with frequencies that lie below the band of noise. Here we see that the masked thresholds follow the frequency characteristic of the noise extremely well and predictably (from critical band values), but do so only so far. How far seems independent of the particular frequencies involved, and thus we are dealing with a mechanism that is not necessarily confined to a certain range of frequencies. Rather, whatever invariance there is appears to have more to do with the difference in db between the maximum and minimum masking or, in other words, a maximum rejection

of between 40 and 50 db. So long as the quiet thresholds are only about 50 db lower than the maximum masked thresholds in the band, no low-frequency masking is seen. But the ear does not seem to be able to maintain a larger difference.

Whatever the mechanism involved, these findings seem to limit the generality of the critical-band as descriptive of auditory masking to either wide-band noise or, in the case of narrow bands, to frequencies that lie within or slightly below (within one octave) the band. It may be that the ear itself is introducing extraneous noise, outside of the specified band limits, but this is irrelevant since predictions of masking, based on the critical band, have to do with measurements of noise before it reaches the ear.

We cannot refrain from one attempt to account for this "remote" masking.[14] The envelope of a band of noise shows irregular changes which are random both in amplitude and in time, for the frequencies within the band. So long as such noise feeds a linear circuit, the output will contain only those frequencies that are in the band. If the level is sufficiently high so that, for example, rectification and thus detection occur, then the randomness of the envelope itself will be detected and we could observe frequencies other than those in the band.

This tentative hypothesis will serve as the basis for further study. It has promise but suffers from at least one serious difficulty. If the resulting detected signal had a spectrum even so broad as a white noise, one would expect constant masked thresholds throughout the frequency range,[5] but not constant masking. This consideration leads us to prefer a second interpretation, much less precise, that involves the possibility that a certain level of stimulation, without regard to the position of the center of its activity in the frequency domain, is sufficient to render a certain portion of the auditory system in-

[14] This explanatory suggestion resulted from discussions with members of the Physiology Laboratory of our Research Department, particularly Dr. Deatherage, Dr. Davis, and Dr. Eldredge.

capable of further response. Relevant physiological data may determine whether or not this view can be either accepted or rejected.*

[* The phenomenon of *remote masking* that was originally described in this paper was subsequently elaborated and explained in the following series of papers: "Physiological evidence for the masking of low frequencies by high," *J. Acoust. Soc. Am.* **29,** 132–137 (1957) by B. H. Deatherage, H. Davis, D. H. Eldredge; "Remote masking in selected frequency regions," *J. Acoust. Soc. Am.,* **29,** 512–514 (1957) by B. H. Deatherage, R. C. Bilger, D. H. Eldredge; "Intensive determinants of remote masking," *J. Acoust. Soc. Am.,* **30,** 817–824 (1958) by R. C. Bilger; "Binaural effects in remote masking," *J. Acoust. Soc. Am.,* **30,** 827–832 (1958) by I. J. Hirsh and M. Burgeat; "Additivity of different types of masking," *J. Acoust. Soc. Am.,* **31,** 1107–1109 (1959) by R. C. Bilger; and "Remote masking in the absence of intra-aural muscles," *J. Acoust. Soc. Am.,* **39,** 103–108 (1966) by R. C. Bilger. RCB, IJH]

34

Changes in Bone–Conduction Thresholds Produced by Masking in the Non–Test Ear

DONALD D. DIRKS
CAROLYN W. MALMQUIST

DONALD D. DIRKS, Ph.D., is Associate Professor of Surgery, Head and Neck Division, Center for Health Sciences, University of California, Los Angeles
CAROLYN W. MALMQUIST is Research Audiologist, School of Medicine, University of California, Los Angeles

Wegel and Lane (1924) were among the first investigators to report changes in threshold on the test ear when a masking tone was delivered simultaneously to the non-test ear at low-intensity levels. Since this early observation, other investigators (Zwislocki, 1953; Ingham, 1957; Sherrick and Mangabeira-Albernaz, 1961; Treisman, 1963) have also reported shifts in threshold due to masking in the contralateral ear. Usually the effect is referred to as "central masking" and implies that the changes in threshold are mediated through a central nervous system mechanism. Obviously, such shifts in threshold should not be confused with those resulting from the introduction of a masking sound in the same ear as the test tone or from the influence of cross masking, both of which produce peripheral masking.

Although some experimenters (Palva, 1954; Naunton, 1957; Liden, Nilsson, and Anderson, 1959) have noted the effects of central masking on bone-conduction measurements, most investigators have been concerned with changes in air conduction. Two recent exceptions, however, were the experiments by Studebaker (1962) and by one of the present investigators (Dirks, 1964). In the former study, shifts in

Reprinted by permission of the authors from *J. Speech Hearing Res.*, **7**, pp. 271–278 (1964).

threshold from measurements at the frontal bone were described as the masking level was increased in the non-test ear. The author observed larger shifts in the bone-conduction thresholds as a result of central factors than were previously reported for air-conducted tones by Wegel and Lane (1924). In the investigation by Dirks (1964), bone-conduction threshold sensitivity via the mastoid process decreased by 4 to 5 dB when wide or narrow bands of noise were presented to the non-test ear via an insert receiver at an effective level (Z) of 30 dB. Comparable thresholds measured at the frontal bone shifted by 7 to 8 dB.

There was no reason to assume that central masking factors would be greater when measurements were made from the test ear via frontal bone conduction than those obtained with the vibrator at the mastoid process. But the larger changes in the frontal bone-conduction thresholds were an impressive result since they occurred at five test frequencies, under two masking conditions (broad and narrow band masking) and with each of two different bone vibrators. An explanation by Studebaker (1962) and later by one of the present authors (Dirks, 1964) suggested that the unmasked thresholds via the frontal bone represented equal stimulation of each ear and were thus binaural. When adequate masking was presented to the non-test ear, however, the bone-conduction threshold was monaural. In other words, the shifts in the frontal bone threshold due to masking in the non-test ear were the result of central factors plus the loss induced by changing from binaural to monaural stimulation.

It was proposed in the latter study (Dirks, 1964) that the contribution of the non-test ear to the mastoid bone-conduction threshold in the quiet unoccluded condition was ordinarily less than the contribution of the non-test ear under the comparable frontal bone condition. If this proposition were true, the effect of masking the non-test ear would alter the threshold, obtained with the vibrator on the opposite mastoid process, due primarily to central masking factors. Therefore, it would be anticipated that a comparably greater change would take place when masking the non-test ear for measurements via the frontal bone than for those at the mastoid process. The investigation of the above theory provided the primary impetus for the present study.

Our investigation was accomplished by two experiments. In the first experiment, the changes in air-conduction and bone-conduction (mastoid and frontal bone placement) thresholds on the test ear were compared as various levels of noise were delivered to the non-test ear. In the second investigation, an attempt was made to evaluate the aforementioned hypothesis which was offered in explanation for the greater shifts in the threshold when testing from the frontal bone.

EXPERIMENT I

Subjects

Ten normal hearing subjects were used in this investigation. The mean age of the subjects was 23 years with a range in age from 18 years to 35 years. The 10 subjects selected included two males and eight females. A normal test ear in this experiment was

defined by the ability to pass a pure-tone audiometric screening test at a hearing level of 10 dB at the experimental frequencies of 500, 1 000, and 4 000 cps.

Apparatus

All experimental data were collected by use of a Bekesy-type automatic audiometer (Grason-Stadler, Model E800). For air conduction stimulation, the output of this audiometer was terminated in a TDH-39 earphone which was mounted in an MX41/AR cushion. The same automatic audiometer was employed as the source for the bone-conduction stimuli. For this presentation, the output was fed to a Radioear B-70A hearing-aid type vibrator fixed on the head with a conventional headband. For both air and bone-conduction thresholds, pulsed tones were used. The interruption rate for the pulsed tone was 2.5 ips with a rise-decay time of 25 msec, and the rate of attenuation change was 2.5 dB per sec. The acoustic output of the pure-tone channel as developed in a 6 cc coupler Bruel and Kjaer DB (0160) was calibrated before the experiment and weekly during the testing session. No systematic variations in the output were observed during the experimental period.

The source for the noise channel was a thermal noise generator (Grason-Stadler, Model E5539A). The output of the generator was passed through a resistive network which fed a variable filter system (Allison, Model 25). From the filter system, the noise signal was delivered to a speech audiometer (Grason-Stadler, Model 162) and terminated in an insert receiver (Beyer, type DT 507). The speech audiometer was employed here as an attenuation system. A standard interrupter switch was inserted between the thermal noise generator and the filter system for ease in threshold testing.

One of three narrow bands of thermal noise was used in the present experiment. The dials on the filter system were selected to insure a series of bands which more than encompassed the critical band widths around the test frequencies of 500, 1 000, and 4 000 cps. Specifically, the resultant bands of noise around the center frequencies of 500 and 1 000 cps were 300 cps wide, while the band width around 4 000 cps was 350 cps. The rejection rate of the filter unit was 30 dB per octave according to the manufacturer's specifications. The over-all acoustic output of each experimental noise band as developed in a 2 cc coupler (Bruel and Kjaer, type DB 0135) was measured weekly. Daily calibration checks were performed by recording the voltage developed at the terminals of the DT 507 receiver.

All the data for this investigation were collected with the subject seated in a double-walled audiometric booth. The test equipment was housed in a room adjacent to the audiometric booth.

Procedure

Each subject was tested during three experimental sessions. In one session, air-conduction thresholds at each experimental frequency were obtained in quiet and then with the appropriate narrow band of thermal noise in the non-test ear. At any test frequency, the earphones were not removed until the thresholds in quiet and at each experimental noise level were measured.

In the remaining two experimental sessions, bone-conduction thresholds were measured. During one session, the vibrator was located at the frontal bone; during the other session the vibrator was placed on the mastoid process. Initially, bone-conduction thresholds were obtained in quiet with both ears unoccluded. Then the insert receiver was fitted to the non-test ear, and bone thresholds were measured as the experimental masking level increased. Once the bone vibrator was affixed to the skull, it was not removed until the measurements at any test frequency were completed. The order of successive test sessions was randomly varied for each subject.

Thresholds also were obtained in quiet with the non-test ear occluded by the insert receiver. These thresholds were not reported

since they reflected responses from the occluded non-test ear. In this study, our interest was focused on the shifts in threshold from the quiet unoccluded condition.

However, as a supplementary measure, the subjects were asked to localize the test tone after each threshold tracing. In the quiet occluded condition, the tone was localized to the non-test ear, but as the level of the masking noise increased above a sensation level of 20 dB, all subjects reported that the tone was heard on the test side.

Most subjects employed in the present experiment had had previous experience in tracing their thresholds via Bekesy audiometry. In the few cases where the task was unfamiliar, the subjects were given thorough practice sessions.

For the masking conditions, the narrow band of noise which encompassed the particular pure-tone stimulus was always presented to the non-test ear. A threshold of audibility for the appropriate band of noise was established in two dB steps by the method of limits. Bone-conduction thresholds were measured on the test ear with the noise signal presented to the non-test ear at levels of 20, 40, 60, and 80 dB above the threshold for the particular band of noise. At each noise level the subject traced his or her threshold pattern for the pure-tone signal for a 40-sec period. The midpoints between the peaks and troughs of the excursions were considered to be the thresholds. Rest periods of one to two minutes were interspersed between the presentation of each noise signal.

Results and Discussion

Table 34-1 summarizes the mean shifts in air and bone-conduction thresholds which occurred as one of the three experimental bands of noise was presented to the non-test ear. The same results are shown in graphic form in Figure 34-1 for the changes in threshold at 500 cps, in Figure 34-2 for 1 000 cps, and in Figure 34-3 for 4 000 cps.

The functions which appear in Figures

TABLE 34-1. MEAN THRESHOLD SHIFT FOR AIR AND BONE-CONDUCTION STIMULI PRODUCED WITH NARROW-BAND
NOISE IN THE CONTRALATERAL EAR

	Frequency (cps)/Test Condition								
	500			1 000			4 000		
Sensation Level		B.C.			B.C.			B.C.	
of Noise (dB)	A.C.	Mastoid	Frontal	A.C.	Mastoid	Frontal	A.C.	Mastoid	Frontal
20	.2 *	.5	−1.4	1.2	.9	.9	.6	.6	1.8
40	1.8	2.9	5.8	3.0	4.5	7.1	2.2	1.6	3.6
60	3.6	5.0	8.1	4.5	5.9	9.0	3.1	2.1	4.6
80	7.2	7.8	10.9	8.8	10.6	14.1	6.2	7.3	10.5

* Threshold shift = threshold with masking − threshold in quiet.

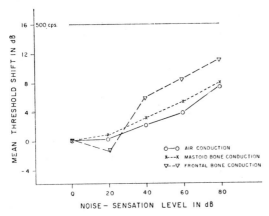

Figure 34-1. Mean threshold shift of a 500 cps tone for air- and bone-conduction stimuli produced with narrow-band noise in the contralateral ear.

34-1, 2 and 3 demonstrate three noteworthy features. First, as the level of the noise in the non-test ear increases, there is a small but gradual shift in the threshold of the test ear. This result is in good agreement with the observations by Studebaker (1962) for measurements at the frontal bone. Second, comparable changes were observed for air-conduction and bone-conduction thresholds when the latter were measured with the vibrator positioned on the mastoid process. Third, shifts from frontal bone measurements were greater than corresponding air or bone-conduction thresholds via the mastoid process. The last finding, of course, supports earlier reported observations (Dirks, 1964).

In Figures 34-1 and 34-2, it should be noted that at a sensation level of 20 dB, shifts in

the thresholds at 500 and 1 000 cps from frontal bone stimulation were either less than or equal to the changes in threshold for air and bone conduction at the mastoid process. The similarity of the changes in threshold was probably due to the fact that the occlusion effect caused by the insert receiver in the non-test ear was not overcome completely at the 20 dB sensation level. In this instance, some thresholds were responses from the occluded non-test ear and, thus, introduced a contaminating factor in the results at this low masking level. When the masker was delivered to the non-test ear at a sensation level of 40 dB or more, the responses were from the test ear.

At each sensation level and for the fre-

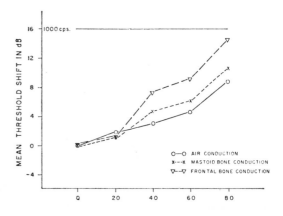

Figure 34-2. Mean threshold shift of a 1 000 cps tone for air- and bone-conduction stimuli produced with narrow-band noise in the contralateral ear.

quencies tested, standard deviations were computed. They ranged from .5 to 2.3 dB for the air-conduction thresholds, from 1.5 to 5.6 dB for the bone-conduction thresholds at the mastoid process, and from 1.2 to 4.8 dB for the bone-conduction thresholds at the frontal bone. In general, the standard deviations for bone conduction at any experimental noise sensation level were slightly larger than comparable standard deviations for air-conduction thresholds.

The present results are in agreement with the previous observations (1964) that greater shifts occur from frontal bone measurements than from comparable air or bone-conduction responses at the mastoid as masking is presented to the non-test ear. Thus, the proposition suggested earlier as an explanation for this phenomenon was now investigated in detail.

EXPERIMENT II

This experiment was designed to investigate the above proposition that the additional shifts in the frontal bone thresholds resulted because of the change from a binaural threshold in quiet to a monaural threshold in the masking condition.

Six of the subjects who were employed in the previous experiment were used in this investigation. The equipment employed was identical to that used in Experiment I.

Procedure

On the assumption that the original proposition was correct, it was reasoned that if the responses to bone-conduction stimulation at the frontal bone became monaural in the quiet condition, the shifts due to central masking would be similar to those resulting from air or bone conduction via the mastoid process. Thus, the test ear of each subject was plugged with commercially available wax-impregnated cotton (Flent Anti-Noise Stopple). For the experimental subjects, the

earplug induced an average loss by air conduction of 17 dB at 500 cps, but an average increase in sensitivity of 15 dB by bone conduction via the frontal bone.

During the test session, air-conduction thresholds were measured in quiet with the earphone fitted over the earplug. Bone-conduction thresholds were obtained in quiet with the test ear plugged. In the quiet condition, thresholds by air or bone conduction via the mastoid process or frontal bone were responses from the plugged test ear only since the non-test ear remained open. Additional thresholds were traced while a

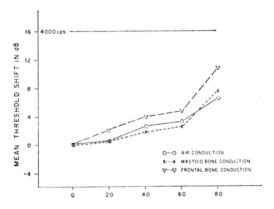

Figure 34-3. Mean threshold shift of a 4 000 cps tone for air- and bone-conduction stimuli produced with narrow-band noise in the contralateral ear.

narrow-band noise, encompassing the frequencies around 500 cps, was delivered to the non-test ear at levels of 40, 60, and 80 dB above the threshold for the noise. Shifts in these monaural thresholds due to the contralateral masker were measured with the insert receiver in the non-test ear as in the first experiment.

Results

The results of the experiment are shown graphically in **Figure 34-4.**

The significant result was the almost identical shifts in threshold which occurred for the three types of experimental stimulation. These shifts in the test-ear thresholds were considered to be essentially the result of central masking factors and no longer influenced by the possibility of changing from binaural to monaural stimulation. Thus, the present data supported the original proposition.

Consider also the threshold shifts for the bone-conducted stimuli in Figure 34-4 with the comparable changes in bone thresholds at 500 cps from Figure 34-1. It was found that the changes in threshold with the vibrator placed on the mastoid were similar in both experiments, but decreased shifts were obtained for frontal bone measurements at all

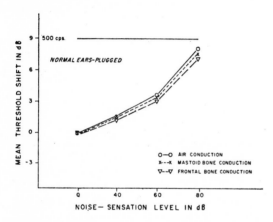

Figure 34-4. Mean threshold shift of a 500 cps tone for air- and bone-conduction stimuli produced with narrow-band noise in the contralateral ear (test ear occluded).

masking levels in the second experiment. This result also demonstrated that the shifts in the frontal bone threshold, reported in Figure 34-4, were due to central masking factors and were not affected by changes from binaural to monaural stimulation as in Figure 34-1.

The data from these experiments would indicate that on normal listeners with ears unoccluded there is less contribution to a binaural threshold in quiet when measurements are made from the mastoid process than from the frontal bone. The authors wish

to emphasize that this attenuation factor, when present, is small and, therefore, does not negate the principle that masking the non-test ear is essential for accurate bone-conduction measurements.

SUMMARY

Two experiments concerning the effects of central masking are reported.[1] In Experiment I, 10 subjects with normal hearing were tested by air and bone-conduction stimuli via the mastoid process and frontal bone as various levels of narrow-band noise were presented to the contralateral ear. For the experimental frequencies of 500, 1 000, and 4 000 cps, small increases in threshold shift were observed as the intensity level of the noise was increased. The changes for air-conduction and bone-conduction thresholds at the mastoid process were similar, but the shifts in threshold via frontal bone conduction were always greater than comparable mastoid measurements. It was suggested that the additional shift in threshold observed for frontal bone measurements was the result of changing from binaural stimulation in quiet to monaural stimulation during the masking condition.

The above proposition was tested in Experiment II. The test ears of six subjects were plugged, and tests were made at 500 cps as in Experiment I. Thus, the bone-conduction sensitivity in quiet was increased, and the contribution to the threshold from the opposite ear was eliminated. When noise was presented to the non-test ear, the threshold shifts by air conduction and by bone conduction from either vibrator placement were found to be similar. Thus, the results supported the proposition that the additional threshold shifts from the frontal bone, noted in Experiment I, were essentially explained by the changes from binaural stimulation in quiet to monaural stimulation when masking.

[1] This research was supported by USPHS Grant NB-04019.

REFERENCES

Dirks, D., Bone conduction measurements. *Arch. Otolaryng.*, **79,** 594–599 (1964).

Ingham, J. G., The effect upon monaural sensitivity of continuous stimulation of the opposite ear. *Q. J. exp. Psychol.*, **9,** 52–60 (1957).

Liden, G., Nilsson, G., and Anderson, H., Narrow band masking with white noise. *Acta Otolaryng.*, **50,** 116–124 (1959).

Naunton, R. F., Clinical bone conduction audiometry. *Arch. Otolaryng.*, **66,** 281–298 (1957).

Palva, T., Masking in audiometry. *Acta Otolaryng.*, suppl. 118, 156–172 (1954).

Sherrick, C. E., and Mangabeira-Albernaz., P. L., Auditory threshold shifts produced by simultaneously pulsed contralateral stimuli. *J. acoust. Soc. Amer.*, **33,** 1381–1385 (1961).

Studebaker, G. A., On masking in bone conduction testing. *J. Speech Hearing Res.*, **5,** 215–227 (1962).

Treisman, M., Auditory unmasking. *J. acoust. Soc. Amer.*, **35,** 1256–1263 (1963).

Wegel, R. L., and Lane, C. E., The auditory masking on one pure tone by another and its probable relation to the dynamics of the inner ear. *Phys. Rev.*, **23,** 266–285 (1924).

Zwislocki, J., Acoustic attenuation between the ears. *J. acoust. Soc. Amer.*, **25,** 752–759 (1953).

35

Interaural Attenuation and Cross–Hearing in Air–Conduction Audiometry

JOSEPH B. CHAIKLIN

JOSEPH B. CHAIKLIN, Ph.D., is Professor of Audiology, University of Minnesota

DEFINITION OF TERMS

A frequent problem in air-conduction audiometry is the undesired transfer of intense stimuli from one ear to the other. As the stimuli cross the head they are attenuated (i.e. weakened), hence the term "interaural attenuation" (IA) has been used to refer to reduction of a signal's intensity as it passes between ears by one means or another. For example, a 60 db (SPL) 1000 cps tone presented to one ear may be subjected to 55 db IA before it reaches the other ear as a 5-db (SPL) signal and will stimulate hearing there only if the cochlea receiving it is sensitive to 5-db signals. When IA is increased, a stronger signal is required to reach the opposite ear; when IA is decreased, a weaker signal is required.

A term sometimes confused with IA is "interaural threshold difference" (often "interaural difference") which refers to threshold differences between ears at the same frequency. "Cross-hearing," "transcranial hearing" and "shadow hearing" are terms used to describe sensation resulting from stimuli crossing the head during air-conduction audiometry. A shadow curve is an air-conduction threshold curve that results from cross-hearing.

Reprinted by permission of the author from *J. aud. Res.*, **7**, pp. 413–424 (1967).

EXPLANATIONS FOR CROSS-HEARING

There has been considerable interest in identifying the route or routes signals follow in cross-hearing. According to Békésy (1948) the bow of the earphone headset does not appear to be a significant route, at least for dynamic earphones in rubber cushions. Békésy concluded that around-the-head (air-conduction) leakage is the primary cross-hearing mechanism in air-conduction audiometry, but most authors appear to favor a through-the-head (bone-conduction) explanation (Feldman, 1963; Fletcher, 1953; Littler, Knight, and Strange, 1952; Sparrevohn, 1946; Studebaker, 1962; Wegel and Lane, 1924; Zwislocki, 1953).

Feldman (1963) found that when unilaterally deaf subjects had both ears covered with TDH-39 phones in MX-41/AR cushions, they evidenced 5- to 15 db less mean IA at 125, 250 and 500 cps and approximately 1 db less at 1000 cps (personal communication) than they did when the better ear was open. If cross-hearing had been by air conduction in this range, signals leaking around the head should have been attenuated further by the phone over the better ear and thus IA should have increased rather than decreased. Feldman attributed this reduction of low-frequency IA to the occlusion effect's apparent enhancement of sensitivity for low-frequency stimuli crossing the head by bone conduction (Goldstein and Hayes, 1965; Naunton, 1957). On the other hand, he found approximately 9 db increased IA at 4000 cps (the only other frequency sampled) in the covered state, a finding he attributed to the phone blocking air-conduction leakage around the head.

NORMATIVE DATA

Interaural attenuation norms are important in evaluating the need for masking in air-conduction audiometry, in estimating maximum permissible masking levels for air- and bone-conduction audiometry and in evaluating test validity.

Previous literature reflects sizeable differences among IA estimates at specific frequencies. For example, Sparrevohn's (1946) report of 57 db IA at 8000 cps contrasts sharply with Zwislocki's (1953) mean value of 74 db reported in his Figures 3–6.

A variety of factors may account for some of the differences referred to above, but earphone and external canal variables are among the most prominent. For example, IA can be increased by using insert phones (Feldman, 1963; Studebaker, 1962) or by deep plugging of the external canal of the nontest ear (Zwislocki, 1953). It can be increased, also, by decreasing the size of the stimulus phone, thus reducing the area of the head stimulated (Feldman, 1963; Studebaker, 1962; Zwislocki, 1953), by increasing the volume of air under the nontest earphone, and, perhaps, by plugging the ear canal of the test ear (Tschiassny, 1952).

Measurement method and subject selection may account for some interstudy differences. For example, Zwislocki (1953) had normal-hearing listeners judge when a strong signal presented to one ear reduced the loudness of a weak signal presented 180° out of phase to the other ear. He found generally higher IA than Miller (1959) and Feldman (1963) found for monaurally deaf patients. Possibly a major source of these normative differences

is inherent intersubject variability (Sparre-vohn, 1946).

Previous reports on IA have usually been limited to relatively few points in the audiometric range and often have failed to describe measurement procedures adequately. The purposes of the present study were to extend previous data by sampling IA under two conditions at all octave and inter-octave points available on the typical clinical audiometer and to relate the findings to clinical considerations.

METHOD

Subjects

Subjects were three female and two male college students with total unilateral deafness. Their ages ranged from 18 to 23 years, with a mean of 19 years. Four had hearing sensitivity in the better ear within ±5 db of zero HL (ISO 1964) for most of the audiometric range and one had a 30 to 40 db loss above 3000 cps. Mumps in early childhood was the probable etiology for four subjects and etiology was unknown for the other. Otoscopic examination and history for each subject's better ear were negative. Pure-tone Stenger results were negative. Hearing in the poorer ear was ruled out with white noise masknig.

General Plan

After conventional pure-tone audiometry, history and otoscopy each subject was scheduled for two additional test sessions (five to ten days apart) consisting of two sets of threshold measurement for each ear at the 11 audiometric frequencies from 125 cps through 8000 cps. Thresholds were measured with Békésy procedure under two conditions: first, with both ears covered by TDH-39 earphones in MX-41/AR cushions, and second, with both ears covered as in the first condition, but with an individually-made medium-soft plug extending into the bony external meatus of the better ear. The plug produced 40 to 50 db attenuation for most air-conduction signals delivered to the better ear and also reduced the occlusion effect to negligible values by occupying most of the external canal. Interaural attenuation values with the plug in place may be considered roughly analogous to values obtained with some conductively impaired patients (those without an occlusion effect). Data for the "phones only" condition may be viewed as representative of results obtained with mild sensory-neural impairment of normal hearing.

In each condition (plug *vs* no plug) the better ear was tested first. The following order was used for each set of threshold measurements for each condition: 125 cps, 250 cps, 500 cps, 750 cps, 1000 cps, 1500 cps, 2000 cps, 3000 cps, 4000 cps, 6000 cps, 8000 cps, 125 cps, 250 cps, 500 cps and 1000 cps. Both sessions started with practice tracking, first at 1000 cps for one minute and then at 500 cps for one minute.

Stimuli were 250-msec tone pulses with 20-msec rise-decay time, separated by 250-msec silent intervals, and delivered for 30 seconds at each frequency at an attenuation rate of 4 db per second. Threshold was defined as the mean of the pen excursion midpoints.

Apparatus

The system used to measure thresholds consisted of the following components in sequence: Hewlett-Packard 201 CR audio oscillator, Grason-Stadler 829C Electronic Switch, Grason-Stadler E 3262A Recording Attenuator, MacIntosh MC 30 amplifier, Hewlett-Packard 350-B Step Attenuator, Telephonics TDH-39 earphones in MX-41/AR cushions and a Grason-Stadler subject switch with which subjects controlled stimulus intensity. Impedance-matching transformers were used when necessary. Subjects were seated in an Industrial Acoustics Company 1202-A test booth. The experimenter and equipment were located outside the booth. During test conditions the booth had a sound level of 23 db on the A-Scale and 48 db on the C-Scale of a Bruel and Kjaer 2203 Sound Level meter. The input to the earphones was

monitored with a Ballantine 300B vacuumtube voltmeter. Earphone output was checked periodically with a Bruel and Kjaer Model 158 audiometer calibration unit with a NBS type 9A coupler.

RESULTS

The data reported below are from the second test session. The first session served to accustom subjects to the experimental task and to reduce practice effects in the second session.

Table 35-1 summarizes mean thresholds (rounded to the nearest 1-db interval) for each ear with and without the plug in the better ear, differences between means for each condition, and dispersion data. Figure 35-1 shows mean threshold data for each condition plotted in SPL re 0.0002 microbar. Mean IA for each condition can be visualized in Figure 35-1 by noting the differences between plotted points for the better and poorer ears. Similarly, differences between the plugged and phones only conditions can be observed by comparing mean points for the two poorer ear curves. Means above 300 cps do not include data from the subject who had elevated thresholds above 3000 cps. An inspection of Table 35-1 and Figure 35-1 reveals that mean IA varied with frequency and test conditions.

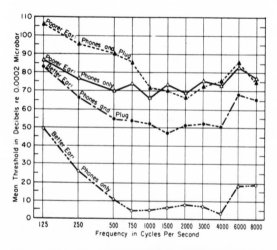

Figure 35-1. Mean thresholds in SPL for each ear with phones only and with phones plus plug in better ear. N = 5 through 3000 cps; N = 4 above 3000 cps.

TABLE 35-1. MEAN THRESHOLDS (RE 0.0002 μBAR) FOR EACH EAR WITH PHONES ONLY AND WITH PHONES PLUS PLUG IN BETTER EAR, AND COMPARISON OF INTERAURAL ATTENUATION (IA) WITH AND WITHOUT PLUG (ALL VALUES ROUNDED TO CLOSEST I-DB INTERVAL). N = 5 THROUGH 3 KC/S; N = 4 ABOVE 3 KC/S

	Frequency (kc/s)										
	.125	.25	.5	.75	1	1.5	2	3	4	6	8
Phones Only											
Deaf Ear Means	87	77	70	74	66	73	69	75	73	83	76
Better Ear Means	49	26	11	5	5	6	8	7	3	18	19
Phones plus Plug in Better Ear											
Deaf Ear Means	106	95	90	85	71	70	67	73	75	85	75
Better Ear Means	83	66	55	54	52	47	51	52	50	68	65
Attenuation Means and Extremes											
IA, Phones Only	38	51	59	69	61	67	61	68	70	65	57
Most IA	45	58	65	71	66	76	72	72	85	76	69
Least IA	32	44	54	62	57	45	55	56	61	56	51
Change in IA with Plug in											
Better Ear	19	18	20	11	5	−3	−2	−2	2	2	−1
Most IA Change	33	31	36	16	14	−7	−4	−14	14	14	−11
Least IA Change	6	10	11	7	3	2	−1	−1	−1	−1	0
IA with Plug in Better Ear	57	69	79	80	66	64	59	66	73	67	56
Most IA	65	75	93	85	79	77	68	81	81	77	59
Least IA	51	66	65	76	56	38	54	54	60	65	52
Attenuation of Plug	34	40	44	49	47	41	43	45	47	50	46
Most Attenuation	37	48	49	54	51	60	48	53	50	63	57
Least Attenuation	29	33	41	46	40	32	38	34	44	38	37

IA with Phones Only

When the ears were covered only with phones mean IA ranged from 38 db at 125 cps to 70 db at 4000 cps; 8 of the 11 means were greater than 58 db. Table 35-1 shows that differences among subjects were greater above 1000 cps for this condition, with the largest difference (31 db) at 1500 cps. The largest differences were well distributed among subjects.

IA with Plug in Better Ear

With the solid plug in the better ear and both ears covered with phones, mean IA increased substantially below 1500 cps; that is, stronger signals had to be applied to the deaf ear to elicit responses in the normal ear. The largest mean increases (18 to 20 db) were at 125 cps, 250 cps, and 500 cps and were probably related to reduction of the occlusion effect present when the better ear was covered only with a phone (Feldman, 1963).

There was a trend toward decreased IA (hence lower cross-hearing levels) above 1000 cps in the plugged condition, but the mean decreases were small and there were large differences among subjects and frequencies, thus underscoring the variable effects of plugging the external canal. Zwislocki (1953) also observed instances of slightly decreased IA above 1000 cps when he plugged the bony external auditory meatus. The reason for these changes is not entirely clear but impedance alteration in the external meatus is a possible explanation.

Clinical Cross-hearing Levels

Figure 35-2 displays mean hearing levels (ISO 1964) for the "phones only" condition to illustrate average audiometric levels at which cross-hearing might occur when a patient's better ear thresholds are very close to Zero hearing level (HL) for most of the audiometric range. The mean HL at which cross-hearing occurred at most frequencies corresponds closely to the interaural differences and IA means. It should be kept in mind, however, that the primary clinical consideration in estimating the likelihood of cross-hearing is the difference between the better ear's best hearing (often bone-conduction thresholds) and the air-conduction level at the poorer ear (Studebaker, 1962). Thus, in a hearing level context, a 250 cps tone presented to a patient's poorer ear at 40 db (ISO 1964) may appear too weak to cause cross-hearing, but if the patient's better ear threshold is −10 db the interaural difference is 50 db, which is within the range of IA values shown in Table 35-1.

Knowledge of the average HLs at which cross-hearing occurs may be less useful clinically than knowledge of the lowest levels at which it occurs. Figure 35-2 contains a composite of the lowest ISO hearing levels at which cross-hearing occurred. Values ranged from 34 db at 125 cps to 60 db at 6000 cps. Figure 35-2 also shows a composite of the highest HLs at which cross-hearing occurred in the "phones only" condition. Values ranged from 47 db at 125 cps to 85 db at 4000 cps. Some of the apparent disparities between the highest and lowest HLs in Figure 35-2 can be understood by comparing the better- and poorer-ear thresholds of individual subjects represented in the composite. This comparison reveals that better-ear thresholds lower than the mean are frequently associated with the lowest poorer-ear levels and *vice versa*.

Attenuation of Plug

The mean attenuation of the ear plugs was 34 db at 125 cps and 40 to 50 db from 250 to 8000 cps. Plug attenuation was fairly homogeneous across subjects with only four deviations from the mean greater than 8 db. All deviations in excess of 8 db were at 6000 and 8000 cps.

Test-retest Agreement

All intrasession retests (125 cps to 1000 cps) for both conditions and both ears were well

within ±5 db of the first measurements. The number of retests that were lower than first tests was nearly equal to the number that were higher. Approximately 20 percent of the retests were identical (i.e. ±.5 db) to first tests. It should be recalled that all tests and retests were conducted with a single phone or plug placement, hence the data do not reflect variability that might result from placement and replacement.

DISCUSSION

Some clinical texts advise masking when the air-conduction interaural threshold difference at any frequency equals or exceeds a uniform criterion level (Newby, 1964; Saltzman, 1949). To the casual observer, this may suggest that IA is uniform at all frequencies, a notion not supported by the data reported above. Furthermore, when the better ear has a conductive component, interaural comparison of air-conduction thresholds is often not meaningful in evaluating IA. In these instances comparison must involve the bone-conduction thresholds of the better ear. If these limitations are kept in mind, however,

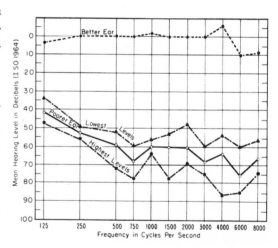

Figure 35-2. Mean thresholds for "phones only" condition plotted in hearing level (ISO 1964) and composites of lowest and highest hearing levels at which tones presented to the poorer ear were heard in the better ear. N = 5 through 3000 cps; N = 4 above 3000 cps.

a single estimate of IA might be useful as a rough guide to deciding when masking must be applied in air-conduction audiometry.

Although no single figure will predict IA at all frequencies for all patients, a single figure could define the lower limits of IA for most frequencies and most patients. An inspection of Table 35-1 reveals that in the 250 to 8000 cps range, the smallest IA values are 44 and 45 db, although most exceed 50 db. This suggests that 45 db may be a reasonable, if somewhat conservative, estimate of the minimum IA that occurs before cross-hearing begins in the 250 to 8000 cps range. At 125 cps, 35 db would be a safer estimate. While these estimates are conservative in terms of the present study's results as well as the results of most previous studies, it is highly probable that additional sampling will reveal patients with less IA than the smallest values reported above. On the other hand, data from this study and other studies suggest that IA usually exceeds the limits proposed above. Consequently, some clinicians may prefer a 50-db estimate for IA in the 250 to 8000 cps range. A 50-db estimate would probably result in error only at isolated frequencies and for relatively few patients.

The use of insert receivers to deliver test stimuli and masking signals has been advocated as a method for increasing IA of stimuli, by reducing the area of the head under the masking phone (Feldman, 1963; Hood, 1960; Studebaker, 1962). It is also possible that a deep insert in the nontest ear may increase IA by reducing the occlusion effect in normal ears or ears with sensory-neural loss. Insert receivers introduce a unique set of problems that have probably discouraged their widespread use. Wide individual variations in canal size, the need to clean the inserts between tests, frequency response limitations of the insert system, and calibration problems are some of the variables that have retarded general adoption of insert receivers.

There has been a tendency to consider the mechanism of cross-hearing in "either-or" terms—either sound crosses the head by air conduction or it crosses by bone conduction.

Clearly, strong air-conduction signals presented to one ear do get to the opposite ear by bone conduction, but they also get there by air conduction. The critical issue, therefore, is the order in which two types of transmission occur. For most of the audiometric range cross-hearing probably proceeds by bone conduction before it occurs by air-conduction, but under special conditions the reverse may be true, at least for a limited portion of the range. Recall, for example, that Feldman (1963) suggested that when the better ear is not covered, cross-hearing occurs at 4000 cps via air-conduction leakage before it occurs via bone-conduction. In the present study, however, above 750 cps mean cross-hearing values with the plug in the better ear were within a few decibels of values without the plug, which suggests that the same processes were probably operating in each condition. Since cross-hearing in the plugged condition was clearly via bone conduction it follows that the minimum levels for around-the-head transmission probably exceed the IA values reported in the present study.

In a recent personal communication Feldman suggested that his 4000 cps results were probably attributable to more intense radiation from the earphone case at 4000 cps than at the other frequencies sampled. Actual measurement of sound radiating from a TDH-39 phone confirms this speculation: There is approximately 20 db greater radiation at 4000 cps and closely adjacent frequencies than at other points usually sampled in audiometry. (Mr. Clayton Mullin of Maico Laboratories, Minneapolis, was kind enough to carry out the physical measurements necessary to clarify this issue.) Further confirmation was obtained by testing two unilaterally-deaf subjects as Feldman had done, first with the better ear covered, then open. Results similar to his were obtained at 4000 cps, but at 1500 cps, 2000 cps, 3000 cps, 6000 cps and 8000 cps there was essentially no difference between the covered and uncovered conditions.

Absolute IA values are a product of many

measurement variables, hence statements about absolute values must relate to specific measurement conditions and specific diagnostic categories. Minimum specifications should include measurement method, the status of both middle ear mechanisms, the status of both external canals, and the type of earphone and cushion used for each ear.

Similarly, changes in IA are relative to specific reference measurement conditions. For example, the fact that low-frequency IA is greater with an insert phone (or plug) in the nontest (better) ear than it is with a standard phone is attributable to the difference in measurement conditions: Low-frequency bone-conduction thresholds tend to be raised by the insert's reduction of the occlusion effect, therefore calculation of IA must relate to the better ear's elevated bone-conduction thresholds. Although hearing level at the poorer ear may appear to increase with the insert, absolute IA may not increase at all when the better ear's bone-conduction status is used to compute IA.

Future study of IA should be directed to expanding data on intersubject variability, particularly to discovering and investigating additional variables that may account for some of this variability. There may be merit, also, in studying the variability of IA in repeated test sessions to determine whether differences between subjects for various measurement conditions are stable differences or merely reflect random intersession variation.

SUMMARY

Interaural attenuation (IA) was investigated in 5 subjects with total monaural deafness. Air-conduction Békésy audiometry was performed at each ear at 11 audiometric frequencies under two conditions—first, with both ears covered by TDH-39 phones in MX-41/AR cushions, and second, with both ears covered as in the first condition but with a deep plug in the meatus of the better ear. Mean IA in the first condition ranged from 38 db at 125 cps to 70 db at 4000 cps; at frequencies below 1500 cps IA means in the plugged condition were 5–19 db higher than means without the plug. The increased IA in the lower frequencies probably was a function of the plugs' reduction of the occlusion effect. It was recommended that 45 db be used as a conservative clinical estimate of minimum IA in the 250–8000 cps range, and that 35 db be used as an estimate at 125 cps. Discussion emphasized variables that affect IA and the importance of specifying measurement conditions and methods.

ACKNOWLEDGMENT

This research was supported by a grant-in-aid from the Graduate School of the University of Minnesota.

REFERENCES

1. Békésy, G. v. Vibration of the head in a sound field and its role in hearing by bone conduction. *J. Acoust. Soc. Amer.*, 1948, 20, 749–760.

2. Feldman, A. S. Maximum air-conduction hearing loss. *J. Speech Hearing Res.*, 1963, 6, 157–163.

3. Fletcher, H. *Speech and Hearing in Communication.* Princeton: D. Van Nostrand, 1953, 157–159.

4. Goldstein, D. P. and Hayes, C. S. The occlusion effect in bone conduction hearing. *J. Speech Hearing Res.*, 1965, 8, 137–148.

5. Hood, J. D. The principles and practice of bone conduction audiometry: A review of the present position. *Laryngoscope*, 1960, 70, 1211–1228.

6. Littler, T. S., Knight, J. J. and Strange, P. H. Hearing by bone conduction and the use of bone-conduction hearing aids. *Proc. Royl. Soc. Med.*, 1952, 45, 783–790.

7. Miller, M. H. Transmission loss across the skull in a patient with known total monaural deafness. *Laryngoscope*, 1959, 69, 100–102.

8. Naunton, R. F. Clinical bone-conduction audiometry. *Arch. Otolaryngol.*, 1957, 66, 281–298.

9. Newby, H. A. *Audiology.* New York: Appleton-Century Crofts, 1964, pp. 98–99.

10. Saltzman, M. *Clinical Audiology.* New York: Grune & Stratton, 1949, p. 155.

11. Sparrevohn, U. R. Some audiometric investigations of monaurally deaf persons. *Acta Otolaryngol.*, 1946, 34, 1–10.

12. Studebaker, G. On masking in bone-conduction testing. *J. Speech Hearing Res.*, 1962, 5, 215–227.

13. Tschiassny, K. The mechanism of shadow hearing. *Arch. Otolaryngol.*, 1952, 55, 22–30.

14. Wegel, R. L. and Lane, C. E. The auditory masking of one pure tone by another and its probable relation to the dynamics of the inner ear. *Phys. Rev.*, 1924, 23, 266–285.

15. Zwislocki, J. Acoustic attenuation between the ears. *J. Acoust. Soc. Amer.*, 1953, 25, 752–759.

36

Clinical Masking of the Non-Test Ear

GERALD A. STUDEBAKER

GERALD A. STUDEBAKER, Ph.D., is Associate Professor, University of Oklahoma Medical Center

The application of a masking noise to the nontest ear is a daily clinical activity. Yet many audiologists know far less about masking procedures than about any other commonly used clinical technique. Clinical masking procedures often consist of unsystematic guesswork for which there is little or no logical defense.

Current texts (Davis and Silverman, 1961; Glorig, 1965; Jerger, 1963; Newby, 1964; O'Neill and Oyer, 1966; Sataloff, 1966) used in beginning and intermediate audiology classes imply by omission that little, or nothing, appears in the journals on the subject of clinical masking. The procedures given in these texts are often presented without reference and, in some instances, the procedures contradict available evidence. The bibliography at the end of this discussion is presented, in part, to illustrate that there is a substantial body of literature on, or closely related to, clinical masking. A review of these references reveals that there are, indeed, some areas of disagreement. However, on many important procedural aspects there is substantial consensus among those who have studied masking methods most thoroughly.

DEFINITIONS

Masking is best defined operationally as an elevation in the threshold of one signal

Reprinted by permission of the author from *J. Speech Hearing Dis.*, **32**, pp. 360–371 (1967).

produced by the introduction of a second signal. The first signal is called the maskee or the test signal and the second signal is called the masker. The level to which the threshold of test signal is shifted by the masker is the effective level of the masker. Effective level can be expressed in sound pressure level, hearing level, or any other level depending upon the reference above which the level of the test signal is expressed. The effective level of a masker at a given intensity level varies across different test signals. That is, a given noise intensity elevates the thresholds of various test signals to different intensity levels.

An efficient masker is one which produces a high effective level at a given intensity level. A given masker may be a more efficient masker of some test signals than others.

Minimum masking equals masker intensity minus effective level (effective level equals the level of a just masked test signal). When the masker is expressed in effective level, minimum masking equals 0 dB. Alternatively, minimum masking may be defined as the masking level which is just sufficient to mask the test signal in the ear to which the masker is presented.

Maximum masking is the masker level at the masked ear which is just insufficient to mask the test signal in the test ear. It is also equal to minimum masking plus interaural attenuation plus the test signal level at test ear cochlea.

Interaural attenuation is the reduction in the physical intensity of an acoustic signal in passing from a transducer on one side of the head to the opposite cochlea.

THE MASKING NOISE

It is generally agreed (Denes and Naunton, 1952; Hood, 1960; Liden, Nilsson, and Anderson, 1959a; Sanders and Rintelmann, 1964; Studebaker, 1962, 1964; Zwislocki, 1951) that narrow-band noises which center at the test signal frequency are the most efficient maskers of pure tones; that is, they produce a given effective level with the least intensity and, therefore, the least loudness. The use of narrow-band noises offers the further convenience that each band can be calibrated in effective level independently. Thus, the numerical masking dial reading equals the test signal intensity that will be just masked at all test tone frequencies.

Palva (1954, 1958) and Palva and Palva (1962) opposed the trend toward the use of narrow-band noises. However, his principal objection is that the gain in efficiency over broad-band noise is not sufficient to justify the additional cost and complexity of narrow-band noise generators. But, narrow-band noise generators have become relatively inexpensive and, in fact, simplify the clinical procedure by permitting the calibration of the noise in effective level for each test tone frequency.

Before clinical masking can begin, it is necessary to determine the minimum masking level for each masker and test signal combination used in the evaluation of patients. A satisfactory procedure is the following one. Introduce the masker and the test signal into the same ear by a single earphone. Each signal must be independently controlled by its own attenuator. With most two-channel clinical audiometers, this is accomplished with ease. The simple combining network shown in Figure 36-1 can be used with portable audiometers or independent noise sources. This network reduces the output of

the earphone by 8 or 9 dB. The reduction is equal for all frequencies and for both masker and test signal. The minimum masking levels obtained, therefore, are unaffected by the network.

The next step is to obtain the threshold of each test signal in the presence of various levels of the appropriate masker in the same ear. Six to 10 subjects with normal hearing

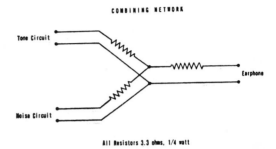

Figure 36-1. A combining network for the purpose of directing test signal and masker to the same earphone. A loss of 8 or 9 dB can be expected with this network.

or with known sensori-neural hearing loss may be used. Minimum masking for a particular test signal and masker combination is equal to the difference between noise level and test signal threshold in the presence of that noise, averaged across subjects and noise levels.

Figure 36-2 illustrates the relationship between masker level and test signal threshold when the test signal frequency is within the noise frequency band. This condition is highly desirable because a one to one relationship between noise level and test signal threshold is observed with this relationship. As Figure 36-2 shows, low levels of masker produce some threshold elevation. As the noise level is increased, the rate of threshold elevation increases until a given increment in noise level produces an equal increment in threshold. The difference between the two signals (minimum masking) then remains constant for all higher noise levels within the expected variability of all threshold measurements. In determining minimum masking levels, it is necessary to exclude the curvilinear portion of the curve from the calculation. Inclusion of these results produces an overestimation of masking efficiency.

Calibration of the noise source is essential when a broad-band noise is used. However, narrow-band noise generators calibrated in effective level should be similarly checked for accuracy since the clinician must assume the responsibility for the calibration of the equipment he uses.

WHEN TO MASK?

Virtually all audiology texts (Glorig, 1965, p. 117; Jerger, 1963, p. 251; Newby, 1964,

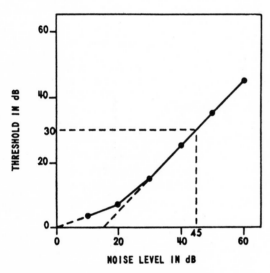

Figure 36-2. The relationship between masker level and test signal threshold when the test signal frequency is within the noise band. Minimum masking equals 15 dB in this example.

p. 76; O'Neill and Oyer, 1966, p. 64; Sataloff, 1966, p. 305) which discuss clinical procedures state or imply that during air-conduction testing masking should be applied to the opposite ear whenever the difference between ears exceeds a specified number of decibels, usually 40 or 50 dB. Hood (1960) also makes this statement. However, available research (Konig, 1962 a and b; Littler, Knight, and Strange, 1952; Luscher and Knnig, 1955; Naunton, 1960; Palva, 1954,

1958; 1962, 1964; Zwislocki, 1951, 1953) indicates that this rule is inadequate and can result in significant error.

It is impractical to discuss here whether air conduction or bone conduction is the pathway of least attenuation of an earphone-presented signal to the opposite cochlea of a normal listener (Zwislocki, 1953). However, when the opposite ear exhibits a conductive loss, there is little question that bone conduction is the pathway of least attenuation, because the conductive loss raises the attenuation in the air-conduction pathway around the head and into the opposite ear by the amount of the air-bone gap (Naunton, 1960; Studebaker, 1962, 1964). In clinical practice, the clinician must assume that an earphone-presented signal reaches the opposite cochlea by passing through the bones of the head. The air-conduction threshold of the opposite ear, therefore, is irrelevant to the determination of when to mask.

Either one of two rules may be applied in air-conduction testing. Palva (1954, 1958) and Palva and Palva (1962) proposed masking the opposite ear whenever the air-conduction presentation level exceeds the smallest expected interaural attenuation value (usually 40 dB). The application of this rule results in unnecessary masking at times but never results in failure to mask when required. A second acceptable rule (Studebaker, 1964) is to mask the opposite ear whenever the air-conduction presentation level at the test ear exceeds the bone-conduction threshold of the opposite ear by more than the smallest expected interaural attenuation value (usually 40 dB). Application of the first rule results in some unnecessary masking. The second occasionally requires a return to air-conduction testing after the completion of bone-conduction testing. However, use of either rule enables the clinician to avoid the errors which must result from the use of a simple comparison of air-conduction to air-conduction.

Both preceeding rules specify test-signal presentation level and not the apparent threshold of the tested ear. In threshold finding procedures, these two values will not differ greatly. However, in suprathreshold presentations it is apparent that the presentation level is the significant variable. For example, in speech discrimination testing, masking should be used whenever the *presentation level* is more than 40 dB above the bone-conduction threshold of the opposite ear (40 dB is used because average interaural attenuation for speech is about 50 dB). When speech is presented to the poorer ear at 40-dB SL, contralateral masking is almost always indicated. This is particularly true when the discrimination score of the tested ear is below that of the opposite (better) ear. Speech arriving at the opposite ear (at presentation level minus interaural attenuation) may be more intelligible than the speech arriving at the tested ear; or, the speech signal at the better ear may contribute enough to improve the apparent test ear discrimination score, even though the sensation level at the opposite ear is considerably less than that at the test ear.

Masking should be applied to the opposite ear during SISI testing on the poorer ear whenever the signal arrives at the nontest ear at a level of 25- to 30-dB HL or above; that is, a presentation at the test ear of about 70-dB HL or more. In tone-decay and Bekesy testing, the opposite ear should be masked when the presentation level is more than 40 dB above the opposite ear bone conduction threshold or, if following Palva's rule, whenever the presentation level is above 40-dB HL.

During bone-conduction testing, most investigators (Hood, 1960; Konig, 1962b; Liden, Nilsson, and Anderson, 1959b; Luscher, and Konig, 1955; Naunton, 1957; Palva, 1958; Sataloff, 1966; Studebaker, 1962, 1964; Zwislocki, 1951) agree that the decision when to mask must not depend upon the difference between the bone-conduction thresholds of the two ears. The very small interaural attenuation of vibrator-presented signals makes it impossible to use an interear comparison for this purpose.

One widely used procedure for determining when to mask and which ear to mask during bone-conduction tests is based on the Weber test (Liden, Nilsson, and Anderson, 1959b; Markle, Fowler, and Molonquet, 1952; Naunton, 1960). If the patient lateralizes the Weber test tone to one ear, the masking noise is applied to that ear. If the tone is reported to be in the center of the head, masking is not used. Clinical experience and research evidence (Fournier, 1954; Konig, 1962b) indicate that lateralization results can be misleading. Even the advocates of this procedure suggest that lateralization should be disregarded if the results appear improbable (Liden, Nilsson, and Anderson, 1959b; Naunton, 1957).

Another commonly applied rule states: "Always mask when testing by bone conduction." While this rule obviously never results in a failure to mask when needed, it does result in considerable wasted effort since it is unnecessary to mask the opposite ear when the unmasked bone-conduction threshold of the tested ear is already as poor as the air-conduction threshold of the same ear. Therefore, a more efficient rule is to apply masking to the opposite ear during bone-conduction tests whenever an air-bone gap is observed.

Placement of the vibrator at the forehead does not change this procedure. The clinician simply assumes that the unmasked threshold obtained from the forehead represents the unmasked bone-conduction threshold of each ear.

HOW MUCH MASKING?

Clinical masking is basically an effort to avoid the presentation of too much or too little noise. Avoidance of improper masking intensities requires consideration of a number of factors, including the test signal level, effective level, interaural attenuation, occlusion effect, and the air-bone gap of each ear. Few clinicians find it feasible to manipulate this number of variables in day-to-day clinical practice. Therefore, various writers have presented procedures designed to simplify the clinician's task. Unfortunately, the simplest procedures provide the greatest opportunity for error. For example, the use of a single masking noise intensity level (Harbert and Sataloff, 1955; Hawkins and Stevens, 1950; Hood, 1960) must result in over- and under-masking in many cases. The masking effectiveness of a given level of saw-tooth or white noises varies as a function of test-signal frequency by 30 dB or more (Sanders and Rintelmann, 1964). This factor, plus the influence of the hearing loss in each ear,

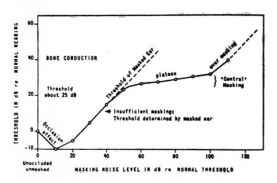

Figure 36-3. An example depicting the course of the apparent bone-conduction threshold as a function of noise level. Assumed are normal hearing for the masked ear and about a 30 dB actual bone-conduction threshold for the test ear.

requires frequent adjustments of masker intensity. The procedure is improved substantially if the proposed single level is a single effective level rather than a single intensity level. However, even under this condition adjustments must be made when the presentation level exceeds 40-dB HL by bone conduction and about 80-dB HL by air conduction.

Another widely used procedure (Liden, Nilsson, and Anderson, 1959b; Markle, Fowler, and Molonguet, 1952; Naunton, 1957) is based upon lateralization of the test tone. As mentioned earlier, the noise is applied to the ear to which the tone is lateralized in the Weber test. The masker level is increased until the patient reports that the test signal has shifted from the masked ear to the tested ear. While this procedure appears adequate

in most cases, it does depend upon the judgment of the patient. Even those who have used this method, express an unwillingness to rely upon it exclusively in all instances (Liden, Nilsson, and Anderson, 1959b; Naunton, 1957).

Threshold shift is the basis for a number of solutions to the clinical masking level problem. Three of the methods based on this phenomenon are presented in the next section. Figure 36-3 illustrates threshold shift in a hypothetical patient. In the figure the course of the apparent bone-conduction threshold of one ear is plotted as a function of noise level in the opposite ear. It is assumed, in this example, that the actual bone-conduction threshold of the test ear is above the bone-conduction threshold of the ear to be masked, that interaural attenuation is 0 dB, and that the masked ear is normal. Without masking in the opposite ear, threshold is obtained at 0-dB HL. Threshold improvement is noted due to the occlusion effect when an earphone is placed on the ear to be masked. Low noise effective levels increase the apparent threshold, because threshold in this instance is determined by the masked ear. As the noise level is increased further, the threshold of the masked ear is elevated above that of the test ear. Threshold is then determined by the test ear. Since the noise is not yet strong enough to mask the test ear, further noise increases produce little threshold increase, forming a plateau in the masking curve (a slight increase is seen due to central masking). When the noise level is increased further, the noise crosses the head with sufficient intensity to elevate the threshold of the tested ear, again increasing the observed threshold. This procedure was labeled a "control test" by Zwislocki (1951). Hood (1960) labeled the shifting threshold "shadowing," and the point of change to the plateau as the "change-over" point.

A number of factors influence minimum and maximum masking levels. The first factor is the presentation level of the test signal. The second is the interaural attenuation of the

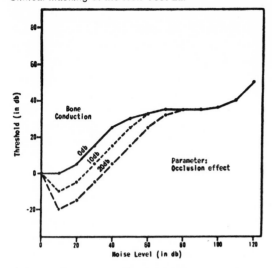

Figure 36-4. The relationship between masker level and apparent bone-conduction threshold for occlusion effects of three magnitudes on the masked ear. Assumed are normal hearing for the masked ear and about a 35 dB actual bone-conduction threshold for the test ear.

test signal for each mode of presentation. The third is the noise level required to mask the test signal. The fourth is the occlusion effect. The fifth are the air-bone gaps exhibited by each ear.

The test signal presentation level is simply the audiometer dial setting. Interaural attenuation for earphone-presented stimuli ranges from about 45 dB at low frequencies to about 65 dB at the highest frequencies. Interaural attenuation for vibrator-presented stimuli ranges from about 0 dB to 250 Hz to about 15 dB at 4000 Hz (with forehead placement interaural attenuation is, in effect, 0 dB at all frequencies). The third factor, effective level, was discussed earlier.

Considering only these factors for a moment, it is apparent that the least masking one can use is an effective level equal to the presentation level minus interaural attenuation (of the test signal to the masked cochlea). The greatest permissible level is an effective level equal to the presentation level plus the interaural attenuation (of the masking noise to the test ear). The occlusion effect and air-bone gap complicate this picture.

The influence of the occlusion effect is illustrated in Figure 36-4. The occlusion effect, produced by placing an earphone over the ear to be masked, increases the intensity of the test signal at that ear (it does not modify cochlear sensitivity). Therefore, the minimum-masking intensity is increased by the amount of this factor. An air-bone gap in the masked ear also increases the minimum required level. The conductive loss decreases the intensity of the noise reaching the cochlea to be masked, but does not decrease the test-signal level arriving from the test ear side.

Both occlusion effect and masked ear air-bone gap increase the minimum required level but do not affect the maximum permissible level. Thus, each decreases the size of the plateau. However, the two factors are mutually exclusive and do not summate as illustrated in Figure 36-5. It is apparent that a large masked ear air-bone gap reduces the plateau to the vanishing point under some circumstances (i.e., during bone-conduction testing and also during air-conduction testing if the test ear also exhibits an air-bone gap).

An air-bone gap on the tested ear affects

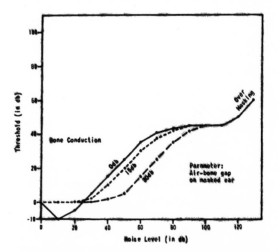

Figure 36-5. The relationship between masker level and apparent bone-conduction threshold with air-bone gaps of three magnitudes on the masked ear. Assumed are normal bone-conduction thresholds for the masked ear and about a 45 dB actual bone-conduction threshold for the test ear.

the maximum permissible masking when the test signals are presented by earphone. With no air-bone gap in the test ear, maximum masking during air-conduction tests equals the test-signal level, plus the interaural attenuation of the masking noise. That is, the noise can be presented safely at effective levels up to 40 dB above the test signal level. A conductive loss in the test ear reduces the test signal level but not the noise level at the test cochlea. Therefore, the maximum permissible level is decreased by the amount of the air-bone gap. In the case of an air-bone gap of about 45 to 50 dB or more, the maximum permissible level for air-conduction tests is equal to the maximum level for bone-conduction tests. It is for these reasons that the "masking dilemma" described by Naunton (1960) occurs with bilateral conductive losses and why it applies equally to both air- and bone-conduction tests.

A further consideration in the development of a clinical procedure is intersubject variability. It is not satisfactory to use the measures of central tendency for interaural attenuation, effective level, or occlusion effect values. The value used for interaural attenuation should be the smallest value expected across subjects. The effective-level value should be as low as expected across subjects when low effective levels are used. Occlusion effect, on the other hand, should always be assumed to be as high as expected with any subject. Only by considering the appropriate extreme of each distribution, is the clinician reasonably assured that he is not over or under masking.

THRESHOLD SHIFT PROCEDURES

A usable clinical procedure must be devised either to avoid or compensate for each of the factors discussed above. Each of the following three masking methods do this or can be so adapted by slight modification.

A procedure based solely on the threshold shift observation was first presented by Hood in 1957. His procedure is as follows: First, find the unmasked threshold. Second, apply a masking noise to the nontest ear at an effective level of 10-dB SL. If no threshold shift is observed, threshold is the value obtained without contralateral masking. If the apparent threshold increases, then raise the noise in 10-dB steps, finding threshold at each step until further increases result in no further threshold shifts. The threshold of the tested ear is the value which does not increase with noise level.

This procedure has the following advantages:

1. The procedure involved is simple and requires a minimum of calculation.
2. The noise levels used are not loud.
3. Masking of air-conduction tests can be carried out without a knowledge of the bone-conduction thresholds.

Disadvantages:

1. The procedure, as originally presented, does not compensate for the occlusion effect. (The occlusion effect should be added to the first noise level used. The value used must be at least as large as the largest occlusion effect expected across individuals and not an average value.)
2. Intersubject variability of effective level and of the occlusion effect may, in individual cases, be sufficient to produce undermasking at the low effective levels used. Therefore, masking should be at least applied at two levels to iusure that the 10-dB SL effective level is not insufficient.
3. If more than the lowest levels are used, there is danger of overmasking in the presence of an air-bone gap in the masked ear. While other procedures have the same limitation, this method does not give the clinician the information necessary to recognize the danger of overmasking.

A second procedure is one reported by Luscher and Konig in 1955 based on earlier work by Zwislocki (1951). This method was published by Konig in English (1962b). With this method, an audiometer is used which automatically presents to the nontest ear a narrow-band noise which centers on the test tone. The noise level is coupled to the test-signal attenuator so that the noise level at the opposite ear is always just above the test-signal level, minus interaural attenuation, plus occlusion effect. A secondary attenuator is used to increase the noise level above this value in order to compensate for an air-bone gap in the masked ear. In practice, the masking is presented at a just-sufficient level automatically, except for the addition of the masked ear air-bone gap by the examiner. The masked ear conductive component is estimated when testing the first ear by bone-conduction by noting the difference between the apparent bone-conduction threshold of the tested ear obtained with the first contra-lateral masking level and the air-conduction threshold of the masked ear. It is recom-mended by Luscher and Konig (1955) that an additional 5 to 15 dB be added to com-pensate for individual variability and that, if there is any doubt, threshold shift procedures should be carried out using 5-dB noise level steps.

Advantages:

1. The procedure is largely automatic and simple to use in practice.
2. The occlusion effect and air-bone gap are considered.
3. The noise levels used are not loud.

Disadvantages:

1. The use of low effective levels requires additional noise-level increases of 5 to 15 dB, nullifying some of the advantage of the automatic procedure.
2. Special equipment is required.

A method published by the present writer in 1964 based on Zwislocki's and Luscher and Konig's work is as follows. First, the unmasked threshold is obtained. Second, a noise is presented at an effective level of 40 dB above the bone-conduction threshold of the tested ear. Third, the noise is increased by an amount equal to any observed threshold shift. If a sizable air-bone gap is observed in the masked ear, a threshold shift procedure is used with the calculated noise level as the starting point. Threshold is the presentation level which does not shift upon masker appli-cation or masker-level increase.

Advantages:

1. The 40-dB effective level produces rela-tively large threshold shifts avoiding the sometimes equivocable outcomes associated with low effective-level presentations.
2. The occlusion effect and smaller masked ear air-bone gaps need not be considered.
3. The noise level is always at a level equal to the interaural attenuation, minus 40 dB, below the smallest average maximum-masking level.
4. The procedure can be used with auto-matic equipment of the type used by Luscher and Konig (1955).

Disadvantages:

1. The basis for the procedure is more diffi-cult to understand.
2. The noise levels used are relatively loud.
3. It is necessary to have bone-conduction results before precise masking levels for air-conduction tests can be determined.

SUMMARY

In contrast to the impression gained from audiologic texts, a considerable body of literature exists on the subject of clinical masking. Most writers now agree that narrow-band noise is the most satisfactory for masking pure-tone test signals. However broad-band noises are still required for the masking of speech signals.

Masking should be applied to the nontest ear when testing by air-conduction whenever the test-signal presentation level exceeds the bone-conduction threshold of the nontest ear by 40 dB or more. When testing by bone-conduction, masking should be applied to the nontest ear whenever an apparent air-bone gap is observed in the tested ear.

Various methods have been proposed to determine the proper masking intensity. Of these, those based on the threshold shift phenomenon seem most satisfactory. Three methods based on this phenomenon are presented including the major advantages and disadvantages of each. The Luscher and Konig procedure requires equipment not

generally found in this country. The Hood method is the simplest of the two remaining procedures. This method has disadvantages associated with the use of low effective levels (as does the Luscher and Konig procedure). The present writer has presented a method which uses higher effective levels in order to solve these problems. This procedure can be used equally well with both air- and bone-conducted stimuli and with suprathreshold, as well as threshold, test-signal presentations.

BIBLIOGRAPHY

Burgemeestre, A. J., Auditory masking in continuous audiometry. *Acta Otolaryng.*, **43**, 506 (1953).

Békésy, G., A new audiometer. *Acta Otolaryng.*, **35**, 411 (1947).

Davis, H., and Silverman, S. R., *Hearing and Deafness*. New York: Holt, Rinehart, and Winston (1961).

Dean, C. E., Audition by bone conduction. *J. acoust. Soc. Amer.*, **2**, 281 (1930).

DeBoer, E., Clinical masking. *Pract. ORL.*, **24**, 351 (1962). (*dsh* #72, Jan. 1963).

Denes, P., and Naunton, R. F., Masking in pure tone audiometry. *Proc. roy. Soc. Med.*, **45**, 790 (1952).

Dirks, D., Bone conduction measurements. *Arch. Otolaryng.*, **79**, 594 (1964).

Dirks, D., and Malmquist, C., Changes in bone-conduction thresholds produced by masking in the non-test ear. *J. Speech Hearing Res.*, **7**, 271 (1964).

Dirks, D. D., and Malmquist, C., Shifts in air-conduction thresholds produced by pulsed and continuous contralateral masking. *J. acoust. Soc. Amer.*, **37**, 631 (1965).

Dirks, D. D., and Norris, J. N., Shifts in auditory thresholds produced by ipsilateral and contralateral maskers at low intensity levels. *J. acoust. Soc. Amer.*, **40**, 12 (1966).

Elpern, B., and Naunton, R. F., The stability of the occlusion effect. *Arch. Otolaryng.*, **77**, 376 (1963).

Feldman, H., Masking the test-tone by the test-tone. *Inter. Aud.*, **1**, 240 (1962). (*dsh*, #1031, July 64).

Fletcher, H., Auditory patterns. *Rev. modern Physics*, **12**, 47 (1940).

Fournier, J. E., The "false-bing" phenomenon. Some remarks on the theory of bone conduction. *Laryngoscope*, **64**, 29 (1954).

Glorig, A., *Audiometry: Principle and Practice*. Baltimore: The Williams & Wilkins Co. (1965).

Goetzinger, C. P., Proud, G. O., and Embry, J. E., Masking and bone conduction. *Acta Otolaryng.*, **54**, 287 (1962).

Harbert, F., Masking levels for clinical use. *Arch. Otolaryng.*, **66**, 214 (1957).

Harbert, F., The clinical masking level. *Ann. Oto. Rhino. Laryng.*, **67**, 332 (1958).

Harbert, F., and Sataloff, J. A., Clinical applications of recruitment and masking. *Laryngoscope*, **65**, 113 (1955).

Hardy, W. G., Masking in testing for otosclerosis. In H. F. Schuknecht (Ed.), *Otosclerosis*. Boston: Little-Brown, 199 (1962).

Hart, C., and Naunton, R. F., Frontal bone conduction tests in clinical audiometry. *Laryngoscope*, **71**, 24 (1961).

Hawkins, J. E., and Stevens, S. S., The masking of pure tones and of speech by white noise. *J. acoust. Soc. Amer.*, **22**, 6 (1950).

Hood, J. D., The principles and practice of bone conduction audiometry. A review of the present position. *Proc. roy. Soc. Med.*, **50**, 689 (1957), and *Laryngoscope*, **70**, 1211 (1960).

Huizing, E. H., Bone conduction. The influence of the middle ear. *Acta Otolaryng. Supp.*, **155** (1960).

Jerger, J., *Modern Developments in Audiology*. New York: Academic Press (1963).

Jerger, J., Tillman, T. W., and Peterson, J. L., Masking by octave bands of noise in normal and impaired ears. *J. acoust. Soc. Amer.*, **32**, 385 (1960).

Jerger, J., and Wertz, M., The indiscriminate use of masking in bone-conduction audiometry. *Arch. Otolaryng.*, **70**, 419 (1959).

Konig, E., On the use of hearing-aid type earphones in clinical audiometry. *Acta Otolaryng.*, **55**, 331 (1962b).

Konig, E., The use of masking noise and its limitation in clinical audiometry. *Acta Otolaryng. Supp.*, **180**, 1 (1962b).

Liden, G., Nilsson, G., and Anderson, H., Narrow band masking with white noise. *Acta Otolaryng.*, **50**, 116 (1959a).

Liden, G., Nilsson, G., and Anderson, H., Masking in clinical audiometry. *Acta Otolaryng.*, **50**, 125 (1959b).

Littler, T. S., Knight, J. J., and Strange, P. H., Hearing by bone conduction and the use of bone conduction hearing aids. *Proc. roy. Soc. Med.*, **45**, 783 (1952).

Luscher, E., and Konig, E., Die Vertaubung des Gegenhores bei audiometrischen Bestimmerng der Knochenlertung. *Arch. Ohr.–Nas. u. Kehlk.–Heilk*, **168,** 68 (1955).

Markle, D. M., Fowler, E. P., Jr., and Molonquet, H., The audiometric Weber test as a means of determining the need for and the type of masking. *Ann. Oto. Rhino. Laryng.*, **61,** 888 (1952).

Martin, F. N., Bailey, H. A. T., Jr., and Pappas, J. J., The effect of central masking on threshold for speech. *J. aud. Res.*, **5,** 293 (1965).

Menzel, O. J., Masking noise in audiometers. *EENT Monthly*, **43,** 93 (1964).

Miller, M. H., Clinical application of paired masking enclosures in pure tone air and bone conduction testing. *Arch. Otolaryng.*, **69,** 315 (1959).

Miller, M. H., Transmission loss across the skull in a patient with a known total monaural deafness. *Laryngoscope*, **69,** 100 (1959).

Naunton, R. F., Clinical bone conduction audiometry. The use of frontally applied bone-conduction receiver and the importance of the occlusion effect in clinical bone-conduction audiometry. *Arch. Otolaryng.*, **66,** 281 (1957).

Naunton, R. F., A masking dilemma in bilateral conduction deafness. *Arch. Otolaryng.*, **72,** 753 (1960).

Newby, H. A., *Audiology*. New York: Appleton-Century-Crofts (1964).

O'Neill, J. J., and Oyer, H. J., *Applied Audiometry*. New York: Dodd, Mead & Company (1966).

Palva, T., Masking in audiometry. With special reference to the non-thermal type of noise. *Acta Otolaryng. Supp.*, **118,** 156 (1954).

Palva, T., Masking in audiometry, Further studies. *Acta Otolaryng.*, **49,** 229 (1958).

Palva, T., and Palva, A., Masking in audiometry. III. Reflections on the present position. *Acta Otolaryng.*, **54,** 521 (1962).

Saltzman, M., and Ersner, M. S., Masking and shadow hearing in bone conduction. *Arch. Otolaryng.*, **51,** 809 (1950).

Sanders, J. W., and Rintelmann, W. F., Masking in audiometry. *Arch. Otolaryng.*, **80,** 541 (1964).

Sataloff, J., *Hearing Loss*. Philadelphia: J. B. Lippincott Co. (1966).

Shuel, J., Masking in pure tone audiometry. Its use and its limitations. *J. Laryng.*, **72,** 959 (1958).

Studebaker, G. A., On masking in bone-conduction testing. *J. Speech Hearing Res.*, **5,** 215 (1962).

Studebaker, G. A., Clinical masking of air- and bone-conducted stimuli. *J. Speech Hearing Dis.*, **29,** 23 (1964).

Veniar, F. A., Individual masking levels in pure tone audiometry. *Arch. Otolaryng.*, **82,** 518 (1965).

Watson, N., and Gales, R., Bone conduction threshold measurements: Effects of occlusion, enclosures, and masking. *J. acoust. Soc. Amer.*, **14,** 207 (1943).

Welsh, L. W., and Welsh, J. J., Clinical problems in masking. *Arch. Otolaryng.*, **73,** 342 (1961).

Zwislocki, J., Acoustic attenuation between the ears. *J. acoust. Soc. Amer.*, **25,** 752 (1953).

Zwislocki, J., Eine verbesserte Vertaubungsmethode fur die Audiometrie. *Acta Otolaryng.*, **39,** 338 (1951). *Trans. Beltone Inst. Hear. Res.*, No. 19, April 1966.

37

The Principles and Practice of Bone-Conduction Audiometry

J. D. HOOD

J. D. HOOD, Ph.D., D.Sc., is Director of the Medical Research Council Audiology and Neuro-Otology Unit, National Hospital, London, England

Whereas the technique of air conduction audiometry is well established, the basic principles of bone conduction audiometry are still far from being generally understood. In consequence, the tests are still too often inefficiently performed and hence fail to provide the vital diagnostic information which is their purpose.

As will be shown, this disappointing state of affairs is quite unnecessary, and requires for its correction no more than a rational standardization of our technical equipment and test procedures, whereby proper use is made of the considerable body of acoustic and physiological knowledge now at our disposal.

An essential requirement with all bone conduction tests is the exclusion of the untested ear by means of an efficient masking sound, so that all threshold readings can be validly related to the tested ear. In order to understand how this requirement arises, we need to know first certain facts concerning the transmission of air and bone conducted sounds across the head; second, the physical characteristics of a sound which confer upon it maximum efficiency for the masking of pure tones of specified frequency.

The facts relating to sound transmission across the head are conveniently studied in

Reprinted by permission of the author from *Laryngoscope*, **70**, pp. 1211–1228 (1960).

subjects with normal hearing in one ear and complete deafness of the other.

The results obtained are shown in Figure 37-1. The calibrated columns are taken to represent the available hearing capacity of each ear; the solid column at the left represents total deafness of the right ear. Positive responses to the test tones of different levels above normal threshold are indicated in this and succeeding figures by serrated lines. If an air-conducted sound of 50 db is applied to the right, or deaf ear, it will be heard in the left ear at threshold intensity. Similarly, a sound of 80 db applied to the right ear will be heard in the left ear at a level some 30 db above threshold. The reason for this is that sound from an air-conduction receiver is transmitted across the skull with an interaural attenuation of the order of 50 db. By contrast, the interaural attenuation for sound from a bone conduction receiver applied to the right mastoid is negligible, and the sound will be heard at the left ear with a loss of only a few decibels.

In the lower half of Figure 37-1 are shown the pure tone audiograms of the right and left ears for air and bone conduction carried out without masking. They indicate normal hearing for the left ear, and a severe conductive deafness for the right ear. In agreement with this, the classical tuning fork tests applied to the right ear lead us into that well-known pitfall of clinical practice, the false negative Rinné; in fact, for the reasons given, the threshold readings, both for air and bone conduction, obtained for the right ear and shown in the audiograms, are false readings derived from the left or untested ear. In the case of air conduction, owing to the comparatively high interaural attenuation of 50 db, such false readings are obtained only when the stimulus intensity exceeds this level. Clearly

ear be raised by any amount above 5 db, a receiver on the right mastoid will give false normal readings derived from the opposite untested ear; hence the rule that *all* bone conduction tests require the exclusion by an air-conducted masking sound of the untested ear. A variety of masking noises has been devised to serve this purpose. A few, like those described by Zwislocki (1951), or Denes and Naunton (1952), are efficient, but of the

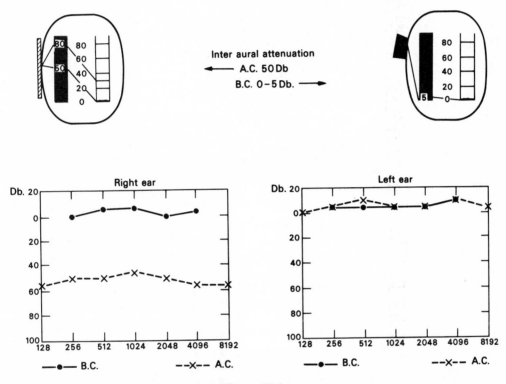

Figure 37-1.

enough, true readings would result with any degree of deafness of the right ear below this level; hence the rule that when the difference in the air-conduction thresholds of the two ears exceeds 50 db the readings for the worst ear cannot be relied upon, unless the better ear is excluded by masking.

In the case of bone conduction, however, the situation is much more difficult. Here the interaural attenuation is negligible, and hence, if the bone-conduction threshold of the right

majority it can only be said that they raise the threshold of the masked ear in some vague unspecified manner.

In order to understand what makes a masking sound efficient, it is helpful to consider first the masking of pure tones by white noise, that is to say, noise having a flat frequency spectrum covering the whole audible frequency range with equal sound energy per cycle. In Figure 37-2 is shown the elevation of the threshold of a pure tone of

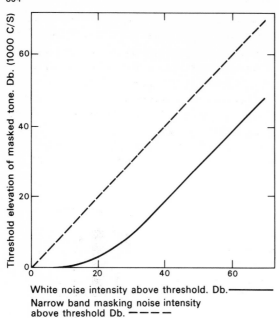

White noise intensity above threshold. Db. ——————
Narrow band masking noise intensity
above threshold Db. — — — —   Figure 37-2.

1,000 cycles in the presence of white noise. The noise intensity is expressed in decibels above normal threshold, and it will be seen that below the 20 db level it produces negligible masking of the pure tone. Above this level there is an incremental equivalence in decibels of masking and of masking noise intensity. At any masking level, therefore, the loudness of the white noise will be much in excess of the pure tone, since its intensity will at all times be some 20 db higher.

This brings us to the first important requirement of a masking noise, namely, high masking efficiency which Denes and Naunton have defined as "good masking ability, but minimal loudness." Clearly, white noise does not conform to this ideal; nevertheless, it is superior to some of the masking noises incorporated in many commercial audiometers. A typical example is shown in Figure 37-3. The masking noise is modified mains hum, its intensity level in decibels above normal threshold is shown on the horizontal scale, and on the vertical scale the resulting threshold elevation of various pure tones. It will be seen that for frequencies above 1,000 cycles masking is grossly inefficient. At 4,000 cycles no masking

at all is produced below an intensity level of some 50 db at which point it is already becoming unpleasantly loud to the subject.

Having considered these examples of inefficient masking sounds, we will consider next how we set about our task of designing what we really require, that is to say, sounds which have the maximum possible efficiency for the masking of the limited range of specified pure tones, which are conventionally used for bone-conduction audiometry. Here, as usual, we turn for guidance to some of Fletcher's (1940) early work upon frequency discrimination, loudness and masking, which led him to define the existence of certain so-called critical frequency bands. Their significance lies in the fact, first, that in any masking noise only those frequencies within a certain critical band centered around the pure tone contribute to its masking, and second, when the tone is just audible against the background of noise, the total acoustic power of the components within the band is the same as that of the pure tone. The principles are illustrated schematically in Figure 37-4. This shows noise bands of varying widths centered about a single pure tone which is just audible in their presence.

The acoustic energy, both in the bands and in the pure tones, is represented by the enclosed area of each. Band A is only three cycles wide, and since its total energy is the same as that of the pure-tone, the energy per cycle of the noise is only one-third that of the pure tone. Band B is five cycles wide. Once again, its total energy is the same as that of the pure tone, which thus has five times as much energy as each cycle of the band. The width of Band C is that of the critical band, and yet again the total energy in the band is equal to that of the pure tone.

In bands D and C the noise spectrum extends beyond the critical band, so that the total energy of the bands is much increased. Since, however, it is only the energy in the critical band which contributes to the masking, these noise bands possess no greater masking power, and the energy level of the just masked pure tone remains the same. In other words, those components outside the critical band, while they may have the effect of making the noise very much louder, contribute nothing to its effective masking power. This provides us with the theoretical basis for the concept of high masking efficiency; clearly our first objective must be to remove as much as possible of these unnecessary components.

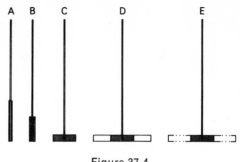

Figure 37-4.

Are we likely to gain anything from the use of band widths which are only a fraction of the critical band, as for example in Band B? Apart from the fact that to do so would present very difficult technical problems of sound filtering, we should gain nothing in efficiency and, in addition, would be faced with the added difficulty of the tonal similarity of the pure tone and the masking noise which might result in some confusion to the patient. If, however, the band width of the masking noise is extended to correspond roughly to that of the critical band, as in Band C, then we find that though masking sound and pure tone are identical in pitch, they are still readily distinguishable, and hence are not confused by the subject tested.

The critical band widths for the various frequencies are shown in Figure 37-5. As will be seen, they are of the order of only a hundred cycles wide. It would be technically impossible to produce noise bands to these specifications, nor, as will be shown, is this necessary.

In Figure 37-6 is shown schematically the equipment we have used for obtaining narrow bands of noise, having the masking efficiency required. A white noise generator is followed in turn by a number of filters of high selectivity centered around each of the pure tones normally used in bone conduction audiometry, followed in turn by an attenuator calibrated in steps of 10 db. Each of the filters can be selected by means of a switch, and passes only a very narrow band of frequencies.

The selectivity curve for the band centered at 1,000 c/s, which is typical of the other

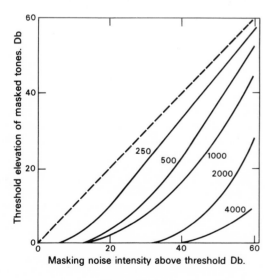

Figure 37-3.

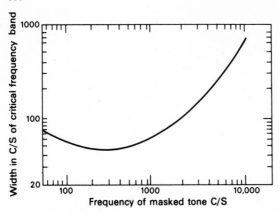

Figure 37-5.

curves, is shown in Figure 37-7. At the center, the two vertical lines give the measure of the width of the critical band. The curves extend somewhat beyond the critical band at the base; nevertheless, the maximum energy in the band is centered within the two parallel lines.

The dotted line in Figure 37-2 illustrates the high masking efficiency obtained with this band.

In contrast to the masking effect of white noise, there is 100 percent masking efficiency. The curve begins at zero, and there is an exact one-to-one relationship between noise level and masked threshold. Thus, if the noise is raised 20 db, the pure tone threshold is raised by an identical amount, and so on. All the noise bands are similar in this respect, and we regard it as one of their most important features. Thus, if it is desired to raise the threshold of a pure tone by, say 40 db, it becomes a simple matter of raising the intensity level of the noise band by exactly the same amount. The practical importance of this is best illustrated by considering the simple application of these

noise bands to the technique of bone conduction tests.

Figure 37-8 is a schematic illustration of the rationale of the procedure employed at the Otological Research Unit, and referred to for convenience as the "shadowing" technique. Let there be a pure nerve deafness of 40 db of the subject's right ear to be tested, and no loss of hearing of the left ear; as before, the columns of each side are taken to represent the available hearing, and are calibrated in decibels. The solid portion of the left column represents the nerve deafness of the right ear. A bone conducted sound at normal threshold intensity applied to the right mastoid is heard in the subject's left ear. This provides us with the first point on the graph shown below, in which the masking intensity at the left ear

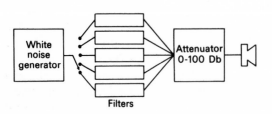

Figure 37-6.

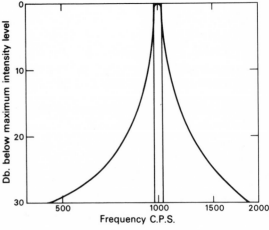

Figure 37-7.

is plotted on the horizontal scale and the bone-conduction threshold responses on the vertical scale.

Now, as shown in Figure 37-8, the masking noise at a level of 10 db applied to the left ear raises its threshold for the bone conducted test tone by 10 db. In the same way,

by the right as well as the left ear. A further intensity increase of the masking noise to 50 or 60 db will further raise the threshold of the left ear alone, leaving the test tone to be heard by the right ear alone without further elevation above its true threshold value, 40 db. The true threshold for the right ear will thus be

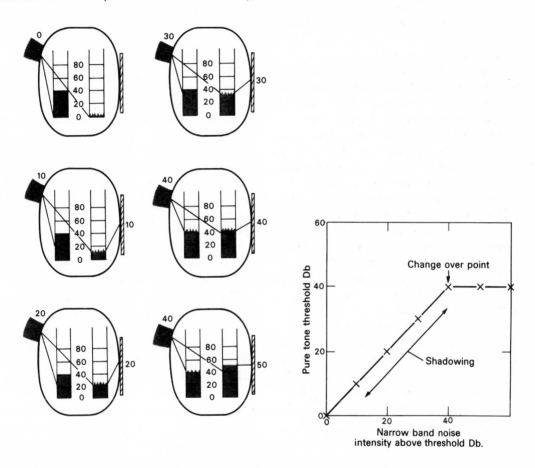

Figure 37-8.

increases in masking noise intensity of 20 or 30 db will bring about increases of identical magnitude in the threshold values for the test tone. Reference to the graph shows, up to this point, this step by step correlation, the "shadowing" effect between the intensities of masking noise and test tone thresholds. When, however, the masking noise reaches the 40 db level it will be seen that the bone conducted test tone will be heard at threshold

shown at a point on the graph, referred to as the "change-over" point, at which the slope of the curve changes from 45 degrees and becomes horizontal. In the case being considered, the change-over point occurs at 40 db. If, extending the argument, the deafness of the tested ear had been 50, 60 or 80 db identical values of masking noise intensity would have been required to reach the "change-over" points. In all cases, true threshold readings would be obtained.

The essential steps of the test procedure are thus:

1. The demonstration of the "shadowing" effect. This establishes that both masking noise and test tone are confined to the untested ear.

2. The identification of the "change-over" point. This establishes the true threshold of the tested ear.

The case analyzed in Figure 37-8 is one of comparative simplicity in that the unilateral deafness was of the "nerve" type. In unilateral deafness of the conductive type, however, we are confronted with a situation of considerably greater difficulty. This arises, as will be shown, from the fact that the interaural attenuation of an air-conducted masking sound does not exceed some 50 db.

The situation is illustrated in Figure 37-9.

Here, the subject has normal hearing of the right, or tested ear, and a pure conductive deafness of 50 db of the left ear. This is indicated by the solid area adjoining the calibrated column which represents the inner ear hearing capacity of the left ear, reduced in B and C by masking.

In ascertaining the bone-conduction threshold of the right ear we must, as usual, apply an air-conducted masking noise to the left ear. Here a serious difficulty arises, since before this noise can become effective its intensity must reach 50 db, the amount of the conductive deafness. At this intensity it will just overcome the interaural attenuation for air-conducted sound, and begin to exert a masking effect upon the right ear as well as the left. If the intensity of the masking noise be further increased in steps of 10 db, a "shadowing" effect will occur, and the bone-conduction thresholds, derived equally from the two ears, will rise *pari passu.* In this instance, however, the "shadowing" effect will continue indefinitely, and no "change-over" point will be reached.

The underlying difficulty is clearly to be found in the fact that the interaural attenuation of the air-conducted masking noise has a limit of some 50 db. What is needed, therefore, is some means of extending this limit, and providing a zone of masking noise intensities which will be above the air-conducted threshold of, and at the same time confined to, the left ear. Within this zone, the "shadowing" procedure could be applied, and the absence of a "shadowing" effect would then prove that bone-conduction threshold readings were derived from the right ear, and could be accepted as valid.

The manner in which such an increase of the interaural attenuation can be accomplished stems from a brief report on the use of insert receivers which appeared in the Report of the Electro-Acoustics Committee "Hearing Aids and Audiometer," 1947. In this it was suggested that the acoustic linkage between the two ears which occurs when any air conduction receiver is used

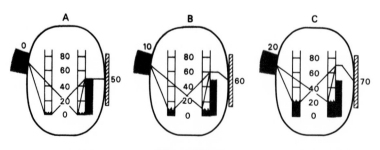

Figure 37-9.*

[* It should be noted that masking generally is not required to assess the better ear's bone-conduction sensitivity in a unilateral hearing loss like the one illustrated in Figure 37-9. This has been included merely to emphasize, in a simple form, the problems of overmasking which have to be borne in mind when dealing with hearing losses of a more complicated kind in which conductive deafness is a prominent feature. JDH]

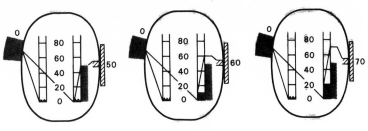

Figure 37-10.

arises from the vibrations imparted to the skull at the air-bone interface bounding the receiver. Both Littler, et al. (1952) and Zwislocki (1953) have carried out further studies, and it has been shown that the vital factor affecting the attenuation is the area of the head exposed to the air conducted sound waves. Thus, the smaller the area the greater the attenuation, and in the limiting case when an insert receiver is used, thus presenting the smallest possible surface to the skull, the interaural attenuation increases to a figure as high as 90 db.

As Littler, et al. (1952) so ably pointed out, the practical importance of this finding is considerable, making possible as it does the accurate determination of bone-conduction thresholds in the presence of conductive deafness well beyond the limit of 50 db. This is illustrated in Figure 37-10. Masking noises of intensities up to 90 db are applied to the left ear by means of a rubber-tipped-insert receiver without fear of cross conduction to the right ear.

Thus, at any intensity between 50 db, the air-conduction threshold of the left ear, and 90 db, the masking noise will be effective in the left ear alone. If we now apply the "shadowing" procedure, and make step by step changes of masking intensity within this range, they will be found to leave unaltered the bone-conduction threshold readings. In other words, the "shadowing" effect is absent, and the threshold reading, o db, can be accepted as valid for the right ear.

When the deafness is bilateral, and of the mixed conductive and nerve type, bone-conduction tests may be greatly complicated,

and indeed it is only within certain limits that accurate results are then obtainable.

An audiometrician needs to know what these limits are, and it is fortunately possible to define them with reasonable accuracy. The situation is analyzed in the cases shown in Figures 37-11 (A, B and C). In 37-11-A the subject has a nerve deafness of 60 db of the right ear and conductive deafness of 30 db of the left. In order to establish the bone-conduction threshold of the right ear, the usual masking noise must be applied to the left, and owing to the conductive deafness its minimum effective intensity will be 30 db. Above this point shadowing will occur, as shown in the graph (A); that is to say, both masking noise and test tone will be confined to the left or untested ear. When the masking intensity reaches the 90 db level, its true masking effect upon the left ear will be restricted to 60 db by the conductive deafness and the test tone will now be heard at threshold in the right ear as well as in the left. This is the critical change-over point, and beyond it a further increase of masking intensity to 100 db, the maximum practicable level, will raise the threshold of the left ear by a further 10 db while leaving unaffected at 60 db that of the right ear. This, therefore, will be its true threshold.

Two factors determine the results thus obtained. First, 100 db is accepted as the maximum intensity of masking noise which it is practicable to use for clinical tests. With this the critical change-over point occurs at a level 10 db lower, 90 db, and to this it is convenient to refer as the maximum critical masking intensity. Second, the threshold of

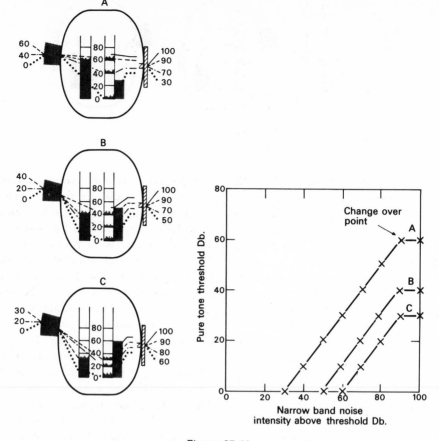

Figure 37-11.

the tested ear can be determined only if it lies at or below the level of masking induced by the maximum critical masking intensity in the untested ear.

Now, in Case 37-11-A this level is reduced by 30 db, the amount of the conduction deafness and hence, 60 db is the maximum measurable elevation of the bone-conduction threshold of the right ear. From this we may derive the limiting formula:

Maximum measurable bone-conduction threshold = 90 — conductive deafness (db) of opposite ear.

The application of the test procedure to the three cases A, B and C, represented in Figure 37-11, is shown in the graph.

In all three the amount of the nerve deafness of the tested ear is the maximum

measurable according to the limiting formula. Thus:

Case A   60 db   (90–30).
Case B   40 db   (90–50).
Case C   30 db   (90–60).

In each case the true threshold is given by the change-over point which occurs at the maximum critical intensity, 90 db of masking noise.

Although for simplicity of explanation the cases shown in Figure 37-11 have been selected to exhibit conductive deafness alone of the untested ear and nerve deafness alone of the tested ear, accurate bone-conduction tests are still possible within the limits of the formula when the deafness, of either one or both ears, is of the mixed type. This is illustrated in Figure 37-12. In the right ear there is a conductive deafness of 40 db with a nerve deafness of 60 db. The air-conduction audiogram thus shows a loss of 100 db. In the left ear there is a conductive deafness of 30 db with a nerve deafness of 50 db. The air-conduction audiogram thus shows a loss of 80 db. With no masking noise applied to the left ear the bone-conduction threshold reading is 50 db, derived, in fact, from the left ear, though this cannot be specified at this stage of the test.

This reading remains constant with increase of masking noise intensity up to 80 db. With the masking intensity increased to 90 db, however, and still confined at this level to the left ear, the threshold reading is increased to 60 db and remains unchanged when the masking intensity is further increased to 100 db. As shown in the graph, "shadowing" occurs between the 80 and 90 db levels of masking noise intensity with the "change-over" point at 90 db. It follows that up to the 80 db level of masking noise intensity, the threshold reading, 50 db, must be derived from the left ear; further, that at and above the 90 db level, the threshold reading, 60 db, is derived from the right ear. Subtraction of these bone-conduction losses

from the air-conduction losses gives the amounts of the conductive deafness, thus:

> Right ear   100 − 60 = 40 db.
> Left ear   80 − 50 = 30 db.

In each case, the amount of the nerve deafness is the maximum which can be measured according to this formula. Thus for the right ear:

60 db (amount of nerve deafness) = 90 − 30 (amount of conductive deafness of left ear).

For the left ear:

50 db (amount of nerve deafness) = 90 − 40 (amount of conductive deafness of right ear). As will be seen from the foregoing analyses, the use of the maximum efficiency masking technique described in this communication brings within the resolving power of air and bone-conduction audiometry all but the few exceptional cases which lie beyond the bounds of the limiting formula.

In all cases, however, careful attention should be given to the fundamental features of the test procedure which is outlined as follows:

1. Establish the air-conduction audiogram of both ears in the normal way with masking, if necessary, of the untested ear,

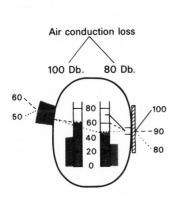
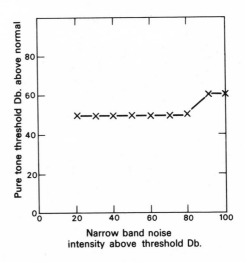

Figure 37-12.

i.e., when the difference in the hearing loss between the two ears exceeds 50 db.

2. Find the bone-conduction threshold with the bone-conductor applied to the mastoid of the tested ear without masking of the untested ear.

3. Apply the masking noise of the appropriate band to the untested ear by means of an insert receiver and find a bone-conduction threshold reading.

4. Apply the "shadowing" procedure thus: Increase the level of the masking noise by 10 db above threshold and retest the bone-conduction threshold. If the bone-conduction threshold is raised by 10 db increase the masking intensity by another 10 db and repeat. Continue this procedure until the point is reached at which the bone conduction remains constant with further additional incremental steps of 10 db of the masking noise. This is the "change-over" point, and

gives the true bone-conduction threshold of the tested ear.

Suggestions for the improvement of standard equipment tend to encounter two kinds of objections: first, that they involve excessive technical difficulties; second, that the solution they offer is far from complete, and hence further development should be awaited.

Neither of these objections appears to be applicable in the present situation. No serious difficulties attend the generation or application of the masking sounds described; and as for further developments, these cannot be expected since in many respects the efficiency obtained is 100 per cent, at which level an ample reserve is provided for the attainment of practically all the clinical results which are required. It is, therefore, to be hoped that the methods described will find useful application in improving the design of standard audiometric equipment.

REFERENCES

Denes, P., and Naunton, R. F.: *Proc. Roy. Soc. Med.*, 45:790, 1952.

Fletcher, H.: *Rev. Mod. Physiol.*, 12:47, 1940.

Littler, T. S.; Knight, J. J., and Strange, P. H.: *Proc. Roy. Soc. Med.*, 45:783, 1952.

Zwislocki, J.: *Acta Oto-Laryngol., Stockh.*, 39:338, 1951; *Jour. Acoust. Soc. Amer.*, 25:752, 1953.

38

Individual Masking Levels in Pure–Tone Audiometry

FLORENCE A. VENIAR

FLORENCE A. VENIAR, Ph.D., is Associate Professor, Douglass College, Rutgers University

The function of the audiologist is twofold (1) to assess the hearing deficit of the individual and (2) to determine, if possible, the locus (or loci) of pathology from which the deficit arises.

While bone-conduction audiometry gives a measure of inner ear deficit (or of cochlear reserve), the difference between air-conduction (AC) and bone-conduction (BC) sensitivity gives a measure of middle ear deficit. (An air-conducted signal passes through the outer and middle ear before entering the inner ear. The bone oscillator, on the other hand, stimulates the inner ear directly. Thus, assuming the outer ear is normal, any difference in sensitivity to AC vs BC stimulus is attributed to middle ear loss.) The problem of assessing bone conduction lies in the fact that it is difficult to stimulate one ear without simultaneously stimulating the other. Thus, a measure of bone conduction of the tested ear may be an indirect measure of the sensitivity of the nontest ear. In order to "block" the nontest ear while the other is being tested, we introduce a sound (usually some type of noise) into the nontest ear. This is known as clinical masking.

The greatest problem in clinical masking is to select a level of noise that will effectively mask the nontest ear without interfering with the sensitivity of the test ear. The reported relationship between threshold shift in the test ear and noise increase in the normal

nontest ear (*1*, *2*) is depicted in the generalized curve (Figure 38-1). The first shift, *A*, is taken to indicate insufficient masking; the plateau, *B*, appropriate masking; and the final shift, *C*, overmasking.

Several investigators (Feldman [*1*], Studebaker [*2*], Naunton [*3*]) have developed formulations and procedures to facilitate the selection of the appropriate noise level for effective masking so that thresholds might be obtained without tracking the entire function. Assumptions underlying the formulations seem to be (1) that only one plateau exists; (2) that this plateau represents true threshold; (3) that knowing the amount of noise needed to mask normal ears, we can extrapolate to the patient who has either middle ear or inner ear deficits, or both; (4) that individual differences in response characteristics, in motivation, and in "central noise" effects are nonexistent, negligible, or noncontrollable.

In our practice, however, these assumptions were not borne out. More than one plateau was often obtained in a single function. In one patient alone, more than one plateau was obtained in each function at four different frequencies (Figure 38-2). Since more than one plateau exists, uncertainty remains as to which plateau truly represents threshold.

Secondly, in several patients asymptotic straight line functions (ie, plateaus neither preceded nor followed by a rise) were obtained throughout the noise range. Such a

Reprinted by permission of the author from *Arch. Otolaryngol.*, **82,** pp. 518–521 (1965).

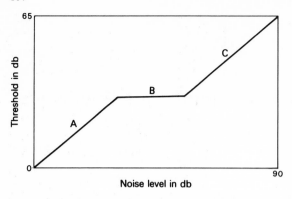

Figure 38-1. Threshold shift in test ear plotted as a function of level of noise introduced into normal nontest ear.

plateau might indicate a true threshold or might, just as well, indicate insufficient masking of the contralateral ear even at 90 db of noise.

Thirdly, noise constituting effective masking in a normal ear cannot be extrapolated to an ear with losses. The very pattern of loss changes the quality and effectiveness of white noise (Denes and Naunton [4], Zwislocki [5]).

And finally, persons respond so differently to the mere introduction of noise in the test situation, that some control for its effect must be included in the procedure.

It was from the recognition of these problems that our present procedure evolved. Briefly, the procedure involves the determination of a minimum effective masking level (MEML) for each person at each frequency. MEML is found by introducing the masking stimulus into the *same* ear that is receiving the AC signal at threshold intensity. The noise intensity is increased in steps of 10 db until

it just obliterates the signal. (This is an accepted experimental technique for masking of pure tone.) It is this obtained MEML which is used initially to mask the ear when the BC threshold of the opposite (test ear) is being validated. The rationale is as follows: if the obtained BC threshold for the test ear were valid, ie, if the tone were perceived in the test ear, it would not be affected by the MEML presented to the nontest ear.

On the other hand, if the obtained BC threshold of the test ear were spurious, ie, were not a true measure of that ear, but rather an indirect (or attenuated) measure of the nontest ear, MEML presented to the nontest ear would render the previous BC "threshold" stimulus at the test ear imperceptible. Threshold sensation in the nontest ear is the same regardless of the nature of the stimulus which evokes that sensation. It is assumed, therefore, that MEML required to mask that threshold sensation remains constant.

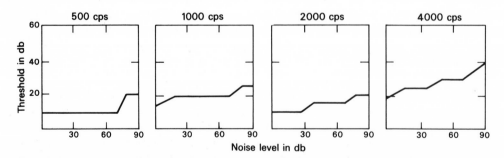

Figure 38-2. Threshold shift in test ear as a function of level of noise introduced into nontest ear at four different frequencies.

A detailed description of the procedure follows.

PROCEDURE

We obtain AC and BC thresholds in the conventional way.[1] We mask for BC thresholds whenever a difference of 10 db or more exists between AC and BC thresholds of the same ear. Let us assume that such a difference was found in the right ear at 2 kc. We would proceed as follows:

1. Give instructions to the patient. "In this test you will again be listening for a pulsating tone. However, this time you will also hear a noise that sounds like rushing wind. Try to ignore the noise. Keep your finger up as long as you continue to hear the pulsating tone. The very moment you lose the pulsating tone, lower your finger. You will sometimes hear the pulsating tone in one ear; sometimes in the other. Don't be concerned with which ear is hearing it. *Just be sure that your finger is up for as long as you hear the pulsating tone, and comes down the very moment you do not hear it.*"

2. Place the headphone on the nontest (left) ear and the bone oscillator on the test (right) ear.

3. Using an interrupted 2 kc signal, determine AC threshold in the nontest ear. (The original value is not used since the intensity of signal required to elicit a threshold sensation under these conditions may be different from what it is when two headphones are used.)

4. With the interrupted signal continued at threshold intensity, introduce noise to the same ear. Gradually, increase the noise (in steps of 10 db) just until the signal is no longer perceptible. This is the minimum effective masking level.

5. Discontinue stimulation of the nontest ear.

6. Using an interrupted 2 kc signal through the oscillator, determine BC threshold in the test ear. A new threshold value is determined since the intensity of signal required to elicit a threshold sensation under these conditions may be different from what it is when neither ear is covered.

7. With the interrupted signal continued at threshold intensity in the test ear (via the bone oscillator) reintroduce noise into the nontest ear at the MEML determined in step 4, above. *If with this amount of masking of the nontest ear the BC signal is still perceptible, we accept the originally obtained threshold as the true threshold.*[2] If the BC signal is not perceptible with this amount of noise in the nontest ear, we proceed as follows:

8. Gradually increase the intensity of the BC signal until it is again just perceptible (new threshold).

9. Increase level of noise 10 db to nontest ear. If threshold shifts again, continue steps 7 and 8 until a plateau is reached, ie, until there is ho change in threshold for two consecutive levels of noise (10 db apart) and accept that as the true threshold.

The advantages of the described procedure are the following:

1. The first plateau obtained may be accepted as the true threshold of the tested ear making further masking at that frequency unnecessary. Since masking was begun at the MEML of the nontest ear, we are assured that we have sufficient noise to avoid undermasking. In addition, because we do not add 30 to 50 db of noise to MEML as a starting point, there is less danger of fatigue/or of overmasking, or both.[3]

2. Determining MEML enables us to determine when the limit of noise (90 db) is insufficient to mask the nontest ear. In such

---

[1] Our equipment includes the Beltone Audiometer, model 15B, with white noise generator having a maximum sound pressure output of 108 db RE 0.0002 dyne/cm².

[2] We accept the original BC threshold that was obtained before placing the headphone on the masked ear, since it is free of any occlusion effect so introduced.

[3] Griesman (6) found evidence of vasospasm, increase of sludge, and jamming of the conjunctival blood vessels two minutes after an 80 second exposure to noise at 65 db. Changes in the conjunctival vessels are thought to reflect similar labyrinthine changes. Since nothing is reported regarding the recovery time following such exposure, it seems desirable to avoid exposure to intense noise as much as possible.

TABLE 38-1. A CASE OF COMPLETE UNILATERAL SENSORINEURAL LOSS

Thresholds Obtained Without Masking

Air Conduction								Bone Conduction							
Right				Left				Right				Left			
500	1000	2000	4000	500	1000	2000	4000	500	1000	2000	4000	500	1000	2000	4000
60	60	65	75	10	10	5	15	10	15	30	45	10	15	15	25

Thresholds Obtained With Masking

Level of Noise Input in Nontest Ear

db	Air Conduction								Bone Conduction							
	Right				Left				Right				Left			
	500	1000	2000	4000	500	1000	2000	4000	500	1000	2000	4000	500	1000	2000	4000
0	60	60	65	75					10	20	30	40				
20																
30		×70														
40		80								×40						
50	×80	90	×NR	×NR					×30	45	×NR	×NR				
60	90	100							40	55						
70	100	NR							50	60						
80	NR								65	NR						
90									NR							

× Indicates minimum effective masking level obtained when both signal and noise were presented to nontest ear.
NR, no response.

a situation, masking is not attempted, and the error of accepting an unmasked threshold as a masked threshold is eliminated.

3. In determining MEML individually at each frequency, we control for differences in the masking effectiveness of white noise which may be a function of the particular pattern of hearing loss (4, 5).

4. In determining the MEML for the individual person we achieve, as a standard for comparison, a level which includes not only the person's adjustments to "central noise" and his motivational level but also the level of ambient noise in the testing room.

5. The same procedure is applicable regardless of type of noise used, calibration of noise, or level of ambient noise in the testing room. Indeed, the same procedure (except for the fact that both headphones are used) is applicable for determining air-conduction thresholds under masking.

SAMPLE CASE STUDIES

More than 200 veterans have now been tested using this method of masking. Initially, one audiologist (I) was called upon to do the masking whenever it was required. Often, then, the masking was done "blind", ie,

without prior knowledge of the medical findings, indeed, without even seeing the veteran being tested. We shall present two of the records obtained in this manner (ie, with blind masking), one sensorineural and one conductive type loss.

Table 38-1 indicates the thresholds in a case of complete, unilateral, sensorineural loss. Thresholds shifted when masking was introduced at MEML and continued to shift as masking increased.

The medical history of this patient revealed "unsuccessful stapes surgery to the right ear resulting in complete loss unilaterally in addition to unilateral facial paralysis."

The second case (Table 38-2) was selected for presentation because, in a sense, it represents a critical experiment. One might expect masking to fail (ie, to distort the true picture) in the case of a bilateral conductive loss where one ear has a much greater loss than the other. MEML in the poorer ear would be so high (80 or 90 db) that the noise would presumably cross over and interfere with the better ear. Thus, the better ear would behave like a sensorineural loss, with thresholds increasing as MEML is introduced to the contralateral ear. The patient represented in Table 38-2 has a binaural conductive loss with differences of 35 db and 30 db at 500 cps

TABLE 38-2. A CASE OF BINAURAL CONDUCTIVE LOSS

Thresholds Obtained Without Masking

Air Conduction								Bone Conduction							
Right				Left				Right				Left			
500	1000	2000	4000	500	1000	2000	4000	500	1000	2000	4000	500	1000	2000	4000
50	50	40	45	15	20	25	30	−10	−5	5	5	0	0	10	25

Thresholds Obtained With Masking

Level of Noise Input in Nontest Ear

db ↓	Air Conduction								Bone Conduction							
	Right				Left				Right				Left			
	500	1000	2000	4000	500	1000	2000	4000	500	1000	2000	4000	500	1000	2000	4000
0	50	50	40	45					−10	0	5	0	5	0	15	15
20																
30																
40									× −10′		× 5′					
50									−10		5	× 0′				
60	× 50′	× 50′	× 40′	× 45′					−10	× 0′	5	0				
70	50	50	40	45					−10	0	5	0			× 15′	× 25
80	55	55	45	50					−5	5	5	0		× 0	20	25′
90	55	55	50	50					−5	5	10	5	× 5′	0	20	25

× Indicates minimum effective masking level obtained when both signal and noise were presented to nontest ear.

′ In the normal testing situation this would be accepted as the true threshold, and masking would be discontinued.

and 1,000 cps respectively.[4] Masking did not alter the picture of binaural conductive loss at these frequencies. The loss in the left ear at 4,000 cps emerges as sensorineural, a common

[4] Though several cases were found to have larger differences between thresholds, the poorer ear was so poor, that there was insufficient noise in the system to attain the MEML.

finding in a veteran population, especially among those who were exposed to sustained gunfire or artillery fire. The medical history of this veteran included a diagnosis of binaural otosclerosis, and a recent tympanotomy of the left ear revealed "adhesions in middle ear across round window" resulting from previous surgery.

REFERENCES

1. Feldman, A. S.: Clinical Bone-Conduction Testing, part 2, Maico Audiological Library Series, No. 4.

2. Studebaker, G. A.: Clinical Masking of Air- and Bone-Conducted Stimuli, *J Speech Hearing Dis* **29**:23–35, 1964.

3. Naunton, R. F.: Clinical Bone-Conduction Audiometry, *Arch Otolaryng* **66**:281–298, 1957.

4. Denes, P., and Naunton, R. F.: Masking in Pure Tone Audiometry, *Proc Roy Soc Med* **45**:790–794, 1952.

5. Zwislocki, J.: Eine Verbesserte vertäubungsmethode für die Audiometrie, *Acta Otolaryng* **39**:338–356, 1951.

6. Griesman, B.: Vascular Patterns of the Conjunctival Vessels in Cases of Deafness, Tinnitus and Dizziness, presented at the meeting of the American Academy of Ophthalmology and Otolaryngology, 1964, Chicago.

part VI

IDENTIFICATION AUDIOMETRY

The early identification of children with hearing loss is an important concern for a diverse group of professionals, a group that includes audiologists, otolaryngologists, pediatricians, educators, and nurses. Early identification of hearing loss results, ideally, in early diagnosis and medical treatment and in early habilitation including correct amplification, speech and language therapy, lipreading and auditory training, and proper educational placement. The goal of an identification audiometry program for school or pre-school children was stated succinctly in Monograph Supplement No. 9 (1961) of the *Journal of Speech and Hearing Disorders*: "The goal is to locate children who have even minimal hearing problems so that they can be referred for medical treatment of any active ear conditions discovered to be present and so that remedial educational procedures can be instituted at the earliest possible date" (p. 16).

Identification audiometry is only one aspect, albeit a very important one, of a total hearing conservation program. To identify a child with a hearing loss is of little value unless the child is followed, appropriate medical treatment obtained, and needed habilitative measures taken. While numerous studies assess the efficiency of hearing tests used in identifying children with hearing loss, relatively little emphasis has been given thus far to evaluating the efficiency of a total program in hearing conservation.

Downs and Sterritt's article, which describes their procedures for identifying hearing loss in infants, is placed first in this section to underline the need for hearing conservation to begin as early in life as possible. The program elaborated by Downs and Sterritt has not, however, gone unchallenged. Goodhill (1967), for example, has questioned the efficiency of neonatal programs for screening hearing; others are concerned about the high false positive rates, the difficulty in identifying false negatives, and the problems involved in quantifying infants' responses (Goldstein and Tait, 1971). Downs and Sterritt do, nevertheless, describe a program that appears to have worked in practice, and, while further research is needed and is being conducted (Eisenberg, *et al.*, 1964; Eisenberg, 1965; Field, *et al.*, 1967), their work represents an important step in the development of a practical program in neonatal screening.

Downs and Doster have constructed a program that probably does represent, to use their words, ". . . the first large scale hearing screening of children between the ages of 3 and 5 in the United States." We ourselves are convinced that the hearing screening of pre-school children between the ages of two and five represents one of the most neglected aspects of identification audiometry. We are familiar with only a few articles in this area (for example, Leshin, 1960; Griffing, Simonton, and Hedgecock, 1967).

Despite the general availability of audiometric equipment, personnel, and test procedures for conducting hearing screening of school-age children, many school systems continue to place too much reliance on teacher identification of children with hearing problems. In their 1956 article, Geyer and Yankauer demonstrated that this method is inadequate for identification purposes. Far too many children with hearing loss are overlooked while too many children with normal hearing are suspected of hearing loss. The classroom teacher may be able to supplement a good program in hearing screening, but she can never serve as a substitute for a hearing test.

Several factors governed our selection of two chapters from the *Journal of Speech and Hearing Disorders*, Monograph No. 9, entitled "Identification Audiometry." First, the two chapters cover a hearing identification program for school-age children in nearly all of its important aspects, including hearing levels to be used (re the ASA-1951 standard), frequencies to be tested, pass-fail criteria, periodicity of testing, equipment, and personnel. Second, a large number of school systems have adopted many of the recommendations made in the chapters. Finally, we have no strong disagreement with the recommendations and believe them, with a few exceptions, to be as valid today as they were in 1961.

Melnick, Eagles, and Levine, in a well-designed study, evaluated some of the recommendations put forth in the Identification Audiometry monograph. Their findings lend strong support to the recommendations made regarding test frequencies, hearing levels, and pass-fail criteria. They found, for example, that the recommended procedure for screening hearing identified correctly 96 percent of the children, had a false positive rate of 1.5 percent, and had a false negative rate of 2.5 percent. Melnick, Eagles, and Levine state that the purpose of an identification program is not only to identify children with hearing loss but also ". . . to locate children with active ear conditions for medical treatment." They found, however, that the hearing-screening program was grossly inefficient in identifying children with ear disease.

Downs, Doster, and Weaver contend in their article "Dilemmas in Identification Audiometry" that a hearing-screening program cannot be expected to identify children with active or past ear pathology, that it is inappropriate to evaluate the efficiency of a hearing-screening test in these terms, and that ". . . fewer than 1 percent of all the significant hearing problems fall into the class that might be preventable if special techniques other than audiometry were used earlier to detect minor deviations." Downs, Doster, and Weaver also insist that greater attention and effort should be devoted to screening children in kindergarten through the third grade since the vast majority of children with hearing loss can be identified by the time they reach the third grade.

In the late 1950's and early 1960's, considerable attention was given to the concept that screening at a limited number of frequencies (4000 Hz or 2000 and 4000 Hz) would detect children who had hearing loss not only at the frequencies tested but at other frequencies as well. (See Newby, 1964, pp. 218 and 220, for a relatively complete list of articles on limited frequency screening.) Unfortunately, most of the research done on limited frequency screening has had significant methodological shortcomings. As a result, we feel that the definitive study of limited frequency screening has yet to be done. We present Siegenthaler's article here because it highlights some of the factors that must be considered in evaluating limited frequency screening and other hearing-screening tests.

In some large school systems, a group hearing test may be more efficient and more desirable than an individual screening test. In the last article in this section, DiCarlo and Gardner report their evaluation of three group pure-tone hearing tests and, on the basis of their findings, make recommendations on the use of group and individual testing in the schools. In addition, DiCarlo and Gardner present a brief historical overview of group testing of hearing and show the method typically used in evaluating the efficiency of group and individual tests for screening hearing. [See Thorner and Remein (1961) for a more detailed description of procedures that can be used to evaluate the efficiency of hearing-screening tests.]

No mention has been made of identification audiometry in military or industrial programs, mainly because until recently, audiologists were seldom involved in hearing-screening programs in the armed forces or industry. The interested reader is referred to the reference list for some sources on industrial and military audiometry.

REFERENCES

1. American Industrial Hygiene Association. *Industrial noise manual.* Detroit, Mich.: American Industrial Hygiene Association, 1966.

2. Davis, H., Hoople, G., and Parrack, H. O. The medical principles of monitoring audiometry. *Arch. Indust. Health,* **17,** pp. 1–20 (1958).

3. Eisenberg, R. B. Auditory behavior in the human neonate: methodologic problems and the logical design of research procedures. *J. aud. Res.,* **5,** pp. 159–177 (1965).

4. Eisenberg, R. B., Griffin, E. J., Coursin, D. B., and Hunter, M. A. Auditory behavior in the neonate: a preliminary report. *J. Speech Hearing Res.,* **7,** pp. 233–244 (1964).

5. Field, H., Copack, P., Derbyshire, A. J., Driessen, G. J., and Marcus, R. E. Responses of newborns to auditory stimulation. *J. aud. Res.,* **7,** pp. 271–285 (1967).

6. Goldstein, R., and Tait, C. Critique of neonatal hearing evaluation. *J. Speech Hearing Dis.,* 36, 3-18 (1971).

7. Goodhill, V. Detection of hearing loss in neonates. *Arch. Otolaryngol.,* **85,** p. 1 (1967).

8. Griffing, T., Simonton, K., and Hedgecock, L. Verbal auditory screening for pre-school children. *Trans. Amer. Acad. Ophthalmol. Otolaryngol.,* **71,** pp. 105–111 (1967).

9. Leshin, G. A. Pre-school hearing conservation on a state-wide basis. *J. Speech Hearing Dis.,* **25,** pp. 346–348 (1960).

10. Newby, H. A. *Audiology* (2nd ed.). New York: Appleton-Century-Crofts, 1964.

11. Sataloff, J. Industrial deafness. New York: McGraw-Hill, 1957.

12. Thorner, R. M., and Remein, Q. R. Principles and procedures in the evaluation of screening for disease. Public Health Monograph No. 67; Washington, D. C.: Government Printing Office, 1961.

13. Usher, J. R. (Ed.) Problems in military audiometry: A CHABA symposium. *J. Speech Hearing Dis.,* **22,** pp. 729–756 (1957).

39

A Guide to Newborn
and Infant Hearing Screening Programs

MARION P. DOWNS
GRAHAM M. STERRITT

MARION P. DOWNS is Director, Clinical Audiology, and Assistant Professor of Otolaryngology, University of Colorado Medical Center

GRAHAM M. STERRITT, Ph.D., is Associate Professor, Division of Clinical Psychology, University of Colorado Medical Center and Director, McClelland Learning Institute

The screening of newborn infants for hearing problems has been widely urged by otolaryngologists, educators, and audiologists ([1–3]). From the medical point of view, the detection of hearing loss at birth offers both an opportunity for early medical treatment and a source of valuable information on the etiology of hearing problems. From the educational and audiological points of view, early detection provides the opportunity to apply auditory habilitation at an age that is most likely to ensure the optimum development of the hearing function. It is generally agreed ([2]) that detection should be made before the infant is 6 months old so that medical or educational treatment can be initiated. Inasmuch as the newborn nursery is the only place where the entire infant population is conveniently available for screening, it is most feasible to conduct screening tests there. Such screening has found increasing acceptance among pediatricians, who are currently focusing a great deal of attention on all aspects of newborn functioning. To them, the economics of a hearing screening program which will detect deficiencies in 1 child in 2,000 or 3,000 is no less logical than the accepted testing for phenylketonuria (PKU), which detects 1 child in 4,000 to 6,000.

Otolaryngologists will be called upon to supervise, counsel, and monitor the professional conduct of newborn screening programs. For this reason it will be useful to have a description of the procedures of a typical community effort in newborn screening to use as a guide in the conduct of further programs. The program from which the following descriptions are taken has been operating for ten months in one Denver hospital, seven months in three Denver hospitals, and four months in three other hospitals in the Denver area. The techniques that are used were developed at the University of Colorado Medical School and reported by Downs and Sterritt ([4]). Although it has been impossible thus far to determine the validity of the technique, i.e., whether it identifies all the hearing impairments of a given degree that are present at birth, several deaf infants have been identified during the course of the program and are benefiting from the early detection. Whatever technique is used—and better ones may certainly be developed in the future—the experiences gained from this ongoing program should be helpful to anyone contemplating newborn screening.

Reprinted by permission of the authors from *Arch. Otolaryngol.*, **85,** pp. 15–22 (1967).

PURPOSES

The goal of the screening program is to identify newborn infants who may have congenital hearing losses of severe degree (65 to 100 db average), so that their physicians will be alerted to look for hearing problems that can be treated or habilitated early. Many deaf or hard-of-hearing children are not identified until they are 2, 3, 4, or 5 years old, at which points valuable time has been lost in their medical or educational rehabilitation. The general trend among educators and audiologists is to begin habilitative procedures for a hearing-handicapped child just as early as possible, in order to develop what hearing remains and to prevent retardation in speech and language as far as possible.

Another valuable aspect of this program is the acquisition of information regarding the causes of hearing loss. It has been variously estimated that 30 percent to 40 percent of all the sensorineural hearing losses in children are of unknown origin. Because most of the losses have not been detected until long after birth, it has been impossible to tell from retrospective case histories whether the losses were present at birth or whether they developed following birth. The determination of hearing status at birth will thus be of far-reaching medical importance.

PERSONNEL

The hospital board contemplating a screening program acts on the advice and counsel of its otolaryngologists and pediatricians in establishing the program. The immediate supervision of the program and the training of the testers are undertaken by a qualified audiologist. The audiologist need not be in residence at the hospital, but he should be in touch with the testers at all times and should check periodically on the interobserver reliability that obtains among the testers.

The testers need not be professional persons. Intelligent, observant volunteers can learn the techniques as well as professionals. This aspect reduces the cost of the program and makes it economically feasible. Trained volunteers from the Junior League of Denver have been successfully carrying out newborn screening in six Denver hospitals, and trained volunteers from the Hospital Auxiliary have conducted the testing in another hospital. The only requisite is that the testers be good observers who can be trained to categorize the infant responses according to a fairly rigid protocol. During the training, poor observers can be identified and "shaped up" or dropped from the program through interobserver comparison with experienced testers.

The volunteers are prepared to abide by all hospital regulations for gowning, masking, scrubbing, etc. Requirements differ, but can usually be met easily and consistently by the volunteers. One important consideration is that the volunteers become members of the Hospital Auxiliary, in order to meet insurance regulations.

EQUIPMENT

Two light, portable instruments have been developed and standardized for neonate testing. Both were designed by electronics companies to the authors' specifications, and are currently available on the market.

1. The *Vicon Apriton* (A-Z signal generator) produces two acoustic signals: one, a filtered narrow band of white noise peaking at 3,000 cps and containing most of its energy between 2,800 cps and 3,800 cps. presented with optional outputs of 70, 80, 90, or 100 db SPL, measured at 4 inches from the source. This is the criterion signal. The second signal is a white noise stimulus covering the entire frequency range of 100 to 10,000, also presented at 70, 80, 90, or 100 db sound pressure level (SPL). This instrument was used in the original neonate screening study (*4*).

2. The *Rudmose Warblet 300* is a single signal generator producing a 3,000-cps tone that is warbled with an FM duration of ±150 cycles at a 30 to 40 cycle rate, presented with optional outputs of 80, 90, 100 db SPL, measured 10 inches from the source. A comparison in 280 cases (unpublished research by Downs, Ster-

ritt, and Squires, 1965) of the response intensities produced by this instrument with the response intensities produced by the Apriton showed the two instruments to be equally effective in all states except when the infant is asleep; under this condition the Warblet possibly tended to elicit slightly higher intensities of response.

The 3,000-cps signal in both instruments is the criterion test signal, which the infant must respond to in order to be cleared. The reason for employing this type of specific signal is that it differentiates from the normal-hearing child those infants with hearing losses that may be more severe in the high frequencies than in the low. Most congenital losses of significant degree show poorer hearing at 3,000 cps than at 125 or 250 cps (5) and the use of a broadband noise—a bell, a horn, a clacker, or a handclap will produce unwanted responses in such cases. A child with a hearing loss of 75 db (re: audiometric zero) or more at 3,000 cps will not respond to a 90-db SPL signal at 3,000 cps, which would be very close to his threshold. Such a child may well have considerably better hearing at frequencies lower than 3,000 cps, so it is expected that fairly moderate losses may be identified.

The easy portability of the instruments and their placement 4 to 10 inches from the infant's ears make it possible for the testing to be accomplished without any contact with the infant or its crib. Occasionally a crib may have to be moved for more convenient positioning, but no other contact is usually necessary.

LOCATION OF TESTING

The tests are done within the newborn nursery itself, with the testers moving from crib to crib and presenting the sound to each child. In this way there is no disruption of nursery routine. It is doubtful whether any program would be acceptable if it disturbed the nurses' schedules or caused them inconvenience. In the premature nurseries where infants are in Isolettes it is necessary to have the nurses lift up the cover so the horn or speaker can be brought close to the child. However, because of the long stay of infants in the premature

nursery, the frequency of testing of these infants is reduced and does not prove to be bothersome.

The presentation of sound to a child in one crib has not been found to disturb any of the other infants sufficiently to affect the subsequent tests on the others. The horn or loudspeaker that delivers the sound is fairly directional, and loudness levels at a short distance and angle from the horn are considerably attenuated.

TIME OF TESTING

The first consideration in scheduling the testing is that it must conform to the nursery routine. Feeding times, bathing times, etc. must be avoided for the sake of the nursery personnel. The optimum testing time from the testers' point of view is 45 minutes to 1 hour before the next feeding. During this time the child is not in the deep sleep that follows feeding, nor in the fretful stage that immediately precedes the next feeding. If this period can conform with nursery routine, the testing should be scheduled accordingly.

Because of the short confinement stay now prevalent in most hospitals, testing should be done every other day in order not to miss infants whose mothers may be discharged after two or three days.

INFANT STATE

The first thing that should be observed is the pretesting state of the infant. It is important to record the state, because the responses that will be seen occur out of the matrix of the infant's ongoing behavior at the time. As shown on the form in the Figure, the condition of the eyelids, face, and body should be noted. For example, if the eyes are closed and the face and body are quiet, an eyelid response such as an eyeblink or an eye widening can be credited with more confidence than if the response occurs out of random movement. It has been found (4) that it is easier to see responses when the child is quiet or sleeping

INFANT SCREENING TEST OF HEARING

RESPONSE INTENSITY: 1-NONE 2-OBSCURED 3-WEAK BUT CLEAR 4-STRONG 5-PAROXSYMAL

Proj. Case No.	Hosp.	SUBJECT LAST, FIRST NAME	Hosp. Case No.	Sex	Birthdate	Crib or Inc.	Test Date	Feed Times		Ear	Rat-er	Clear Sus.
					9-14 Hr. Born		20-25 Time	Last	Next			
1-6	7		8		15-18	19	26-29	30-33	34-37	38	39	40

1.

STIMULUS				INFANT STATE												RESPONSE								Time	CO-RATER	
F	DB	Dur	Rep	Eyelids			Face						Body			Int.	Type								Name	Indep
				Closed	Droop	Open	Quiet	Suck	Grim	Vocal	Fret	Cry	Quiet	Limbs	Whole		Lid	Widen	Cess.	Limb	Turn	Suck	Mov.			
2	3-5	6	7-8	9	10	11	12	13	14	15	16	17	18	19	20	21	22	23	24	25	26	27	28	29	30	31

2. TEST DATE:

STIMULUS				INFANT STATE												RESPONSE								Time	CO-RATER	
F	DB	Dur	Rep	Eyelids			Face						Body			Int.	Type								Name	Indep
				Closed	Droop	Open	Quiet	Suck	Grim	Vocal	Fret	Cry	Quiet	Limbs	Whole		Lid	Widen	Cess.	Limb	Turn	Suck	Mov.			
2	3-5	6	7-8	9	10	11	12	13	14	15	16	17	18	19	20	21	22	23	24	25	26	27	28	29	30	31

3. TEST DATE:

STIMULUS				INFANT STATE												RESPONSE								Time	CO-RATER	
F	DB	Dur	Rep	Eyelids			Face						Body			Int.	Type								Name	Indep
				Closed	Droop	Open	Quiet	Suck	Grim	Vocal	Fret	Cry	Quiet	Limbs	Whole		Lid	Widen	Cess.	Limb	Turn	Suck	Mov.			
2	3-5	6	7-8	9	10	11	12	13	14	15	16	17	18	19	20	21	22	23	24	25	26	27	28	29	30	31

4. TEST DATE:

STIMULUS				INFANT STATE												RESPONSE								Time	CO-RATER	
F	DB	Dur	Rep	Eyelids			Face						Body			Int.	Type								Name	Indep
				Closed	Droop	Open	Quiet	Suck	Grim	Vocal	Fret	Cry	Quiet	Limbs	Whole		Lid	Widen	Cess.	Limb	Turn	Suck	Mov.			
2	3-5	6	7-8	9	10	11	12	13	14	15	16	17	18	19	20	21	22	23	24	25	26	27	28	29	30	31

5. TEST DATE:

STIMULUS				INFANT STATE												RESPONSE								Time	CO-RATER	
F	DB	Dur	Rep	Eyelids			Face						Body			Int.	Type								Name	Indep
				Closed	Droop	Open	Quiet	Suck	Grim	Vocal	Fret	Cry	Quiet	Limbs	Whole		Lid	Widen	Cess.	Limb	Turn	Suck	Mov.			
2	3-5	6	7-8	9	10	11	12	13	14	15	16	17	18	19	20	21	22	23	24	25	26	27	28	29	30	31

6. TEST DATE:

STIMULUS				INFANT STATE												RESPONSE								Time	CO-RATER	
F	DB	Dur	Rep	Eyelids			Face						Body			Int.	Type								Name	Indep
				Closed	Droop	Open	Quiet	Suck	Grim	Vocal	Fret	Cry	Quiet	Limbs	Whole		Lid	Widen	Cess.	Limb	Turn	Suck	Mov.			
2	3-5	6	7-8	9	10	11	12	13	14	15	16	17	18	19	20	21	22	23	24	25	26	27	28	29	30	31

than where he is awake or fretful. The record of the infant's state is thus useful to anyone examining the records at a later date.

RESPONSES TO BE OBSERVED

The responses of the infants are recorded on the form shown in the Figure. (Instructions for filling out this form are given in Table 39-1.) These represent the classic newborn infant responses to sound. The eyeblink response, or auropalpebral reflex, consists of either a slight or a very exaggerated drawing of the lids to-

TABLE 39-I. INFANT SCREENING TEST OF HEARING TEST FORMS AND INSTRUCTIONS

Infant Screening Test of Hearing, Instructions for Use of the Record Form:

The record form is designed for flexible application to many different clinical and research situations in which the Infant Screening Test of Hearing might be used. The top line contains boxes for identification data on the infant, hospital, and person doing the rating of responses. Each of the following lines, numbered one to six, contains spaces for recording information on a single trial, so that as many as six successive trials with one infant can be scored on a single form. It is probable that some of the information called for on the form will be irrelevant to some applications. When this is the case, the irrelevant boxes can, of course, be left blank. Space has been left at the bottom of the form, and the entire back of the form is blank, so that additional information can be entered.

The small numbers in the left-hand corners of some boxes are to aid a key-punch operator to punch cards for computer tabulation of infant test information. The person administering the Infant Screening Test of Hearing should pay no attention to those numbers.

The form is to be completed as follows:

Identification Data

Project Case No.	As many as six letters or digits, supplied by the project secretary. The same project case number should appear on all records referring to the same infant.
Hospital	A single letter or digit—see hospital code supplied by secretary.
Subject: Last, first name	Any number of letters.
Hospital Case No.	Any number of digits.
Sex	M or F.
Birthdate	It is less confusing to *write* the name of the month, as March 12, 1965, rather than use a number for the month.
Hour born	Designate AM or PM and the hour.
Crib or Incubator	Indicate which the infant is in when tested (C or I).
Test Date	*Write* the name of the month; use numerals for day and year.
Test Time	Designate AM or PM and the hour.
Feeding Times	Designate AM or PM next to the hour—usually obtainable from nursery personnel.
Ear	Indicate if right ear or left ear (R or L) is to be stimulated, depending upon the infant's position.
Rater	One letter—see rater code supplied by secretary.
Cleared or Suspect	Enter when the screening test is completed (C or S).

Test Data

Test No. (1–6)	Printed on test form. If more than 6 tests are given, cross out printed Nos. 1–6 and enter 7–12.
Stimulus	If more than one trial is to be given with no change in the stimulus settings, the stimulus information may be entered once, with an arrow down through the other test-stimulus-setting boxes to indicate that all were the same.
Flat	Enter F = flat, or 3 = 3,000 cps.
Decibels	Enter the intensity setting: 70, 80, 90, or 100.
Duration	Enter 2 if the standard stimulus-duration of approximately 2 seconds is used.
Repetition	Enter 15 if the standard repetition rate of 1 stimulus every 15 seconds is followed.
Infant State	Check the box that best describes the infant's state before the stimulus is applied. Note and score this *before every* stimulus presentation.
Eyelids:	
Closed	Lids remain closed through approximately 10 seconds of prestimulation observation.
Droop	Lids appear "heavy," half open, or slowly opening and shutting.
Open	Lids remain open or blink rapidly but do not droop.
Facial Activity:	
Quiet	None of the facial activity listed below is present.
Suck	Active sucking in air or on digits, etc.
Grimace	Active facial movement without vocalization.
Vocal	Vocal noises such as grunting, not including whimpering or crying.
Fret	Whimpering or weak crying.
Cry	Moderate to strong crying.
Body Movement:	
Quiet	No discernible movement.
Limbs	Movement restricted to one or more limbs.
Whole	Movement of more than two limbs at once.

Response Intensity	Score immediately after *each* stimulus presentation—do not try to record several trials at once.
	Score 1 to 5 according to the scale printed at the bottom of the record form.
No Demonstrated Response to Sound	1. Total or near total inactivity before and during stimulation. 2. The infant is active before the stimulus is applied, obscuring the response— a response *is* seen which *could* be in reaction to the stimulus, but the ongoing activity makes it difficult to be sure.
Demonstrated Responses to Sound	3. There is little ongoing activity, so it is clear that the response was in reaction to the stimulus, even though the response was weak. 4. Any *very* clear response to the stimulus. 5. A very violent response that must involve the whole body.
Response Type:	
Lid	Blinking of the eyelid.
Widen	Eyelids suddenly open wide.
Cessation	Cessation of ongoing activity.
Limb	Jerking of 1 or 2 limbs.
Turn	Turning head or eyes toward (T) or away (A) from loud-speaker.
Suck	Sucking movements.
Movement	Movement of some part of the body or the whole body, but not classifiable as any of the above. Example: stretching of head and neck.
Response Time	Enter O if the response is immediately after onset of the stimulus, or a single digit denoting the approximate number of seconds after onset of the stimulus that the response began.
Co-rater:	
Name	If two people observe the same infant simultaneously, enter the code letter for the other rater.
Independent	It often happens that one rater communicates his judgment to the other, either in words or by facial expressions, etc. Do not check the independence box unless the two raters scored all categories *entirely* independently.

gether. It can be accompanied by a complete facial grimace. Occasionally the eyes will widen noticeably, particularly if they are in a drooping state, and this will represent a kind of arousal response. If the infant is very active, i.e., the limbs are flailing and the head is turning about, the signal may cause a momentary cessation of all movement, indicating a response to the sound. If the infant is sleeping or in a drowsy state, the sound may produce a fluttering or raising of the limbs, most noticeable in the hands. More often than might be expected the infant gives a head turn, either toward or away from the sound source. Sucking activity is elicited occasionally, especially from a background of light sleep. General body movements are sometimes observed in response to the signal, such as shoulder shrugging, stirring from sleep, or stretching of the head and neck. The Moro reflex, or startle, is a classic response in which the entire body jerks and the limbs are drawn toward the midline in a sort of paroxysm. Because of its uniqueness, the Moro response is recorded as a special intensity value rather than as a response type.

The intensity of the responses are recorded on a 5-point scale, as follows:

Nonhearing zone 1 = No response
2 = Questionable
Hearing zone 3 = Slight but definite
4 = Strong
5 = Paroxysmal (Moro response)

The advantages of using an intensity scale such as this are first, it lends itself to research investigations, and second, it is useful in determining interobserver reliability in the training and supervision of observers. The recording of the response type is also useful in the training of observers, as it gives them specific phenomena to look for (Table 39-2). A movie* depicting the various response categories is available for demonstration and training purposes.

PROCEDURE

After following hospital requirements for sterile technique, the testers go into the nursery

[* Two movies demonstrating the techniques are currently available: "Not Cleared for Hearing:" 15 min., color, sound. Price Vowell Associates, 3491 Cahuenga Blvd. West, Suite 2, Hollywood, Calif., 90028. "Auditory Responses of Infants:" 5 min., silent, color. Thorne Films, Inc., 1229 University Ave., Boulder, Colo. MPD, GMS]

area with the testing instrument. In the routine testing, two or three observers watch the responses of each child and record them on individual forms. They group themselves in an advantageous position around the crib and observe the infant for a few moments before presenting the signal. The pretesting state of the infant is recorded before the signal is given. One of the testers then positions the instrument at the prescribed distance from the exposed ear and gives the 90-db signal, usually for a 2-second duration. Immediately, the observers record their judgment of the type and intensity of the response, without communicating their evaluation in any way to the other testers. (The independence of the observations

made tends to be maintained if the testers are asked to record under "Indep", whether or not any communication occurred.) If no response is seen in the opinion of the tester holding the instrument, another presentation is given as soon as recording has been completed and the present state of the infant has been observed. Three to six presentations may be given before the notations are compared. If no one has judged that a response occurred, it is best to move on to the next child, and to return to the first one after all the children in the nursery have been screened. Often there will be several infants who are not cleared in the first series, but who will respond the second or third time tested. If no response is obtained

TABLE 39-2. BABY AUDITORY BEHAVIOR INDEX

Age	Acoustic Signal	Mean Signal Strength for This Age (Re: Audiometric 0)	Expected Response	Level He Listens or Localizes Measured Speech	Startle to Voice
0–6 wk	3,000 cps	78 db (depending on environment noise)* range: 72–84 db †	Eyeblink, Moro's, eye shift or widen, cessation of activity		65 db
	Hand-clap, horn, "kissing sound"	?	Same as above		
6 wks–3¾ mo	3,000 cps	70 db; range: 60–80 db	Eyeblink, quieting, rudimentary head-turn	47 db; range: 45–50 db	65 db
	Noisemaker rattle, horn squeeze toy, bell (6)	?	Eyeblink, quieting, rudimentary head-turn		
4 mo–6¾ mo	3,000 cps	51 db; range: 40–60 db	"Listening" head-turn on lateral plane & beginning localizing below the ear (7)	21 db; range: 13–29 db	65 db
		?	Same as above		
7 mo–8¾ mo	Noisemaker 3,000 cps	45 db; range: 30–60 db	Localization on lateral plane directly to below ear level, indirectly above	15 db; range: 7.5–22.5 db	
		?	Same as above		
9 mo–12¾ mo	Noisemaker 3,000 cps	38 db; range: 20–50 db	Localization directly on lateral and lower plane, and directly above ear level	8 db; range: 1–15 db	65 db
		?	Same as above		
13 mo–15¾ mo	Noisemaker 3,000 cps	32 db; range: 22–42 db	Direct localization on all planes	5 db; range: 0–10 db	65 db
		?	Same as above		
16 mo–20¾ mo	Noisemaker 3,000 cps	25 db; range: 15–35 db	Direct localization on all planes	5 db; range: 4–6 db	65 db
		?	Same as above		
21 mo–24 mo	Noisemaker 3,000 cps	26 db; range: 16–36 db	Direct localization on all planes	3 db; range: 1–6 db	65 db

* These measurements have been made under structured, quiet conditions, not necessarily in sound rooms.

† Standard deviations have been used to calculate the range of responses around the mean that can be expected. This means that 68.26 percent of the cases this age can be expected to respond within the range shown.

to the 90-db signal, 100 db may be used, but its use should be recorded.

During the training program for observers, one of the three testers will be an experienced observer—often the audiologist who is conducting the program. During the early part of the training situation, the experienced person will lead a discussion as to what was seen after each signal presentation. The object of the discussion is to communicate to the novices the ways of looking at the infant's behavior: how to distinguish a response from the child's random activity; how to look for behavior patterns that are peculiar to this child at this time; and how to use the child's pretesting state as a background for the observation of the response. After several sessions of discussion on each child, the three testers will begin to make independent observations and compare them at a later time. A tester who is scoring consistently at variance with the others will again be put through a discussion series. After a few weeks of testing with the experienced observer, any individual who continues to make observations that deviate too far from those of the other testers must be eliminated from the program.

Another method of determining independent observations is to use a white noise masking attachment connected to earphones worn by the observers. The person carrying the instrument will randomly give a signal or no-signal, but each time the button is pressed the masking noise will go into the earphones, so the observers will not know if a signal has been given or not. The notations made after each signal or no-signal will indicate whether the observer is actually seeing a response or whether she is allowing the awareness of the signal presentation to influence her judgment of whether a response was present.

CRITERIA FOR FAILURE AND FOLLOW-UP

An infant who fails to respond (scores 1 or 2 in response intensity) after several presentations of the signal, or after retest at a later time, is marked as "Suspect." His current treatment chart is then stamped with a notation reading:

Not Cleared for
Hearing
Date..............
AP response absent
to 2,500-3,500-cps band
at 90 db SPL

The charts of those who have given responses of 3 or more in intensity are stamped:

Cleared for Hearing
Date..............
AP response present to
2,500-3,500-cps band at
90 db SPL

In those hospitals where an audiologist is in residence, he is immediately notified of a failure and will evaluate the infant again before it leaves the hospital. If his testing continues to show no responses, an appointment is made to bring the child back for further testing at three weeks. If no responses are seen at the second testing, the child is referred for electroencephalographic (EEG) auditory testing if available in the hospital.

In those hospitals where an audiologist is not available, another procedure can be used for follow-up. The volunteers record the name of the doctor in charge of the infant, and after six weeks an inquiry is sent to him as to whether or not the child was cleared for hearing at his six weeks' examination. The private doctor uses his discretion as to how he will test or where he will refer the child.

In those situations where a reporting program on testing for PKU in infants is in operation it may be advantageous to arrange to stamp the results of the hearing test on the same card that is sent to the physicians regarding the PKU test. In this way every physician may receive direct information on every test.

RESULTS

Out of almost 10,000 infants screened in the ongoing program in the Denver area, approximately 150 positives were recorded. Immediate follow-up known to us was obtained on only 30 of these positives at Colorado General Hospital. Two true hearing inpairments were confirmed. In the other hospitals, reporting by the physicians has been only recently instituted because of the experimental nature of the program. The confirmation of two additional hearing-impaired infants has been brought to our attention from these other programs. Thus, at the present time, four infants of the 150 have been tentatively confirmed. Subsequent follow-up of additional suspects may yield additional true positives. Two of the four confirmed positives were infants later found to have histories of congenital hearing loss on both sides of the family; another child proved to have two older deaf siblings with congenital nephritis; the fourth had no positive history that would indicate the etiology of the loss. The latter child has been shown by repeated EEG testing to have a severe hearing loss, and has been wearing a hearing aid successfully since 3 months of age.

These figures illustrate the fact that a great many false positives can be expected in such a program, and that fewer than 3 percent of these will be found to have true hearing impairment. Probably roughly 0.04 percent of the total population will be found at birth to have peripheral hearing impairment. The confirmation of one hearing loss in a child with no positive history indicates that possibly 25 percent of the congenital hearing impairments found will be of unknown etiology and in an otherwise negative history category.

Because of the fact that this program has been in a formative stage, the figures quoted above may not be representative of what will be found after the program has reached maturity.

The number of false positives, although large, does not represent any real problem for the physician, who can determine often by simple tests with the guidance of an otological or audiological examination and by questioning the parents, whether a true loss exists. The parents are not informed of the suspicion unless the loss is confirmed, thereby avoiding unnecessary distress to them.

The instruments used for the newborn screening have also been found useful in screening the older child in a clinical situation. Gross hearing abnormalities can be ruled out in the 4, 6, or 8-month-old child by determining whether localization responses occur when the 3,000-cps signal is presented out of the child's visual field.

SUMMARY

A procedure for a community program of detection of hearing loss at birth has been developed, using trained volunteer workers to do the testing. The instruments that have been designed for this purpose present measurable acoustic signals that will differentiate various hearing losses from normal hearing. The otolaryngologist can encourage and initiate such a program with the assistance of qualified audiologists. Although precise statistics have not been compiled, it is estimated that one child in 2,000 to 4,000 will be found with congenital hearing loss.

The fact that the program may produce a numerically low yield is far outweighed by the benefits to the individual child who will receive the optimum habilitation for his handicap. The low operating costs make the program economically feasible.

REFERENCES

1. The Young Deaf Child: Identification and Management, Proceedings of a Conference Held in Toronto, *Acta Otolaryng* (suppl 206) 1965.

2. Glorig, A.: *Audiometry: Principles and Practice*, Baltimore: The Williams & Wilkins Co., 1965.

3. Watson, T. J.: The Use of Residual Hearing in Education of the Deaf, *Volta Rev* **64**:84, 1962.

4. Downs, M. P., and Sterritt, G.: Identification Audiometry for Neonates: A Preliminary Report, *J Aud Res* **4**:69, 1964.

5. Fisch, L.: The Aetiology of Congenital Deafness and Audiometric Patterns, *J Laryng* **69**:7, 1955.

6. Hardy, J. B.; Dougherty, A.; and Hardy, W. G.: Hearing Responses and Audiologic Screening in Infants, *J Pediat* **55**:382–390, 1959.

7. Murphy, K. P.: Development of Hearing in Babies, *Child and Family* (April) 1962.

40

A Hearing Testing Program for Pre-school Children

MARION P. DOWNS
MILDRED E. DOSTER

MARION P. DOWNS is Director, Clinical Audiology, and Assistant Professor of Otolaryngology, University of Colorado Medical Center

MILDRED E. DOSTER, M.D., M.S.P.H., is Assistant Director, Division of School Health Services, Denver Public Schools

A mass screening program to detect hearing losses in preschool children has been established on a firm basis in the Denver Public Schools.[1] It is believed that this program represents the first large-scale hearing screening of children between the ages of 3 and 5 in the United States. Although technics are still being perfected, all those connected with the program agree that it has demonstrated an effective case-finding procedure for hearing loss in this age group.

The technic, as described in a pilot study reported in the Journal of School Health, March, 1965, consists of the presentation of familiar sounds which have been filtered into designated band widths, 250–750 cycles per second (cps), 1,000–2,000 cps, and 3,000–5,000 cps. The child is oriented to point to pictures representing the sounds he hears at a loud level, and then given a test presentation at a 15 decibel (db) level. Inability to identify any of the sounds in either ear constitutes a

Reprinted by permission of the authors from *Rocky Mt. Med. J.*, **56**, pp. 37–40 (1959).

[1] These authors gratefully acknowledge the cooperation and assistance of Leland M. Corliss, M.D., Director of the Health Service Department, Denver Public Schools; Elizabeth Kaho, Ph.D., Executive Secretary of the Denver Hearing Society; Mrs. Lois Humphrey, Coordinator of the Parent Education and Preschool Department; and Mrs. Frank Spratlen and Mrs. O. R. Birkland, who are cooperative members of the Junior League of Denver.

failure, and the child is rechecked and then scheduled for a threshold audiogram.

The program has been a cooperative project of several Denver agencies. The test was developed by the University of Denver Audiology Department at the suggestion of the Health Service Department of the Denver Public Schools. This was offered routinely each of the last two years to the 2,000–2,500 children in the Parent Education and Preschool Department of the Denver Public Schools. The testing procedure is carried out by volunteers of the Junior League of Denver, with about 30 members devoting many days a week during the year to the project. The contribution of their time by these interested and capable young women is a great factor making for the success of the program, and cannot be over-emphasized. A very important factor for efficient testing is the preparation of the children to "play the game" and identify the common sounds. This has been done by the parent education and preschool teachers and parents who plan toward the testing procedure with the children. There are 79 groups with an enrollment of 20–30 children in each.

The recheck audiograms are conducted at the Denver Hearing Society in their sound-proof room. Testing is done by the staff of the Hearing Society, aided by graduate students of the University of Denver. The criteria for the test were originally established by a committee of otologists representing the Colorado Society of Otolaryngology.

The statistics derived from the 1957–1958 screening of 1,635 children demonstrate the effectiveness of the program. Only 2 percent of the children could not be tested because of unwillingness to cooperate. Seventy-four (4.5 percent) were suspected to have hearing losses and upon final threshold audiograms, 46 (2.8 percent) children were verified to have significant hearing impairments. The criteria for designation of failure on the test was either a 15 db. loss at one frequency or more, and/or two 15 db. differences between air and bone conduction. This latter criterion was established as a result of the findings in the pilot study which indicated that this age child can be expected to have —10 or better hearing, and therefore a 5 db. loss by air conduction would be a significant loss if —10 bone conduction thresholds prevailed.

A further breakdown of the findings revealed the following distribution:

20 percent—nerve loss, mainly in high frequencies.

80 per cent—conductive loss:

    50 percent—high frequency conductive loss.

    48 percent—flat conductive loss.

    2 percent—low frequency conductive loss.

These findings are in agreement with national studies which indicate that 80 percent of the hearing problems of children are of a conductive nature, which may yield to medical treatment. Careful checks in the original pilot study indicated that almost all of the conductive losses which were discovered were either improved or restored to normal with medical treatment. These facts point to the effectiveness and great need for early detection of hearing impairments for this age group.

The breakdown of conductive losses suggests some interesting conclusions. Fifty percent of these losses were high frequency conductive losses, indicative of what has been termed a "mass tilt" type of audiogram. The high frequency tilt is customarily interpreted to indicate the presence of mass in the middle ear. This fact would point to a conclusion that 50 percent of the conductive-type losses in children are caused by a serous or gelatinous mass in the middle ear. The medical implications here are certainly significant.

The Denver Public School program has definitely shown the practicability of testing the hearing of preschool age children by rapid screening methods. It is being continued with the excellent cooperation of the Junior League volunteers and the Denver Hearing Society.

Another group of 1,508 preschool children have been tested during the 1958–1959 school year and 56 (3.7 percent) were found to be in need of follow-up care. A few cases are here summarized to demonstrate the types of cases found by such a program. Complete follow-up studies have not been done to find the degree of improvement after medical care was obtained.

1. Boy of 5 years thought to be slow in speech development because he never sounded "S's," etc., was found to have a bilateral conductive loss of 30 dbs. He is receiving medical treatment and improving in hearing and speech.

2. Girl of 4 years was referred to the family physician with her audiogram denoting about 25 dbs. loss. The physician preferred to wait a year and retest before instituting any definitive care.

3. Boy of 4 years was found defective in one ear. On subsequent otologic examination an atresia of the canal was discovered for which the family has obtained plastic surgery.

4. Girl of 5 years showed a moderate bilateral loss and was taken to the family physician who performed a tonsillectomy and adenoidectomy. Four months later the loss was still present and the mother was concerned that more should be done.

GENERAL CONCLUSIONS

1. In the past four years Denver preschool children have been tested by a new and simple

screening test using "common sounds" filtered and calibrated to allow accurate audiometry.

2. During routine screening the past two years, 3,143 3- and 4-year-olds were tested and 126 (4.0 percent) were suspected of having hearing losses.

3. Parents, physicians, and school need to be more aware of the importance of early attention to the hearing impairments of the preschool age children, when at least 80 per cent can be cured or arrested by adequate medical care.

41

Teacher Judgment of Hearing Loss in Children

MARGARET L. GEYER
ALFRED YANKAUER

MARGARET L. GEYER is Audiologist, Department of Special Education, City School District, Rochester, New York

ALFRED YANKAUER, M.D., M.P.H., is Senior Lecturer, Department of Health Services Administration, Harvard School of Public Health

In many school systems in the United States, the ideal of testing the hearing of each child every year or even every two years cannot be approached (5, 7). Compromises must necessarily be made while maintaining the highest possible case-finding efficiency. Such compromises are often achieved at the expense of children below the third grade level since younger children require more time to test. This has been the case in Rochester, New York (elementary school population 42,000). Children below third grade have been tested only if referred by teachers, whereas children from grades three to seven have been tested biennially.*

Several studies reporting the inaccuracies of teacher-judgments of hearing loss have been made. Most recently, Curry (2, 3) concluded that 'the identification of hard of hearing children should be done by audiometric examination and not by a system of teacher referrals.' However, his study, as well as previous studies, leave certain questions unanswered. How does the accuracy of teacher referrals relate to hearing loss for speech frequencies only, to different degrees of loss, to the proficiencies of different teachers and the size of their classes, to the specificity of observed signs and symptoms, and to educational and medical recommendations made for the children? The present study was undertaken to find answers to these questions.

PROCEDURE

Seven elementary schools of varying socio-economic background were selected for study. A form used by the teachers in previous years for listing their referrals was revised and given to every first and second grade teacher in the seven schools. The teacher was requested to list the name of each child in her grade and to give her opinion of each child's hearing. If she questioned a child's hearing, she was requested to specify the reason or reasons, using the following check-list code.

A. Physical Signs
1. Ear discharge
2. Cotton in ear
3. Tired, strained expression long before day is over
4. Mouth breather
5. Watches lip movements very intently

Reprinted by permission of the authors from *J. Speech Hearing Dis.*, **21**, pp. 482–486 (1956).

[* In 1960, mass screening of kindergarten children was begun and continued until 1964 when a change to first-grade children was made. Currently (1968) all children in the first and the highest elementary grades are screened annually. MLG, AY]

B. Behavior

1. Is inattentive
2. Cocks head toward speaker
3. Fails to carry out spoken directions
4. Asks to have words or questions repeated
5. Lacks clear or distinct speech
6. Has abnormality of voice
7. Is shy and withdraws from group
8. Fails to volunteer in class

C. Complaints

1. Has earache
2. Has buzzing or ringing in ears
3. Has stuffy feeling in ears
4. Hears noises in head

Teachers gave their judgment on the hearing of 1197 children in their grades. One hundred and forty-four children who later were absent for the screening and/or threshold test were eliminated. The number remaining, 1053, was the number considered in this study.

An individual pure tone sweep check test was subsequently given to each of the 1053 children. A Maico F-1 audiometer was used. Each child was screened on five frequencies: 500, 1000, 2000, 4000 and 6000 cps (*4, 6*). The attenuator was set at 20 db. *re* ASA, 1951. If a child failed to hear any one frequency in either ear he was screened out and later given an individual threshold test. These latter tests were given on a Western Electric 6BP audiometer. Six frequencies were used: 256, 512, 1024, 2048, 4096 and 6144 cps. The criterion for determining hearing loss on the threshold test was a 20 db. loss for any two frequencies, or a 25 db. loss for any one frequency, in either or both ears.

All children found to have a hearing loss by these criteria were examined by an otolo-

gist.[1] Medical recommendations were made on the basis of inspection of the nasal passage, pharynx and tympanic membrane. Nasopharyngoscopy was not performed. Educational recommendations were made jointly by the otologist and audiologist.

RESULTS

Eighty-one of the 1053 children screened (7.7 percent) were found to have a hearing loss as defined above (see Table 41-1). Medical or educational recommendations were made for all but 8 of the 81 children. Twenty-four percent of the 1053 children were suspected of hearing loss by teachers. Of the 81 children with loss, 62 percent were unsuspected by teachers, so that if reliance had been placed upon teacher selection three out of five children would have been overlooked. On the other hand, teacher "suspicion" increased the likelihood of finding hearing loss. Twelve percent of the 256 "suspected" children had a hearing loss as compared to only 6 percent of the 797 "unsuspected" children.

The audiograms of the 31 children suspected of hearing loss by teachers were compared with those of the 50 children whose loss was unsuspected. In this analysis only the three speech frequencies were considered: 512, 1024, and 2048 cps. For audiograms showing unilateral loss, the decibel levels at these three frequencies were averaged showing the loss of the poorer ear. In cases of bilateral loss, the better ear average was determined by selecting the lower threshold for each of the three speech frequencies and averaging them. The

[1] Dr. Lawrence J. Nacey, now retired, was Consultant Otolaryngologist, Rochester General and St. Mary's Hospitals in Rochester, New York.

TABLE 41-1. INCIDENCE OF HEARING LOSS ACCORDING TO PRIOR TEACHER JUDGMENT OF HEARING LOSS

Teacher Judgment	Total Examined		Hearing Loss Found		Hearing Loss Not Found	
	Number	Percent	Number	Percent	Number	Percent
Hearing loss suspected	256	24.3	31	38.3	225	23.1
Hearing loss not suspected	797	75.7	50	61.7	747	76.9
Total	1,053	100.0	81	100.0	972	100.0

TABLE 41-2. AVERAGE DB LOSS IN SPEECH RANGE OF 81 CHILDREN WITH HEARING LOSS BY TYPE OF LOSS AND TEACHER JUDGMENT OF LOSS

Average db. Loss in Speech Range (512, 1024, 2048 cps)	Unilateral Loss		Bilateral Loss *	
	Teacher Selected	Not Teacher Selected	Teacher Selected	Not Teacher Selected
5 or under	3	6	1	3
6–10	1	4	2	2
11–15	6	8	3	4
16–20	3	6	1	3
21–25	6	5	1	0
26–30	2	2	0	0
31–35	1	4	0	0
36 and over	0	3	1	0
Total	22	38	9	12

* Better ear average computed by averaging the better score for each of the three speech frequencies.

results of this analysis are shown in Table 41-2. Only two children can be said to have had a moderate bilateral loss at the speech frequencies and both of these were suspected by the teacher. However, in the case of unilateral loss even severe degrees of loss were not suspected.

A second analysis of audiogram findings in the speech range was made in an attempt to see if teachers were more likely to select children with speech range losses than children with losses at high frequencies (see Table 41-3). In this analysis, children were considered

TABLE 41-3. TEACHER JUDGMENT OF HEARING LOSS FOR 81 CHILDREN FOUND ON EXAMINATION TO HAVE HEARING LOSS, ACCORDING TO RESULTS OF EXAMINATION AT SPEECH FREQUENCIES

Teacher Judgment of Hearing	Results of Examination at Speech Frequencies			
	Passed		Failed *	
	Number	Percent	Number	Percent
Suspected of loss	13	38	18	38
Not suspected of loss	21	62	29	62
Total	34	100	47	100

* 20 db. or more loss at two or 25 db. or more loss at one of the three speech frequencies: (512, 1024, 2048 cps).

to have "failed" at speech range frequencies (512, 1024, 2048 cps) if there were losses of 20 db. or more at two speech frequencies or 25 db. or more at one of the three speech frequencies. This analysis showed no relationship between teacher-judgment and failure at speech frequencies even in the case of children with bilateral losses (using same criterion for both ears).

Further analyses were made of the children with hearing losses both at all frequencies tested and at the three speech frequencies in attempts to relate the efficacy of teacher case-finding to sex of child, to individual teachers (analysis by schools), to size of class, and to specific symptoms and signs on the check-list. None of these analyses disclosed any significant relationships.

These results confirm those of previous studies. Teacher-judgments cannot be relied upon as a method of selecting children with a hearing loss. In this study, teachers overlooked 62 percent of the children found to have a loss whereas 88 percent of the children they "suspected" of loss had normal hearing.

Only two children were found with appreciable bilateral loss and both of these children were suspected of loss by their teachers. In the "teacher-suspected" group, the incidence of hearing loss was twice as great as in the group not suspected of loss by teachers. This latter finding is somewhat puzzling since the teacher-selected group had no higher proportion of children with speech-range loss and no special symptoms or signs that distinguished them from the unsuspected group.

Conceivably, if facilities were available to screen only one-quarter of the younger children, there is some advantage in screening the quarter selected by teachers rather than a random quarter. It seems highly unlikely that this point is of any practical importance, however. If a program is already committed to screening one quarter of a given class, the extra effort required to screen the remaining three-quarters is relatively slight.

SUMMARY

Teacher-judgments of hearing loss based upon a check list of symptoms and signs were obtained on 1,053 first and second grade children in seven schools. All children were screened for hearing loss by individual pure-tone sweep check testing. Children failing this screening test were threshold tested and seen by an otologist. Teachers "over-suspected" children to an appreciable extent and failed to suspect 62 percent of the children with a hearing loss. However, the incidence of hearing loss was twice as great in the "teacher-suspected" group as in the "unsuspected" group. No significant relationships were found between the effectiveness of teacher selection and hearing loss at speech frequencies (except when moderately severe), sex of child, size of class, nature of symptoms or signs, or individual teachers and schools.

REFERENCES

1. Carhart, R. Speech audiometry in clinical evaluation. *Acta Otolaryng.*, 41, 1952, 18–42.

2. Curry, E. T. Are teachers good judges of their pupils' hearing? *Excep. Childr.*, 21, 1954, 15–17, 29.

3. Curry, E. T. The efficiency of teacher referrals in a school hearing testing program. *JSHD*, 15, 1950, 211–214.

4. Hirsh, I. J. *The Measurement of Hearing.* New York: McGraw-Hill, 1952.

5. Manual for a school hearing conservation program. Com. on Cons. of Hear. Amer. Acad. Ophthal., Otolaryngol., 1951. (100 First Avenue Bldg., Rochester Minnesota.)

6. Report of the Council on Physical Medicine and Rehabilitation. *JAMA*, 146, 1951, 817.

7. Wilson, C. C. (ed.) *School Health Services.* N.E.A., A.M.A. (N.E.A., Washington, D.C.) c 1953.

42

Identification Audiometry for School–Age Children: Basic Procedures*

* The report from which this article was selected was prepared by the Committee on Identification Audiometry, American Speech and Hearing Association. The report was edited by Frederic L. Darley, Ph.D., and the Chairman of the Committee was William G. Hardy, Ph.D.

GENERAL TEST METHODOLOGY

Identification audiometry in the school-age population is best described in two stages. The first has traditionally been called screening audiometry. It involves the testing in an abbreviated way of large numbers of children resulting in the ready identification of those who have no hearing problems and the tentative identification of those who may have hearing problems. The second stage involves a test of minimal hearing sensitivity; this is a more detailed test by more highly trained personnel with more elaborate equipment. Its purpose is to lead to the final identification of those who should be referred to an otologist, or other physician, for a complete diagnostic work-up.

The first stage of the procedure involves either individual or group limited-frequency testing. Procedural details are presented in this chapter and the next. Only pure tone audiometric procedures are considered. It is strongly recommended that individual pure tone testing be planned for all grade levels whenever possible. Many experts believe that periodic screening on an individual basis is better than an annual screening using group procedures. However, if a choice must be made between group pure tone audiometry or none, group procedures are possible at least at third grade level and above.

Reprinted by permission of the American Speech and Hearing Association from *J. Speech Hearing Dis., Mono. Suppl. No. 9*, pp. 26–34 (1961).

Local considerations having to do with scope of the total program, the ages of the children to be tested, and the amount of time and money available for the program may make it necessary to resort to group methods (*4, 8, 13*). Data from several state programs indicate that group testing is considerably less expensive than an individual screening program: for example, in one state costs for individual pure tone screening run between 25 and 35 cents per capita, whereas group pure tone screening procedures involve a cost of between 15 and 17 cents per child.[1] Figures from the Michigan Hearing Conservation Program indicate that relatively untrained technicians can do accurately between 70 and 80 individual sweep check hearing tests per day; through the use of group pure tone screening procedures between 200 and 250 pupils can be tested per day with comparable accuracy when an adequately quiet testing environment can be achieved. In a community where group hearing testing equipment can be left in one room, the procedure would involve considerable economy. However, where this is not possible, the time spent in setting up and servicing the equipment would no doubt reduce the amount of saving involved in group testing procedures. Group procedures requiring paper and pencil responses can be employed satisfactorily only with children

[1] These data from an unpublished time-cost study conducted by the Hearing Conservation Section, Michigan Department of Health, were reported at the Conference by Courtney D. Osborn.

in the third grade and above. Younger children cannot be relied on to make appropriate responses to this kind of test.

Descriptions of appropriate group testing procedures can be found in standard textbooks. Group procedures using fading numbers are not recommended. Criteria for failure which are presented at the end of this chapter may be applied to group as well as individual techniques using pure tones. Where group procedures are used, the equipment should be carefully calibrated and checked regularly and the results of its use validated against the results of individual hearing testing so that administrators may be sure that the program is functioning with acceptable efficiency.

In the second stage of the process, the threshold test, standardized procedures should be followed. Descriptions of these procedures can be found in standard textbooks (*5, 12*).

It is possible that in the future some of the automatic audiometric techniques mentioned in Chapter V may be adapted for use with school-age children. Administrators of hearing conservation programs may well want to investigate developing automatic audiometric procedures and the variations of use to which they may be put.

ENVIRONMENT

It is useless to carry out the recommended identification audiometric procedures unless the results obtained can be assumed to be valid. Their reliability depends upon three important aspects: the environment in which the testing is done, the equipment used, and the personnel operating the equipment. If there is a breakdown anywhere, the results of the program become meaningless.

A good acoustic environment is necessary. It can safely be said that millions of dollars and thousands of man hours are now being spent on worthless programs simply because space has been utilized because of its convenience rather than because of its suitability for the purpose. If an examiner is screening at 15 db above audiometric zero while the en-vironment induces 20 db of masking, spuriously large numbers of subjects will be identified as having hearing problems and will be referred on to successive stages of the program. Initial expenditure of money for a suitable testing environment results in substantial savings of money spent for the referral of children erroneously thought to have hearing impairment.

The amount of space to be planned for hearing testing will depend upon whether the first stage makes use of group audiometric techniques or whether both stages involve individual testing. Regardless of the type of test used, the testing environment must be one in which valid measurement can be obtained. This requirement necessitates the use of acoustic treatment in all enclosures used for testing.

In existing school buildings appropriate space may conceivably be found and adapted for this use. Past experience suggests that this possibility is often unlikely. Useful space should be located as far away as possible from heating and other mechanical equipment, the school shop, the music room, the typing room, the cafeteria, rest rooms, and other sections where student traffic and regularly scheduled activities can be expected to induce high masking levels. In planning to adapt already existing space or in planning space designed for hearing testing in new construction, administrators will find it advisable to make sound level and spectral analyses in order to determine whether the rooms meet the specifications established by the American Standards Association.[2]

They may also secure the services of acoustical consultants available in nearby universities or industrial establishments. Cox (*2*) has recently defined the minimal noise levels allowable for testing various frequencies at given intensity levels. It is earnestly to be hoped that school boards will come to see the need for specifying the inclusion in each new school building of space planned for the efficient implementation of hearing conservation programs. It is also to be hoped that architects

[2] ASA Standard S3.1-1960, American Standard Criteria for Background Noise in Audiometer Rooms.

who plan the space will give due consideration to the problems involved.

It is likely that the program will demand sound treatment beyond what the usual existing school can provide or what local carpenters can well construct. It is, therefore, strongly recommended that in schools which cannot provide adequately quiet quarters, sound-treated prefabricated booths be purchased and installed. A portable booth which can be conveniently dismantled and set up again is not recommended, as the best of these portable structures achieves only from 20 to 25 db of attenuation in the frequencies tested. A standard sound-treated booth made by a commercial manufacturer which can guarantee at least 40 db attenuation is recommended. Such booths are avilable at a cost of between $1200 and $1500. School boards may find it less expensive to procure mobile testing units—specially constructed buses or trailers—that provide the necessary sound isolation to guarantee reliable test results. Such units are useful, too, for covering large areas of sparse population. In the larger mobile units, group as well as individual testing can be performed.

Only through planning a program in accordance with such stringent criteria for test environment can those responsible for the program be sure that they are measuring the hearing levels of the children and not just the background noise of the school. The required outlay of funds is reasonable and essential. Schools which lack appropriately designed space will find a kind of precedent set by industry. It is an impressive fact that upon the insistence of noise engineers and audiologic and otologic consultants to industry, over 1,000 prefabricated sound-treated booths have now been installed in industrial situations in the United States.

A supervising audiologist will want to make frequent check of the number of individuals identified because of failure in the low frequencies tested. If he finds an inordinate number of failures at 500 cps or below, in cases where normal hearing is found in the higher frequencies, he will know that the screening level he has adopted is inappropriate for use in all frequencies in the testing environment he has.

FREQUENCIES TO BE TESTED

Since a complete threshold test of every child at all frequencies may not be feasible, a selection of certain frequencies must be arrived at through some process of compromise. Certain factors which enter into the making of this compromise must be carefully weighed. These include the time devoted to the initial screening, the time required in the retesting of children who fail to meet the criteria of the initial screening, the realities of the acoustic conditions of the testing environment, and the reliability of instrumentation in the testing of certain frequencies.

At present, definitive data are not available which would make a decision about the frequencies to be tested clear-cut. Data do not exist which incontrovertibly indicate that the extremes of the frequency spectrum should be included, for example, 125 cps and 8000 cps. Similarly there is a lack of incontrovertible evidence that limited frequency testing using only one or two frequencies will result in the identification of an acceptable percentage of hearing losses in a school-age population.

In the absence of these definitive data, it is recommended that no less than four, preferably five, frequencies be tested. *The frequencies recommended for identification audiometry at the school-age level are 500, 1000, 2000, 4000, and 6000 cps.*

There are several reasons why elimination of the lower frequencies is recommended. It is generally agreed that useful clinical information is seldom gained by testing at 125 and 250 cps. It is difficult in most testing environments adequately to combat interfering environmental noise in testing these frequencies.

Some audiologists recommend not including 500 cps in the screening of school-age children. In many testing environments there is considerable masking at 500 cps. There is some evidence to indicate that even under excellent testing conditions the use of 500 cps does not necessarily improve the effectiveness of the screening if 1000 cps is used. A study conducted in one state indicated that when 500 cps was used in the initial screening, almost one-fourth of the total failures on the screening test were due to failures to reach the criterion level on 500 cps only. It was found that if this frequency were eliminated, only 2.2 percent of the medically significant hearing losses confirmed by detailed testing in otological clinics would have been missed; thus 97.8 percent of the medically significant losses would have been identified without testing at 500 cps.[3] On the basis of the economic considerations indicated by such information some programs may very well prefer to omit 500 cps, in this way probably reducing the number of children referred for threshold testing and thus permitting personnel to devote more time to the initial screening of larger numbers of children.

On the other hand, when the hearing testing environment can be made to meet the criteria set forth herein, as can usually be done, it is highly desirable to test at 500 cps. The purpose is to identify as many children with hearing problems as possible, and certain published information (*3*, *9*) supports the view that 500 cps *may* be a critical frequency in identification audiometry for school-age children.

There is no general agreement about which of the higher frequencies should be included in a screening test. There is fairly good agreement that reliable testing at 8000 cps is difficult. It is felt that no audiometer presently available can consistently hold ASA standards at 8000 cps. The response of earphones frequently begins to fall off sharply at 8000 cps and an audiometer is easily put out of calibration at that frequency. The Armed Forces-National Research Council Committee on Hearing and Bio-Acoustics (CHABA) (*14*) has recommended that 8000 cps not be used in identification audiometry.

The inclusion of 4000 and 6000 cps for identification purposes has been widely debated. Some feel that the identification program should be concerned primarily with medically reversible conductive-type hearing losses; therefore testing of the higher frequencies is advised against. Others feel that high frequency hearing losses should be discovered in the intial screening if possible.

It is known that a substantial part of the population demonstrates a dip at 4000 cps. In some cases this dip can be related to environmental noise, for example, the noise of tractors which farm children may drive.[4] Apparently in some individuals the presence of a 4000-cycle dip has little significance, and when serial audiometry is done, no change in the amount of loss is found over a period of years. Since such large numbers of children are found with a 4000-cycle dip, many otologists have indicated that they prefer not to have referred to them children with a loss at only that frequency. Many audiologists feel that it is important to test at both 4000 and 6000 cps; if hearing is normal at 6000 cps, one can dismiss a dip at 4000 cps as of minor significance. However, if a loss is found at 6000 as well as at 4000 cps, there is evidence of a more pervasive involvement and the child should be referred for threshold testing and possibly for an otological examination. In line with this reasoning, some audiologists prefer to screen only at 6000 cps and not at 4000 cps.

It may be restated that no valid data exist supporting the use of a sweep-check hearing test at all frequencies; nor are there adequate data available yet to support limited frequency audiometry using only one or two frequencies (*6*). In programs of preventive medicine, however, if one too early strips his data-gathering down to the minimum, he will fail to answer all of the pressing questions about hearing loss. The procedure of choice, then, is to test more frequencies rather than fewer frequen-

[3] Data taken from unpublished study by Evan Lounsbury, Regional Audiologist, Hearing Conservation Section, Michigan Department of Health. Reported at the Conference by Courtney D. Osborn.

[4] A study in progress, "Incidence of 4000 cps binaural losses in school children," is a research project of the Division of Special Education, Iowa Department of Public Instruction, supported by Research Grant #B-1970 (A), S.D.(A), National Institute of Neurological Diseases and Blindness.

cies until such time as definitive data are available justifying the use of only one or two frequencies.

INTENSITY LEVELS AND CRITERIA FOR FAILURE

Current practices with regard to the use of given intensity levels are based upon recommendations made by the American Academy of Ophthalmology and Otolaryngology in 1943 (7). These recommendations were apparently based on clinical practice and not upon some statistical determination of what would constitute the best screening level and the most appropriate criteria for failure.

In the discussion that follows it is to be remembered that a two-step audiometric procedure is undertaken prior to referral of a child to an otologist. The first step is a four- or five-frequency screening test. (Some audiologists may prefer to insert an immediate re-screening step following this in case of a child's failure to meet the criteria.) The second step consists of a threshold test involving all frequencies. *The criteria for failure apply to both steps.* The first test is designed to yield a considerably larger number of cases than are found in the second step to have a significant hearing loss. The second step is designed to identify those children most appropriately referred to an otologist for a diagnostic examination. The interposition of the second step is designed to prevent unnecessary referral.

Current criteria for referral (*12*, p. 210) specify failure at two of the frequencies tested at a sensation level of 20 db or failure at one frequency tested at a level of 30 db. A 15 db sensation level has been adopted as the screening level for identification audiometry almost uniformly across the country. The historical basis for this choice is that 15 db is a level about two standard deviations above the mean threshold of individuals with normal hearing. A second justification for the use of this level is that disability in understanding speech in some situations begins at about 15 db above audiometric zero.

It is now recommended that practice be altered as follows: *only four frequencies shall be considered in the criteria for referral: 1000, 2000, 4000, and 6000 cps. It is recommended that screening be done at the 10 db level* with reference to the present American Standard audiometric zero *for the frequencies of 1000, 2000, and 6000 cps, and at the 20 db level for the frequency of 4000 cps.* A child would be judged to have failed the screening test and to be a candidate for referral for the next step if he failed to hear the 10 db level at either 1000, 2000 or 6000 cps, or if he failed to hear the 4000-cycle tone at the 20 db sensation level in either ear. It is to be remembered that if screening is done at 15 db, a person who has a 15 db hearing loss is passed. The use of 10 db as the screening level at 1000, 2000, and 6000 cps results in the clear labeling of the person who has a 15 db hearing loss as warranting further attention.*

CHOICE OF EQUIPMENT

Noisy environments can lead to the spurious identification of individuals as having hearing losses. The audiometers themselves may also be responsible for the erroneous identification of apparent losses. To many users of audiometric equipment the instruments are very impressive and seem to imply high reliability. In actuality, many audiometers are relatively unstable and much care must be exerted in their selection and maintenance.

The audiometer to be used in the first stage of identification audiometry should meet the requirements established by the American Standards Association for limited frequency

[* In order to conform to the recommendations made in the monograph on identification audiometry when using either the ISO 1964 standard or the ANSI 1969 standard, screening levels will have to be raised by the amount of the differences between the old ASA 1951 standard and either one of the newer standards. These differences are incorporated in the recommendations made on page 412 by Downs, Doster, and Weaver. It is important to note, however, that the 20 dB screening level recommended by Downs, Doster, and Weaver is approximately *10 dB too high at 600 Hz if the TDH-39 earphone is employed in testing* (see Appendixes D and F in the ANSI 1969 standard). For absolute conformity to the recommendations made in the monograph, we suggest that when using the TDH-39 earphone, a 10 dB (re ANSI 1969) screening level be used at 6000 Hz. Eds.]

audiometers.[5] This equipment allows for the testing by air conduction of five or six frequencies with an output up to 70 or 80 db. It need not provide for masking or for bone-conduction testing. (See also *11*.) The audiometer to be used in the second stage for the obtaining of the threshold audiogram should meet the requirements established by the American Standards Association (*1*) for diagnostic audiometers. (See also *10*.) Such audiometers can, of course, also be used in the first stage of screening.

The purchaser of a new audiometer should request that the manufacturer supply data corresponding to the specifications established by the American Standards Association. The purchaser of audiometric equipment for school testing purposes should be aware of the fact that audiometers are generally most efficient in the measurement of hearing loss of a considerable degree. It is technically easier to make the attenuation linear at levels above audiometric zero than it is at or near audiometric zero. Whereas the otologist will more usually be concerned with measurements in the 40 to 70 db range, personnel working with school-age children will be more concerned with the linearity of audiometers at levels near audiometric zero where measurements of children with normal or near normal hearing are made.

The equipment purchased for individual audiometry should include head sets with two earphones so as to reduce the masking effect of ambient noise. When group testing equipment is purchased, it should provide up to 40 pairs of phones in head sets with cushions. Only one phone of each set need be live, but there should be provision for covering the ear not under test.

Attention should be given to the size of the earphones used with individual children. Especially with the school-age group heads and ears vary greatly in shape and size, and some obtained differences in hearing may be attributed to differences in the fit of earphones.

[5] ASA Standard Z24.12-1952: American Standard Specification for Pure-Tone Audiometers for Screening Purposes. [†Note that this standard as well as the one for diagnostic audiometers referred to below has been replaced by ANSI 3.6-1969. Eds.]

Headbands should provide pressure adequate to hold cushions tightly against the head; headbands providing more degrees of freedom in all directions are to be preferred.

Purchasers of equipment for testing school-age children will be interested in following the progress made in the development of supra-aural muffs; some muffs that have been developed promise to provide an economical answer to problems of masking in environments not specifically planned for hearing testing. It is to be hoped that such muffs will be standard equipment on audiometers in the near future; also desirable is a universal type of cushion appropriate for both children and adults or separate cushions for different age groups tested in the identification audiometry program.

Purchasers of equipment will also be interested in the simplicity of design of the equipment (the types of circuits involved, the number of tubes, etc.), the smoothness of function of the controls, the durability of the chassis, and the convenience of placement of the dials and control levers. Audiometers of desired ruggedness and stability with a variety of special features are available but obviously at greater cost to the consumer. Suffice it to say that the inexpensive audiometer ordinarily purchased for use in the testing of school-age children may well be relatively unstable and requires the constant vigilance of the user if valid results are to be obtained from it.

MAINTENANCE OF EQUIPMENT

The person in charge of the hearing testing program should have a clearly stated policy of what the individual audiometrist is expected to do with regard to maintenance of the equipment and what he is expected not to do. The audiometrist who daily operates the equipment should be responsible for testing of tubes; the replacement of earphone cords, fuses, and line cords; and the biological calibration of the audiometer daily to detect any marked shift at given frequencies. He should periodically listen to each phone to be sure that it is operating and to determine whether increasing the intensity 5 db results in corresponding changes in loudness. The audiometrist, who knows his own audiogram, should check his hearing daily and at least bi-weekly check the audiometer with a group of individuals not noise-exposed and known to have normal hearing. Personnel should be warned against soldering joints and replacing the earphones from one audiometer with those from another.

Beyond this first-echelon maintenance, it will be helpful to have some kind of independent evaluating agency available to users of audiometers for consultation on calibration procedures. If local demands are great enough, calibration check centers should be established by departments of health to serve programs within states or within still larger regions. Several new devices are being developed which will be useful for checking the calibration of earphones in the field without returning them to the factory. The critical point in calibration of audiometers is the intensity output at various frequencies. Four companies now offer calibration equipment which can be purchased for use in a regional or state calibration center. Such equipment can be used to determine whether an individual audiometer needs to be returned to the factory and can also be used to check on the adequacy of factory calibration.

In the absence of such an evaluating agency a supervising audiologist would be responsible for making the next level check, to determine whether an audiometer needs a factory overhaul. It is strongly recommended that an audiometer should be returned to the factory (or factory-designated regional center) for calibration check, re-calibration, and any necessary repair after every four months of use or, if this is not possible, after six

months of use, and in any case no less frequently than once each calendar year.

SUMMARY

Identification audiometry for school-age children consists of mass screening of large numbers followed by a test of hearing sensitivity for those suspected of having hearing problems. Mass screening may be done by individual or group screening methods. Individual screening is more accurate but more costly.

Quiet environment is essential for reliable hearing testing. Testing rooms should be acoustically treated. It is recommended that schools purchase commercial sound-treated booths, which are available at reasonable cost.

The frequencies recommended for identification audiometry at the school-age level are 500, 1000, 2000, 4000, and 6000 cps. It is recommended that screening be done at the 10 db level (with reference to the present American Standard audiometric zero) for the frequencies of 500, 1000, 2000, and 6000 cps and at the 20 db level for the frequency of 4000 cps. It is recommended that the criteria for failure be failure to respond to the 10 db level at 1000, 2000, or 6000 cps or to the 20 db level at 4000 cps.

Equipment should meet the requirements established by the American Standards Association for limited frequency and diagnostic audiometers. Equipment should be properly calibrated and maintained. Independent regional calibration check centers should be established where needed by departments of health. Calibration checks of audiometers should be made after each four months of use and in no case less frequently than once a year.

REFERENCES

1. *American Standard Specification for Audiometers for General Diagnostic Purposes* (ASA Z24.5-1951, approved March 21, 1951). Reprinted in Hirsh, I. J., *The Measurement of Hearing*. New York: McGraw-Hill, 1952, pp. 321–327.

2. Cox, J. R., How quiet must it be to measure normal hearing? *Noise Control*, 1, 1955, 25–29.

3. Farrant, R. H., The audiometric testing of children in schools and kindergartens, *J. aud. Res.*, 1, 1960, 1–24.

4. Harris, J. D., Group audiometry. *J. acoust. Soc. Amer.*, 17, 1945, 73–76.

5. Hirsh, I. J., *The Measurement of Hearing*. New York: McGraw-Hill, 1952.

6. House, H. P., and Glorig, A., A new concept of auditory screening, *Laryngoscope*, 67, 1957, 661–668.

7. Hughson, W., and Westlake, H., Manual for program outline for rehabilitation of aural casualties both military and civilian. *Trans. Amer. Acad. Ophthal. Otolaryngol.*, *Supplement*, 48, 1943–44, 3–15.

8. Johnston, P. W., The Massachusetts hearing test. *J. acoust. Soc. Amer.*, 20, 1948, 697–703.

9. Lawrence, C. F., and Rubin, W., The efficiency of limited frequency audiometric screening in a school hearing conservation program. *Arch. otolaryng.*, 69, 1959, 606–611.

10. Minimum requirements for acceptable pure tone audiometers for diagnostic purposes. *J. Amer. med. Ass.*, 146, May 19, 1951, 255–257. Reprinted in Hirsh, I. J., *The Measurement of Hearing*. New York: McGraw-Hill, 1952, pp. 304–310.

11. Minimum requirements for acceptable pure tone audiometers for screening purposes. *J. Amer. med. Ass.*, 144, Oct. 7, 1950, 465. Reprinted in Hirsh, I. J., *The Measurement of Hearing*. New York: McGraw-Hill, 1952, pp. 311–313.

12. Newby, H. A., *Audiology*. New York: Appleton-Century-Crofts, 1958.

13. Nielson, S. F., Tonaudiometermethode zur Gruppenuntersuchung des Gehörs des Schulkinder. *Acta otolaryng.*, 32, 1944, 263–283.

14. The medical principles of monitoring audiometry. *AMA Arch. ind. Health*, 17, 1958, 1–20.

43

Identification Audiometry for School–Age Children: Implementing the Program*

* The report from which this article was selected was prepared by the Committee on Identification Audiometry, American Speech and Hearing Association. The report was edited by Frederic L. Darley, Ph.D., and the Chairman of the Committee was William G. Hardy, Ph.D.

PERIODICITY OF TESTING

Practices and philosophies vary with regard to the frequency with which hearing tests should be administered to children in the school-age group. Some audiologists feel that the ideal program involves testing every child every year. Because of the fact that such a practice involves large numbers of people and the outlay of large amounts of money, many kinds of compromises have been suggested. Perhaps the most reasonable compromise is dictated by two considerations: (1) detection of hearing loss is particularly important in the younger part of the school-age population; if a child fails an early screening test, there is reasonable probability that he will fail subsequent tests; (2) some children constitute special referrals for hearing testing outside of the routine periodicity of tests.

In newly-established programs an effort should be made to test all of the children during the first school year. Thereafter an adequate program includes aggressive attention to the possibility of hearing problems in the early years in school. This can be implemented by *annual testing in kindergarten and grades 1, 2, and 3. Less frequent testing can be planned in subsequent school years, but no child should experience more than a three-year interval between tests from grades 4 through 12.*

Some programs prefer to operate a screening program in such a way that children will be tested once every two years, for example, in grades 1, 3, and 5, or 2, 4, and 6, plus one test at high school level. More important than to schedule hearing testing in certain grades every year is to insure that no child fails to have his hearing tested at least every two or three years. Accounting, then, should be *by child* rather than *by grade*.

Extension of periodical hearing testing into the high school age is recommended. Because of the tendency for otosclerosis to appear late in school-age, it is important that high school students be tested in grade 10, 11, or 12.

The time of year at which the identification audiometric program is conducted should be selected with care. Clinical findings indicate that there are important differences between the results of tests given at different times of the year. Some have suggested that hearing testing should be done in the "worst" season of the year with regard to hearing conditions. There are perhaps two seasons of the year when the prevalence of hearing problems increases significantly: the so-called "cold" season in mid-winter, extending through January and February, and the allergy season, the time and duration of which will vary in different parts of the country. There are always difficulties in designing a program which identifies the maximal number of problems during both seasons. Ideally a child should not have his hearing tested at the same season on successive hearing tests.

The most reasonable compromise would

Reprinted by permission of the American Speech and Hearing Association from *J. Speech Hearing Dis., Mono. Suppl. No. 9*, pp. 35–44 (1961).

seem to be to test hearing as early in the school year as possible. The supervisor of the program must exercise judgment in deciding how best to use the personnel available to him. He may choose to consolidate his hearing testing personnel and have them move as a group into a school to accomplish the complete routine hearing testing in the briefest possible time, moving on successively to other schools, and thus accomplish the total identification program within a matter of weeks or months rather than stretch it out over the entire year.

In addition to the routine periodicity discussed above, an adequate program should include opportunity for immediate testing of the following types of children (*1*):

(1) All pupils who are new to the individual school or to the school district.

(2) Pupils discovered by previous tests to have a hearing impairment.

(3) Children with delayed or defective speech.

(4) Pupils returning to school after a serious illness.

(5) Pupils enrolled in adjustment or remedial classes or programs.

(6) Pupils who appear to be retarded.

(7) Pupils having emotional or behavior problems.

(8) Pupils referred by the classroom teacher for hearing testing for any reason.

RECORDS

Records of hearing testing through the school-age years should be made a part of the child's general health record. Space should be provided for recording information from a series of audiograms over the school years, with the dates of the tests, the recommendations, and the follow-up.

Such records should be kept as long as is reasonable. Some school systems, having limited storage space, keep the records no longer than they are required to keep them, usually three years after the child's graduation from school. When records are maintained by state health departments, the period is often three years beyond the limit of children's programs, which typically deal with individuals up to age 21.

Medical personnel, vocational rehabilitation personnel, and personnel in military service and industry who have access to records of hearing testing done during the school-age years would find these helpful as reference audiograms in relationship to subsequent hearing tests. School or health agencies can turn such records over to the families of the children involved, particularly if they suggest that the child had had some history of hearing loss.

It seems obvious that if current hearing test records are to be maximally useful, they should be available to medical and educational personnel as well as to parents. They should be used in the planning of educational programs as well as in programs of health. The school and public health nurse, physicians, and school and community speech clinicians should all have the opportunity to scrutinize these records in connection with their various programs.

PERSONNEL

Identification audiometry with school-age children usually requires personnel at two levels, supervisory and technical. A supervising audiologist should hold the certificate in hearing of the American Speech and Hearing Association or at least meet the academic and practicum requirements for that certificate. He has responsibility for selecting the most appropriate procedures for testing the particular population to be studied; selecting, training, and supervising audiometrists; referring certain children for more complex audiological study; supervising equipment calibration; discussing test results with otologists; educating various segments of the public in acceptance of the program of identification audiometry; following up on referrals; and in general carrying out the entire sub-program of identification audiometry.

At the second level are audiometrists capable of performing both individual and group screening tests and individual threshold tests. If possible these audiometrists should have at least one college-level course in audiometry, including supervised practice in testing. More detailed academic training than this is certainly desirable but in some cases even less training may have to be accepted if enough personnel are to be available to man a program.

Prescribed training might well consist of a short course lasting from two to six weeks: approximately one-half of the time would be devoted to basic information about hearing and hearing impairment and the instrumentation used in hearing testing; the other half would be devoted to supervised practice in testing. Such an intensive course would give relatively little attention to the neurology and physiology of hearing, to testing by bone conduction, and to the use of speech audiometry, GSR audiometry, and tests for malingering and psychogenic deafness. Trainees would practice using the audiometer on many individuals with different hearing characteristics, all under close supervision. Such short courses may be offered in universities and colleges or by the staffs of state departments of health.

Short courses of the type described have been successfully used in military service (for example, U.S. Navy, six weeks, 108 hours; Walter Reed Hospital, two weeks, 80 hours) and elsewhere (Michigan Department of Health, six weeks, 180 hours). The whole question of training programs for persons of limited responsibility has for some years been under consideration by the American Speech and Hearing Association. Guidelines regarding the scope of such courses have recently been published (2). There is agreement that it is desirable that the course be presented over a period of several weeks, as opposed to a concentrated two- or three-day institute.

How many audiometrists will be needed to implement a program for testing school-age children? One state department of health has found that an audiometrist handling the first two stages of the program and using a combination of group and individual testing can reasonably test a school population of between 10,000 and 12,000 children per school year. If the program requires a test only every other year rather than every year, the audiometrist can handle a population of about 24,000.[1] A similar program in another state has reported comparable figures, an audiometrist serving between 12,000 and 15,000 children per school year, the exact number depending upon the distance covered by the audiometrist and the amount of travel involved.[2] In a third state reimbursement regulations recently drafted prescribe that an audiologist shall serve a population of from 12,000 to 13,000. The audiometrist in this program is envisioned as serving a population of 4,000 children, but his work is described as only part-time work in the first and second stages of testing.[3]

There is some difference of opinion about the type of personnel who should be selected for work as audiometrists. Their job, involving as it does frequent repetition of certain basic operations, does not allow for much creativity. Individuals with substantial training in audiology may find such employment unattractive for an extended period. On the other hand, if progress is to be made in hearing conservation programs around the country and if usable research data are to emerge from these programs, close attention must be given to the competence of those doing the work. Only an adequately trained person knows the implications of being careless.

Speech clinicians and registered nurses may, when they have had appropriate training, be competent to handle the first-stage screening and the second-stage threshold examination. But if they are used for these purposes, the skills which they were primarily trained to employ will be wasted. As a matter of economy, then, people other than nursing and speech correction personnel

---

[1] Data reported by Courtney D. Osborn.
[2] Reported by George J. Leshin.
[3] Reported by Dale S. Bingham.

are customarily selected to handle the first two stages.

Volunteer personnel (housewives, retired school teachers) who are intelligent, highly motivated to do this sort of service, tactful, insightful in observing children's behavior, and capable of working easily with children as well as amenable to the suggestions of the supervisor, may be selected and trained. If such selection is done with discretion, problems of frequent turnover of personnel may be obviated. Where such persons are employed, administrative procedures should be set up and maintained to see that they are prevented from making evaluations and decisions which they are not competent to make; they should be prevented from doing more than first- and second-stage hearing testing.

The success of the entire hearing conservation program rests upon the validity of the hearing measurement done in the first two stages, and this validity rests importantly upon the competence of the personnel doing the testing. Efforts should continually be made, then, to help them maintain high standards of performance and to provide expert supervision to insure the validity of their results.

REFERRAL PROCEDURES

It is difficult to discuss the procedures of identification audiometry without making some reference to the steps which must follow. It has been stated that the program of hearing testing should provide for adequate medical consultation. Certainly the final steps in the appraisal and management of individuals identified as probably having hearing impairment should be in the hands of medical personnel most competent to give the children the care they need. An otological examination of such children is not just a desirable feature which hopefully can be arranged but is a requirement if the program is to be effective.

The procedures adopted in order to accomplish this goal vary from locality to locality.

In some communities the results of the two-stage identification process are studied by an audiologist in the central municipal or county or state administrative headquarters of the hearing conservation program. In some programs he alone does not make the decision about subsequent referrals but makes it together with an otological consultant. Such joint professional review of each case is particularly desirable since it permits a careful weighing of all previous data about the child's hearing together with pertinent information from the case history. As a result of this third step, a decision is finally made that a given child should have a comprehensive evaluation of his hearing, comprising a diagnostic audiological workup and an otological examination.

Some programs have developed a plan, approved by local or regional medical groups, to make such referrals directly to otologists. In other programs procedures involve an initial referral to the child's family physician, who may accept responsibility for the care of the child if he feels himself competent to do so or who may, in turn, refer the child to an ear, nose, and throat specialist. Throughout the country hearing conservation programs are increasingly endeavoring to communicate to pediatricians and general practitioners the urgency of the problems involved. Moreover, some programs have made excellent use of public health or school nurses to help parents understand the reason for the referrals that are made and to help them make and keep appointments for further audiological and otological examinations.

In every hearing conservation program problems inevitably arise concerning the number of referrals for medical examination created by identification audiometry. Efforts should obviously be made to avoid referring for complete audiological and otological workups large numbers of children who turn out to have no medically or educationally significant hearing loss. *Educators and physicians alike, however, agree that as a matter of general principle it is better to err on the side of over-referral than it is to take a chance with under-referral and thus neglect to secure necessary medical treatment for children who need it.* Cooperation among educational, audiological, and medical personnel in organizing and implementing hearing conservation programs is necessary in creating an understanding of the intent of the total program and of the possibility that occasionally children will be referred who are found to possess no significant hearing problem.

When it has been determined that a child has a significant hearing loss as a result of the sequence of referrals described above and when necessary medical and surgical treatment and follow up have been provided, there is one further important step to be taken. The audiological and medical findings of the otologist must be conveyed to the parents and to other persons who are particularly concerned with the management of the child. The special education supervisor, the speech clinician, and the classroom teacher must be apprised of the child's needs and encouraged to meet them as comprehensively as possible. Appropriate entry should be made in the child's school health record so that a continuing program of care can be insured.

PROGRAM EVALUATION

Administrators of programs of identification audiometry will naturally be concerned as to whether the expenditure in terms of personnel, time, and money is warranted and whether the program is yielding the desired results. Only by constant scrutiny of the results of ongoing programs can weaknesses be perceived, corrective steps be taken, and maximal usefulness be derived.

One way in which such a continuing evaluation can be made is by a comparison of the results emerging from the various stages of the process. Several steps are involved: first a validation of the first screening test by comparison of it with the results of the second-stage threshold examination; a further validation of the results of the first two

stages is provided in the third-stage processing of the results by a professionally capable person in the field of audiology, ideally together with a professionally capable person in the field of otology, who can state on what basis they made a decision for further referral or not; a third validation is provided by the final clinical report made by the otologist who accomplishes the comprehensive otological examination. Careful analysis of the information yielded by this succession of tests indicates whether an efficient program of preventive medicine is being carried out.

There is another kind of evaluation which the administrator may want to make. The total number of audiograms produced in either the first or the second stage or both can be translated into a distribution of hearing losses. If the distribution deviates substantially from the distribution that one expects for a normal population, the administrator will be interested in examining into the testing environment, the calibration of audiometers, and the procedures used by individual testers.

SUMMARY

In newly-established programs all children should be tested during the first school year. Thereafter children should be tested annually in kindergarten and grades 1, 2, and 3. Less frequent testing can be planned in subsequent school years, but no child should have more than a three-year interval between tests from grades 4 through 12. Provision should be made for immediate testing of new pupils, pupils returning to school after a serious illness, those presenting special adjustment problems, and those referred by teachers specifically for hearing testing.

Records of hearing testing should be made a part of the child's general health record and made available to medical and educational personnel responsible for the child's welfare. Such records should be turned over to the child or his family upon his graduation from school.

Supervisors of identification audiometry

programs should be trained audiologists holding the certificate in hearing of the American Speech and Hearing Association. Audiometrists administering screening and threshold tests should have training and supervised practicum in these procedures. A minimum training program is suggested.

All testing procedures should be followed by medical, audiological, and educational evaluation so that each child's needs may be identified and steps taken to meet these needs.

REFERENCES

1. *Hearing Testing of School Children.* Sacramento: Calif. State Dept. of Educ., 1954.

2. Report of Committee on Short Courses in Audiometric Techniques. *Trans. Amer. Acad. Ophthal. Otolaryngol.*, 63, 1959, 852–853.

44

Evaluation of a Recommended Program of Identification Audiometry with School-Age Children

WILLIAM MELNICK
ELDON L. EAGLES
HERBERT S. LEVINE

WILLIAM MELNICK, Ph.D., is Associate Professor, Department of Otolaryngology, The Ohio State University

ELDON L. EAGLES, M.D., is Deputy Director, National Institute of Neurological Diseases and Stroke, Bethesda, Maryland

HERBERT S. LEVINE, Sc.D., is Head, Biostatistics Department, Montefiore Hospital and Medical Center, New York City

Identification audiometry refers specifically to the case-finding aspects of a hearing conservation program. It does not refer to making a specific diagnosis, to medical treatment, or to rehabilitation. An important part of such a program is early case-finding. In order to establish general guidelines to resolve the confusion regarding audiometric procedures for case-finding programs, the National Conference on Identification Audiometry was convened in Baltimore in May, 1960. The work of this conference resulted in a monograph on identification audiometry, one chapter of which presented a proposal of basic procedures in a program of identification audiometry for school-age children (Hardy, 1961, pp. 26–34). The purpose of the investigation being reported here was the evaluation of some of those procedures.[1]

Reprinted by permission of the authors from *J. Speech Hearing Dis.*, **29,** 3–13 (1964).

[1] This investigation was supported in part by Grant B-2375 from the National Institute of Neurological Diseases and Blindness to the Subcommittee on Hearing in Children, Committee on Conservation of Hearing of the American Academy of Ophthalmology and Otolaryngology. Additional support was provided by a grant from the U.S. Children's Bureau through the

Test programs for school-age children often involve testing large numbers of children by an abbreviated or screening method. From the results of one screen, children are selected for another screen from which a final selection is made of candidates for more detailed testing of hearing. The purpose of the testing program is the identification of children who should be referred to a physician for a complete diagnostic examination. These are children who have hearing less sensitive than a selected criterion hearing level as shown by the threshold hearing test.

The pure-tone sweep check, probably the most preferred screening technique, has been performed most often at a level of +15 dB for the test frequencies which are routinely used during a threshold test, i.e., 125, 250, 500, 1000, 2000, 4000, 6000, and 8000 cps. The number and choice of frequencies varies among screening programs, and there have been recommendations for using one or two frequencies for screening. The National Conference on Identification Audiometry made

Commonwealth of Pennsylvania Department of Health to the University of Pittsburgh.

the following recommendations regarding screening procedures:

(1) Testing should be conducted in acoustically treated test rooms.

(2) The frequencies recommended for identification audiometry at the school-age level are 500, 1000, 2000, 4000, and 6000 cps.

(3) The frequencies 500, 1000, 2000, and 6000 cps should be screened at 10 dB and at 20 dB for the frequency 4000 cycles.

(4) The criteria for failure should be failure to respond at 10 dB at 1000, 2000, or 6000 cps or at the 20-dB level at 4000 cycles.

(5) The same failure criteria should apply to both the screen and the pure-tone threshold test.

These are the recommendations that the present study attempts to evaluate. The recommended procedures differ mainly in two respects from those which have been used in testing school children. First, the screening level for the sweep check has been uniformly 15 dB re audiometric zero. Second, failure at two of the test frequencies has required the child to have a pure-tone threshold test. In some instances the child might have been tested a second time before a threshold measurement was made. Criteria for failure has specified threshold sensitivity at a level of 20 dB or greater at two frequencies, or 30 dB or more for any one frequency. These levels have been based on adult test results and sensitivity norms which are themselves under question.

The recommended procedures advise a +10-dB screening level in order to identify children who begin not to hear at +15 dB, the level at which hearing impairment for speech may begin. The less stringent requirement of +20 dB at 4000 cps suggests that a loss of this magnitude at this frequency has less significance than it would have at other frequencies.

The use of the new screen level requires testing in an environment quieter than any usually found in schools. A quiet part of a school building is no longer acceptable. The use of acoustically treated test rooms is specifically recommended.

SUBJECTS

Eight hundred and eighty children from kindergarten through the eighth grade of four elementary schools in the Pittsburgh public school system participated in the study. These children were functioning as normal public school pupils with no apparent hearing problems at the time of the test. They were participants in a larger Pittsburgh hearing study (Jordan and Eagles, 1961) and had experienced hearing testing prior to this investigation. No use was made of information from medical histories.

ENVIRONMENT

Both the screening and the threshold tests were performed in a double-walled test room, Industrial Acoustics Model 1202. Sound sampling has shown that the ambient noise levels were well below the levels described as criteria for background noise in audiometer test rooms by the American Standards Association (1960).

EQUIPMENT

Audivox 8-B audiometers with Western Electric 705A earphones and associated sponge rubber cushions were used for testing. An additional 40 dB of attenuation was provided by an auxiliary attenuator. The equipment was calibrated monthly to meet the American Standard specifications. The equipment and environment are described in more detail by Eagles and Doerfler (1961).

TECHNICIANS

Four female test technicians performed the audiometric tests. These women were trained and had considerable experience in performing the test techniques used in the Pittsburgh hearing study. Each technician was assigned a permanent school location and performed both the sweep check and the threshold examinations for children attending that school.

TEST TECHNIQUES

Sweep Check

The test frequencies were 500, 1000, 2000, 4000, and 6000 cps, and were presented in that order. The screening level was set at 20 dB for 4000 cycles and at ten dB for the other frequencies. One ear was tested completely before shifting to the other ear. The duration of the tone varied between one and three seconds at each frequency. The criterion for failure was no response at any one of the test frequencies for either ear. Only one presentation per ear was made of a test frequency.

Threshold Test

A serial method of limits was used. The test tone was started at 40 dB and reduced in steps of ten dB until the subject failed to respond. The intensity was then increased by 5-dB steps until response was obtained. The tone was again reduced ten dB and a 5-dB ascent was presented. This procedure continued until a point was reached which produced a response in two out of three ascending trials. If there was no response at the initial 40-dB level, the tone intensity was increased until a response was obtained or until the maximum output was reached. When a response was given, the procedure continued in the way just described. Only the ascending trials were used in determining the threshold hearing levels. The thresholds at 250 and 8000 were obtained in addition to those frequencies presented in the sweep check. In the analysis only those tones common to both types of test were investigated.

PROCEDURE

The child was instructed to raise his hand whenever he heard the tone and to keep his hand up as long as the tone was heard. This mode of response was the same for both the pure-tone sweep check and the threshold test. The child then entered the test room, the earphones were placed by the technician, and the testing was begun. The first test performed was the sweep check. If the child passed the first screen, he was immediately tested by the threshold technique. The child who failed the sweep check was dismissed at this point and scheduled for a second test session the following school day. The second test period involved another sweep check and then, regardless of whether the child failed or passed, a threshold test was performed.

All of the children who were tested by the sweep check and the threshold tests within a particular week were examined by an otolaryngologist sometime during that same week.

Although the second sweep check is not part of the recommendations of the Conference on Identification Audiometry, this procedure is often used in present hearing testing programs. It was used here in order to evaluate its effectiveness in reducing the number of false failures.

The criteria used to define a failure did not follow precisely the recommendations of the conference. Because of anticipated problems in obtaining a quiet environment and consequently of masking, the conference did not include 500 cps for consideration of failure and referral. The quiet environment was available for this study, and prior large-scale experience in testing children did not indicate a particular problem with 500 cps. Therefore, criteria were established that defined a failure as no response at 10 dB for 500, 1000, 2000, or 6000 cps, and at 20 dB for 4000 cps.

RESULTS AND DISCUSSION

A comparison of the results of the first sweep check with those of the threshold technique

TABLE 44-1. COMPARISON OF THE PERFORMANCE ON THE FIRST SWEEP-CHECK SCREEN AND ON THE THRESHOLD TEST

| | First Sweep Check | | |
	Passed	Failed	Total
Threshold Test			
Passed	666	51	717
Failed	18	125	143
Total	684	176	860

TABLE 44-2. COMPARISON OF THE PERFORMANCE ON THE SECOND SWEEP-CHECK SCREEN AND ON THE THRESHOLD TEST OF CHILDREN WHO FAILED THE FIRST SCREEN

| | Second Sweep Check | | |
	Passed	Failed	Total
Threshold Test			
Passed	38	13	51
Failed	3	122	125
Total	41	135	176

is shown in Table 44-1. Twenty of the participating children who could not be tested reliably were excluded from the study, and the total number of children available for analysis was thus reduced from 880 to 860. The test results were judged unreliable if the child did not perform according to test instruction and if the child's responses were inconsistent with the presentation of the test signals. The twenty unreliable subjects were distributed throughout the age range and were found to have no abnormalities upon otoscopic examination.

Table 44-1 shows that 51 children or 29 percent of the 176 who failed the initial screen, passed the threshold test. These 51 subjects represent the false positives, i.e., those who would have been needlessly referred for further audiometric testing on the basis of an initial screen and who, therefore, represent one form of inefficiency. The 18 subjects who passed the initial screen but failed the threshold test are called the false negatives. They are children who possibly might have a hearing problem but were missed by the first sweep-check screen, reflecting another type of inefficiency of screening methodology.

The number of false positives can be reduced by a second screening; but in the case where only the failures of the first sweep check are given a second screening, the number of false negatives can only be kept the same. When failures on the initial screen were rescreened and the result compared with the threshold test, Table 44-2, the number of false positives was reduced to 13, or only seven percent of the initial failures. Three of the initial failures passed the second

screening but failed the threshold test. Of the 135 who failed both screens (Table 44-2), 122 or 90.4 percent were shown to fail the threshold test also. Had only one screen been used (Table 44-1) only 71 percent of the screening failures, 125 of 176, would have failed the threshold as well. (The second screening reduced the over referrals by almost ten percent.)

A more intensive investigation of the audiometric performance of the children showed that among the 21 false negatives uncovered by both screenings, in 15 cases the child failed the threshold at only one frequency and by just one (five dB) intensity step. The six remaining children showed thresholds less sensitive than the criterion at two frequencies and again usually by five or ten dB (one or two steps).

Out of the total of 51 false positives, 38 children failed the first screen, but passed both the second screen and the threshold test (Table 44-2). Thirty-one of these 38 children failed the first sweep check at only one frequency in one ear. The difference in performance between the two screens could be attributed to variability acceptable in this type of test situation. Differences of five dB are given little significance in clinical test-retest results and yet could have produced failure of one screen with success in passing another. This much difference can result from variables other than a decrease in hearing sensitivity and could well have been an attention or a motivation problem. This is especially so when only one frequency is involved. Failure at only one frequency was seen among the remaining 13 false positives who failed both screens but passed the threshold test

(Table 44-2). Nine out of the 13 who failed the first screening, and ten out of 13 who failed the second screening did so at only one frequency in one ear. In this particular sample of children, 41 of the 51 false positives, or 80 percent could have been eliminated if the criterion for failure were changed to failure at any two test frequencies in either ear rather than failure at any one frequency. Failure at 500 cycles did not contribute greatly to the number of false positives. In only three of the 51 cases was 500 cycles the sole failing frequency. In those children who failed all three of the tests, the same picture regarding performance at 500 cps was seen. Three subjects failed the first screen at 500 cycles and one child on the second screen.

The two screens showed relatively good agreement with each other. Among the 122 children who failed both, there was complete agreement in 60 cases. Thirty-two cases differed at one frequency, and the remaining 30 children differed at more than one frequency. The second screen agreed more closely with the threshold failures than the first. There was complete agreement for 71 out of 122 children, while for the first screen, this was true in only 49 cases. The greater agreement was due probably to the fact that the second screen and threshold

tests were given consecutively on the same day, thus reducing the possibility of variation not only in the subjects' hearing sensitivity but in other conditions of the subject, environment, tester, and equipment.

Table 44-3 shows the number of failures

TABLE 44-3. NUMBER OF FAILURES AT EACH FREQUENCY FOR THE 122 CHILDREN WHO FAILED * BOTH SCREENS AND THE THRESHOLD TEST. CLASSIFIED BY TEST TECHNIQUE AND EAR

Test Technique	500	1000	2000	4000	6000
Right Ear					
First Screen	31	40	41	35	61
Second Screen	31	39	34	31	56
Threshold	28	38	37	29	60
Left Ear					
First Screen	31	40	47	33	57
Second Screen	29	38	47	36	41
Threshold	24	37	37	29	58

* Failure criteria for screening tests was no response at 10 dB re American audiometric zero for 500, 1000, 2000, and 6000 cps and 20 dB at 4000 cps. Failure on the threshold tests was indicated by a threshold higher than 10 dB at 500, 1000, 2000, and 6000 cps and 20 dB at 4000 cps.

for each screen as well as for the threshold examination at each frequency. Among the 122 children who failed all three tests, the greatest number of failures occurred at 6000 cps. The larger value of the failure criterion for 4000 cps (+20 dB) produced

TABLE 44-4. A COMPARISON OF PASS-FAIL PERFORMANCE ON TWO SCREENINGS USING PURE-TONE SWEEP CHECK, AND A PURE-TONE THRESHOLD TEST FOR CHILDREN CLASSIFIED BY AGE

Year Age of Child	Total		Passed First Screen *				Failed First Screen but Passed Second				Failed Both Screens			
			Passed Threshold		Failed Threshold		Passed Threshold		Failed Threshold		Passed Threshold		Failed Threshold	
	No.	Pct.	No.	Pct.	No.	Pct.	No.	Pct.	No.	Pct.	No.	Pct.	No.	Pct.
4	2	0.2	2	0.3	—	—	—	—	—	—	—	—	—	—
5	28	3.3	20	3.0	—	—	—	—	—	—	1	7.7	7	5.7
6	131	15.2	111	16.7	3	16.7	1	2.6	—	—	3	23.1	13	10.6
7	116	13.5	87	13.1	2	11.1	6	15.8	1	33.3	1	7.7	19	15.6
8	106	12.3	82	12.3	2	11.1	2	5.3	1	33.3	1	7.7	18	14.8
9	75	8.7	51	7.6	4	22.2	6	15.8	—	—	2	15.4	12	9.8
10	101	11.7	78	11.7	1	5.6	4	10.5	—	—	2	15.4	16	13.1
11	97	11.3	77	11.6	2	11.1	3	7.9	—	—	1	7.7	14	11.5
12	116	13.5	95	14.3	2	11.1	9	23.7	—	—	1	7.7	9	7.4
13	60	7.0	43	6.4	1	5.6	6	15.8	1	33.3	—	—	9	7.4
14	25	2.9	17	2.6	1	5.6	1	2.6	—	—	1	7.7	5	4.1
15	3	0.3	3	0.4	—	—	—	—	—	—	—	—	—	—
Total	860	100.0	666	100.0	18	100.0	38	100.0	3	100.0	13	100.0	122	100.0

* Not given second screen.

TABLE 44-5. DISTRIBUTION OF PASS-FAIL PERFORMANCES BY CHILDREN ON THE SCREENING AND THRESHOLD TESTS, CLASSIFIED BY TYPE OF OTOSCOPIC FINDING

Otoscopic Finding in One or Both Ears	Total		Passed First Screen *				Failed First Screen but passed Second				Failed Both Screens			
			Passed Threshold		Failed Threshold		Passed Threshold		Failed Threshold		Passed Threshold		Failed Threshold	
	No.	Pct.	No.	Pct.	No.	Pct.	No.	Pct.	No.	Pct.	No.	Pct.	No.	Pct.
No Abnormality	610	70.9	497	74.6	10	55.6	24	63.2	1	33.3	11	84.6	67	54.9
Unsatisfactory Visibility	123	14.3	89	13.4	3	16.7	6	15.8	1	33.3	0	0.0	24	19.7
Evidence of Active Pathology	27	3.1	10	1.5	2	12.5	2	5.3	0	0.0	0	0.0	13	10.6
Evidence of Past Pathology	100	11.6	70	10.5	3	16.7	6	15.8	1	33.3	2	15.4	18	14.8
Total	860	100.0	666	100.0	18	100.0	38	100.0	3	100.0	13	100.0	122	100.0

* Not given second screen.

numbers of failures more consistent with those seen at 500, 1000, and 2000 cps. If a +20-dB criterion had also been adopted for 6000 cps, the number of failures for the threshold examination at that frequency would have been reduced almost 50 percent.

The subjects varied in age from four to 15 years. It was possible that the age factor may have been an important influence in causing inconsistencies between screening and threshold test results. To investigate this possibility the failures were tabulated as a function of age. As Table 44-4 shows, however, there were no obviously consistent patterns in the age distributions which would indicate a systematic influence of the age variable for these children.

The Monograph on Identification Audiometry states that the purpose of the audiometric testing ". . . is to lead to the final identification of those who should be referred to an otologist, or other physician, for a complete diagnostic work-up" (Hardy, 1961, p. 26). "The goal is to locate children who have even minimal hearing problems so that they can be referred for medical treatment of any active ear conditions discovered to be present and so that remedial educational procedures can be instituted at the earliest possible date" (Hardy, p. 16).

Thus, the purpose of audiometric testing is two-fold. Initially, it is to locate children with decreased hearing sensitivity and, secondly, to locate children with active ear conditions for medical treatment. It has been assumed that the group with decreased hearing sensitivity would contain those children in need of medical attention.

To evaluate this second function of the identification program, an otolaryngological examination was given to all the children who participated, regardless of audiometric test results. The results of the otoscopic portion of the examination are shown in Tables 44-5 and 44-6.

Some definition of the otoscopic categories appears in order. The category of "unsatisfactory visibility" resulted from the fact that the physicians were not permitted to remove cerumen or any other substance which may have occluded the auditory canal. The "evidence of active pathology" category consisted of those children with inflammation or discoloration of the tympanic membrane, perforation with and without discharge, bulging, and retraction if the last finding occurred in combination with other signs which were considered evidence of acute or chronic otitis media. The category called "evidence of past pathology" included instances of scars, decreased mobility, calcium plaques, and retraction of the tympanic membrane when it was a single sign.

There was a considerable proportion of each audiometric performance classification without apparent otoscopic abnormality or unsatisfactory visibility (Table 44-5). These children, if referred to an otologist, might be

TABLE 44-6. CHILDREN WITH DIFFERENT TYPES OF OTOSCOPIC FINDINGS CLASSIFIED BY PERFORMANCE ON THE SCREENING
AND THRESHOLD TESTS

Otoscopic Findings in One or Both Ears	Total		Passed First Screen *				Failed First Screen				Failed Both Screens			
			Passed Threshold		Failed Threshold		Passed Threshold		Failed Threshold		Passed Threshold		Failed Threshold	
	No.	Pct.	No.	Pct.	No.	Pct.	No.	Pct.	No.	Pct.	No.	Pct.	No.	Pct.
No Abnormality	610	100.	497	81.5	10	1.6	24	3.9	1	0.2	11	1.8	67	11.0
Unsatisfactory Visibility	123	100.	89	72.4	3	2.4	6	4.9	1	0.8	0	0.0	24	19.5
Evidence of Active Pathology	27	100.	10	37.0	2	7.4	2	7.4	0	0.0	0	0.0	13	48.0
Evidence of Past Pathology	100	100.	70	70.0	3	3.0	6	6.0	1	1.0	2	2.0	18	18.0
Total	860	100.	666	77.4	18	2.1	38	4.4	3	0.3	13	1.5	122	14.2

* Not given second screen.

considered over-referrals by him. Of the 122 children who would be referred on the basis of having failed all three tests, 67 or 54.9 percent would be found with no otologic abnormality.

The category of most interest is that of active pathology. There were 27 cases in the entire group examined, only 13 of which would have been referred for a diagnostic examination because of a failure on all three tests. Thus, the 13 children with active pathology who failed the hearing tests represent 48 percent of the total, while 52 percent were falsely labelled as negative at some point in the hearing testing program and lost to referral. Even more interesting is the fact shown in Table 44-6, that 12 of the 27 cases, or 44 percent, passed the more carefully conducted threshold test. The audiometric program would have referred for a diagnostic work-up two out of seven children observed with inflammation of the tympanic membrane, one out of two children with acute otitis media, six out of 13 children with chronic serous otitis media, and four out of five with perforation and discharge.

The children with evidence of past infection should be identified as well as possible in a hearing conservation program in order to provide these children with more careful and perhaps more frequent monitoring of their hearing sensitivity and the physical condition of their ears. Some of these children may have been identified by historical infor-

mation. Since this study did not make use of medical histories, this factor cannot be evaluated. From the results solely from hearing testing, Table 44-6 shows the test program to be less successful at identifying these children. Seventy percent passed both the initial screening and the threshold test. This is not surprising since many of the children return to levels of hearing sensitivity which are considered normal from the clinical point of view.

When the more liberal criteria for failure of the threshold test which has served in past programs, i.e., two frequencies with a hearing level of 20 dB or one frequency with a level of 30 dB or more, are used, only one additional child identified as having active pathology would have been missed. The change in the failure criteria to the more stringent levels did not apparently improve the identification of the children with otologic abnormality.

Following the completion of the threshold test, each child was questioned about his status with regard to colds, earaches, and ear discharge at the time of the test. Little positive information resulted from the children's responses. The children who failed all three tests showed a slightly higher percentage of colds at the time of the test or during the preceding week than other children. It was hoped that a history of respiratory illness might account for inconsistent results between the two screens, but this had little apparent effect.

Twenty-seven of 860 children reported earaches in one or both ears, but only seven of the 27 failed the three audiometric tests. Fourteen of the 27 showed negative otoscopic findings. There were eight cases of reported ear discharge, five of which were present in the failing group. Out of the eight, four were reported to have no abnormality by the otolaryngologists. The reliability of the cold, earache, and ear discharge information is questionable.

The results of this study show that the recommended screening program was successful in characterizing the hearing sensitivity of the participating public school children. Of the 860 children, 96 percent were correctly identified as having either normal or decreased hearing sensitivity when a threshold test was used for validation. The screening test incorrectly indicated normal hearing sensitivity in 2.5 percent of the children who subsequently were shown to have some hearing loss by the threshold measurement. The remaining 1.5 percent were falsely identified as having decreased hearing sensitivity by the screenings.

A second screening for those children who failed, reduced the number of children incorrectly labelled as failures by about 74 percent. The screening program was made more effective by using failure on two sweep checks as an indication for more thorough threshold testing.

The use of the audiometric test results to identify those children with otologic problems was not adequate. Almost half of the cases with active pathology and probably in need of immediate medical attention were missed.

Seventy percent of the children with evidence of past otological difficulty were not identified. These findings are similar to those reported by Jordan and Eagles (1961). Changes in the criteria for failure of the sweep check and threshold tests to lower hearing levels did not rectify the situation.

The frequency most often failed by the children was 6000 cps. Changing the criterion for failure to the more liberal 20 dB on the threshold test would keep the number of failures at 6000 cps consistent with those at the other test frequencies. A similar change in the failure criterion for this frequency on the screening tests would probably produce the same effect, although this is not known since it was not done. In the quiet environment used for testing in this study, 500 cycles did not present any particular problem for the children who were tested. This study was not designed to evaluate a one- or two-frequency screen; and, therefore, no speculation concerning this aspect was made.

SUMMARY

The recommended program of the National Conference on Identification Audiometry for identification audiometry with the school-age child was applied to 860 children in four public elementary schools. The test program was successful in finding those children with a reduced hearing sensitivity. The hearing test results, both for the screening and the threshold test procedures, did not adequately identify children with otoscopic evidence of active or past ear pathology.

REFERENCES

American Standard Criteria for Background Noise in Audiometer Rooms, S 3.1. New York Amer. Standards Assoc., 1960.

Eagles, E. L., and Doerfler, L. G., Acoustic environment and audiometer performance. *J. Speech Hearing Res.* 4, 1961, 149–163.

Hardy, William G. (General Chairman), National Conference on Identification Audiometry Committee, Identification audiometry. *J. Speech Hearing Dis.* Monograph Suppl. 9, 1961.

Jordan, R. E., and Eagles, E. L., The relation of air conduction audiometry to otological abnormalities. *Ann. Otol. Rhin. and Laryng.*, 70, 1961, 819–827.

45

Dilemmas in Identification Audiometry

MARION P. DOWNS
MILDRED E. DOSTER
MARLIN WEAVER

MARION P. DOWNS is Director, Clinical Audiology, and Assistant Proffessor of Otolaryngology, University of Colorado Medical Center
MILDRED E. DOSTER, M.D., M.S.P.H., is Assistant Director, Division, of School Health Services, Denver Public Schools
MARLIN WEAVER, M.D., is Assistant Clinical Professor, University of Colorado Medical Center

Recent articles on identification audiometry have highlighted dilemmas for schools and other agencies conducting hearing conservation programs. The first dilemma concerns procedures and standards: shall the agencies continue to follow the recommendations of the National Conference on Identification Audiometry (1960) that a 10 dB level be used in their screening programs; or shall they attempt to identify, without regard to hearing level, all children who have active or past ear pathology, as suggested by Melnick, Eagles and Levine (1964) and by Jordan and Eagles (1961)? These latter reports found that not only does a 10 dB screening level fail to identify those children with otoscopic evidence of past or present ear pathology, but that even a 0 dB screening level would fail to identify all ear diseases. The implication is that audiometric screening programs as presently conducted fail to meet the goals and responsibilities of the agencies undertaking them.

The second dilemma concerns the frequency of conducting screening programs and the number of grades that should be screened: shall the agencies continue to screen throughout the grades, every two or three years, as

Reprinted by permission of the authors from *J. Speech Hearing Dis.*, **30**, pp. 360–364 (1965).

suggested by the National Conference on Identification Audiometry (1961), or shall they cover the lower grades more intensively and minimize screening in the upper grades, as indicated in a report by Corliss and Watson (1961)? The latter study demonstrated that at least 85 percent of all hearing problems that evolved during the school years were detected in screening by or during the third grade. There appears to be a law of diminishing returns operative in the screening process, and a sense of practicality demands that this factor be examined.

From the respective viewpoints of an audiologist, a school health physician and an otolaryngologist, the authors have been greatly concerned with the confusion resulting from the above studies. The discussion which follows undertakes to provide a few guidelines for interested agencies.

PROCEDURES AND STANDARDS

The criticisms implicit in the studies of Melnick, Eagles and Levine (1964) and Jordan and Eagles (1961) were anticipated by Downs and Doster (1958) and by Hildyard, Stool and Valentine (1963). These reports demonstrated that indeed young children can be expected to have extremely good bone conduction thresholds, and that normal air conduction thresholds did not preclude the presence of either air-bone gaps or ear pathology.

Melnick and Eagles' (1964) figures explicitly point up the problem: 52 percent of all children with active pathology were not identified by audiometric procedures, and 70 percent of those with evidence of past ear diseases were not identified by pure tone tests. These authors concluded that audiometric procedures do not adequately identify children with otoscopic evidence of active or past ear pathology.

The criticisms implied by the above studies rest on the premise that the primary goal of school hearing programs is the detection of active or past ear disease, whether accompanied by hearing loss or not. This premise must be carefully examined before we fall into the error of castigating present programs for their inadequacies. What, actually, are the stated goals of agencies conducting screening programs? The most representative statement of goals has been made by the Joint Committee on Health Problems in Education, of the NEA and the AMA (1964):

> From the point of view of school health services, primary responsibilities are an awareness of the importance of early recognition of suspected hearing loss, especially in the primary grades; intelligent observation of pupils for signs indicative of hearing difficulty; organization and conduct of an audiometric screening survey; and a counseling and follow-up program to help children with hearing difficulties obtain diagnostic examinations, needed treatment, and such adaptations of their school program as their hearing condition dictates.

This statement of purpose is concerned with a hearing level that is adequate for communication purposes—not with minor ear pathologies that can only be detected otoscopically. No agencies concerned with school testing have ever stated otherwise.

We can assume that a 10 dB screening level fulfills the goal of identifying hearing that is adequate or inadequate at the time of testing. The question that remains is whether such identification is effective in maintaining the adequate hearing that is now present in ears with minor pathologies. Does the presence of positive ear pathology, unaccompanied by significant hearing loss, presage the development of more significant ear pathology and concomitant communication problems, in large enough numbers to justify an all-out effort in the field of preventive medicine in ear disease?

The predominant active middle ear pathology which may progress into a hearing loss without the obvious symptoms of hearing deficit, pain, or discharge, is that of chronic serous otitis media. This condition is characterized by the accumulation of a gluey residue in the middle ear in association with occlusion of the eustachian tube following acute otitis media that is not completely resolved. Such cases are often found with normal air conduction levels, but with significant air-bone gaps when both air and bone conduction are tested. If the gluey residue is allowed to remain, it may consolidate, affecting the function of the ossicular chain and other middle ear structures. The resultant hearing loss may be difficult to correct medically or surgically, and it is these cases which concern otologists interested in preventive measures. However, the development of irreversible middle ear changes is difficult to predict and the frequency, though low, is ill-defined.

Similarly, it is not possible to estimate the number of children with evidence of past infection who can be expected to have recurrent ear problems that will throw them into the positive hearing loss group. It is quite probable that the pathologies in such cases would eventually fall into the categories of inflammation of the tympanic membrane, acute otitis media, and perforation and discharge—all of which would be identified by the symptoms of hearing loss, pain or discharge. Such cases would probably not be progressive unless unattended in their active state, or unless they were to develop into serous otitis. They do not therefore constitute a large group of sub-clinical ear conditions which may cause irreversible hearing loss such as the serous otitis condition.

Although no estimates are available on the actual numbers that need concern us, we can look at the results of on-going hearing surveys and determine how many children who pass screening tests in their early years show up with hearing losses later on. The study of Corliss and Watson (1961) reviewed the individual pure tone screening program of the Denver Public Schools since 1947, in which a 15 dB screening level was used. They showed that only 15 percent of all the eventually significant ear problems developed after the third grade had been reached. When one considers that a large proportion of the 15 percent new cases must have been caused by the more obvious etiologies—not progressive serous otitis—it follows that only a relatively small number of previously undetected cases need concern us. Melnick, Eagles and Levine (1964) found fewer than half of their active cases to have chronic serous otitis media, and 48 percent of these were detected by the pure tone screening testing. Projecting their own figures it seems reasonable to conclude that fewer than 1 percent of all the significant hearing problems fall into the class that might be preventable if special techniques other than audiometry were used earlier to detect the minor deviations.

How far should a program go to single out so small a number of cases for preventive treatment? To accomplish the otoscopic screening suggested by Melnick, Eagles and Levine (1964), qualified otolaryngologists would have to examine annually the ears of every school child in order to detect those few whose progressive involvement may be prevented. The economics of such a program approaches absurdity.

An alternative step to insure identification of more of the ear pathologies would be to institute annual threshold audiometric tests of every school child. Requisite to such a program would be sound-isolated rooms and

well-trained audiologists. The former are expensive; the latter both expensive and scarce. The economics of this kind of program precludes its implementation in the foreseeable future.

A third possibility would be to institute a tuning fork testing program as suggested by Hildyard, Stool and Valentine (1963). This procedure would be a practical one if audiologists and trained volunteers were able to conduct the tests with validity and reliability, but we are not too sanguine about the prospects of developing this skill in enough people to make wide-scale testing feasible.

It seems we are left only the status quo, with which we must live for a while—and it is not at all a bad prospect. The primary concern of education programs is to screen out pupils with deviations in hearing that affect classroom communication. Certainly, all agencies should attack vigorously the medical problems of school children in their Hearing Conservation programs, and should conduct all screening testing as meticulously as possible. But we urge the agencies to feel confident that a routine screening program in schools using a 10 dB criterion,* with a stoutly pursued medical follow-up procedure, satisfies the responsibilities incumbent upon them. If any further expenditure were justified, it would be to assure that every child found in the screening programs be brought to consultation with an otolaryngologist—for herein lies one of the greatest weaknesses of present programs. Melnick, Eagles and Levine do us a great service in allowing us to recognize the limitations of our programs, but we will do better to concentrate on the present weaknesses than to attempt

[* *As of 1968, the authors are currently recommending that when audiometers are calibrated to the ISO 1964 Standard, the following criteria be used:*

500	1000	2000	4000	6000
25 dB	20 dB	20 dB	25 dB	20 dB

We suggest a 25 dB screening level be used at all frequencies tested when a high level of noise is a chronic condition in the screening environment. Further, if 500 Hz is the only frequency failed, the screening level here can be raised to 30 dB. MPD, MED, MW]

questionable and impractical extensions of programs.

FREQUENCY OF SCREENING AND GRADES SCREENED

We come now to the obverse of the coin: is it possible that screening programs are actually wasting time and effort in unproductive testing in the upper grades? In Corliss and Watson's analysis (1961) of school screening records on 14,800 tenth graders, only 31 (0.21 percent) were cases that had not been detected in the lower grades. Many hours—probably over 300—were required to detect these 31 previously unknown cases, or about 50 days of screening and audiometric testing. This is indeed a high price to pay for such a low yield—particularly when the study demonstrated that 63 percent of all the hearing defects were detected at age five in kindergarten, and 85 percent by the third grade. Certainly any agency must consider the cost of a program in relation to its yield, and these diminishing returns in testing the upper grades should be scrutinized carefully. Would it be more profitable to screen more intensively and finely in kindergarten and in grades 1, 2, and 3, and to minimize testing in the upper grades? The Denver Public Schools, on the basis of the above study, have elected to test only to the seventh grade; beyond that, testing is made only of new students, previous screening failures, and parent, physician, and teacher or nurse referrals. Other school systems with different types of testing equipment, personnel, small student bodies, etc., may find it feasible to extend their programs to the upper grades, but many will find it impractical to do so on the basis of low yield.

CONCLUSIONS

Although agencies may vary considerably in their approaches to the problems we have discussed, we feel it is reasonable to make the following recommendations:

1. The presently recommended screening level of 10 dB† adequately fulfills the goals and responsibilities of educational programs at the present time.

2. The medical aspects of the hearing problems of school children should be attacked vigorously, with special emphasis on obtaining examination by an otolaryngologist of every child found to have a hearing problem.

3. More intensive search should be concentrated on the lower grades, where the largest percentage of hearing problems occur, and consideration may be given to relaxing the search in the upper grades.

[† See previous footnote.]

REFERENCES

Corliss, L., and Watson, J., A school system studies the effectiveness of routine audiometry. *J. Health, Phys. Ed. Rec.* of NEA, March, 1961, 27.

Darley, F. L., Identification audiometry. Monograph Supplement, *J. Speech Hearing Dis.*, 9, 1961, 1–68.

Downs, M., and Doster, M., A hearing testing program for pre-school children. *Rocky Mt. Med. J.*, 56, 1959, 37–39.

Hildyard, V. H., Stool, S., and Valentine, M., Tuning fork tests as aid to screening audiometry. *Arch. Otolaryng.*, 78, 1963, 151–154.

Jordan, R. E., and Eagles, E. L., The relation of air conduction audiometry to otological abnormalities. *Ann. Otol. Rhin.*, 70, 1961, 819–827.

Melnick, W., Eagles, E. L., and Levine, H. S., Evaluation of a recommended program of identification audiometry with school-age children. *J. Speech Hearing Dis.*, 29, 1964, 3–13.

Report of the committee for hearing conservation of the school health section of the American Public Health Association and the American School Health Association. *J. School Health*, 24, #5, 1959, 171–186.

Wilson, C. C., School Health Services. *Publication of the Joint Committee on Health Problems in Education of the N.E.A. and the A.M.A.*, 1964.

46

Evaluating School Hearing Testing Procedures

BRUCE M. SIEGENTHALER

BRUCE M. SIEGENTHALER, Ph.D., is Director, Speech and Hearing Clinic, Pennsylvania State University

In a recent paper comparing a two-frequency and a five-frequency technique for public school screening, it was reported that the two-frequency procedure was simpler, faster to administer, and less fatiguing for the tester. The report also indicated that the two-frequency method was less reliable, but that it could be administered in a familiar classroom environment and was less distracting to young children, less advanced preparation was needed to administer the two-frequency screening method, and it did not disrupt class schedules as much as the five-frequency procedure (Norton and Lux, "Double Frequency Auditory Screening in Public Schools," *J. Speech Hearing Dis.*, *25*, 1960, 293–299). All these are important reasons for using two-frequency screening as the method of choice.

However, the data leading to some of these conclusions deserve further consideration, especially as they relate to time required for testing. According to the data reported, an ordinary classroom (of approximately 33 children) could be screened by the two-frequency method in 10 to 15 minutes and by the five-frequency method in 20 to 40 minutes. Assuming an even distribution among classrooms, the 1046 subjects in the study would be found in 32 classrooms. (Although there probably was not equal distribution of subjects among classrooms inasmuch as some were in special classes, the assumption is

Reprinted by permission of the author from *J. Speech Hearing Dis.*, **26**, pp. 291–294 (1961).

adequate for present purposes.) In view of the time range given, a reasonable average screening time per classroom is 13.5 minutes for the two-frequency method and 30 minutes for the five-frequency method. Thus, 432 minutes would be required for the two-frequency screening and 960 minutes would be required for the five-frequency screening of 32 classrooms. On the basis of these data, the two-frequency method has a time advantage of more than 1 to 2 over the five-frequency method for the screening of 1046 children.

However, a school testing program intends to detect children with hearing problems as verified according to threshold testing. Therefore, an evaluation of testing time for a procedure must take into account the total time required to identify children with hearing losses.

According to the Norton and Lux data, among the 196 children who failed the two-frequency screening 103 were false positives (did not have hearing loss confirmed by follow-up testing) and 93 had hearing loss confirmed; among the 164 children who failed the five-frequency screening 76 were false positives and 88 had confirmed hearing loss.

When school children with screening test failures are followed up, a common procedure is to do a recheck screening test and to give a threshold test only when it is evident that the child has failed the second screening. Rechecks should be done in a quiet room separate from the classroom. Time is required to move the child to and from the test room and special care should be taken on the recheck. A reasonable minimum time is two minutes in which to recheck (by screen test only) a child who failed the initial screening and to confirm that he does not have a loss. If this time of two minutes is applied to the number of false positives mentioned above, 206 minutes would be required to recheck false positives from the two-frequency screening, and 152 minutes would be required to recheck false positives from the five-frequency screening.

A reasonable time for follow-up of a child with hearing loss (screening to the point of failure and thresholds by air conduction on two ears) is 15 minutes, assuming an expert tester and cooperative child. Thus, 1395 minutes would be required to retest the 93 children with loss according to the two-frequency screening method, and 1320 minutes would be required to retest the 88 children with loss according to the five-frequency screening method.

By adding the various times involved an estimate of total testing time for each of the screening methods is obtained (Table 46-1).

TABLE 46-1. TESTING TIMES IN MINUTES USING TWO SCREENING METHODS FOR 1046 CHILDREN

	Two-Frequency Screening	Five-Frequency Screening
Screening	432	960
Recheck of false positives	206	152
Threshold testing	1395	1320
Total minutes	2033	2432
Total hours	33.9	40.5

These values show the two-frequency screening method to have a 6.6 hour advantage and the time ratio between the two-frequency program (screening plus rechecks and thresholds) and the five-frequency program is about four to five. This ratio is of a somewhat different order than that implied by the approximately 10 to 15 minutes per classroom for two-frequency screening versus 20 to 40 minutes per classroom for five-frequency screening mentioned earlier.

However, the above does not give a definitive comparison of the two methods. According to the two-frequency method 103 children were false positives; by the five-frequency method 76 children were false positives. The time spent rechecking a false positive child is wasted not only for the tester but also for the child and for school personnel such as teachers who must arrange for the child's recheck. Although the total time for the case finding based on the two-frequency screening was less, the amount of time wasted by this method was greater than for the five-frequency method. (On the other hand, it can be argued that the longer time for screening by the five-frequency method during which a classroom is disturbed offsets the greater disturbance caused by the more rechecks required by the two-frequency method.)

Further considerations also ought to influence the evaluation of a hearing testing program. For example, it would be an unusual situation in which 32 classrooms were contained in the same school building. Ordinarily the tester must travel from one school to another; this travel time would be approximately the same for any screening method. If a constant amount of time for moving from school to school is added to the total testing time for each of the two screening methods, the absolute time difference would remain. But the relative time differential would be reduced. Furthermore, saving in time for screening must be evaluated in terms of the total program; that is, completion of testing at one site an hour in advance of the testing time required for testing by another method does not necessarily mean that this hour can be used to accomplish testing at another site.

Efficiency of a screen procedure in terms of case finding is also of interest. The two-frequency screening was reported to be 98 percent as accurate as the five-frequency screening, but the data used to arrive at the accuracy value were not indicated. However, it was indicated that among the 1046 screening tests administered the two-frequency procedure had 942 accurate tests and the five-frequency procedure had 964 accurate tests. The percentage ratio between these two numbers is 97.72, and it may be assumed this was the basis for the 98 percent accuracy given to the two-frequency screening. (Unfortunately, the data do not indicate whether all of the 942 children were included in the 964 children, and it is difficult to know the total number of children among the 1046 with hearing loss. Among 1046 children screened, 21.9 percent (229) were reported to have failed threshold testing. This appears to be a very high proportion of failures.)

The procedure for computing 98 percent accuracy for the two-frequency procedure is questionable. Assume a sample of 100 children among whom five have hearing loss. Screening method A with follow-up testing results in the final detection of four who have hearing loss, and screening method B with follow-up results in the detection of three with loss. Method A has 99 accurate tests, and method B has 98 accurate tests. Method B should not, in this writer's opinion, be considered 98.99 percent as accurate as method A (98 accurate tests divided by 99 accurate tests) because, although speed and convenience are important factors when evaluating a hearing testing procedure, the factor of primary concern is the detection of children who have aural difficulty. (The above type of error in evaluating the efficiency of a screening method has been committed by other researchers.) Accuracy ratings of a case finding procedure should be strongly weighted in terms of accuracy of discovering children with ear trouble, and this means the child with an aural problem is

the unit to be considered. Thus in this hypothetical example, method B is 75 percent as accurate as method A because it detected three-fourths as many children with hearing loss as method A.

The intent of the present note is not to denigrate what is an interesting and informative article by Norton and Lux. Rather, the the intent is to express the viewpoint that the value of a school hearing testing program does not reside in time taken for screening only, but is related to total time required to complete the case finding of individuals among the group of interest. The total lapsed time to accomplish a testing program should be considered. Furthermore, the evaluation of a testing method should emphasize the proportion of persons with hearing loss detected, and not be limited to considering the total sample of individuals tested or total number of accurate tests.

Other factors which also should be considered involve cost of equipment and convenience of operation, maintenance and calibration of the equipment especially with respect to battery testing and replacement, acoustic conditions for testing and the effects of different testing environments on obtained results, total amount of disturbance to the school or work programs of individuals tested, and reactions of school personnel or employers to the testing procedures. Although none of the studies so far reported (including one by the present writer) has taken into account such a wide range of factors or has attempted to measure objectively a number of them, a final decision regarding double-frequency screening or other screening methods should be dependent on consideration of these numerous aspects.

47

The Efficiency of Three Group Pure–Tone Screening Tests for Public School Children

LOUIS M. DiCARLO
ERIC F. GARDNER

LOUIS M. DiCARLO, Ed.D., is Chairman, Department of Speech Pathology and Audiology, Ithaca College

ERIC F. GARDNER, Ed.D., is Chairman, Psychology Department, Syracuse University

INTRODUCTION

The successful prosecution of an adequate medical and educational program for children with impaired hearing rests on an early and systematic detection of hearing loss.[1,2] Early in the century, Goldstein (3), returned from Europe where he studied with the famous otologist, Urbantschitsch, and devoted himself to the study of the problems of deafness, especially among children. In the early twenties, Fowler and Fletcher (2), and others became interested in the preventive aspects of hearing impairment and were instrumental in the development of the phonograph audiometer. Goldstein and Fowler advocated early detection of hearing impairment, medical rehabilitation, and educational habilitation of school children in an effort to reduce the incidence of adult deafness and alleviate the the educational obstacles confronting children with irreversible hearing loss. They recognized the magnitude of the problem and the need for a quick and accurate measurement of auditory performance with stimuli of some known acoustic value. From crude simple tests including coin-clicks, tuning forks, and voice, emerged pure-tone audiometry, and more recently speech audiometry for the evaluation of hearing performance. Lindenberg and Fowler (9), have indicated that pure-tone audiometry "is the only known method from which capacity to hear speech can be calculated." This generalization has face validity but can be questioned in many instances. Speech audiometry permits the calculation of hearing loss for speech directly and is definitely related to pure-tone audiometry of 500, 1000, and 2000 cycles.

The 4A phono-audiometer group screening test for hearing was introduced in the New York State Public Schools in 1924 (4). New York State made mandatory the testing of public school children in 1938 (8). Many states have passed legislation requiring periodic testing and reporting of children with hearing impairments. Since hearing tests of large

Reprinted by permission of the authors from *Except. Child.*, **24**, pp. 351–359 (1958).

[1] The writers express their indebtedness to Monsignor James E. Callahan, superintendent of the parochial schools of Syracuse, New York, for permission to use the entire population of St. Vincent's School. Thanks are also extended to Virginia G. Harris, M.D., director of bureau of child health, and Ada K. Perry, R.N., supervisor of school nursing, in the Syracuse Parochial Schools for their cooperation in the organization and prosecution of the testing.

[2] Grateful appreciation for his help, is expressed to Philip W. Johnson, M.D., of the Massachusetts Department of Public Health. He provided the Audivox 7 BP and tray of Western Electric #716-A receivers, which were used throughout the entire experiment.

populations require time and often may become prohibitive financially, the search *for the most efficient* group screening test has continued to the present day. Nevertheless this quest for *the best* screening test has proved unrealistic.

West (*17*), Gardner (*3*), Johnston (*6, 7*), and others, have critically evaluated the phono-audiometer group test and have revealed this test may not screen out individuals with high frequency loss. This phenomenon has been true in the writers' experiences. The failure of the speech tests to screen out high frequency losses may be due to the individual's ability to capitalize on fragmentary speech cues. Speech is resistant to a good deal of distortion. Furthermore, most of the sound pressure levels for the vowels lie below 1000 cycles and individuals listening to numbers with an attitudinal set will make a high degree of correct guesses on the basis of the vowel sounds. In addition, the phono-audiometer test is quite susceptible to interfering ambient noise levels. The test consequently fails many individuals with normal hearing. Other sources of failure on this test are lack of coordination, language, and writing ability. Mentally retarded and motor handicapped children experience difficulty with this test.

Gardner (*3*), Harris (*5*), Johnston (*6, 7*), Munson (*11*), Myers (*12*), Nielsen (*13*), adapted individual pure-tone audiometric methods to group testing. Myers, Harris, and Fowler (*12*), concluded: "It would appear that in terms of completeness and accuracy of results, a group method of pure-tone audiometry is feasible in a reasonably alert population." Lindenberg and Fowler (*9*), Gardner (*3*), and Newhart (*15*), and others, have advocated pure-tone individual sweep-check as an efficient method for screening populations. By inspection this method would appear to be the best and where time and economy are not factors, this is probably the most efficient test for screening. Nevertheless, individual pure-tone screening has certain disadvantages: It is more time consuming than group tone. Yankauer, Geyer, and Chase (*18*) evaluated three screening methods including group phonograph, group pure-tone, and individual pure-tone tests. They tested 2,404 elementary school children from grades three to seven. The individual pure-tone test required 1.9 minutes, as against .9 minutes for group pure-tone, and 1.4 minutes for the group phonograph test. They concluded that the individual pure-tone screening was superior to the other two methods. Both Gardner (*3*), and Munson (*11*), found group pure-tone testing a satisfactory techinque for testing young children. In the beginning the equipment cost was considered prohibitive. Johnston (*6*) devised the Massachusetts Pure Tone Screening Test for testing the Massachusetts school population. He later modified his test to make it more efficient with an accuracy approaching that obtained in individual screening tests.[3] Johnston (*7*) contended this method had certain advantages over his previous test. First grade children could be tested by this new technique. There was no need for paper or pencil. The tester employed the same principles as he would use in sweep-check, the method was faster, and less fatiguing. Where Gardner (*3*) used pulses, Johnston (*6*) first used pure-tone stimuli of selected intensities. In the first test (*6*) the subject indicated whether he heard the stimuli by marking the yes or no option on his paper. In the later test (*7*) the children raised their hands. Johnston (*7*), later converted the instrument so that one intensity level was used for the screening frequencies.

DiCarlo and Gardner (*1*), employed a modified form of the Massachusetts Test (*6*) in screening 1754 incoming students at Syracuse University in September 1951. One hundred and twenty-seven individuals (88 males and 39 females) failed the group test and an approximate 12 percent (188 students

---

[3] Instructions for the Group Pure Tone Hearing Test, Massachusetts Department of Public Health, Division of Maternal and Child Health, Vision and Hearing Conservation Section.

—99 males and 89 females) random sample of the remaining 1627 subjects passing the group test, were given individual audiometric tests. They concluded "in terms of time, cost, and the results, the Massachusetts Pure Tone Group Test if modified, and when administered under the conditions . . . provides a very efficient testing tool for hearing testing of university populations." These results led the writers to extend this screening procedure to elementary school populations.

A period of trial with a number of school systems indicated that while the modified form of the Massachusetts Test was satisfactory with college populations, it did not appear to be an efficient instrument for testing school children in the first, second, and third grades. It was considered advisable to modify the test further by pulsing the tones instead of using the yes and no option. Pulsing the tone shortened the test and since no reading was involved, it was our belief the test could be successfully extended to the first grade.

PRESENT STUDY

Permission was obtained from Monsignor James E. Callahan, superintendent of the Syracuse parochial schools, to test an entire school containing children in kindergarten through grades eight. St. Vincent's School, comprising 519 children, was selected for the study. The first consideration was the establishment of a satisfactory criteria for passing and failing the test. Johnston (6), calibrated his system by the loudness balance technique. His ultimate values were to provide a 15 decibel signal level for screening purposes. In his later test (7), he modified the equipment so that one setting permitted a 15 decibel signal level for all of the frequencies. Kaiser (8), suggested 15 decibels as a satisfactory passing criterion. Newby (14) and Peterson (16), advocated a 20 decibel criterion. In his first test, Johnston (6), used 512, 1,024, 4,096, and 11,584

cycles. In the later test, he used six frequencies: 250 to 6000 cycles.[4]

PROCEDURES

The three group and the individual pure tone tests were administered to all children from kindergarten through grades eight. In testing the school population we followed Johnston's instructions.[5] In our testing procedures we modified the signal frequencies to five instead of six and used 250, 500, 1000, 2000, and 6000 cycles. A second modification was applied to our pulse tone presentations. We used the modified Massachusetts Test as employed by DiCarlo and Gardner (1), a pulse tone, and Johnston's (7) test. These three group tests were all evaluated against pure-tone audiometry. Individuals failing any one frequency in any group test were considered to have failed the test. The criteria for failing the individual pure tone test was established as 15 decibels for two frequencies, and 20 decibels for one frequency.

The following are the mean ambient noise levels of the testing rooms calculated on readings with the General Radio Sound Level Meter, Type 1551A, with setting at the A position:

Group testing room	42 db
Testing room 1	36 db
Testing room 2	38 db
Testing room 3	40 db
Testing room 4	40 db

These means are the results of 10 readings at different intervals of the day in each room, taken under conditions similar to those of the testing situation. A total of 519 students, or 1038 ears, were tested. The apparatus for the two group test was set up in one part of the auditorium, while the Johnston's 7PB Audivox audiometer and a tray of Western Electric #716-A receivers which he loaned us for the experiment, was set up in another part of the

[4, 5] Personal communication.

INDIVIDUAL TESTS

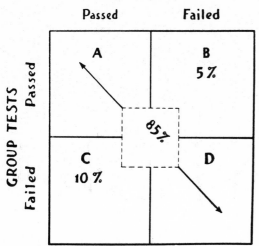

Figure 47-1. Accepted hypothetical criterion values representing agreement in classification of individual and group tests.

ANALYSIS

The analysis employed in this investigation is similar to that used by DiCarlo and Gardner (*1*). Figure 47-1, represents the accepted hypothetical criteria of values suggested by Newby (*14*). A criterion that misclassifies 10 percent of the hearing losses erroneously may be accepted providing that the errors are committed on the group tests. A margin of error in terms of failure to detect hearing at five percent might be considered. With respect to Cell C, the 10 percent criterion would be acceptable although the closer this limit approaches zero, the better would be the test instrument. The same rationale applies to Cell B. Certainly in Cell B the instrument should be as close to zero as possible. Consequently a new criterion suggested itself which is represented in Figure 47-2. Of the 1,038 ears tested it was felt that the five percent in Cell B should be reduced to two percent. Figure 47-2 shows the hypothetical distribution of the agreements and disagreements between the individual and the group tests. This investigation purported to compare the group audiometer tests to the individual thresholds at five frequencies.

Table 47-1 represents the distribution and

auditorium. The equipment used for the modified Massachusetts and the pulse tone tests comprised the Maico Pure Tone Audiometer Model F-1, with 40 matched receivers and adapter. Method for calibrating the receivers was the same employed by DiCarlo and Gardner (*1*).

Individual tests were administered with two ADC Model 50-C2, and two Audivox 7BP audiometers. The noise levels outside the testing rooms were kept at a minimum by the directive of the school authorities and the co-operation of the entire school personnel. Virginia G. Harris, school physician, and Ada K. Perry, supervisor of school nursing in the Syracuse parochial schools, organized the school testing program and were instrumental in eliminating any activities that might interfere with the testing. The noise element in the testing situation was kept at a minimum by the monitors who directed the subjects to and away from the testing rooms. In the group tests, modified Massachusetts and the pulse tone, the tester listened through one of the receivers to ascertain the optimum testing conditions. Pretest instructions and demonstrations were given to the children.

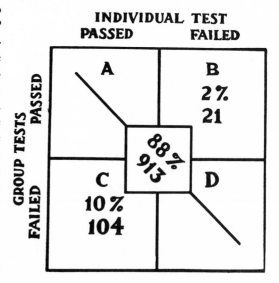

Figure 47-2. Suggested new hypothetical criterion values for representing agreement in classification of individual and group tests for 1038 ears.

TABLE 47-1. VALUES REPRESENTING AGREEMENT AND
DISAGREEMENT IN CLASSIFICATION BETWEEN MODIFIED
MASSACHUSETTS, PULSE TONE, JOHNSTON'S, AND INDIVIDUAL
TESTS FOR 1038 EARS

Test	Cell	Passed both group and individual tests	Failed both group and individual tests	Passed group but failed individual tests	Failed group but passed individual tests
	Cell	A	D	B	C
Modified	N	727	68	8	235
Mass. Test	%	70	7	1	22
Pulse tone	N	788	68	8	174
Test	%	76	7	1	16
Johnston's	N	906	68	11	53
Test	%	87	7	1	5

classification of responses in categories of agreement and types of disagreement of the results for 1,038 ears. The modified Massachusetts test agrees in 795 individuals, eight individuals passed the group and failed the individual test while 235 children passed the individual but failed the group test. For the pulse tone test, 856 individuals agree, eight passed the group test but failed the individual test while 174 children passed the individual but failed the group test. For Johnston (7) test, there is agreement on 974 children. 11 passed the group but failed the individual test while 53 passed the individual but failed the group test. Table 47-1 presents the actual distribution of the performances in the different cells. Examination of the distribution reveals that in all three group tests, Cell B values are lower in the actual test results than the hypothesized criteria. The values for Cell C, however, are much higher for the modified Massachusetts and the pulse tone tests, than the postulated criteria. Cell C values for the modified Massachusetts test were 22 percent and for the pulse tone test 16 percent. In both these tests the values are greater than the hypothesized criteria and reveal that too many ears would be needlessly retested. Of the 1,038 ears tested with Johnston's (7) test, 53 ears or five percent, failed the group test but passed the individual test. This value is much lower than the hypothesized value. For all three tests the Cell B values are much lower than the two percent hypothesized for the test. The modified Massachusetts test and the pulse tone test failed to detect hearing loss in eight

individuals, which comprised less than one percent of the total population. The Johnston (7) test failed to detect 11, or one percent, which is still lower than the hypothesized values. Any test instrument devoid of error would approximate zero. Nevertheless one percent is as low a margin of error as might be expected under the most satisfactory testing conditions.

The modified Massachusetts test agreed 77 percent in passing and failing individuals on group and individual tests. The pulse tone test agreed 83 percent in passing and failing individuals on the group and individual tests. Both these values are less than 88 percent, and are therefore inferior to the hypothesized criteria. Johnston's (7) test, agreed 94 percent in passing and failing on the group and individual tests. This value was superior to the hypothetical criteria. Analysis of the total test results reveals the Johnston (7) test resulted in extended agreement with the hypothetical criteria, while the disagreement categories were much lower than the hypothetical limits.

Chi-squares were computed for the data in Table 47-2. Table 47-2 presents the chi-

TABLE 47-2. CHI-SQUARE, DEGREES OF FREEDOM, AND
PROBABILITY VALUES FOR EACH TEST (N = 1038)

Test	Cell	Observed frequency	Theoretical frequency	Chi-square	Degrees of freedom	p
Modified	AD	795	913	188.31	2	.001
Mass.	B	8	21			
	C	235	104			
Pulse tone	AD	856	913	58.72	2	.001
	B	8	21			
	C	174	104			
Johnston's	AD	974	913	33.82	2	.001
	B	11	21			
	C	53	104			

square, degrees of freedom, and probability values for the three tests. The chi-square value for the modified Massachusetts test was 188.31, which with 2 degrees of freedom resulted in a probability value of less than .001 percent. The chi-square value for the pulse tone test was 58.7, with a probability value of less than .001 percent. The chi-square for Johnston's (7) tests, of 33.8, also gives a probability value of less than .001 percent. The chi-square values for the modified Massachusetts and pulse tone tests, indicated agreement between the group and the individual tests only in Cell B as being better than would be considered acceptable on the basis of the critical limiting values defined by the postulated criteria. While Table 47-2 reveals a relationship between these two group tests and the individual test as greater than could be possible by chance factor, inspection of the obtained percentages reveal that for Cells A, C, and D, the results are much poorer than the hypothesized criteria. It was considered desirable to analyze statistically the relationship between the obtained results and the hypothesized criteria.

Table 47-3 presents the critical ratios for

TABLE 47-3. CRITICAL RATIOS FOR DIFFERENCES BETWEEN PERCENTAGES OF OBSERVED AGREEMENT AND A PRIORI THEORETICAL PERCENTAGES OF AGREEMENT (N = 1038)

Test	Cell	Observed percentage	Theoretical percentage	Critical ratio	p
Modified Mass.	AD	76.59	88.00	11.30	.001
Pulse tone	AD	82.47	88.00	5.48	.001
Johnston's	AD	93.83	88.00	5.77	.001

the differences between percentages of observed agreement and the a priori theoretical percentages of agreement for 1,038 ears. The critical ratio values of 11.30 for the modified Massachusetts test and 5.48 for the pulse tone test, and 5.77 for the Johnston (7) test, the probability values are less than .001 percent. Nevertheless while these critical ratios indicate significant differences between the tests, the modified Massachusetts and the pulse tone tests are significantly inferior to the hypothesized criteria, while the Johnston (7) test, is significantly better than the hypothesized criteria.

Since both the modified Massachusetts and the pulse tone tests did not appear to be satisfactory instruments, it was decided to analyze the data further by eliminating certain children. All children from kindergarten through the third grade were deleted for the modified Massachusetts test, and all children in kindergarten and first grade were deleted for the pulse tone test. Table 47-4 presents the

TABLE 47-4. CLASSIFICATION OF RESPONSES OF 624 EARS TESTED BY THE MODIFIED MASSACHUSETTS WITH GRADES KINDERGARTEN THROUGH THIRD DELETED, PULSE TONE WITH KINDERGARTEN AND FIRST GRADE DELETED FOR 826 EARS, AND INDIVIDUAL TESTS

Test	Tests agree	Passed group but failed individual tests	Passed individual but failed group tests
Modified Mass. with Grades Kindergarten thru Third deleted	570	5	49
Pulse tone with Kindergarten and First Grade deleted	775	7	44

classification of responses of 624 ears tested by the modified Massachusetts test with kindergarten through third grade deleted, and the pulse tone for 826 ears, with kindergarten and first grade deleted, and individual tests. Table 47-5 indicates values representing agree-

TABLE 47-5. VALUES REPRESENTING AGREEMENT AND DISAGREEMENT BETWEEN THE MODIFIED MASSACHUSETTS, WITH GRADES KINDERGARTEN THROUGH THIRD DELETED (N = 624), PULSE TONE WITH KINDERGARTEN AND FIRST GRADE DELETED (N = 826), AND INDIVIDUAL PURE TONE TESTS

Test		Passed both group and individual tests	Failed both group and individual tests	Passed group but failed individual tests	Failed group but passed individual tests
Modified Mass. with Grades Kindergarten thru Third deleted	Cell	A	D	B	C
	N	527	43	5	49
	%	84.4	6.9	.8	7.9
Pulse tone with Kindergarten and First Grade deleted	Cell	A	D	B	C
	N	723	52	7	44
	%	87.5	6.3	.9	5.3

ment and disagreement between the modified Massachusetts test with kindergarten through third grade deleted, for 624 ears, and the pulse tone test with kindergarten and first grade deleted, for 826 ears and individual pure-tone tests.

With the kindergarten through third grade

children deleted, Cells A and D in the modified Massachusetts test account for 91.3 percent of all the population, while Cell B represents 5 children or .8 percent of children failing detection, and Cell C shows 49 or 7.9 percent of the children failing the group but passing the individual test. The pulse tone test indicates 93.8 percent of the population accounted for in Cells A and D with .9 percent of the children in Cell B, and 44 or 5.3 percent of the children in Cell C. All of these values are better than the hypothesized criteria.

Table 47-6 exhibits the chi-square, degrees

TABLE 47-6. CHI-SQUARE DEGREES OF FREEDOM, AND PROBABILITY VALUES FOR MODIFIED MASSACHUSETTS, WITH GRADES KINDERGARTEN THROUGH THIRD DELETED (N = 624), AND PULSE TONE WITH KINDERGARTEN AND FIRST GRADE DELETED (N = 826)

Test	Cell	Observed frequency	Theoretical frequency	Chi-square	Degrees of freedom	p
Modified Mass. with Grades Kindergarten thru Third deleted	AD	570	549	8.45	2	.05
	B	5	13			.015
	C	49	62			
Pulse tone with Kindergarten and First Grade deleted	AD	775	727	26.56	2	<.001
	B	7	16			
	C	44	83			

of freedom, and probability values, for the modified Massachusetts and the pulse tone tests. Table 47-7 reveals the critical ratios for the differences between percentages of the modified Massachusetts test with kindergarten through third grades deleted, and the pulse tone with kindergarten and first grade de-

TABLE 47-7. CRITICAL RATIOS FOR DIFFERENCES BETWEEN PERCENTAGES OF THE MODIFIED MASSACHUSETTS, WITH GRADES KINDERGARTEN THROUGH THIRD DELETED (N = 624), AND PULSE TONE WITH KINDERGARTEN AND FIRST GRADE DELETED (N = 826)

Test	Cell	Observed percentage	Theoretical percentage	Critical ratio	p
Modified Mass. with Grades Kindergarten thru Third deleted	AD	91.35	88	2.58	.01
Pulse tone with Kindergarten and First Grade deleted	AD	93.82	88	5.15	<.001

leted. A critical ratio value of 2.58 indicates a significant difference at the 1 percent level for the modified Massachusetts test, while for the pulse tone test a critical ratio of 5.1 reveals a significancy at the .001 percent level of confidence.

Table 47-8 shows the obtained proportions

TABLE 47-8. OBTAINED PROPORTIONS IN CATEGORIES B AND C FOR EACH TEST, WITH CRITERION VALUE FOR CELL B = 2 PERCENT, AND CELL C = 10 PERCENT

Test	Cell B	Cell C
Modified Mass.	.77%	22.64%
Pulse tone	.77%	16.76%
Johnston's	1.06%	5.11%
Modified Mass. with Grades Kindergarten thru Third deleted	0.8%	7.85%
Pulse tone with Kindergarten and First Grade deleted	.82	5.33%

for Category B and C for each test with criterion value for Cell B of two percent, and Cell C of 10 percent. Analysis of the results would indicate that the modified Massachusetts and the pulse tone tests, fail an exceedingly greater number of children than the hypothesized criteria. Johnston's (7) test, gives values much better than those of the hypothetical limits for the entire school population, while the modified Massachusetts test with kindergarten through third grade deleted, and the pulse tone test with kindergarten and first grade deleted, appear to be satisfactory at these levels.

Table 47-9 indicates the limits for obtained proportions in Cell C at five percent and one percent levels. On the basis of the results obtained, the limits for the obtained propor-

TABLE 47-9. LIMITS FOR OBTAINED PROPORTIONS IN CELL C AT 5 PERCENT AND 1 PERCENT LEVELS

Test	5%		1%	
	Lower	Upper	Lower	Upper
Modified Mass.	20.09	25.19	19.31	25.97
Pulse tone	14.21	19.13	13.43	20.09
Johnston's	3.35	6.87	2.81	7.41
Modified Mass. with Grades Kindergarten thru Third deleted	5.50	10.20	4.78	10.92
Pulse tone with Kindergarten and First Grade Deleted	3.29	7.37	2.65	8.01

tions in Cell C at the five percent and one percent levels reveal that the modified Massachusetts and the pulse tone tests are inferior to the hypothesized criteria, while the modified Massachusetts test with kindergarten through third grade deleted, is satisfactory at the lower end of the five percent and one percent levels but unsatisfactory at the upper levels of the five percent and one percent levels. The Johnston (7) test and the pulse tone test with the kindergarten and first grade deleted, satisfy the conditions of the hypothesized criteria.

DISCUSSION

A comparison of the actual results of the three group tests with the hypothesized criteria revealed that in all three tests the actual results as indicated by the critical ratios was significantly different than could be expected by chance. The results of the modified Massachusetts test and the pulse tone test, were much poorer than the Johnston (7) test when administered to the entire school population. The Johnston (7) test results were much better than the a priori established criteria. In all three tests the Cell B values were satisfactory and much better than the criteria, but the modified Massachusetts and the pulse tone tests, were inferior instruments to the Johnston (7) test and to the established hypothetical values. The Johnston (7) test succeeded quite accurately in separating subjects with significant hearing losses from those with essentially normal hearing. In addition, the test failed only five percent of the population which was 50 percent lower than the hypothesized value. The Johnston (7) test nevertheless, did have a higher distribution in Cell B than either the modified Massachusetts or the pulse tone test, even though the number was minimized. While the value in Cell B would be more satisfactory if it were zero, it is very questionable whether this value would ever be obtained without imposing more stringent restrictions upon the criteria. Such further restriction might reduce the distri-

bution in Cell B but would also increase disproportionately the distribution in Cell C. Examination of the score sheets revealed that the distribution in Cell C for the modified Massachusetts test was due to the failure of children in the kindergarten, first, second, and third grades with the preponderance of failures in kindergarten, first and second grades This would appear reasonable when one considers that children in kindergarten, first, and second grades have had little experience with reading and writing. The task also proved too difficult for a good number of the third grade students. The investigation also indicated that the pulse tone was more suitable for children in the second and third grades, than the modified Massachusetts test. The experience with the test also indicated that first grade children could do fairly well with the test if instead of using numbers they were permitted to make a mark every time they heard a tone. When the examiner moved from one frequency to another, he would say "circle." The children would circle the numbers of marks and move to the next space. Figure 47-3 represents a score sheet used for children in the first, second and third grades.

The elimination of kindergarten through third grades for the modified Massachusetts test reduced the number of ears to 624. When the chi-square and the critical ratios were computed, this test was also significantly better than the hypothesized criteria at the one percent level. When the kindergarten and first grade were eliminated from the pulse tone test, this reduced the number of ears to 826, but the test results revealed that the pulse tone test was significantly better at less than the .001 percent level. Tables 47-8 and 47-9 revealed that for Johnston's (7) test, and the modified Massachusetts with kindergarten through third grades eliminated, and pulse tone test with kindergarten and first grades eliminated, the results were significantly better than the a priori criteria. This would indicate that the modified Massachusetts test is a satisfactory test for testing children from the fourth grade upward, while the pulse tone test would accomplish the same task with children from the second grade upward. In this respect, Johnston's (7) test effectively screened all the children from kindergarten up.

Analysis of the per pupil testing time indicated that Johnston's (7) test, which tested 10 children at once, required a greater amount of time. The testing time per child with Johnston's (7) test was 55 seconds, while the testing time for the modified Massachusetts test, testing children from the fourth grade up, was 21 seconds, and the testing time for the pulse tone test testing children from the second grade was 12.5 seconds. In terms of time, Johnston's (7) test requires almost more than twice as much time as the modified Massachusetts test, and almost five times greater time than the pulse tone. The per pupil testing time for pure tone screening was 2.1 minutes. An evaluation of the results indicated that in terms of time, the pure tone takes longer to administer while the pulse tone required the least time of all the tests.

In many schools today, group pure-tone testing can be successfully administered since most of these schools have rooms for music instruction which are usually pretty quiet. The school authorities would be willing to sacrifice activities for a day or two, but not for any longer period. While pure-tone screening would appear to be the best test, satisfactory conditions for administering the test are difficult to maintain for a long time. On the other hand, an efficient group test could easily be included as part of the regular activities of a school in which all school personnel participate. Evaluation of the results clearly establishes that the Johnston's (7) test more closely approximates the efficiency of pure-tone individual screening but in terms of economy and time, it is less efficient than either the modified Massachusetts with grades kindergarten through third eliminated and the pulse tone with kindergarten and grade one eliminated. A new method of scoring which permits children to write in marks makes the test applicable to first graders. The results establish also the possibility of a combination of

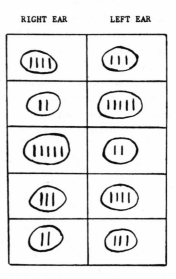

RIGHT EAR   LEFT EAR

Figure 47-3. Score sheet employed in recording responses by first, second, and third grade students.

techniques to provide the best screening results. The writers believe that the following combination provides the best approximation:

1. Johnston's (7) group pure-tone screening for kindergarten and first grade children.

2. The pulse tone group pure tone screening for children from the second grade up.

Another satisfactory combination would be to employ:

1. Pure-tone screening for the kindergarten.

2. Johnston's (7) group test for the first grade.

3. Group pulse tone testing for the children from second grade up.

Another effective combination but not as efficient as either the first two alternatives would be:

1. Pure-tone screening for kindergarten.

2. Pure-tone pulse tone for grades one, two and three.

3. The modified Massachusetts for grades four, up.

These combinations do not require change in equipment.

Furthermore Lutz (*10*) has demonstrated September and October, March and April to be the most propitious months while January and February the worst for testing.

The evaluation of the results also indicates that either one of these three combinations can be applied to a successful testing program in elementary schools. The efficiency will depend upon: (1) a carefully planned administration of the program which reflects the cooperation of the school authorities with the entire school personnel participating; (2) adequate structuring of the test situation and (3) most important of all as indicated, a relatively quiet room.*

[* Since the publication of this study the senior author has tested an additional 25,000 children employing group pure-tone audiometry. The author's philosophy has not changed, although some modification in methodology has occurred. The preferred method, whenever feasible, is individual pure-tone screening. But in large and even in small school populations, contingent upon spatial, temporal, economic, and personnel factors, group pure-tone testing programs conducted under conditions stressed in this article have many advantages to recommend them. In the case of youngsters who have not learned to handle writing responses and associate them with auditory stimuli, the Johnston Massachusetts method may include a larger number of children per group if classroom teachers

CONCLUSION

Analysis of the findings indicate that pure-tone group screening testing is feasible, reliable, and efficient for screening elementary school populations when carried out under the conditions out-lined in the study. In terms of time, cost and results, the combination of Johnston's (7) pure tone group test for kindergarten and first grade and the group pulse tone for grades two and up appears to offer the best combination.

first give the children practice in raising the hand and in using small masks which cover the eyes to eliminate responses to movement rather than to auditory stimuli. Years of testing have consistently revealed that children who are discovered to have hearing loss in the first three or four grades continue to be rediscovered each year, while the rest of the school population remains normal—suggesting that yearly testing of the entire school population may not be necessary. Provisions for testing children who contract respiratory and other infectious ailments that may affect hearing should be automatic immediately upon the youngsters' return to school. Moreover, each high school student should be tested prior to graduation (11th or 12th grade), since in some cases early signs of otosclerosis begin to become manifest at that age. In measuring ambient noise levels of testing rooms the C reading on the sound level meter may be more appropriate. Finally, in testing the first four grades (group or individual) and in any other individual testing, volunteer personnel, unless qualified, should not perform the actual testing. LMD, EFG]

REFERENCES

1. DiCarlo, L. M., and Gardner, E. F., "The Efficiency of the Massachusetts Pure-Tone Screening Test as Adapted for a University Testing Program." *Journal Speech and Hearing Disorders*, 18, June 1953, 175–82.

2. Fowler, E. P., and Fletcher, H., "Three Million Deafened School Children: Their Detection and Treatment." *Journal American Medical Association*, 1926, 87:1877.

3. Gardner, M. B., "A Pulse Tone Technique for Clinical Audiometric Threshold Measurements." *Journal Acoustic Society America*, 19, 1947, 592–99.

4. Goldstein, M. A., "Problems of the Deaf." *The Laryngoscope Press*, 1933, St. Louis.

5. Harris, J. D., "Group Audiometry." *Journal Acoustic Society America*, 17, 1945, 73–76.

6. Johnston, P. W., "The Massachusetts Hearing Test." *Journal Acoustic Society America*, 20, 1948, 697–703.

7. Johnston, P. W., "An Efficient Group Screening

Test." *Journal Speech and Hearing Disorders*, 17, 1952, 8–12.

8. Kiser, B., "A Demonstration of Group Audiometer Tests." *Journal Speech Disorders*, 5, 1940, 151–52.

9. Lindenberg, P., and Fowler, E. P., Jr., "Genetal Practice, Industrial Military, and School Audiometry." *New York State Journal of Medicine*, 52, December 1952, 2897–2902.

10. Lutz, K. R., "Seasonal Variations in Hearing Screening Results." *Exceptional Children*, 22, November 1955, 67–68, 84.

11. Munson, W. A., "Trial Tests of Pulsing Tone Audiometers." Unpublished research memo 20871-2, Bell Telephone Labs., 1937.

12. Myers, C. K., Harris, J. D., and Fowler, E. P., Jr., "The Feasibility of Group Audiometry." *Industrial Medicine*, 17, July 1948, 245–52.

13. Neilsen, S. F., "Group Testing of School Children

by Pure Tone Audiometry." *Journal Speech and Hearing Disorders*, 17, 1952, 4-7.

14. Newby, H. A., "Evaluating the Efficiency of Group Screening Tests of Hearing." *Journal Speech and Hearing Disorders*, 13, 1948, 236-40.

15. Newhart, H., "A New Pure Tone Audiometer for School Use." *Archives Otolaryngology*, Chicago, 48, 1938, 129-36.

16. Peterson, G. E., "The Pure Tone Screen Test of Hearing." *Journal Speech Disorders*, 9, 1944, 114-120.

17. West, R., "A Critique of the Rationales of Tests of Hearing." *Journal Speech Disorders*, 5, 1940, 19-24.

18. Yankauer, A., Geyer, M. L., and Chase, H. C., "Comparative Evaluation of Three Screening Methods for Detection of Hearing Loss in School Children." *American Journal Public Health*, 44, January 1954, 77-82.

part VII

PROBLEMS IN MEASUREMENT

The articles in this section were selected to illustrate some of the more common problems encountered in the "routine" measurement of hearing. The articles also serve to alert the clinician to the constant need to ask questions of himself: "What am I doing?" "Why am I doing it?" "What do the results mean?" This type of self-questioning behavior is one of the characteristics that distinguish the audiologist from the technician.

In the lead article Simmons and Dixon emphasize the need to ask the patient a very simple question: "What do you hear?" The answer to this question, as they so well illustrate, may have important diagnostic implications. The more general point, of course, is that the clinician must direct questions not only to himself but to the patient as well. Simmons and Dixon's article should help to reverse ". . . the increasing tendency toward substitution of the techniques of electronic audiometry for careful questioning of patients with hearing loss."

"Do you feel it or do you hear it?" is the question to which Nober addresses himself in his article on pseudoauditory bone-conduction thresholds. At high output levels in bone-conduction testing, the patient may respond to tactile sensation rather than to auditory sensation. Nober describes this phenomenon in deaf children, discusses a method for identifying pseudoauditory bone-conduction thresholds, and points out the diagnostic implications of knowing whether the patient has "felt" the tone or heard it. In a later article, Nober (1967) demonstrated that vibrotactile thresholds can be obtained for air conduction as well as for bone conduction.

The next two articles are related to the question "What do you see?" and emphasize the importance of looking at the patient's ears and ear canals prior to testing. Ventry, Chaiklin, and Boyle first reported the audiometric discrepancies and threshold variability associated with the collapse or closure of the external auditory canal caused by earphone pressure. Hildyard and Valentine, in a later study, showed that collapse of the ear canal is more common than had been recognized and stressed the diagnostic significance of a discrepancy between tuning fork tests (a positive Rinne) and an audiometric air-bone gap.

Naunton's paper points out the difficulties involved in determining true bone-conduction thresholds with standard techniques when there is a large air-bone gap and a bilateral loss of sensitivity for air conduction. This very problem has led to various alternatives to standard bone-conduction audiometry (see the Jerger and Jerger article and the Tillman article in PART II), but in the majority of clinical settings, Naunton's dilemma is not Naunton's alone.

Sataloff presents a number of problems commonly encountered in routine audiometry. Among them are the use of adequate masking, the type of masking noise employed, the problem of masking when there are large air-bone gaps, and the fact that reliable test results do not mean that the results are valid. Sataloff urges (as we do) the need for the clinician to keep an "open mind" in evaluating hearing test results.

In the last selection, Dixon and Newby deal with the problem of functional hearing loss in children. They discuss some of the behavioral characteristics of such children, describe typical test findings, and suggest techniques that can be used to resolve the audiometric discrepancies. Unfortunately, we do not know much more about functional hearing loss in children today than we did when Dixon and Newby's article was written more than 10 years ago.

We have not included an article on the audiometric problems associated with functional hearing loss in adults, mainly because most articles on this subject tend to focus only on selected aspects of the problem. Detailed treatment of functional hearing loss is contained elsewhere in two publications, both of which have extensive reference lists (Chaiklin and Ventry, 1963; Ventry and Chaiklin, 1965).

REFERENCES

1. Chaiklin, J. B., and Ventry, I. M. Functional hearing loss. In J. F. Jerger (Ed.), *Modern developments in audiology*. New York: Academic Press, 1963. Pp. 76–125.

2. Nober, E. H. Vibrotactile sensitivity of deaf children to high intensity sound. *Laryngoscope*, **77**, pp. 2128–2146 (1967).

3. Ventry, I. M., and Chaiklin, J. B. (Eds.) Multidiscipline study of functional hearing loss. *J. aud. Res.*, **5**, pp. 179–272 (1965).

48

On the Importance of the Question: What Do You Hear?

F. BLAIR SIMMONS
RICHARD F. DIXON

F. BLAIR SIMMONS, M.D., is Associate Professor of Otolaryngology, Stanford University School of Medicine

RICHARD F. DIXON, Ph.D., is Director, Division of Speech Pathology and Audiology, University of North Carolina at Greensboro

The utilitarian ubiquitousness of the audiometer has advanced clinical otology more than any tool of recent times, nor does its promise for the future seem dim. Yet this very success breeds danger—failure to appreciate the audiometer's innate limitations. The audiometer is not a substitute for clinical acumen. It cannot, for example, ask the patient what he hears during a test. The situation demands only that the subject respond by raising a finger or pressing a button, etc.

Our concern for this rather obvious fact lies in the observation that there seems to be an increasing tendency toward substitution of the techniques of electronic audiometry for careful questioning of patients with hearing losses. (Observe, for example, the number of audiograms published without comment about the patient's subjective observations of sounds in general, or even comments relevant to the audiometric tones themselves.) Perhaps this trend is due to the authoritarian appeal of lines on a graph, or to the convenience of relegating hearing testing to an office technician, or perhaps to failure to appreciate the severity of the audiometer's limitations in certain cases. Whatever the cause, the trend definitely seems to exist and can lead to diagnostic error.

Reprinted by permission of the authors from *Arch. Otolaryngol.*, **80,** pp. 167–169 (1964).

Through the medium of a particular case, this article attempts to underscore one type of error that can occur. During this man's audiometric evaluation, he dutifully "raised his finger," through virtually every common clinical test. Yet, after many hours of testing, the most significant characteristic of his hearing loss remained unknown because not one examiner asked the question: *What do you hear?*

A 61-year-old male amateur musician and hi-fi enthusiast was in good health and was aware of no particular hearing problem until 12:45 PM on August 5. Then while driving his car, he felt slightly light-headed and noted a severe hearing loss in his right ear. Two hours later he was examined by a resident otolaryngologist who described the patient's complaints: ". . . a sudden onset of hearing loss, rushing tinnitus and unsteady sensation involving the right ear." Except for the hearing loss, the neurological examination was normal. There was, however, a past history of a mild bilateral hearing loss and a vague vestibular disturbance five years earlier.

Figure 48-1 shows the audiogram taken by the resident immediately prior to the patient's admission to the hospital with a working diagnosis of "vascular spasm." Intravenous histamine therapy was initiated after consultation with a member of the clinical staff. Approxi-

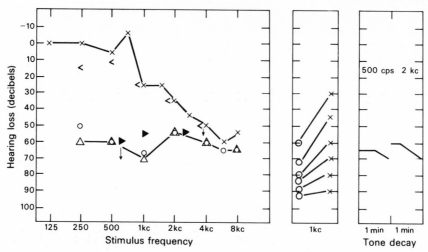

Figure 48-1. Pure tone audiogram, 1 kc binaural alternate loudness balance, 500 cps and 2 kc tone decay measurements obtained shortly after right-sided hearing loss.

mately three hours after admission, a second audiogram was taken (unchanged), and the other measurements shown in Figure 48-1 were obtained. Speech discrimination was poor (as estimated by running speech and a few words of one syllable). Vestibular examination by electronystagmography showed a type II (Nylen) left-beating positional nystagmus, most marked in the left lateral head position.

At this time, the presence of nearly complete recruitment and minimal tone decay seemed to confirm the admitting diagnosis, a cochlear lesion producing moderately severe damage between 125 and 2000 cps. However, we felt that the supposed etiology of the loss was doubtful because the audiometric evidence strongly suggested a good deal of residual function in the involved apical half of the cochlea. Consequently, causes other than vascular spasm were considered including acute labyrinthine hydrops (edema), intracochlear hemorrhage, and detachment, or rupture, of a scala media structure, cause unknown. (It was assumed that the bilateral high-frequency loss did not directly relate to the acute right-sided loss.)

This diagnostic uncertainty led, in the following 36 hours, to further audiological evaluation during which two more examiners were

involved. Additional information thus obtained is shown in Figure 48-2. The Békésy audiogram and more recruitment studies still suggested an intracochlear lesion. Note that the speech discrimination score was 0 percent.

Not shown in Figure 48-2 are results of at least six pure-tone audiograms, which remained unchanged during three days of hospitalization. Four persons had been involved actively in conducting these hearing studies, and several others had reviewed the results. Yet at no time during the tests had any one actually asked the patient, who was considered an excellent listener, *What do you hear?*

By this time, the patient had made some rather astute observations of his own: All sounds had a high-pitched metalic quality—a ringing sensation. Paper being crumpled sounded like broken glass being stirred in a metal bowl. Rubbing the skin of the ear sounded like rubbing the rim of a wine glass. Speech and other sounds seemed to reverberate in the ear.

These observations seemed a little bizarre, compared to the usual type of subjective dysacousic complaint. It occurred to us that both the patient's observations and the lack of speech discrimination might be explained by an abnormally prolonged damping of sound waves within the cochlea. Subsequently, on the fourth day, some special tests were administered to examine this hypothesis. The results were inconclusive after two hours of testing. Then as a final task the patient was asked to make some differential pitch judgments and *was* asked, What do you hear? The pitch studies proved to be most revealing and added significant information to the understanding of the hearing problem. They suggested, in fact, a lesion completely destroying the apical half of the cochlea.

The patient was completely unable to assign any pitch sensation whatsoever to frequencies in the lower portion of the hearing range tested, 200–730 cps; he noted only a "buzzing" sensation which varied somewhat in loudness. He was first able to assign a pitch to 750 cps but was unable to differentiate it from 1000 cps, except for a slight increase in loudness. At still higher frequencies his difference limen for frequency was also poor, requiring an approximate 10 percent change in frequency.

The point in this story is a simple one. If the question, What do you hear? had been asked during any one of the pure-tone audiograms, a good deal of confused thinking could have been avoided. In retrospect the patient's audiograms were not, in fact, true *pure-tone* measurements at all below 1,000

cps. Rather, they signified the sound level at which he first heard an atonal buzz. This percept was also present for the Békésy tracings, for tone decay, and for SISI tests. Perhaps the most remarkable feat of all was his binaural alternate loudness balance at 500 cps, which was actually a balance between a buzz and a tone. Thus, these scores had one meaning from the audiometric reports, and perhaps quite a different meaning when interpreted in the light of the patient's sensations.

This case is unusual but far from unique. There are at least two other situations involving pure-tone acuity measurements where the patient's sensations have little or no relationship to the intended stimulus. Most clinicians are familiar with instances where patients with sharply falling audiograms hear clicks or noise when high-frequency tones are presented with the interrupter switch. Also an article by Carhart reports an instance where the patient apparently was responding to aural harmonics of the stimulus tones; this was determined only after the clinician investigated the nature of the patient's experience during the test.

The numbers on the frequency dial of an audiometer describe only generally the stimulus presented to the patient. The numbers themselves provide no information concern-

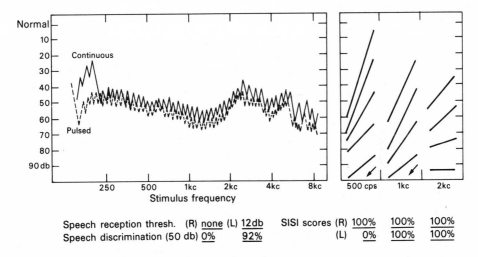

| Speech reception thresh. (R) none (L) 12db | SISI scores (R) 100% 100% 100% |
| Speech discrimination (50 db) 0% 92% | (L) 0% 100% 100% |

Figure 48-2. Continuous and interrupted-stimulus Békésy audiogram of right ear and other test results obtained 24 to 48 hours after hearing loss.

ing harmonics of the stimulus frequency nor existence of possible unwanted transients.

Thus in some instances, the patient's report of the subjective sensation may bear little or no resemblance to the stimulus, the pure-tone audiogram being completed without the patient or the examiner being aware of anything unusual. To record the listener's "yes" response on an audiogram below a specific frequency heading may be misleading. The gap between audiometry and an adequate evaluation of hearing still exists. Perhaps a more persistent use of the question, *What do you hear?* will help to bridge it.

REFERENCE

1. Carhart, R.: Atypical Audiometric Configurations Associated With Otosclerosis, Ann Otol 71:744–758 (Sept) 1962.

49

Pseudoauditory Bone–Conduction Thresholds

E. HARRIS NOBER

E. HARRIS NOBER, Ph.D., is Chairman and Professor of Communication Disorders, University of Massachusetts

Air-conduction thresholds reflect the sensitivity of the auditory mechanism as a functional unit. Bone-conduction thresholds provide essentially the same information but the transmission route bypasses the conductive mechanism. When bone thresholds are ten dB (or more) better than the air thresholds the air-bone gap is considered significant and the quantitative difference represents the impedance of the conductive mechanism. In essence, the specific relationship between the air and bone thresholds will provide data for ascertaining the amount of the hearing loss that can be attributed to impairment in the conductive mechanism and the amount attributed to impairment in the sensory-neural mechanism.

Theoretically, the gap should not occur in cases with pure sensory-neural pathology, but it is not uncommon to obtain a significant low-frequency air-bone gap for subjects with sensory-neural pathology. Indeed, response to bone-conduction stimulation has even been observed with people who consistently failed to yield any response to air-conduction stimulation at maximum intensity. Bocca and Perani (1960) observed this audiologic "absurdity" and contended that "this peculiar behavior of bone thresholds over lower frequencies only concerns the frequencies between 125 and 500 d.v. . . . and are almost never better

Reprinted by permission of the author from *J. Speech Hearing Dis.*, **29,** pp. 469–476 (1964).

than 20–30 db." The dynamics were explained in terms of a primitive vestibular hearing mechanism that was supposedly mediated through the vestibular endings in the saccule and the vestibular endings in the cochlea. They cited phylogenic, anatomic, physiologic, and clinical evidence in support of their theory.

Nober (1963a) presented a study before the International Congress for the Deaf demonstrating the low-frequency air-bone gap in cases with sensory-neural hearing loss. His data suggested tactile exteroception as the mechanism responsible for this phenomenon.

Little experimental attention has been directed to the possibility that this low-frequency air-bone gap observed in cases with sensory-neural pathology may be the result of tactile exteroception. The goal of this study is to explore tactile exteroception as the mediator of invalid bone-conduction responses.

The objectives of this study are to:

(1) confirm that an apparent low-frequency air-bone gap can occur in cases with sensory-neural pathology exclusively;

(2) demonstrate that the low-frequency bone-conduction thresholds responsible for the gap are invalid or "pseudoauditory";

(3) provide additional audiometric criteria to help differentiate between the valid and the invalid bone-conduction thresholds;

(4) demonstrate the existence of bone-conduction thresholds on areas other than the head; that is, "non-auditory" areas;

(5) investigate whether the invalid bone-conduction responses may result from tactile exteroception.

SUBJECTS

Seventy children from the Mill Neck Manor School for the Deaf were divided into three groups according to the kind and degree of hearing loss. One group consisted of 38 partially deaf children with varying degrees of residual hearing; all 38 had medical diagnoses of sensory-neural hearing loss. A second group was composed of 12 totally deaf children also diagnosed as having sensory-neural impairment. This group served as a control for the partially deaf sensory-neural group, as the totally deaf subjects gave no responses to maximum air-conduction stimulation at any frequency. A third group with 20 partially deaf children had medical diagnoses of mixed loss (conductive and sensory-neural). This group represented a population with bone-conduction thresholds that were known to be valid. The effects of a masking noise on valid bone-conduction thresholds and supposed invalid bone-conduction thresholds could then be compared. Finally, 30 children selected from the above three groups were given bone-conduction tests for tactile thresholds on three areas of the body other than the head, that is, on "non-auditory" areas.

METHOD AND PROCEDURE

A Beltone bone-conduction oscillator provided the tones for the auditory and the tactile stimuli at frequencies 250, 500, 1000, 2000, and 4000 cps. All the subjects were conditioned to respond when they "heard" the tones with the oscillator placed on the mastoid process. The test for tactile thresholds on the three non-auditory areas was administered not sooner than sixty days after the auditory tests. Three locations for the tactile non-auditory tests were chosen after a preliminary exploration of several areas of the body. These

were: the fingers (vibrator held between the thumb and forefinger), the ulna (near the elbow), and the clavicle. The subjects were instructed to respond when they perceived a sensation such as a tickle, tingle, vibration, etc.

In general, the "better" ear was used as the experimental ear (see Nober 1963b). Failure to respond at the maximum intensity level was designated as "NR" (no response).

RESULTS AND DISCUSSION

Table 49-1 shows the median air- and bone-conduction thresholds for the three groups. The median air-conduction at 250 cps was 70 dB for the partially deaf sensory-neural group and NR for the totally deaf sensory-neural group. Both groups yielded identical median bone-conduction thresholds of 25 dB. The median air-conduction threshold at 500 cps for the partially deaf sensory-neural group was 80 dB and for the totally deaf sensory-neural group, an NR designation. Again, both groups yielded identical bone-conduction thresholds of 50 dB. Neither of the two groups gave any bone-conduction responses at 1000, 2000, and 4000 cps.

Because the bone-conduction responses of the two sensory-neural groups were similar and the air-conduction thresholds dissimilar it was assumed that the identical bone-conduction thresholds at 250 and 500 cps for the two groups could not be a valid measure of the inner ear sensitivity. It is unreasonable that the inner ear loss could be independent of the air-conduction thresholds as these data would imply if they were valid, especially with such depressed air-conduction thresholds and over a relatively wide range of hearing levels. Consistent bone-conduction responses at frequencies with no air-conduction sensitivity may conceivably occur in cases with a maximum middle ear impedance superimposed on a cochlear pathology. Collectively both pathologic conditions could raise the air-conduction thresholds to exceed the maximum output of the audiometer. In this study, however, the two sensory-neural deaf groups were composed only of subjects who received careful otological examinations that ruled out the probability of any middle ear pathology.

These results and observations indicated that the bone-conduction thresholds reflected something other than auditory sensitivity. The responses given to the stimuli delivered by the bone-conduction oscillator would be more properly termed "pseudo-auditory" responses. They occurred at 25 dB for 250 cps and at 50 dB for 500 cps, but never above the latter frequency. The bone-conduction thresholds of Bocca and Perani (1960) were remarkably similar but were approximately ten dB better at 250 cps, that is, 15 dB; at 500 cps the identical 50-dB threshold was noted.

The confirmation of an invalid low-frequency air-bone gap required the development of some definitive audiometric technique or set of criteria to differentiate valid from invalid bone-conduction thresholds. For this purpose, 20 partially deaf subjects with "mixed" hearing impairment were used. Table 49-1 also shows the air and bone thresholds of this third group. The median values for air-conduction thresholds throughout the entire frequency range used differed by very little from the median values for the partially deaf sensory-neural group. At 250 cps there was a 15-dB difference but the differences were ten dB or less beyond this frequency.

The most important aspect of these data concerned the bone-conduction thresholds.

The median bone-conduction values were 10 dB at 250 cps, 30 dB at 500 cps, and 55 dB at 1000 cps. The hearing levels at 250 and 500 cps showed a marked departure of 15–20 dB from the levels of the two sensory-neural groups. Another feature of the mixed-loss group is that there were responses to bone-conduction stimuli at 2000 and 4000 cps for some subjects although this is not seen from Table 49-1. The NR designation in these two instances indicates that less than half of the subjects responded at 2000 and 4000 cps. This finding was in contrast to results for the two sensory-neural groups where all the subjects failed to respond at any frequency above 500 cps.

The complete lack of response beyond 500 cps is of critical audiologic significance in identifying pseudoauditory bone-conduction responses since no sensory-neural subjects responded above 500 cps. In essence, the 1000 cps frequency becomes the focal point for identifying the pseudoauditory bone-conduction responses.

From the foregoing it was assumed that: (1) the low-frequency bone-conduction responses of the two sensory-neural deaf groups were invalid or pseudoauditory responses, and (2) the bone-conduction responses of the mixed group were valid bone-conduction thresholds that reflected cochlear-neural sensitivity. In order to pursue these two assumptions further two hypotheses were formed and experimentally tested. The first hypothesis asserted that the pseudoauditory bone-conduction thresholds of the partially deaf sensory-

TABLE 49-1. MEDIAN AIR- AND BONE-CONDUCTION THRESHOLDS OF THE THREE EXPERIMENTAL GROUPS. VALUES SHOWN ARE HEARING LEVELS IN DECIBELS RE: AUDIOMETRIC ZERO. NR INDICATES FAILURE TO RESPOND AT MAXIMUM OUTPUT ON THE AUDIOMETER

	Frequency in CPS									
	250		500		1000		2000		4000	
	Air	Bone	Air	Bone	Air	Bone	Air	Bone	Air	Bone
Partially deaf sensory-neural	70	25	80	50	90	NR	95	NR	NR	NR
Totally deaf sensory-neural	NR	25	NR	50	NR	NR	NR	NR	NR	NR
Partially deaf mixed (conductive & sensory neural)	55	10	70	30	85	55	90	NR	90	NR

neural group would not be raised by air-conduction masking. The principle here is that an auditory masking stimulus does not affect non-auditory thresholds. The second hypothesis asserted that the valid bone-conduction thresholds of the partially deaf mixed-loss group would be raised because of the air-conduction masking and in a directly proportional relationship. In this instance it was assumed that the valid bone-conduction thresholds would be affected by the masking noise.

These hypotheses were investigated by giving all the subjects in the partially deaf sensory-neural group and the partially deaf mixed-loss group a masking white noise at an over-all sensation level that exceeded their air-conduction thresholds by approximately 15 dB at 250 cps and 20 dB at 500 cps. Table 49-2 lists the masked threshold increases for

TABLE 49-2. MEAN ELEVATION OF BONE-CONDUCTION THRESHOLDS WITH MASKING

	Frequency in CPS	
	250	500
Partially deaf sensory neural	1.8 dB	2.5 dB
Mixed-loss (conductive and sensory-neural)	* 15.0 dB	* 22.0 dB

* Significant at the 1 percent level of confidence.

the two groups. The partially deaf sensory-neural group had a masked bone-conduction mean increase of 1.8 dB at 250 cps and a mean increase of 2.5 dB at 500 cps. As neither of these slight threshold shifts was statistically significant, according to an analysis of variance, the first hypothesis was accepted. The masked bone-conduction mean threshold shifts for the partially deaf mixed-loss group were 15.0 dB at 250 cps and 22.0 dB at 500 cps. Both of these mean threshold shifts were statistically significant at the one percent level of confidence and so the second hypothesis was accepted. The masked threshold shifts were also proportional to the sensation level of the masking noise.

The results of the masking study lead to the conclusion that: (1) the low-frequency bone-conduction thresholds of the sensory-neural

groups were invalid and manifested pseudo-auditory perceptions that did not reflect the sensitivity of the inner ear; (2) the bone-conduction thresholds of the partially deaf mixed-loss group represented the sensitivity of the inner ear and auditory nerve; (3) pseudo-auditory and auditory bone-conduction responses were differentiated from each other by inspection of the bone-conduction audiogram and by appropriate masking. Furthermore, masked threshold shifts of the auditory responses were proportional to the magnitude of the masking stimulus. These criteria collectively provided adequate audiometric information to ascertain the validity of a low-frequency air-bone gap.

What is the basis for the pseudoauditory low-frequency air-bone gap? Bocca and Perani (1960) discussed a primitive mechanism of vestibular hearing. They supported their theory with vestibular tests that suggested the low-frequency perceptions were associated with an intact vestibular mechanism. They cited instances of labyrinthine dysfunction and concomitant failure to respond to low-frequency bone-conduction stimulation. Perhaps the large amplitude displacement of the bone-conduction oscillator at the low frequencies 250 cps and 500 cps may exceed the tactile thresholds for these frequencies. Indeed, the reciprocal relation of amplitude displacement and frequency (intensity held constant) is commensurate with the results that only the low frequencies 250 and 500 cps were invalid.

In order to explore the possibility of tactile exteroception 30 children were randomly selected from the three groups described above and the same Beltone oscillator was applied to three areas of the body, other than the head (non-auditory). The three non-auditory areas were: (1) the fingers, (2) the ulna, and (3) the clavicle. The bone-conduction oscillator was held between the thumb and forefinger by the subjects and applied to the ulna and clavicle by the examiner.

Table 49-3 shows that the tactile thresholds were 15 dB with respect to audiometric "0"

TABLE 49-3. TACTILE BONE-CONDUCTION THRESHOLDS
FOR THREE TESTED NON-AUDITORY AREAS. VALUES GIVEN
ARE IN DECIBELS RE: NORMAL THRESHOLD LEVELS (OR
AUDIOMETRIC ZERO). NR INDICATES THAT NO RESPONSES
WERE GIVEN AT MAXIMUM OUTPUT OF THE AUDIOMETER

| | Frequency in CPS | | | | |
	250	500	1000	2000	4000
Fingers	15	30	50	NR	NR
Ulna	15	35	NR	NR	NR
Clavicle	15	35	NR	NR	NR

at 250 cps for all three non-auditory areas.
At 500 cps the ulna and clavicle areas both
yielded a 35-dB threshold and the fingers, a
30-dB threshold. There were no tactile responses at 1000, 2000, and 4000 cps for
the ulna and clavicular areas. Ten children,
or one-third, yielded a 50-dB threshold at the
fingers for 1000 cps.

The three non-auditory areas were ten
dB more sensitive than the pseudo-auditory
thresholds at 250 cps and 15–20 dB more sensitive at 500 cps. The importance of these data
is that bone-conduction tactile sensitivity is
better in the non-auditory areas. Consequently,
the bone-conduction thresholds elicited from
the auditory area for 250 and 500 cps have
exceeded the non-auditory tactile thresholds
by 10–20 dB. This leaves considerable latitude
for the possibility of tactile contamination at
the mastoid area. The evidence strongly suggests that tactile exteroception may be the
neurological mechanism for mediating the
pseudoauditory low-frequency bone thresholds.

The controversy of vestibular hearing versus
tactile hearing (exteroception) has more than
academic interest; there is the important
clinical significance of ascertaining the integ-
rity of the labyrinth. Bocca and Perani (1960)
contended that the low-frequency air-bone
gap reflected normal vestibular functioning
and was absent in cases with labyrinthine
pathology. If this is true, then these low-
frequency bone-conduction responses are not
"invalid"; indeed, they would be of diagnostic significance for testing the adequacy of the
vestibular mechanism. On the other hand, if
the responses are tactile as suggested in this
study then perhaps the bone-oscillators should

not be calibrated to exceed the thresholds
given above for 250 and 500 cps.

The ambiguous and inconclusive results
of associating labyrinthine dysfunction with
diagnostic prototypes is well documented in
the literature. Rosenblüt, Goldstein, and
Landau (1960) reported the vestibular responses of deaf and aphasic children relevant
to educational classification, etiologic factors,
hearing level, motor abnormality, and EEG.
Their principal finding indicated a "greater
proportion of abnormal responses among
aphasics than among deaf children." They
concluded that "vestibular tests have negligible
value in the differential diagnosis of auditory
disorders in young children." Similar conclusions were made by Carruthers (1945),
Christoph (1943), and Guilder and Hopkins
(1936). Rosenblüt, Landau, and Goldstein
concluded that "there was a significant relation between the depression of hearing sensitivity and the depression of vestibular responsiveness but not enough to be predictive for the
individual case."

The importance of dependable audiologic
criteria to differentiate the valid from the
invalid low-frequency air-bone gap is critical
to the otologist as his therapy is based on accurate diagnoses. Goodhill and Moncur (1963)
asserted that the "negative Rinne and air-
bone gap are the two diagnostic criteria for
impedance loss." They also directed attention
to the problem of "tactile confusion" but they
were basically concerned with the diagnostic
implication of a valid air-bone gap. They
concluded that the "air-bone gap limited to
the low-frequency area, begins to loom as an
important diagnostic tool not only in 'mixed
deafness' but also in certain cases where the
loss appears to be solely sensory-neural while,
in fact, a conductive component does exist."

Since the low frequency air-bone gap does
have crucial diagnostic implications as Goodhill and Moncur (1963) contend it is imperative that the audiometric validity of bone
conduction be assured. This author hopes
that his study will provide some framework for
the further development of definitive tech-

niques to ascertain the validity of bone-conduction thresholds.

SUMMARY AND CONCLUSION

This study purported to demonstrate an artifactual low-frequency air-bone gap in cases of sensory-neural impairment. Furthermore, an attempt was made to show that the bone-conduction thresholds were "pseudoauditory" perceptions that may be mediated through tactile exteroception. To accomplish this, 50 deaf children ranging in age from 5–14 years were divided into two "sensory-neural" groups according to degrees of impairment. One group consisted of 38 partially deaf children with varying degrees of residual hearing while the second sensory-neural group had 12 totally deaf children who gave no responses to maximum air conduction at any frequency.

Air- and bone-conduction tests were given to all subjects and the results indicated that the bone-conduction thresholds of these two groups were nearly identical; they were 25 dB at 250 cps and 50 dB at 500 cps. None of the subjects in either of these groups gave any bone-conduction responses above 500 cps. Since the medical diagnosis was exclusively sensory-neural, since the bone-conduction thresholds showed little or no variations regardless of the air-conduction levels, and since there were no bone-conduction responses above 500 cps, the air-bone gaps resulting from these thresholds were assumed to be invalid. Perhaps the strongest indication came from the totally deaf groups with no air-conduction responses to maximum stimulation but with bone-conduction thresholds virtually equivalent to the partially deaf subjects.

The contention that the bone-conduction thresholds of the two sensory-neural groups were "pseudoauditory" was pursued further by introducing a third group of 20 partially deaf children who had varying degrees of mixed hearing loss, that is, conductive and sensory-neural. Air- and bone-conduction thresholds were elicited from this group. Although the air-conduction thresholds were similar to the partially deaf sensory-neural group, the bone-conduction thresholds varied markedly in degree and also extended beyond 500 cps. It was then temporarily assumed that the bone-conduction thresholds of this group were valid and reflected true inner ear sensitivity. This assumption was subsequently tested by comparing the bone-conduction thresholds of the partially deaf sensory-neural group with the bone-conduction thresholds of the partially deaf mixed-loss group, in the presence of a masking white noise. The rationale for masking was based on the premise that a masking auditory stimulus would only raise the thresholds of the valid bone-conduction responses (auditory) and not affect the threshold of the pseudoauditory bone-conduction responses (tactile); that is, auditory masking would not affect non-auditory perceptions. Results confirmed the above. The masked bone-conduction thresholds of the mixed-loss group shifted significantly (one percent level) and in proportion to the magnitude of the white noise while the bone-conduction thresholds of the sensory-neural group remained unaltered.

The neurological mediating mechanism for the pseudoauditory responses was studied relative to Bocca's theory of "vestibular hearing" and Nober's theory of "tactile hearing" or "pseudoauditory exteroception." To pursue the possibility of tactile contamination further, 30 subjects were selected from the three groups above to determine the bone-conduction thresholds on three "non-auditory" areas of the body. Results showed the non-auditory bone-conduction thresholds were generally comparable or better than those obtained from the mastoid area. This suggests that tactile exteroception may be the intervening modality of the pseudoauditory bone-conduction responses. Differential diagnosis was also discussed relevant to the clinical and theoretical implications.

The conclusions were that:

a. an artifactual low-frequency air-bone

gap can occur in cases with sensory-neural impairment;

b. the identification of the pseudo-auditory bone-conduction thresholds may be assisted by a symptomatic bone-conduction audio-gram configuration and changes with appropriate masking;

c. the pseudoauditory perceptions may be mediated through tactile exteroceptions.

REFERENCES

Bocca, D. and Perani, G., Further contributions to the knowledge of vestibular hearing. *Acta otolaryng.*, 51, 1960, 260–267.

Carruthers, D. C., Congenital deaf-mutism as a sequela of a rubella-like maternal infection during pregnancy. *Med. J. of Australia*, 32, 1945, 315–320.

Christoph, C. H., Occurrence of congenital family deaf-mutism in six children. *Arch. Otolaryng.*, 38, 1943, 300–320.

Goodhill, V. and Moncur, J., The low-frequency air-bone gap. *Laryngoscope*, 73, 1963, 850–867.

Guilder, R. P. and Hopkins, L. A., Auditory function studies in an unselected group of pupils at the Clarke School for the Deaf: III, relation between hearing acuity and vestibular function. *Laryngoscope*, 46, 1936, 190–197.

Nober, E. H., Pure tone bone-conduction thresholds and tactile exteroception of the deaf: presented at the International Congress of the Deaf, Gallaudet College, Washington, D.C., June, 1963a.

Nober, E. H., Pure tone air-conduction thresholds of deaf children. *Volta Review*, 65, 1963b, 229–241.

Rosenblüt, B., Goldstein, R., and Landau, W., Vestibular responses of some deaf and aphasic children. *Ann. Otol. Rhin., and Laryng.*, 59, 1960, 747–755.

50

Collapse of the Ear Canal During Audiometry

IRA M. VENTRY
JOSEPH B. CHAIKLIN
WILLIAM F. BOYLE

IRA M. VENTRY, Ph.D., is Professor of Audiology, Teachers College, Columbia University
JOSEPH B. CHAIKLIN, Ph.D., is Professor of Audiology, University of Minnesota
WILLIAM F. BOYLE, M.D., is an otolaryngologist in private practice in San Francisco, California

Functional hearing loss may be defined as a decrease in measured auditory acuity without a known organic basis. Usually a diagnosis of functional hearing loss is made when there are significant intratest or intertest disagreements among audiometric assessments of a person's hearing acuity, and medical examination reveals that the discrepancies cannot be attributed to organic pathology, such as otitis media. Thus a diagnosis of functional hearing loss is based on a consideration of audiometric, otological, and other medical findings. Functional hearing loss is usually superimposed upon an organic auditory deficit, in which case it is referred to as a functional overlay. Functional hearing loss without an organic component appears to occur rarely.

One of the most commonly accepted indications of functional hearing loss is pure-tone threshold variability greater than ± 5 db. in the absence of a known organic condition to account for such variability (3–5). There are, however, a number of organic otologic conditions that may produce threshold variability similar to the audiometric variability associated with functional hearing loss. Organically induced threshold shifts have been

Reprinted by permission of the authors from *Arch. Otolaryngol.*, **73,** pp. 727–731 (1961).

attributed to serous otitis media, Ménière's disease, Eustachian tube dysfunction, tinnitus, otosclerosis, infection, and impacted cerumen (1, 2, 5, 6). There appear to be no published reports, however, relating threshold variability to collapse of the external auditory canal by earphone pressure during audiometric evaluation. The 2 cases presented in this article illustrate the audiometric and diagnostic problems associated with collapse of the external auditory canal during audiometry.

REPORT OF CASES

CASE 1.—A 49-year-old white male government employee was referred to the Veterans Administration Hospital in San Francisco for evaluation of an apparent functional hearing loss observed on earlier examinations. The impression of functional hearing loss was based on unexplained threshold shifts of 10 db.–30 db. He gave a history of having told previous examiners that during audiometric evaluation, the pressure of the audiometer earphones "blocked" his hearing. He stated, further, that holding the earphones away from his ear or moving his jaw caused his hearing to be "unblocked."

The patient first became aware of his hearing loss at the age of 32 when he noted tinnitus in both ears and difficulty in hearing conversational speech. The hearing loss progressed and the tinnitus became a persistent ringing sensation of varying pitch. He gives no history of vertigo. He has worn a hearing aid for the past 14 years and stated that without the aid he experiences considerable difficulty in hearing. In noisy environments he has greater difficulty in hearing speech unless people speak louder.

During a 3-year tour of duty in the Air Corps, he had a moderate amount of exposure to aircraft noise but does not relate his hearing loss to this noise exposure. He presents no history of temporary deafness, otalgia, otorrhea, head injury, febrile diseases, or ingestion of ototoxic agents. He had a tonsillectomy and adenoidectomy as a child and a submucous resection in 1949. His mother had a hearing problem at the age of 45 and he has one brother and one sister who had hearing losses that began when they were in their 40's.

Physical examination revealed external auditory canals that were narrowed. The tympanic membranes were intact and freely mobile. Detailed examination (prompted by audiometric inconsistencies and by the patient's unusual report of decreased acuity with earphones in place) revealed that the patient's external auditory canals could be collapsed and completely closed by pressure on the pinna. Normally, the canals are patent.[1] During audiometry, however, pressure on the pinna from the test earphones collapsed the cartilaginous external auditory canal producing threshold shifts (Figure 50-1) similar to the shifts reported as inconsistencies on earlier examinations. In order to maintain the patency of the ear canals during audiometry, plastic tubes 0.5 cm. in diameter were placed in the external auditory canals. This produced test results (Figure 50-1) represen-

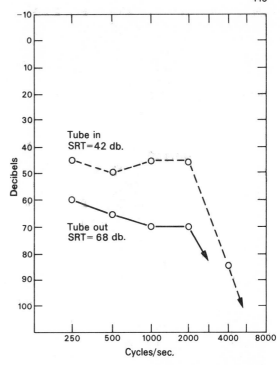

Figure 50-1 (Case 1). Pure-tone thresholds obtained for the right ear with plastic tube in place and with plastic tube removed. With the tube in, galvanic skin response (GSR) results were in excellent agreement with voluntary thresholds. A similar audiometric picture was obtained for the left ear.

tative of the patient's hearing acuity under normal conditions. The remainder of the otorhinolaryngological examination, including labyrinthine function studies, was within normal limits. The diagnosis was deafness, bilateral, mixed conductive, secondary to clinical otosclerosis.

CASE 2.—The second patient, a 62-year-old white male was recently retired from the United States Air Force as a master sergeant. He was referred to the VA Hospital for an outpatient compensation examination. During his initial examination there were unexplained audiometric discrepancies, and, since otological examination revealed no organic factor to account for these discrepancies, he was believed to have a functional component to his hearing problem. He was hospitalized later for a period of observation and re-examination.

[1] Photographs of Case 1's ears were taken but proved inadequate for publication. It was not feasible for him to return for retakes. It should be noted, however, that his ears were very similar in size and shape to Case 2's ears, which are shown in Figures 50-2 and 50-3.

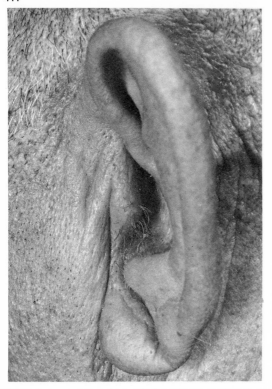

Figure 50-2 (Case 2). The left ear and external auditory canal under normal conditions.

Physical examination revealed clear external auditory canals and slightly thickened, but mobile, tympanic membranes. The left external auditory canal was extremely narrow and sloped sharply upward, starting approximately 1.5 cm. from the canal meatus. Similarly to the first patient, this patient's external auditory canals collapsed when earphones were placed over his ears or when pressure was applied to the pinnae. Figure 50-2 shows the patient's left ear in its normal position and Figure 50-3 illustrates the collapse of the left external canal with pressure applied to the pinna. The audiometric results with the canal open and with the canal closed are shown in Figure 50-4. Inflation of the left middle ear produced no significant threshold shifts. The remaining otorhinolaryngological examination was essentially normal except for a nasal septum

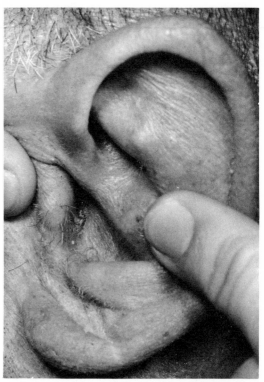

Figure 50-3 (Case 2). Closure of the left external auditory canal produced by pressure on the pinna.

The patient reported that during most of his Air Force career he was exposed to airplane noise at close range, and in the last 10 years of his service he had considerable exposure to jet noise. About 5 years ago he began to notice difficulty in hearing, especially in his left ear. Speech became less clear and in noisy environments he experienced great difficulty in understanding conversation. For the past 15 years he has had persistent, high-pitched tinnitus in his left ear, consisting of a buzzing sensation and, occasionally, the sound of bells. During childhood he had several episodes of ear infections, but none as an adult. At the age of 35 years he incurred a fractured nose. In the period from 1932 to 1949 he had 3 internal and external nasal surgical procedures. He had a tonsillectomy and adenoidectomy at the age of 52. The remainder of the otorhinolaryngological history was negative.

deviation to the right side. The diagnosis was perceptive deafness, right ear, due to acoustic trauma; deafness, left ear, mixed perceptive, perceptive component due to acoustic trauma, and conductive component, etiology undetermined, but possibly due to otosclerosis.

COMMENT

The 2 cases described above demonstrate that, in certain patients, pressure produced by audiometric earphones may result in a collapse of the external auditory canal. This collapse is produced when the earphones compress the pinna against the side of the head which, in turn, moves the pinna forward and causes a compression of the soft cartilaginous portion of the external auditory canal. It is important to note that this compression and the resultant closure of the canal does not in itself cause the audiometric variability. The actual variability appears to be caused by at least 4 factors. The first, and probably most important, factor is movement of the jaw associated with talking, yawning, or other deliberate movement. These jaw movements tend to pull the cartilaginous external canal forward and downward, causing an increase in the patency of the lumen of the external auditory canal. The first patient deliberately opened and closed his jaw in order to "unblock" his hearing. A second factor that may cause threshold shifts is movement of the audiometer earphone itself. Holding the phone slightly away from the ear would remove the pressure from the pinna, thus restoring the patency of the canal. The patient, under this circumstance, might give the unusual report of hearing better with the earphone off the ear. Intertest discrepancies, e.g., a discrepancy between pure-tone average and speech reception threshold, might result if the earphones are removed from the ears (during bone-conduction testing) and repositioned somewhat differently for another portion of the test. The different place-

ment of the phones might result in a significant difference in the size of the lumen of the canal, producing an unexplained intertest discrepancy. Changes in the tension of the earphone headband is a third factor that might produce threshold shifts. During audiometry a significant change in the tension of the headband would alter the pressure of the earphone on the pinna. This, in turn, would result in a different degree of closure of the ear canal. The change in the degree

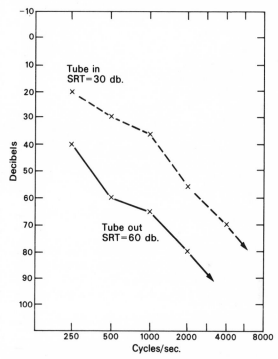

Figure 50-4 (Case 2). Pure-tone thresholds obtained for the left ear with plastic tube in place and with plastic tube removed. With the tube in, audiometric results, including GSR audiometry, were consistent. With the tube out, audiometric results were more variable. A similar audiometric picture was obtained for the right ear.

of closure would produce audiometric inconsistencies. Finally, the audiometric picture might be complicated by inadequate placement of the plastic tubing in the ear canal. In Case 2, shifts in threshold were noted after the plastic tubing was inserted into the canal. Inspection revealed that the tubing had partially slipped out of position and become occluded, again causing variations in acuity. More stable results were obtained by placing a rubber-covered stock ear insert (Figure 50-5) into the canal. In summary, once the external auditory canal has been closed by the pressure of the audiometer earphones, movements of the jaw, placement of the earphones, changes in the tension of the earphone headband, and improper place-

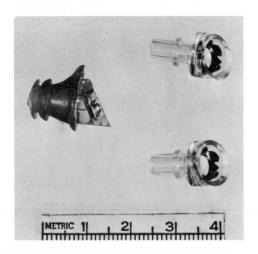

Figure 50-5. Several plastic stock ear inserts that may be utilized to maintain canal patency. The inserts are used with removable rubber tips as shown on the left insert.

ment of the plastic tubing can all cause changes in the size of the lumen of the external auditory canal, resulting in significant intratest and intertest audiometric inconsistencies. It is possible, of course, that some cases of collapsed canals may go undetected if the canal closure is complete and stable.

In such cases there would only be an unrecognized overestimate of the amount of hearing deficit with no intratest or intertest inconsistencies.

It is interesting to note that the 2 cases presented in this article had large lop ears, which suggests that the collapsed ear canal phenomenon may be more prevalent in cases with ears of this type. Unusually narrow external canals were also observed in both cases suggesting that this may be another predisposing factor. The exact incidence of the collapsed ear canal phenomenon is unknown, and further investigation is necessary to determine its occurrence in the hard-of-hearing population. One might speculate, however, that the incidence of complete canal closure is relatively infrequent and partial closure more common. It is difficult to state the amount of canal closure necessary to produce audiometric problems, although it seems reasonable to assume that nearly complete closure would be required.

SUMMARY

Two cases are presented to illustrate a previously unreported condition—collapse of the external auditory canal caused by audiometer earphone pressure—that may account in some cases, for previously unexplained intratest and intertest audiometric inconsistencies. Failure to recognize this condition may lead to an erroneous diagnosis of functional hearing loss. Medical histories, audiometric results, photographs, and comments are presented.

REFERENCES

1. Coates, G. M.; Schenck, H. P., and Miller, M. V., editors: Otolaryngology, Vol. 1, Hagerstown, Md., W. F. Prior Company, Inc., 1956.

2. Fowler, E. P., Jr., editor: Medicine of the Ear, New York, Thos. Nelson & Sons, 1947.

3. Johnson, K. O.; Work, W. P., and McCoy, G.: Functional Deafness, Ann. Otol. Rhin. & Laryng. 65:154–170 (March) 1956.

4. Newby, H. A.: Audiology: Principles and Practice, New York, Appleton-Century-Crofts, Inc., 1958.

5. Sataloff, J.: Industrial Deafness, New York, McGraw-Hill Book Company, Inc., 1957.

6. Williams, H. L.: Ménière's Disease, Springfield, Ill., Charles C Thomas, Publisher, 1952.

51

Collapse of the Ear Canal During Audiometry

VICTOR H. HILDYARD
MILTON A. VALENTINE

VICTOR H. HILDYARD, M.D., is Clinical Professor of Otolaryngology, University of Colorado Medical Center
MILTON A. VALENTINE, Ph.D., is Professor of Speech Communication, Oregon State University

The report by Ventry, Chaiklin, and Boyle of 2 cases of collapse of the external auditory canal during audiometry (*1*) serves to emphasize a previously more or less neglected phenomenon and also to underline the importance of close professional interaction between otologist and audiologist. We began an investigation of the phenomenon of ear canal collapse during August, 1960. We were prompted to an investigation of this phenomenon more by observed and unexplained discrepancies between tuning fork observations and audiometric test results than by the inconsistencies in test results referred to by the previous writers.

The possibility of ear canal collapse during audiometry was first suggested to us by a number of cases in which air-conduction bone-conduction gaps indicated by routine audiometry exceeded 20 db. but were not accompanied by negative Rinne responses when tuning forks were used. When a plastic stopple of the type used in preliminary hearing-aid evaluations was introduced into the ear canal, the differences were reduced or, in some cases, disappeared altogether.

The present study is based upon 48 cases of ear canal collapse during audiometry observed between August, 1960, and Septem-

Reprinted by permission of the authors from *Arch. Otolaryngol.*, **75**, pp. 422–423 (1962).

ber, 1961. In general, these findings support those of Ventry et al. However, certain differences were observed in the present investigation, and a somewhat more complete description of the phenomenon is possible on the basis of the larger number of cases here considered.

METHOD OF OBSERVATION

Experience during the early phase of the investigation indicated that several observations might suggest the possibility of complete or partial collapse of the ear canal. The first and most reliable of these observations was the air-conduction bone-conduction gap mentioned earlier in combination with positive Rinne responses. The second, somewhat less reliable in our experience, was the inconsistency of test results mentioned by Ventry et al. A third indication of possible canal collapse was the clinical observation of discrepancy between the patient's responses to speech when the earphones were and were not in place. Whenever one or more of these indications was present, the patient was retested using routine audiometric techniques and then retested again with the introduction of the plastic ear stopple.

SUMMARY OF RESULTS

A total of 48 cases of collapse of the ear canal during audiometry were discovered in the course of the 13-month observation period. This represents about 4 percent (4.05 percent) of the patients seen for audiometric testing.

The average improvement in air-conduction threshold obtained by the introduction of the stopple was 9.6 db. when all patients and all frequencies were considered. At the various frequencies studied, the average improvements were as follows: at 500 cps—6.2 db.; at 1,000 cps—7.3 db.; at 2,000 cps—11.4 db.; and at 4,000 cps—6.9 db. The modal or typical case, however, showed improvements as follows: at 500 cps—9.4 db.; at 1,000 cps—10.7 db.; at 2,000 cps—14.6 db.; and at 4,000 cps—9.9 db. The range of improvements shown at individual frequencies after the introduction of the stopple was as follows: at 500 cps—20 db. gain to 5 db. loss; at 1,000 cps—25 db. gain to 10 db. loss; at 2,000 cps—30 db. gain to 10 db. loss; and at 4,000 cps—20 db. gain to 5 db. loss. In no case in which the introduction of the stopple caused a loss was that loss present at all frequencies. In other words, in a few cases the introduction of the stopple might cause a given patient to appear to have a greater air-conduction bone-conduction gap than previously shown at 1 or even 2 frequencies, but in no case was such an increased gap present "across the board."

The age of patients who improved with the stopple procedure proved to be a skewed distribution emphasizing the older age groups. The mean age was 52.8 years, the modal age 64 years, and the age range from 8–76 years. Only 5 patients were younger than 30, while 8 were over 65, and 10 between 65 and 70 years of age.

No particular pattern of diagnosis other than that presumed to characterize the general population was revealed. The numbers of patients who improved with the stopple procedure with particular diagnoses were as follows: otosclerosis 15; presbyacusis 9; Ménière's disease 6; sensorineural 4; perceptive losses (toxic) 3; otitis media 3; noise-induced loss 2; dislocated incus 2; hemotympanum, epitympanitis, labrynthitis, and normal hearing, 1 each.

With the cases studied, collapse of the canal might occur as follows: in both ears, 28 cases; in 1 ear, 20 cases. It should be noted, however, that not all patients were affected at all frequencies. In 17 cases, patients were affected at 3 frequencies only; 5 were affected at 2 frequencies only, and 2 patients at 1 frequency only. The frequency most commonly affected—47 times out of 48—was 2,000 cps.

Of the cases studied, only 12, or 25 percent, failed to repeat the retest audiogram (without stopple) within 5 db. of the initial test. And of these cases, only 9 showed inconsistency of response during the initial testing.

Of the cases studied, 7 showed the "large, lop ears" noted by Ventry et al.

COMMENT AND SUMMARY

The cases summarized here indicate that collapse of the external ear canal during audiometry may lead to spurious audiograms. The error in these audiograms may be sufficient to affect the diagnosis and treatment of a given patient.

The presence of a collapsed canal does not necessarily reveal itself by inconsistency of response; tuning fork tests and clinical observation are necessary checks on audiometry.

Apparently the phenomenon of collapse of the ear canal during audiometry is somewhat more common than the initial report by Ventry, Chaiklin, and Boyle indicated.

The average error introduced by collapse of the canal appears to be of the order of 10 to 15 db. and it is greatest at 2,000 cps. Thus, an improvement of 10 db. or more at 2,000 cps when a stopple is introduced and the patient retested by routine audiometry should provide a reliable sign of a collapsed canal.

Partial collapse or collapse affecting only some frequencies is possible but not typical.

Careful professional interaction and clinical observation by both otologist and audiologist are again emphasized by the appearance of this phenomenon.

REFERENCE

1. Ventry, I. M.; Chaiklin, J. B., and Boyle, W. F.: Collapse of the Ear Canal During Audiometry, Arch. Otolaryng. 73:727–731 (June) 1961.

52

A Masking Dilemma in Bilateral Conduction Deafness

RALPH F. NAUNTON

RALPH F. NAUNTON, M.D., is Professor of Surgery and Chairman, Otolaryngology, University of Chicago

There are theoretical grounds for believing that, in testing the hearing of some subjects with bilateral conduction deafness, it is impossible adequately to mask the hearing of the opposite ear without at the same time masking the hearing of the test ear.

Discussion of this problem will be facilitated by a preliminary definition of a number of familiar audiological terms.

DEFINITIONS

Test Ear

The ear whose performance is under investigation in a monaural hearing test.

Opposite Ear

The ear whose performance is *not* under investigation in a monaural hearing test.

Auditory Stimulus

Any sound, simple or complex, fed to a listener's ear during a hearing test.

Test Stimulus

The auditory stimulus to whose presence or arrival a listener's response is being examined during a hearing test.

Reprinted by permission of the author from *Arch. Otolaryngol.*, **72,** pp. 753–757 (1960).

Overheard Stimulus

Any auditory stimulus fed into one ear will also stimulate the other ear; the stimulus may, for the sake of clarity of definition, be said to travel from the transducer (headphone, loudspeaker, bone-conduction receiver, etc.) into one ear then "across the head" to the other ear. The stimulus "crossing" the head and arriving at the other ear may still be of sufficient magnitude to evoke a sensation of hearing at that ear; the stimulus is then said to be overheard. It has been shown that when air-conduction receivers are in use, the overheard stimulus "crosses" largely by bone conduction (*1*).

Mask Ear

Under some circumstances in monaural hearing tests the opposite ear must be actively prevented from hearing a test stimulus "crossing the head" from the test ear; this end must be achieved in such a way that the performance of the test ear remains unaffected. Taking an analogy from the telephone company, detection of the overheard test stimulus is prevented by creating a "busy line" state—the opposite or overhearing ear being kept busy listening to another auditory stimulus. The hearing of the opposite ear for the test stimulus "crossing" the head is said to be masked, and that ear is thereafter described as the *mask ear*.

Masking Stimulus

The auditory stimulus referred to above that keeps the mask ear in a busy line state. The masking stimulus will usually be an electronically generated noise whose audible character will be clearly different from that of the test stimulus (tone or speech). The masking stimulus operates by raising the threshold of the mask ear for the test stimulus, the magnitude of the masking stimulus required to insure a "busy line" effect being dependent upon the magnitude of the overheard test stimulus. In subsequent discussion it will be assumed that, for any given test stimulus, "X" db. of masking stimulus will raise the threshold of the mask ear by "X" db. (i.e., "X" db. of masking stimulus will be assumed to have a *masking effect* of "X" db.).[1]

Interaural Attenuation

In "crossing" from one ear to the other an auditory stimulus will usually be reduced in intensity (or attenuated) en route. This intensity reduction (in decibels) is described as the "interaural attenuation"; its magnitude will depend upon the frequency of the stimulus and the type of transducer (headphone, loudspeaker, bone-conduction receiver, etc.) delivering the stimulus to the head. The test stimulus and the masking stimulus are both auditory stimuli and both will "cross the head," being attenuated by the amount of the interaural attenuation en route. Masking will be required when a test stimulus is overheard; but the masking stimulus will "cross the head" and, if it is overheard by the test ear to a sufficient extent, will mask the test ear and distort the hearing test results.

INDICATIONS FOR MASKING

The situations in air conduction tests where masking is required are often described by

[1] It should be noted that this relation between the intensity of the masking stimulus and its masking effect,

quoting the simplest type of masking problem, the case with a large (40 to 50 db. or more) disparity between the air conduction losses in a listener's two ears. This description, correct as far as it goes, is based upon the general recognition that when using standard headphones the interaural attentuation is approximately 50 db. There are other cases where masking is desirable but where there may, for example, be as little as zero difference between the two ears.

Application of available information to two theoretical situations will clarify the "indications for masking" and illustrate a theoretical dilemma.

The rule, quoted above, indicates that, in this theoretical case, the right ear must be masked when the air-conduction thresholds of the left ear are determined because there is a disparity between the air-conduction thresholds of the two ears of more than 40 or 50 db. It is, however, more practical to arrive at the same conclusion by what may appear to be an unnecessarily laborious process of deduction. Thus the sound entering the left ear or test ear when its threshold is reached is 55 db.; this sound will "cross the head," losing 50 db. en route, and will be heard by the right or opposite ear at a level of 5 db. (It is assumed that the interaural attenuation is 50 db. and that the bone-conduction hearing of the right ear is normal.) Masking is therefore necessary to exclude the right ear from the test.

The maximum amount of masking that can be delivered to the right or mask ear without raising the threshold of the test ear can similarly be deduced. Any masking stimulus entering the mask ear will "cross the head," losing 50 db. en route, since the interaural attentuation is 50 db.; but, if the test ear is to remain unaffected by it, the masking stimulus must be at 0 db. (re normal threshold) when it reaches the test ear; if it arrives at 0 db., having lost 50 db. en route, it must have started at 50 db. The maximum

while being near true for narrow band noises (2), does not hold for the commonly used broad-spectrum white noise.

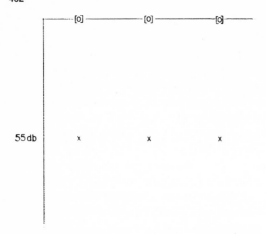

Figure 52-1. Stylized pure-tone audiogram of theoretical case Type 1: unilateral conduction deafness.

permissible intensity of the masking stimulus entering the right or mask ear must therefore be 50 db. above normal threshold.

The masking effect of this 50 db. masking stimulus will be 50 db. because the air conduction threshold of the mask ear is normal (*see* section above, "Definitions": Masking Stimulus).

Three conclusions have thus been reached concerning the theoretical case, Type 1:

1. The right ear must be masked when the air conduction threshold of the left ear is determined.

2. No more than a 50 db. masking stimulus may be used for this purpose.

3. The masking effect of the 50 db. masking stimulus will be 50 db.

The steps described leading to the 3 conclusions above appear to be laborious, but the process is often a very necessary one, both in carrying out hearing tests and in interpreting their results; with very little practice these steps become far easier to apply than to describe.

A second type of theoretical situation may be examined in the same way.

The 55 db. test stimulus entering the left ear or test ear at its threshold will "cross the head" and stimulate the opposite ear at a level of 5 db. (i.e., 55 − 50 db.). The bone-conduction threshold of the opposite ear is assumed to be normal; therefore the test stimulus will be overheard by the opposite ear at a level of 5 db. Masking is therefore necessary, when testing the left ear, to exclude the right ear from the test.

Any masking stimulus entering the right or mask ear (regardless of the state of air-conduction or bone-conduction hearing in the mask ear) will "cross the head" losing 50 db. en route; but, if the test ear is to remain unaffected by it, the masking stimulus must be at zero db. (re normal threshold) when it reaches the test ear. If it arrives at 0 db. (re normal threshold) when it reaches the test ear, having lost 50 db. en route, it must have started at 50 db. The maximum permissible intensity of the masking stimulus entering the mask ear must therefore be 50 db. above normal threshold.

The masking effect of this 50 db. maximum masking stimulus will, however, be zero because the air-conduction threshold loss of the mask ear is 55 db.; thus the masking stimulus will not be heard by or elevate the threshold of the mask ear.

Three conclusions have been reached concerning the theoretical case, Type 2:

1. The right ear must be masked when the threshold of the left ear is determined.

2. No more than a 50 db. masking stimulus may be used for this purpose.

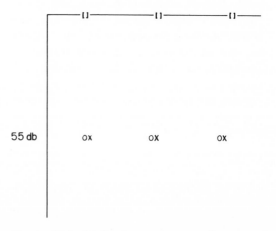

Figure 52-2. Stylized pure-tone audiogram of theoretical case Type 2: bilateral conduction deafness.

3. The masking effect of the 50 db. masking stimulus will be zero.

Theoretical case Type 2 thus serves to illustrate a theoretical dilemma where masking is necessary but impossible to achieve without at the same time affecting the test ear.

It will be recognized that the general type of audiogram illustrated in theoretical case Type 2 is commonly found in otosclerosis and other types of bilateral middle ear deafness and that the dilemma, if in fact it does occur, will be found in clinical cases of this type. The existence of the dilemma will be proven if, in a clinical case, a masking stimulus fed to one ear masks both ears simultaneously and to equal extents.

EXPERIMENTAL INVESTIGATION

The intensity of a broad-spectrum white noise masking stimulus required to mask a 500 cps tone, 10 db. above the listener's threshold of hearing for that tone, was determined for a group of 20 adults suffering from bilateral otosclerosis. The air-conduction losses of the patients tested in this series ranged between 25 and 65 db. at 500 cps.

Matched PDR 10 receivers covered with small rubber cushions were used for all tests. Complete unmasked air- and bone-conduction threshold audiograms were first made; then measurements of the threshold of hearing for a 500 cps pulsed tone, in the presence of noise, were made under each of two conditions. Each listener's two ears will

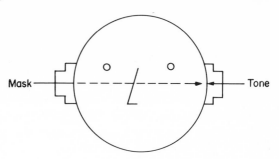

Figure 52-4. Test condition B.

be identified as Ear 1 and Ear 2 for purposes of description.

Condition A (Figure 52-3): Pure tone and white noise mixed and fed to Ear 1. Experimental measurement: Intensity of white noise required to mask a 500-cps tone 10 db. above the threshold of Ear 1. Condition B (Figure 52-4): White noise delivered to Ear 1; pure tone delivered to Ear 2. Experimental measurement: Intensity of white noise required to mask a 500-cps tone 10 db. above the threshold of Ear 2.

It can be stated, on the basis of the preceding discussion, that the audiometric dilemma illustrated theoretically in case Type 2 will have been demonstrated practically if, in the experimental investigation outlined, examples occur where little or no difference can be found between the intensities of the direct (Condition A, Figure 52-3) and overheard (Condition B, Figure 52-4) masking stimuli required to mask the 10 db. 500 cps tones.

RESULTS

The differences observed in the 20 experimental subjects between the intensities of the direct and the overheard masking stimuli required to mask the 10 db. test stimuli at the two ears were as follows:

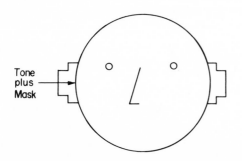

Figure 52-3. Test condition A.

24.6 db.	17.4 db.	8.4 db.	3.8 db.
23.4	16.9	8.3	3.1
20.1	15.0	8.1	2.6
19.3	14.8	7.8	− 3.7
17.5	13.6	4.8	−12.4

Positive values indicate that the ear receiving the masking stimulus directly, mixed with the tone, required less noise to mask the 10 db. tone than the opposite ear required when receiving the masking stimulus by conduction "across the head"; negative values indicate the reverse, that the masking stimulus fed directly to one ear was masking the opposite ear by cross conduction more effectively.

COMMENT

The investigation described has served to indicate that an audiometric dilemma, predicted on a theoretical basis, does in fact occur in clinical cases of otosclerosis. There clearly are cases within the group studied conforming with the theoretical case Type 2 in which a masking stimulus fed to one ear masks the opposite ear to an almost equal extent. There were two cases where a masking stimulus fed to one ear produced a greater masking effect on the opposite ear than on the ear receiving the mask directly.

The figures listed can, without introducing any serious error, be assumed to represent the differences between the *masking effects* produced at a listener's two ears by a masking stimulus fed to one ear. Clearly, if this assumption is made, the experimental results indicate that it would be impossible in practice to carry out a monaural hearing test on approximately half of the subjects examined because any stimulus used to produce a useful degree of masking in the mask ear will also mask the test ear. The magnitude of this problem will be increased as above-threshold and bone-conduction tests are attempted because the overheard test stimuli will be greater and will require more intense masking stimuli to prevent their being heard by the untested ear.

The limiting factor in the theoretical and practical problems discussed is the interaural attenuation, whose value is determined by the nature of the headphones or other devices used to deliver auditory stimuli to the listeners' ears during audiometric testing. Zwislocki (*1*) has examined this aspect of the problem in detail and indicated that the acoustical isolation between a listener's ears (interaural attenuation) depends upon the area of contact between the listener's head and the headphone or other device delivering the auditory stimuli; when this area of contact is large (e.g., in orthodox headphones) the interaural attenuation is poor; when the area is small (e.g., when sound-conducting tubes are inserted into the external meatuses) the interaural attentuation will be considerably increased. The dilemma whose occurrence has been demonstrated will be overcome to a considerable degree if masking stimuli are delivered to the mask ear by means of a sound-conducting tube held in the external meatus rather than by an orthodox headphone, because the resulting increase in interaural attenuation will reduce the risk of cross conduction of the masking stimulus. An additional advantage will accrue if air-conduction test stimuli are delivered by a similar system in that there will be fewer occasions when masking is required.

It should be reemphasized that the interaural attenuation, although frequency dependent, is not otherwise related to the type of auditory stimulus "crossing the head." For this reason the interaural attenuation is unaffected by the use of narrow-band masking stimuli in place of broad band white noise; there are advantages in the use of narrow-band noises (*2*), but increased interaural attenuation is not one of them.

It should also be noted that, in examining the need for the use of masking in a clinical hearing test, the determining factor is the difference between the air-conduction threshold of the tested ear and the bone-conduction threshold of the opposite or untested ear.

SUMMARY

There are theoretical grounds for believing that in some subjects with bilateral middle ear deafness it is impossible adequately to mask the hearing of the untested ear without at the same time masking the hearing of the tested ear. Measurements of the masking effect of white noise made on a series of 20 listeners with bilateral otosclerosis have indicated that the problem is encountered in practice and is therefore more than a theoretical concept without foundation in fact.

REFERENCES

1. Zwislocki, J.: Acoustic Attenuation Between the Ears, J. Acous. Soc. America 25:752–759, 1953.
2. Denes, P., and Naunton, R. F.: Masking in Pure Tone Audiometry, Proc. Roy. Soc. Med. 45:790–794, 1952.

53

Pitfalls in Routine Hearing Testing

JOSEPH SATALOFF

JOSEPH SATALOFF, M.D., is Professor of Otology, The Jefferson Medical College of Philadelphia

An appreciation of the problems of validity and reliability of hearing tests has always been important; as middle ear surgery for deafness becomes more frequent, these problems become increasingly serious.

The routine hearing tests currently used by practicing otologists are usually air- and bone-conduction audiometry, tuning fork tests, and less frequently, speech reception and discrimination tests. In most instances the results of these tests lead to an accurate diagnosis. Occasionally, however, they can be highly misleading. It is the purpose of this presentation to call attention to some of the pitfalls encountered in routine hearing tests. In order to describe some of these pitfalls, a series of illustrative cases has been selected. Most of them are from my clinical practice and some reflect personal errors.

Figure 53-1 shows the audiogram of a patient who was referred with a diagnosis of right-sided conductive deafness and advised to have a stapes mobilization. The lack of lateralization with a tuning fork is not uncommon in long-standing unilateral deafness. In the same patient's audiogram, shown in Figure 53-2, it is evident that with more accurate testing and adequate masking there is in reality a total loss of hearing in the right ear as the result of mumps labyrinthitis during infancy. The caloric studies were normal. This case emphasizes the importance

This article has been revised from the original and is reprinted by permission of the author from *Arch. Otolaryngol.*, **73**, pp. 717–726 (1961).

of adequately masking out the good ear while testing the bad one and the need for masking when using tuning forks. If the physician had masked the left ear when he tested bone conduction in the right, he would have found no response to bone conduction and recognized a sensorineural rather than a conductive loss.

The type of masking noise used and its intensity are most important. The audiogram in Figure 53-3, for example, reveals residual hearing for air and bone conduction in the right ear when the left is unmasked. It would appear from these results that the loss in the right ear is mostly conductive. When 80 db. of white noise is used for masking the left ear, it becomes evident there is actually no useful residual hearing in the right ear, either by bone or air conduction. It is notable that when only 60 db. of masking is used during bone-conduction testing, there is still a reasonable response to bone conduction, up to and including 2,000 cps, even though the right ear is totally deaf as the result of severe head trauma. With white noise masking it is difficult to obliterate completely the responses at the low tones of 500 and 250 cps. These tones can be masked out, however, by using narrow-band noise or douching the ear.

While the need for masking is well recognized for air-conduction and bone-conduction audiometry, its importance in speech reception and discrimination testing has often been overlooked. The test results in Figure 53-4 are from a 24-year-old man whose

JOSEPH SATALOFF, M. D.
1721 PINE STREET   PHILADELPHIA, PA. 19103

HEARING RECORD

NAME _____   AGE 41

AIR CONDUCTION

| | | | RIGHT | | | | | | | | LEFT | | | | | |
DATE	Exam.	LEFT MASK	250	500	1000	2000	4000	8000	RIGHT MASK	250	500	1000	2000	4000	8000	AUD.
11-15-57			50	55	60	60	65	70		0	-5	0	5	5	0	

BONE CONDUCTION

| | | | RIGHT | | | | | | | LEFT | | | | | |
DATE	Exam.	LEFT MASK	250	500	1000	2000	4000		RIGHT MASK	250	500	1000	2000	4000	AUD.
11-15-57			0	5	5	5	5			0	-5	-5	0	5	

SPEECH RECEPTION

DATE	RIGHT	LEFT MASK	LEFT	RIGHT MASK	FREE FIELD	MIC.

DISCRIMINATION

DATE	% SCORE	TEST LEVEL	LIST	LEFT MASK	% SCORE	TEST LEVEL	LIST	RIGHT MASK	EXAM.

HIGH FREQUENCY THRESHOLDS

| | | RIGHT | | | | | | LEFT | | | | |
DATE	4000	8000	10000	12000	14000	LEFT MASK	RIGHT MASK	4000	8000	10000	12000	14000

RIGHT		WEBER	LEFT		HEARING AID		
RINNE	SCHWABACH		RINNE	SCHWABACH	DATE	MAKE	MODEL
					RECEIVER	GAIN	EXAM.
					EAR	DISCRIM.	COUNC.

REMARKS

Figure 53-1. Audiogram of patient referred as having a conductive hearing loss in right ear. Note that in right ear, bone conduction was better than air conduction; lack of lateralization with a No. 512 tuning fork.

only complaint was hearing loss in the right ear. With adequate masking, this loss was found to be quite severe and neural in origin. Recruitment was absent and caloric studies suggested a right acoustic neuroma that was confirmed at surgery.

It is interesting to note that during speech reception testing, the threshold in the right ear was 48 db. when the left ear was unmasked, but changed to no response with adequate masking in the left ear. This latter finding, of course, was consistent with the other findings.

Adequate masking is particularly essential with speech discrimination tests since they are done at above-threshold levels. The patient represented by the audiogram in Figure 53-5 had a right acoustic neuroma proved at surgery. During speech discrimination testing, at an intensity of 90 db., he repeated 90 percent of the phonetically balanced word list when the right ear was tested without masking the left. This was, of course, an unexpected result in view of the type of hearing loss present and its etiology. When an 80 db. mask was used in the left ear,

JOSEPH SATALOFF, M. D.
1721 PINE STREET   PHILADELPHIA, PA. 19103

HEARING RECORD

NAME _____   AGE *41*

AIR CONDUCTION

			RIGHT							LEFT						
DATE	Exam.	LEFT MASK	250	500	1000	2000	4000	8000	RIGHT MASK	250	500	1000	2000	4000	8000	AUD.
11-15-57			50	55	60	60	65	70		0	-5	0	5	5	0	
11-15-57		WN 80dB	75	80	↓	↓	↓	↓								

BONE CONDUCTION

			RIGHT						LEFT					
DATE	Exam.	LEFT MASK	250	500	1000	2000	4000	RIGHT MASK	250	500	1000	2000	4000	AUD.
11-15-57			0	5	5	5	5		0	-5	-5	0	5	
11-15-57		WN 80dB		40	45	↓	↓							

SPEECH RECEPTION / DISCRIMINATION

			SPEECH RECEPTION					DISCRIMINATION	RIGHT				LEFT			
DATE	RIGHT	LEFT MASK	LEFT	RIGHT MASK	FREE FIELD	MIC.		DATE	% SCORE	TEST LEVEL	LIST	LEFT MASK	% SCORE	TEST LEVEL	LIST	RIGHT MASK	EXAM.

HIGH FREQUENCY THRESHOLDS

	RIGHT						LEFT					
DATE	4000	8000	10000	12000	14000	LEFT MASK	RIGHT MASK	4000	8000	10000	12000	14000

RIGHT		WEBER		LEFT		HEARING AID		
RINNE	SCHWABACH			RINNE	SCHWABACH	DATE	MAKE	MODEL
						RECEIVER	GAIN	EXAM.
						EAR	DISCRIM.	COUNC.

REMARKS

Figure 53-2. Audiogram of same patient as in Figure 53-1. More accurate testing and adequate masking revealed a sensorineural hearing loss. Right ear with masking: AC > BC. Patient denied hearing tuning fork with masking on left ear.

however, only 46 percent of the words were discriminated, a finding consistent with the other tests.

One of the major pitfalls in hearing testing occurs when attempting to mask an ear in which there is conductive deafness present. Figure 53-6 represents an interesting case in which the right ear was mobilized but without any improvement in hearing, and subsequently caloric studies revealed it to be a completely dead ear. In all likelihood, this ear had no residual hearing, even before the surgery. The good preoperative speech reception and discrimination reported in the right ear were doubtless due to insufficient masking in the left. If adequate masking had been applied to the left ear, the speech reception and discrimination would probably have been unobtainable and the surgery would not have been done. In patients of this type, there is always the danger that a stapes mobilization or fenestration surgery will be performed on an ear that has no useful residual nerve potential. Speech discrimination testing is particularly useful when used with adequate masking in helping to decide the amount of residual hearing left in a patient who has a bilateral conductive hearing loss.

The terms "reliability" and "validity" have special significance in hearing testing. Hearing tests are "reliable" when they give consistent results on repeated testing; they are "valid" when the test results represent an accurate measurement of the patient's hearing. The first 4 hearing levels in Figure 53-7 show severe and quite consistent deafness. This patient gave the same hearing level on numerous other tests performed by other testers and using different techniques. While these tests may have been reliable in the sense that they were reproducible, they were really not valid. Actually, this patient had excellent hearing but suffered from functional deafness, as confirmed by means of a psychogalvanic skin resistance test and by later routine audiometry.

A cardinal pitfall in hearing testing is for the otologist to have fixed, inflexible ideas. Some of these ideas may be based upon premises not yet established or with many exceptions. One example is the tendency to

JOSEPH SATALOFF, M. D.
1721 PINE STREET   PHILADELPHIA, PA. 19103

HEARING RECORD

NAME _____   AGE **52**

AIR CONDUCTION

DATE	Exam.	LEFT MASK	RIGHT 250	500	1000	2000	4000	8000	RIGHT MASK	LEFT 250	500	1000	2000	4000	8000	AUD.
5-10-58			50	65	65	90	↓	↓		0	15	15	30	55	40	
		WN 80dB	↓	100	↓	↓	↓	↓								

BONE CONDUCTION

DATE	Exam.	LEFT MASK	RIGHT 250	500	1000	2000	4000	RIGHT MASK	LEFT 250	500	1000	2000	4000	AUD.
5-10-58			10	20	25	35	↓		5	10	15	25	40	
		WN 60dB	10	25	40	50	↓							
		WN 80dB	40	45	↓	↓	↓							

SPEECH RECEPTION

DATE	RIGHT	LEFT MASK	LEFT	RIGHT MASK	FREE FIELD	MIC.

DISCRIMINATION

DATE	RIGHT % SCORE	TEST LEVEL	LIST	LEFT MASK	LEFT % SCORE	TEST LEVEL	LIST	RIGHT MASK	EXAM.

HIGH FREQUENCY THRESHOLDS

DATE	RIGHT 4000	8000	10000	12000	14000	LEFT MASK	RIGHT MASK	LEFT 4000	8000	10000	12000	14000

RIGHT RINNE	SCHWABACH	WEBER	LEFT RINNE	SCHWABACH	HEARING AID		
					DATE	MAKE	MODEL
					RECEIVER	GAIN	EXAM.
					EAR	DISCRIM.	COUNC.

REMARKS

Figure 53-3. Audiogram of patient showing (in error) residual hearing for air and bone conduction in the right ear when the left is unmasked. Note that 60 db. of masking was inadequate in bone-conduction testing.

JOSEPH SATALOFF, M. D.
1721 PINE STREET   PHILADELPHIA, PA. 19103

HEARING RECORD

NAME _____   AGE **24**

AIR CONDUCTION

			RIGHT								LEFT						
DATE	Exam.	LEFT MASK	250	500	1000	2000	4000	8000	RIGHT MASK	250	500	1000	2000	4000	8000	AUD.
6-24-55			65	60	50	55	60	10		5	0	0	0	0	5	
		80dB	80	70	65	60	60	15								
		100dB	80	80	85	75	65	20								
9-19-55			65	50	60	60	65	40		10	5	5	0	-5	5	
		80dB	↓	100	100	100	100	80								

BONE CONDUCTION

			RIGHT								LEFT					
DATE	Exam.	LEFT MASK	250	500	1000	2000	4000		RIGHT MASK	250	500	1000	2000	4000	AUD.
6-24-55		WN 80dB	40	60	↓	70	70								

SPEECH RECEPTION / DISCRIMINATION

DATE	RIGHT	LEFT MASK	LEFT	RIGHT MASK	FREE FIELD	MIC.		DATE	% SCORE	TEST LEVEL	LIST	LEFT MASK	% SCORE	TEST LEVEL	LIST	RIGHT MASK	EXAM.
9-19-55	48		4														
	↓	80dB															

DISCRIMINATION   RIGHT   LEFT

HIGH FREQUENCY THRESHOLDS

	RIGHT							LEFT					
DATE	4000	8000	10000	12000	14000	LEFT MASK	RIGHT MASK	4000	8000	10000	12000	14000	

RIGHT		WEBER		LEFT		HEARING AID		
RINNE	SCHWABACH			RINNE	SCHWABACH	DATE	MAKE	MODEL
						RECEIVER	GAIN	EXAM.
						EAR	DISCRIM.	COUNC.

REMARKS

Figure 53-4. Audiogram of patient complaining only of hearing loss in the right ear. At surgery a large acoustic neuroma was found on the right side. Note effect of masking on speech reception in the right ear.

conclude that high-tone hearing loss or reduced bone conduction always means sensorineural damage. Figure 53-8 shows that this is not always the case. This patient had a hemotympanum as a result of head trauma. When resolution occurred, both air and bone conduction returned to normal.

Another example of the need to keep an open mind is demonstrated in Figure 53-9. I had always held the fixed impression that because of their physical characteristics, hearing aids could not produce acoustic trauma. For this reason when the youngster

whose hearing chart is shown in Figure 53-9 complained that his hearing was getting progressively worse, I promptly ordered a long series of investigative studies, including endocrine studies, eye grounds, a general medical examination, etc. This youngster was 3 years of age at the time of his first visit. A hearing aid was fitted to his left ear and was worn daily for the next 4 years.

It was only after all the studies were reported normal that I removed the hearing aid from the left ear, and the child's hearing returned to its original level. It can be seen from this Figure that each time the hearing aid was removed the hearing returned to its original level. When the hearing aid was replaced the hearing was again adversely affected. Interestingly enough, amplification for the right ear did not cause reduced sensitivity in that ear.

No discussion of hearing is complete nowadays without some mention of otosclerosis or stapes mobilization. The case described in Figure 53-10 demonstrates a serious pitfall in interpreting hearing tests. This 67-year-old woman required coercion by her family to consult me. She refused to try or wear a hearing aid and communicated mostly in writing for many years. Repeated hearing tests confirmed an almost total loss of hearing in both ears, but a somewhat better response with bone-conduction testing. Only after considerable pressure from the family did I agree to explore the middle ear and to attempt to mobilize the stapes if this were indicated. The stapes was found to be very fixed, but mobilized quite readily, with pres-

JOSEPH SATALOFF, M. D.
1721 PINE STREET   PHILADELPHIA, PA. 19103

HEARING RECORD

NAME _____   AGE **47**

AIR CONDUCTION

DATE	Exam.	LEFT MASK	250	500	1000	2000	4000	8000	RIGHT MASK	250	500	1000	2000	4000	8000	AUD.
					RIGHT							LEFT				
11-10-57			25	45	65	60	75	85		10	15	30	35	50	45	
		WN 80dB	25	45	70	65	80	80	WN 80dB	10	15	30	35	50	35	

BONE CONDUCTION

DATE	Exam.	LEFT MASK	250	500	1000	2000	4000		RIGHT MASK	250	500	1000	2000	4000	AUD.
					RIGHT							LEFT			
11-10-57			30	25	45	60	75			10	20	30	40	55	
		WN 80dB	–	50	–	–	–		WN 80dB	–	10	30	45	55	

SPEECH RECEPTION

DATE	RIGHT	LEFT MASK	LEFT	RIGHT MASK	FREE FIELD	MIC.
11-10-57	60					

DISCRIMINATION

DATE	% SCORE	TEST LEVEL	LIST	LEFT MASK	% SCORE	TEST LEVEL	LIST	RIGHT MASK	EXAM.
			RIGHT				LEFT		
11-10-57	90	90dB	Pb						
	46	90dB	Pb	WN 80dB					

HIGH FREQUENCY THRESHOLDS

DATE	4000	8000	10000	12000	14000	LEFT MASK	RIGHT MASK	4000	8000	10000	12000	14000	
			RIGHT							LEFT			

RIGHT		WEBER		LEFT		HEARING AID		
RINNE	SCHWABACH			RINNE	SCHWABACH	DATE	MAKE	MODEL
						RECEIVER	GAIN	EXAM.
						EAR	DISCRIM.	COUNC.

REMARKS

Figure 53-5. Audiogram of patient with a right large acoustic neuroma proved at operation. Cold caloric test showed no response on right, perverted response on left (horizontal instead of rotary nystagmus with head forward), absence of sensitivity reactions. Note the absence of recruitment and poor discrimination with opposite ear masked.

JOSEPH SATALOFF, M. D.
1721 PINE STREET   PHILADELPHIA, PA. 19103

HEARING RECORD

NAME _____   AGE **64**

AIR CONDUCTION

DATE	Exam.	LEFT MASK	250	500	1000	2000	4000	8000	RIGHT MASK	250	500	1000	2000	4000	8000	AUD.
11-14-58		WN 80dB	70	60	80	80	95	65		55	55	55	65	↓	↓	
RIGHT STAPES MOBILIZATION																
4-6-59		WN 80dB	70	65	75	85	↓	↓								
4-6-59		INTENSE MASKING	70	80	↓	↓	↓	↓								

BONE CONDUCTION

DATE	Exam.	LEFT MASK	250	500	1000	2000	4000	RIGHT MASK	250	500	1000	2000	4000	AUD.
11-14-58			25	30	50	↓	↓		10	25	40	45	↓	
4-6-59		INTENSE MASKING	40	↓	↓	↓	↓							

SPEECH RECEPTION / DISCRIMINATION

DATE	RIGHT	LEFT MASK	LEFT	RIGHT MASK	FREE FIELD	MIC.	DATE	% SCORE	TEST LEVEL	LIST	LEFT MASK	% SCORE	TEST LEVEL	LIST	RIGHT MASK	EXAM.
11-14-58	80		60				11-14-58	84	100 dB		NO MASK					
4-6-59	↓	INTENSE MASKING	60				4-6-59	↓			INTENSE MASKING					

DISCRIMINATION — RIGHT — LEFT

HIGH FREQUENCY THRESHOLDS

DATE	4000	8000	10000	12000	14000	LEFT MASK	RIGHT MASK	4000	8000	10000	12000	14000	

RIGHT		WEBER		LEFT		HEARING AID			
RINNE	SCHWABACH			RINNE	SCHWABACH	DATE	MAKE		MODEL
						RECEIVER	GAIN		EXAM.
						EAR	DISCRIM.		COUNC.

REMARKS

Figure 53-6. Audiogram of patient with otosclerosis who had an unsuccessful right mobilization performed. Subsequently, caloric tests on right gave no response, and it is probable that the right ear was out prior to surgery. Note difficulty in masking left ear.

sure on the incus. A marked improvement in hearing occurred in both ears after stapes mobilization surgery. Interestingly enough the patient still refuses to wear a hearing aid because she feels her hearing has been restored to normal (despite my restrained efforts to correct her impression).

This exercise pointedly demonstrates that just because a patient gives no response at the maximum intensity of the audiometer it does not necessarily mean that the ear is dead. It merely means that the patient's hear-

ing at that frequency is beyond the limits of the audiometer.

Figure 53-11 reveals another instance of a 69-year-old woman who had a practically "dead ear" according to routine audiometry and yet responded well to stapes mobilization indicating very useful residual hearing.

Another patient, Figure 53-12, had a successful stapes mobilization in her left ear, and it appears that her hearing has been excellently restored to an almost normal level. It should be noted, however, that the patient's masked discrimination score was 94 percent preoperatively and between 42 percent and 60 percent postoperatively, so that while this patient may show a much improved hearing threshold, she discriminates less postoperatively than preoperatively. The patient is not nearly as satisfied as the surgeon, who fails to appreciate the importance of maintaining good discrimination. We need to bear in mind that threshold audiometry does not always give a good description of how the person gets along in everyday hearing.

When we review critically the causes for most of the pitfalls presented in this series, we find several underlying factors: (1) reliance on a single threshold and failure to obtain repeatedly consistent hearing tests; (2) inadequate masking and (3) failure to keep an open mind while interpreting results of hearing tests. If more attention is paid to these factors in everyday practice it should result in more valid and reliable hearing tests.

JOSEPH SATALOFF, M. D.
1721 PINE STREET   PHILADELPHIA, PA. 19103

HEARING RECORD

NAME _____   AGE **21**

AIR CONDUCTION

			RIGHT							LEFT						
DATE	Exam.	LEFT MASK	250	500	1000	2000	4000	8000	RIGHT MASK	250	500	1000	2000	4000	8000	AUD.
2-2-59			60	60	70	80	75	60		60	55	75	75	75	60	
2-2-59			60	55	70	80	70	65		55	60	75	75	70	70	
2-6-59			55	60	70	75	70	65		60	60	75	70	75	70	
2-10-59			65	60	65	75	75	65		60	60	70	75	70	70	
2-10-59			10	10	20	←—PGSR—→				10	5	10				
2-10-59			0	0	5	5	10	20		0	0	10	20	25	20	

BONE CONDUCTION

			RIGHT						LEFT					
DATE	Exam.	LEFT MASK	250	500	1000	2000	4000	RIGHT MASK	250	500	1000	2000	4000	AUD.
2-2-59			↓	↓	↓	↓			↓	↓	↓	↓		
2-2-59			↓	↓	↓	↓			↓	↓	↓	↓		

SPEECH RECEPTION / DISCRIMINATION

SPEECH RECEPTION							DISCRIMINATION	RIGHT				LEFT				
DATE	RIGHT	LEFT MASK	LEFT	RIGHT MASK	FREE FIELD	MIC.	DATE	% SCORE	TEST LEVEL	LIST	LEFT MASK	% SCORE	TEST LEVEL	LIST	RIGHT MASK	EXAM.
INCONSISTENT RESULTS																

HIGH FREQUENCY THRESHOLDS

	RIGHT							LEFT					
DATE	4000	8000	10000	12000	14000	LEFT MASK	RIGHT MASK	4000	8000	10000	12000	14000	

RIGHT		WEBER	LEFT		HEARING AID		
RINNE	SCHWABACH		RINNE	SCHWABACH	DATE	MAKE	MODEL
					RECEIVER	GAIN	EXAM.
					EAR	DISCRIM.	COUNC.

REMARKS

Figure 53-7. Audiogram of patient with functional deafness. Former tests were not valid, although they gave repeatedly consistent thresholds. The speech reception and discrimination tests were inconsistent with the audiograms.

JOSEPH SATALOFF, M. D.
1721 PINE STREET   PHILADELPHIA, PA. 19103

HEARING RECORD

NAME _____   AGE _____

AIR CONDUCTION

DATE	Exam.	LEFT MASK	250	500	1000	2000	4000	8000	RIGHT MASK	250	500	1000	2000	4000	8000	AUD.
7-55	WN		30	35	35	30	55	65		10	10	5	10	0	10	
9-55			10	5	5	0	0	0								

(RIGHT / LEFT)

BONE CONDUCTION

DATE	Exam.	LEFT MASK	250	500	1000	2000	4000		RIGHT MASK	250	500	1000	2000	4000		AUD.
7-55	WN		20	20	20	25	40									

(RIGHT / LEFT)

SPEECH RECEPTION

DATE	RIGHT	LEFT MASK	LEFT	RIGHT MASK	FREE FIELD	MIC.

DISCRIMINATION   RIGHT   LEFT

DATE	% SCORE	TEST LEVEL	LIST	LEFT MASK	% SCORE	TEST LEVEL	LIST	RIGHT MASK	EXAM.

HIGH FREQUENCY THRESHOLDS

DATE	4000	8000	10000	12000	14000	LEFT MASK	RIGHT MASK	4000	8000	10000	12000	14000	

(RIGHT / LEFT)

RIGHT		WEBER	LEFT		HEARING AID		
RINNE	SCHWABACH		RINNE	SCHWABACH	DATE	MAKE	MODEL
					RECEIVER	GAIN	EXAM.
					EAR	DISCRIM.	COUNC.

REMARKS

Figure 53-8. Post-traumatic hemotympanum. When resolution occurred, air and bone conduction returned to normal.

JOSEPH SATALOFF, M. D.
1721 PINE STREET   PHILADELPHIA, PA. 19103

HEARING RECORD

NAME _____   AGE **7**

AIR CONDUCTION

DATE	Exam.	LEFT MASK	RIGHT 250	500	1000	2000	4000	8000	RIGHT MASK	LEFT 250	500	1000	2000	4000	8000	AUD.
5-10-52			25	55	60	70	90		AID ON	15	40	50	50	45		
6-7-54										70	↓	↓	↓	↓		
6-21-54									AID OFF	50	70	85	85	75		RINGING TIN.
9-4-54										30	55	60	55	50		
10-2-54									AID ON	25	50	60	55	50		
11-20-54										60	85	95	85	70		
12-4-54									AID OFF	30	50	60	60	50		
4-2-55									AID ON	25	60	85	80	80		SUDDEN RINGING
4-8-55									AID OFF	15	50	60	60	50		PERSIST RINGING
9-4-56	AID	ON	25	50	65	70	85		AID ON	55	↓	↓	↓	↓		
9-14-56			25	50	65	70	85			60	90	↓	↓	↓		
10-13-56			15	45	60	65	85		AID OFF	20	50	60	70	60		
1-20-57			20	45	65	70	90		AID ON	25	45	65	70	70		
4-6-57			15	40	60	75	↓			55	↓	↓	↓	↓		
9-2-57			20	45	70	70	↓		AID OFF	↓	45	40	75	↓		

BONE CONDUCTION

DATE	Exam.	LEFT MASK	RIGHT 250	500	1000	2000	4000		RIGHT MASK	LEFT 250	500	1000	2000	4000		AUD.

SPEECH RECEPTION							DISCRIMINATION		RIGHT			LEFT			
DATE	RIGHT	LEFT MASK	LEFT	RIGHT MASK	FREE FIELD	MIC.	DATE	% SCORE	TEST LEVEL	LIST	LEFT MASK	% SCORE	TEST LEVEL	LIST	RIGHT MASK	EXAM.

REMARKS

Figure 53-9. In this case, the hearing aid produced acoustic trauma.

JOSEPH SATALOFF, M. D.
1721 PINE STREET   PHILADELPHIA, PA. 19103

HEARING RECORD

NAME _____   AGE 67

AIR CONDUCTION

			RIGHT								LEFT					
DATE	Exam.	LEFT MASK	250	500	1000	2000	4000	8000	RIGHT MASK	250	500	1000	2000	4000	8000	AUD.
9-17-56			90	95	85	90	↓	↓		85	↓	↓	↓	↓	↓	
9-27-56			90	95	90	90	↓	↓		85	↓	↓	↓	↓	↓	
11-5-56			55	60	65	↓	80	95		75	85	↓	↓	↓	↓	
12-6-56			50	55	55	70	75	55		80	80	90	90	90	↓	
1-31-57			45	50	45	75	65	65		65	75	75	75	90	↓	
2-14-57			50	55	45	75	70	45		60	70	70	70	75	↓	

RIGHT STAPES MOBILIZATION, 10-31-56   BONE CONDUCTION   LEFT STAPES MOBILIZATION, 1-25-57

			RIGHT							LEFT					
DATE	Exam.	LEFT MASK	250	500	1000	2000	4000		RIGHT MASK	250	500	1000	2000	4000	AUD.
9-17-56			40	30	40	50	55			15	35	35	50	45	
1-31-57			35	30	25	↓	55			10	20	35	50	45	

SPEECH RECEPTION

DATE	RIGHT	LEFT MASK	LEFT	RIGHT MASK	FREE FIELD	MIC.
2-14-57	58		86			

DISCRIMINATION

		RIGHT				LEFT			
DATE	% SCORE	TEST LEVEL	LIST	LEFT MASK	% SCORE	TEST LEVEL	LIST	RIGHT MASK	EXAM.
2-14-57	44	88			68	98			

HIGH FREQUENCY THRESHOLDS

	RIGHT						LEFT					
DATE	4000	8000	10000	12000	14000	LEFT MASK	RIGHT MASK	4000	8000	10000	12000	14000	

RIGHT		WEBER		LEFT		HEARING AID		
RINNE	SCHWABACH			RINNE	SCHWABACH	DATE	MAKE	MODEL
						RECEIVER	GAIN	EXAM.
						EAR	DISCRIM.	COUNC.

REMARKS

Figure 53-10. Audiogram of patient for whom stapes mobilization proved effective, after repeated hearing tests confirmed an almost total loss of hearing in both ears.

JOSEPH SATALOFF, M. D.
1721 PINE STREET   PHILADELPHIA, PA. 19103

HEARING RECORD

NAME _____   AGE **69**

AIR CONDUCTION

			RIGHT								LEFT					
DATE	Exam.	LEFT MASK	250	500	1000	2000	4000	8000	RIGHT MASK	250	500	1000	2000	4000	8000	AUD.
1-28-58			75	80	↓	90	↓	↓		40	40	55	55	70	55	
2-6-58	c̄	Pack.	40	70	90	90	↓	↓		40	40	55	60	75	55	
2-13-58			40	55	55	50	75	↓		40	45	55	55	70	55	

RIGHT STAPES MOBILIZATION, 2-5-58   BONE CONDUCTION

			RIGHT								LEFT					
DATE	Exam.	LEFT MASK	250	500	1000	2000	4000		RIGHT MASK	250	500	1000	2000	4000		AUD.
1-28-58		WN 80dB	10	30	50	50	↓			20	30	45	55	↓		

SPEECH RECEPTION / DISCRIMINATION

DATE	RIGHT	LEFT MASK	LEFT	RIGHT MASK	FREE FIELD	MIC.		DATE	% SCORE	TEST LEVEL	LIST	LEFT MASK	% SCORE	TEST LEVEL	LIST	RIGHT MASK	EXAM.
1-28-58	95																

DISCRIMINATION   RIGHT   LEFT

HIGH FREQUENCY THRESHOLDS

		RIGHT						LEFT					
DATE	4000	8000	10000	12000	14000	LEFT MASK	RIGHT MASK	4000	8000	10000	12000	14000	

RIGHT		WEBER		LEFT		HEARING AID			
RINNE	SCHWABACH			RINNE	SCHWABACH	DATE	MAKE		MODEL
						RECEIVER	GAIN		EXAM.
						EAR	DISCRIM.		COUNC.

REMARKS

Figure 53-11. A practically "dead ear" according to routine audiometry responded well to stapes mobilization in this case.

JOSEPH SATALOFF, M. D.
1721 PINE STREET   PHILADELPHIA, PA. 19103

HEARING RECORD

NAME   AGE

AIR CONDUCTION

			RIGHT								LEFT						
DATE	Exam.	LEFT MASK	250	500	1000	2000	4000	8000	RIGHT MASK	250	500	1000	2000	4000	8000	AUD.
9-15-59			45	45	45	50	↓	↓		65	70	65	65	85	75	L. Tube
9-16-59										10	25	60	65	↓	75	
9-18-59										55	50	50	60	90	75	
9-21-59										15	15	30	45	90	75	
10-1-59										15	15	5	30	85	75	

BONE CONDUCTION

			RIGHT							LEFT					
DATE	Exam.	LEFT MASK	250	500	1000	2000	4000		RIGHT MASK	250	500	1000	2000	4000	AUD.
9-15-59			-10	-10	-10	25	50			-5	0	-5	15	55	

SPEECH RECEPTION

DATE	RIGHT	LEFT MASK	LEFT	RIGHT MASK	FREE FIELD	MIC.
9-15-59		64				
9-21-59		34				
10-1-59		12				

DISCRIMINATION

		RIGHT				LEFT			
DATE	% SCORE	TEST LEVEL	LIST	LEFT MASK	% SCORE	TEST LEVEL	LIST	RIGHT MASK	EXAM.
9-15-59					94	90dB		max	
9-16-59					42	64dB		max	
10-1-59					60	42dB		max	

HIGH FREQUENCY THRESHOLDS

	RIGHT							LEFT					
DATE	4000	8000	10000	12000	14000	LEFT MASK	RIGHT MASK	4000	8000	10000	12000	14000	

RIGHT		WEBER		LEFT		HEARING AID			
RINNE	SCHWABACH			RINNE	SCHWABACH	DATE	MAKE		MODEL
						RECEIVER	GAIN		EXAM.
						EAR	DISCRIM.		COUNC.

REMARKS

Figure 53-12. Audiogram of patient with hearing restored almost to normal level in left ear after a stapes mobilization. But, note reduced discrimination.

54

Children with Nonorganic Hearing Problems

RICHARD F. DIXON
HAYES A. NEWBY

RICHARD F. DIXON, Ph.D., is Director, Division of Speech Pathology and Audiology, University of North Carolina at Greensboro

HAYES A. NEWBY, Ph.D., is Director, Division of Speech and Hearing Science, University of Maryland

INTRODUCTION

Hearing problems which are not correlated with actual pathology of the hearing mechanism have been referred to variously as "functional" losses of hearing, "psychogenic" losses, or "malingering." From the audiologist's point of view, none of these terms is completely satisfactory. "Functional" is frequently used in other contexts to refer to a loss of function which may be on an organic basis, and thus it is probably not the proper term to apply to a hearing problem which may have no organic correlate. "Psychogenic" and "malingering" refer to the presumed absence or presence of a conscious element of feigning as a part of the symptom-picture. While the psychiatrist may be able to differentiate between an unconscious variety of hearing loss, which might be considered as a conversion reaction or so-called hysterical deafness, and the conscious type of assumed loss, which is properly termed malingering, the audiologist is usually in no position to make this kind of judgment. From the audiologist's—and perhaps the otologist's—standpoint, a better term to encompass all forms of assumed hearing loss would be "nonorganic." Such a term obviously means that the pathological condition

Reprinted by permission of the authors from *Arch. Otolaryngol.*, **70,** pp. 619–623 (1959).

of the hearing mechanism is in doubt, and it does not attempt to identify the hearing problem as being of the conscious or the unconscious variety. As a matter of fact, to be strictly accurate, the audiologist should probably refer to nonorganic hearing *problems* rather than to nonorganic hearing *losses*, because some patients appear to have no hearing handicap except in the examination situation.

In recent years, as audiologic diagnostic methods have been refined, it has become apparent that nonorganic hearing problems are more prevalent among the adult population than had previously been assumed. Audiology centers concerned with the testing of veterans for compensation purposes are required to employ a battery of tests designed to discover the presence of nonorganic problems and to enable the examiner to determine the true organic threshold of each individual patient. In such centers, the incidence of nonorganic problems among the veteran population tested has been estimated at from 20 percent to 40 percent. Johnson, Work, and McCoy (*1*) have reviewed the literature and discussed the increase in the incidence of nonorganic hearing problems in military and veteran populations as familiarity with this type of difficulty has become more widespread. A nonorganic hearing problem, however, may range from a situation in which all of the patient's assumed hearing loss is nonorganic in nature to the situation in which a genuine loss exists but the patient exaggerates the true extent of his hearing problem.

As more audiologists and otologists have become involved in examining claimants in medicolegal cases, the presence of non-organic hearing problems in nonveteran populations is also being discovered to a greater degree. While there are instances of such problems among adults which are not concerned with monetary compensation, these cases are relatively rare. It is commoner to find financial considerations closely tied in with the individual patient's misleading performance on certain auditory tests.

Nonorganic hearing problems may exist in children as well as in adults. In the case of children, the motivation for assuming a hearing loss is almost never associated with monetary compensation. In fact, without considerable additional study of a psycho-diagnostic nature, it is not possible to establish in most cases just what motivates children to behave in the test situation as if they were hard of hearing. It behooves school audiometrists, school psychologists, teachers, administrators, and others who are concerned with the health programs in the schools to be aware of the possibility of the existence of nonorganic hearing problems in children of school age.

Over the past two years, some 40 children with significant nonorganic hearing problems have been examined at the San Francisco Hearing and Speech Center. The purpose of this paper is to discuss some findings pertaining to these 40 children and to describe the procedures which seemed to be the most effective in demonstrating true acuity.

DESCRIPTION OF SUBJECTS

The 40 children who constitute the subjects of this discussion ranged in age from 6 to 18 years, with a mean age of 10.9 years. Thirty-one of the children were female and nine were male. In all 40 cases the audio-

gram furnished by the referral source indicated a suspected marked bilateral hearing impairment when, in fact, our examination eventually revealed the hearing to be within normal limits in each ear.

Twelve children had a history suggesting previous disease of the middle ear and, perhaps, previous hearing loss of an organic nature. Fourteen were receiving special help in school, such as lip-reading instruction, auditory training, and preferential seating. Two children were in special classes for the hard of hearing, and one was in a class for the deaf. One child had been furnished with a hearing aid. It should be noted that in the case of most of these children there was no indication in the referral information to suggest that the hearing loss was not as represented on the accompanying audiograms. In fact, 16 of the children were referred to the Hearing and Speech Center specifically for a hearing aid evaluation.

Most of the children seemed to be performing well academically, to be intellectually normal, and were without noticeable emotional disturbances. Nine children displayed symptoms which might be related to their "hearing problems." These symptoms included functional articulatory speech disorders, and—according to parental reports—strong sibling rivalry, persistent enuresis, anxiety reactions, possible nonorganic visual difficulties, and lack of satisfactory academic progress. It should be reemphasized, however, that children with any symptoms or history of psychological significance were definitely in the minority—less than 25 percent of the total group. On the basis of our own observations, we cannot state why these children performed as they did on hearing tests. We can only report how they did behave, and how we were able to establish that their hearing was normal.

TESTING PROCEDURES

It was noted that during their initial interview, 39 of the 40 children were able to follow normal conversation with no difficulty.

Typically, parents reported that in their observations the children usually did not behave as if they were hard of hearing. In almost every case, poor hearing had not been suspected by the parents until this possibility had been pointed out to them by the results of pure-tone tests, usually performed in the school situation. Apparently it was only in a testing situation that all of the children demonstrated hearing problems. It was curious that only a few previous examiners had noted inconsistencies between the children's responses to conversation and their hearing test results.

At the Hearing and Speech Center, pure-tone tests routinely precede speech audiometry. In the case of these 40 children, it became apparent very quickly that their responses to the pure-tone stimuli were grossly inconsistent with their behavior in a conversational situation. Typically, these children would profess average threshold levels between 40 and 60 db. at all frequencies. Their audiograms tended to be "flat" in configuration and with equal losses by air and by bone conduction. Figure 54-1 is a typical initial audiogram. Note that this loss pattern bears a striking resemblance to the curve of the most comfortable listening level for normal ears.

At this point, it should be mentioned that serial pure-tone audiograms, even widely

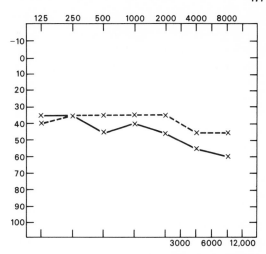

Figure 54-2. Test-retest reliability for the same ear of one child later found to have normal hearing.

spaced in time, do not necessarily provide sufficient variation to make one suspect a nonorganic hearing problem. Although we had no opportunity to estimate the ability of these children to give consistent erroneous thresholds from day to day, we were frequently provided with medical and school records indicating good test-retest reliability, sometimes over a long period of time. Figure 54-2 illustrates one child's ability to maintain consistent false thresholds over an interval of six weeks. The thresholds of the opposite ear showed equally small variations. This child was later found to have normal hearing in each ear.

After examining a few of these children, it became apparent that the speech reception threshold (SRT) was almost always closer to normal levels than the pure-tone thresholds. We recommend, therefore, that at the first indication one may be dealing with a nonorganic problem in a child—for example, the impression gained in the initial interview—monaural, live-voice speech audiometry be employed. The method by which one obtains the child's SRT is important. We found that best results were obtained when the SRT was approached from below, that is, by use of an ascending technique. The use of a descending or an ascending-descending method usually resulted in establishing a false SRT,

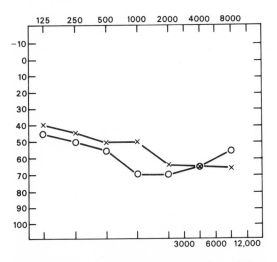

Figure 54-1. Typical initial audiogram for children with nonorganic hearing problems.

and the task of measuring the true organic threshold became more difficult.

It is usually necessary to spend considerable time—and to exercise a great deal of patience—in obtaining the child's SRT. Starting at maximum attenuation, the examiner presents 6 to 10 spondee words, interspersed with such comments as, "I know it's very soft, but you must try hard to repeat these words." If the child fails to respond, the intensity of the signal is increased by 5 db. and the examiner tries again, coaxing the child to respond at almost every word. Occasionally, the examiner may insert a question, such as, "Will you take off the earphones now?" to see if any reaction is observed to indicate that the child heard the question. Also, it may be possible to engage the child in a conversation on a topic that the examiner knows is of particular interest to the child. Thus, one child who would not repeat a spondee word at any sensation level was willing to talk about her pet dog and answer the examiner's questions when the hearing-loss dial was set at 5 db.

With the use of an ascending method and considerable urging of one kind and another, we were able to establish SRT's of 10 db. or better in each ear in 33 of the 40 children. Thus, for most of the children, it was possible to rule out any marked hearing loss by the use of speech-reception measurements. Incidentally, it was unusual to find one of these children manifesting any significant loss of speech discrimination ability. Thirty-four of the children scored 90 percent or better in each ear on discrimination tests administered at levels well above previously established thresholds.

In a few of the children, normal hearing could not be shown by either speech audiometry or conventional pure-tone techniques. It was then necessary to use such special tests as PGSR and delayed feedback measurements to obtain valid estimates of organic thresholds. But even in these cases, before any special testing was done, there were indications of normal hearing. These were usually found in the subject's responses to conversational voice

when he was not aware that he was being tested.

At the conclusion of each examination session, after normal hearing had been established by one method or another, a final attempt was made to secure valid pure-tone thresholds, that is, pure-tone thresholds which would agree reasonably well with the speech audiometric results, or the results of special tests such as PGSR and delayed feedback. The subjects were told that the pure-tone test was being repeated because it was obvious that they had misunderstood the directions on earlier tests, or had made a mistake in judging why they should respond. Sometimes they were told that they would hear a different kind of tone which would be easier to hear than the previous ones used. Then, either a warbled tone or a pulsed tone would be employed. Valid final audiograms were obtained in the case of 33 of the children. It was possible to obtain valid thresholds with some children even when they did not respond *correctly* to the number of pulses presented. These children, after being instructed to count the number of tones they heard, would wait until a series of pulses had been presented and then blandly respond with the wrong number. But the very consistency of their responding with a number after each series of pulses, even though the intervals between presentations were widely varied, argued for the fact that they were hearing the tones. Although, as stated earlier, it is not within the audiologist's province to determine the relative consciousness of motivation in patients displaying nonorganic problems in hearing-test situations, there does seem adequate reason to believe that some of these children wilfully and deliberately attempted to deceive the examiner.

In some respects children with nonorganic hearing problems are similar in their behavior to adults with such problems, and in some respects they are dissimilar. Both children and adults tend to respond to incidental conversation in a manner that is inconsistent with their test results. Both may present a history of previous middle ear problems, but pure-tone test results that are characteristic of perceptive losses. In the test situation, however, the adult will generally exhibit some degree of loss for speech stimuli, even though the speech audiometric results may not be reasonably consistent with the pure-tone results, whereas most children will respond with valid thresholds to speech audiometry, provided the techniques suggested earlier are employed.

SUMMARY AND CONCLUSIONS

In discussing our experience at the San Francisco Hearing and Speech Center with 40 children who had nonorganic hearing problems, it has been our intention to point out that children with normal hearing, like adults, will sometimes perform on hearing tests as if a hearing loss were present. We found this tendency to be considerably more marked in girls. Children with such problems typically do not show difficulty in understanding conversational speech. While they are likely to exhibit grossly erroneous pure-tone responses, most of them will give normal speech-reception scores when time-consuming modifications of standard speech audiometric procedures are employed. A child's consistency on serial pure-tone audiograms in itself

does not rule out the possibility that he has a nonorganic hearing problem. While speech audiometry will yield valid results in most cases, in some instances it will be necessary to resort to special test procedures, such as PGSR and delayed feedback, in order to obtain valid organic thresholds. In most cases it is possible to obtain a final pure-tone audiogram which represents the child's actual hearing levels. The reasons why a child will demonstrate a nonorganic hearing problem in a test situation are obscure but apparently are not, as with adults, associated with pecuniary gain.

It is our hope that audiometrists, educators, and health authorities who deal with hearing-impaired children will be alert to observe that some children who fail school hearing tests may actually be exhibiting hearing problems of a nonorganic nature. On the basis of our observations, we recommend that children who fail school hearing tests not be placed in special classes or be regarded in any way as hearing-impaired children until the organicity of their hearing problems has been established through proper audiological study. We also suggest that nonorganic hearing problems deserve the attention of psychiatrists and psychologists in order to determine why some children behave in an aberrant fashion while having their hearing assessed.

REFERENCE

1. Johnson, K. O.; Work, W. P., and McCoy, G.: Functional Deafness, Ann. Otol. Rhin. & Laryng. 65:154–170 (March) 1956.

appendix

AMERICAN NATIONAL STANDARD
SPECIFICATIONS FOR AUDIOMETERS *

American National Standard

An American National Standard implies a consensus of those sub-stantially concerned with its scope and provisions. An American National Standard is intended as a guide to aid the manufacturer, the consumer, and the general public. The existence of an American National Standard does not in any respect preclude anyone, whether he has approved the standard or not, from manufacturing, marketing, purchasing, or using products, processes, or procedures not conforming to the standard. American National Standards are subject to periodic review and users are cautioned to obtain the latest editions.

CAUTION NOTICE: This American National Standard may be revised or withdrawn at any time. The procedures of the American National Standards Institute require that action be taken to reaffirm, revise, or withdraw this standard no later than five years from the date of publication. Purchasers of American National Standards may receive current information on all standards by calling or writing the American National Standards Institute.

Published by

American National Standards Institute, Inc
1430 Broadway, New York, New York 10018

———

Copyright 1970 by the American National Standards Institute, Inc

Printed in USA

S2M270/450

Contents

American National Standard
Specifications for Audiometers

1. Scope and Purpose

The audiometers covered by this specification are devices designed for use in determining the hearing threshold level of an individual, in comparison with a chosen standard reference threshold level, primarily for the purpose of identification of hearing deficiencies of the individual.

The purpose of this specification is to insure that tests of the hearing of a given individual ear on different audiometers of a given class complying with this specification, shall give substantially the same results under comparable conditions, and that the results obtained shall represent a true comparison between the hearing threshold level of the individual ear and the standard reference threshold level.

Effective September 1, 1970, this standard replaces three previous American National Standard specifications: Audiometers for General Diagnostic Purposes, Z24.5-1951; Pure-Tone Audiometers for Screening Purposes, Z24.12-1952; and Speech Audiometers Z24.13-1953.

Prior to 1965, many laws and administrative rules and regulations relating to the impairment of hearing, to minimum requirements for hearing in military service, to audiometric screening levels in school systems, to admission to schools for the deaf, etc, were written in terms of decibels, usually without explicit statement of any reference level. In addition, unwritten practices under certain other laws have been developed for expressing permanent hearing disability in terms of decibels relative to audiometric zero. It should be clear that the intent in all such situations was to refer to ANSI Z24.5-1951. Furthermore, it should be clear that the intent was always to specify a particular set of physical sound pressure levels that the listener would or would not be able to hear or at which screening tests should be carried out. The adoption of the Table 2 of this standard must not be interpreted as altering these previously implied physical sound pressure levels for specific purposes. These sound pressure levels can be expressed equally well on the scale of Table 2, and it is hoped that each organization will redefine its laws, rules, regulations or practices in terms of the levels of Table 2. Until this is done, however, all levels measured by the scale of Table 2 must be translated to the ANSI Z24.5-1951 scale before the law, rule, regulation or practice in question is applied. In this way, the original intent will be preserved in each case.

Similar conversions to ANSI Z24.5-1951 values shall be made before applying the specifications as to hearing loss mentioned in American National Standard Method for the Measurement of Real-Ear Attenuation of Ear Protectors at Threshold, Z24.22-1957, and also the specifications in American National Standard Criteria for Background Noise in Audiometer Rooms, S1.3-1960.

Audiometric measurements may be made either by the use of pure tones or by the use of spoken material. This differentiates two general classes of audiometers: (1) the pure tone audiometer, and (2) the speech audiometer. Changes of test material and of sound pressure level, and the recording of results, may be performed automatically. An audiometer may be equipped to serve both as a pure tone audiometer and as a speech audiometer.

2. Definitions

2.1 Pure Tone Audiometer. An electroacoustical generator which provides pure tones of selected frequencies and of calibrated output.

2.1.1 *Wide Range Audiometer.* A pure tone audiometer which covers the major portion of the human auditory range in frequency and in sound pressure level. It includes one or two air-conduction earphones, a bone vibrator, a tone switch, and facilities for masking the opposite ear during testing by air conduction or by bone conduction. The wide range audiometer is intended primarily for clinical and diagnostic purposes, or for the measurement of the hearing thresholds of children.

2.1.2 *Limited Range Audiometer.* A pure tone audiometer which is more restricted than a wide range audiometer in its ranges of frequency and of sound pressure level but, for air conduction tests, produces at least tones of 500, 1000, 2000, 3000, 4000, and 6000 Hz, with levels from 10 dB to at least 70 dB re standard reference threshold level. Facilities for bone conduction measurements and for masking may be omitted. The limited range audiometer is intended for measuring the hearing threshold levels of adult populations such as those found in industry.

2.1.3 *Narrow Range Audiometer.* A pure tone audiometer which is more restricted than a limited range audiometer in its ranges of frequency and sound pressure levels.

2.2 Speech Audiometer. Provides spoken material at controlled sound pressure levels, and includes an acoustoelectric source, an amplifier, control means, and earphones. The acoustoelectric source may be a live voice with microphone, or may be a disc, magnetic or other record with a suitable pick-up. Facilities for masking shall be included. No facilities for bone conduction tests are required.

2.3 Limited Range Speech Audiometer. A speech audiometer designated as a Limited Range Speech Audiometer is more restricted in its range of sound pressure level than one designated simply as a Speech Audiometer. Facilities for masking need not be included.

2.4 Group Audiometer. One with which the acoustic material, either pure tones or speech material, is presented to a group of persons simultaneously by a procedure in which each individual may give reliable information as to the test items that are heard.

2.5 Hearing Threshold Level (of an Ear). The amount in decibels by which the threshold of audibility for that ear exceeds a standard audiometric threshold.

2.6 Sound Pressure Level of an Audiometer. As used in this standard, the rms sound pressure level developed by the audiometer earphone in a coupler conforming to Fig. 1, although a coupler not conforming to Fig. 1 may be used if suitable comparison data are available.

3. General Requirements

3.1 General. The frequencies of pure tones generated shall be indicated in hertz and the

hearing threshold levels shall be indicated in decibels.

The audiometer shall have a nameplate giving the manufacturer's name, the model, the serial number, the voltage and frequency of the power supply to be used, and the power consumed by the audiometer. On a battery powered audiometer, means shall be provided for test of the proper condition of the battery supply.

3.2 Earphones. For tests by air conduction, the subject's ear which is not under test shall be covered either by a dummy earphone or by an operable earphone. If two operable earphones are provided for alternative testing of the two ears, as by means of switching arrangements on the audiometer, the output of each earphone must meet the specifications. If the two earphones are not permanently connected to the audiometer, color coding or mechanical arrangements shall be provided to assure the connection of each earphone to its intended circuit. Each earphone shall be equipped with an earphone cushion for contact with the head of the subject (see Fig. 2).

3.3 Headbands. There shall be provided a spring headband which is adequate to hold the earphones against the ears to provide a satisfactory seal.

3.4 Shock Hazard. Audiometers shall be free of shock hazard. A shock hazard shall be considered to exist at an exposed part if the open circuit potential to ground or to another exposed part is more than 30 volts rms and the current through a 1500 ohm resistor is more than 5 milliamperes.

It is recommended that where a power line operated audiometer is to be used with other power line operated devices or in an operating room, the line cord be of the three-wire type with the third wire to provide an electrically conductive connection from the audiometer chassis to the metal conduit of the power line.

3.5 Warm-up Time. For those specifications in which the warming up of the audiometer may be a factor, the audiometer shall meet the specifications after an initial warm-up time of 30 minutes.

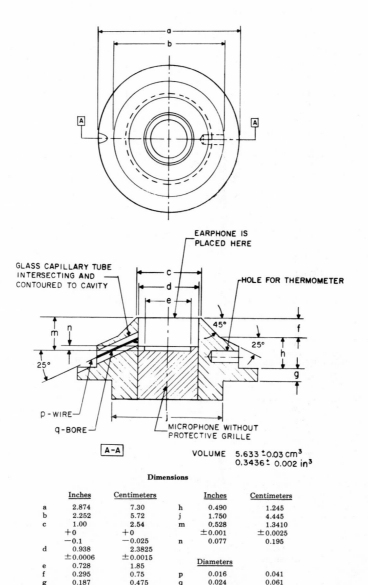

Fig. 1
National Bureau of Standards 9-A Coupler

VOLUME   5.633 ±0.03 cm³
          0.3436 ± 0.002 in³

Dimensions

	Inches	Centimeters		Inches	Centimeters
a	2.874	7.30	h	0.490	1.245
b	2.252	5.72	j	1.750	4.445
c	1.00	2.54	m	0.528	1.3410
	+0	+0		±0.001	±0.0025
	−0.1	−0.025	n	0.077	0.195
d	0.938	2.3825			
	±0.0006	±0.0015		**Diameters**	
e	0.728	1.85			
f	0.295	0.75	p	0.016	0.041
g	0.187	0.475	q	0.024	0.061

9

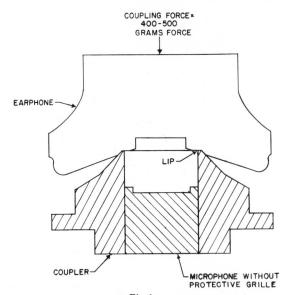

COUPLING FORCE =
400 - 500
GRAMS FORCE

EARPHONE

LIP

COUPLER

MICROPHONE WITHOUT
PROTECTIVE GRILLE

Fig. 1a
Schematic Drawing Showing Method
of Assembly in Use of the NBS 9-A Coupler

4. Requirements for Pure Tone Audiometers

4.1 Test Tones for Wide Range Audiometers
  4.1.1 *Frequencies*. Tones of at least the following definitely identified frequencies shall be produced for both air-conduction and bone-conduction measurements: 250, 500, 1000, 1500, 2000, 3000, and 4000 Hz, and also 6000 and 8000 Hz for air-conduction measurements. Additional frequencies are optional.

  4.1.2 *Accuracy of Tone Frequencies*. Each of the above frequencies generated by the audiometer shall be within three percent of the indicated frequency, except as noted in 4.3.

  4.1.3 *Purity of Tones*. The sound pressure level of any harmonic of the fundamental shall be at least 30 dB below the sound pressure level of the fundamental. Measurements for compliance with this requirement shall be made at the fundamental frequencies of 4.1.1 and the output levels shown in Table 1.

Table 1
Output Levels

Frequency Hz	Minimum Upper Limit of Hearing Threshold Level, dB
125*	70*
250	90
500	100
750*	100*
1000	100
1500	100
2000	100
3000	100
4000	100
6000	90
8000	80

*125 and 750 are not required frequencies but they are given with their appropriate levels.

4.1.4 *Sound Pressure Levels*
  4.1.4.1 *Range and Intervals of Dial Readings of Hearing Threshold Level*. Dial readings of hearing threshold level shall have a mini-

10

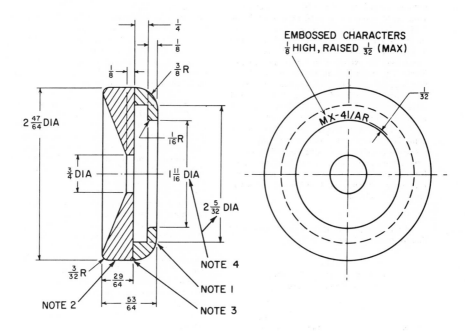

NOTES:

(1) Base material; Buna-S rubber.
(2) Cap material; sponge neoprene.
(3) Base (Note 1) and cap (Note 2) shall be securely bonded together by use of a suitable cement or other approved means.
(4) Durometer readings (Shore A): 20 ± 5 for the front cap; 40 ± 5 for the back base.
(5) Finished cushion shall withstand, without appreciable deterioration, an oxygen bomb test at a pressure of 300 psi and a temperature of 70°C for 48 hours.
(6) Dimension of the base may be modified to adapt to a chosen earphone.
(7) All dimensions are in inches.
(8) Tolerance, $\pm^1/_{64}$ inch.

**Fig. 2
Earphone Cushion (MX-41/AR)***

*From information from U.S. Signal Corps and Bell Telephone Laboratories.

11

mum range of from 0 dB to the values given in Table 1, by intervals of 5 dB or less, with the 0 dB setting at each frequency corresponding to the reference threshold sound pressure levels given in Table 2. If desired, this minimum range may be extended to lower and higher levels. The measured difference between two successive designations of hearing threshold level shall not differ from the dial-indicated difference by more than (1) three-tenths of the dial interval measured in decibels, or (2) 1 dB, whichever is larger. Measurements for compliance with this requirement shall be made electrically at the input to the earphone, with the earphone attached to a coupler conforming to Fig. 1, or the earphone may be replaced by a dummy load which simulates the earphone electrically.

4.1.4.2 *Standard Reference Threshold Sound Pressure Levels.* See Table 2.

Table 2
Standard Reference Threshold
Sound Pressure Levels

Frequency Hz	Standard Reference Threshold Sound Pressure Levels Decibels Relative to 0.0002 Microbar
125	45.5
250	24.5
500	11
1000	6.5
1500	6.5
2000	8.5
3000	7.5
4000	9
6000	8
8000	9.5

NOTE 1: The reference threshold sound pressure level for intelligible speech from an earphone is 19 dB above 0.0002 microbar, measured in accordance with 5.3, and based on 50 percent intelligibility of spondee words.

NOTE 2: These standard reference threshold sound pressure levels apply to the use of the Western Electric Type 705-A earphone and the National Bureau of Standards 9-A coupler (see Fig. 1); the associated condenser microphone being used without a protective grille.

4.1.4.3 *Accuracy of Sound Pressure Levels.* The sound pressure produced by an earphone as referred to the standard reference level shall not differ from the indicated value of sound pressure level at any reading of the hearing threshold level dial by more than 3 dB

at the indicated frequencies of 250 to 3000 Hz inclusive, by more than 4 dB at 4000 Hz, nor by more than 5 dB at frequencies above or below this range. Measurements for compliance with this requirement may be made by combining an acoustical measurement of sound pressure level at a 70 dB setting with voltage measurements at other settings.

4.1.4.4 *Standard Reference Threshold Levels for Other Earphones and Couplers.* The standard reference threshold levels of Table 2 may be transferred to values which are applicable to such other earphones as are adapted for pressure measurements on the National Bureau of Standards 9-A coupler (see Fig. 1). This is done by a "loudness balance" procedure. The respective signal voltages required by the standard earphone of Table 2 and the other earphone to produce equally loud tones are determined from judgments made by a group of not less than six subjects having otologically normal ears, by alternate listening or balancing. This loudness balance shall be done at a level of 20 to 40 dB above the zero reference threshold. If signal voltages of the above determined ratio are then applied to the respective earphones when attached to the standard coupler, there may be determined what pressure generated in the coupler by the second earphone corresponds to the standard reference pressure generated by the original earphone. To obtain standard pressure values applicable to a type of coupler other than that on which Table 2 is based, but which is approved as an American National Standard, a direct comparison may be made of the pressures generated in the two couplers by the standard earphone of Table 2 with a given voltage applied to the earphone. For an earphone and a type of coupler both of which are different from those of Table 2, the two suggested procedures may be combined to obtain applicable standard pressure values. Separate determinations must be made for each frequency.

4.2 Test Tones for Limited Range and Narrow Range Audiometers. The frequencies of the test tones produced and identified in a limited range audiometer shall be as given in the definition (see 2.1.2), and those in a narrow range audiometer shall be selected from the frequencies given in 4.1.1. The purity of the test tones shall meet the requirements of 4.1.3. The sound pressure levels shall meet the requirements of

4.1.4, except that the range of hearing threshold level readings may be more restricted, as specified in 2.1.2 and 2.1.3.

4.3 Variation in Method of Presentation of Test Tones. A pure tone audiometer may be designed to supply sounds over a continuous frequency range instead of at discrete frequencies. Such an audiometer shall have identified on it such frequencies in its range as are listed in 4.1.1, with an accuracy of 5 percent in the indicated frequency values, shall meet the requirements of 4.1.3 as to purity of tones and shall meet the requirements of 4.1.4 as to sound pressure levels within its range, using reasonable interpolations for values of reference levels at the intermediate frequencies. These interpolations may be made graphically.

4.4 Noise During Test

4.4.1 *Sound from Test Earphone.* Any sound from the test earphone, other than the desired test signal, shall not be of such a magnitude as to affect the threshold judgment of any properly instructed subject.

4.4.2 *Sound from Second Earphone.* Any signal from the earphone not being used for test purposes shall have a sound pressure level at least 10 dB below the hearing threshold reference level, except that it need not be more than 70 dB below the signal from the "on" earphone.

4.4.3 *Other Unwanted Sound.* Any sound due to the operation of audiometer controls during the actual listening test, or to radiation from the audiometer, shall be inaudible at each setting of the hearing threshold level dial up to and including 50 dB. The test for this requirement shall be made by a subject having normal hearing, wearing a pair of disconnected earphones and located at the recommended test position, the electrical output of the audiometer being absorbed in a resistive load equal to the impedance of the earphone at 1000 Hz.

NOTE: This limitation on noise from controls would apply to any noise which could furnish a clue which would influence the test results. It is not intended to apply to a mechanism such as a detent on the frequency switch, any noise from which would occur when the subject is not actually being tested.

4.5 Tone Switch. A tone switch is required on manual wide range and limited range audiometers, and is optional on other pure tone audiometers. The tone switch is for optional presentation of the tone signal to the subject by the operator, and its operation shall be such as to establish and eliminate the tone without producing audible transients or extraneous frequencies. The time required for the sound pressure level to rise from −20 dB to −1 dB re its final steady value shall not be less than 0.02 second and not more than 0.1 second, and the time required for the sound pressure level to decay by 20 dB shall be not less than 0.005 second and not more than 0.1 second.

The steady output voltage level in the "Off" position shall be at least 50 dB below its steady voltage in the "On" position, or at least 10 dB below that corresponding to the Zero Hearing Threshold Level, whichever of these two levels is the higher.

The operation of the tone switch shall not cause the output voltage level operating the earphone to attain at any time a value more than one dB above its steady state.

The tone switch shall be of the "normally off" type, although it is recommended that it be also adapted to "normally on" operation. It may also be arranged to operate automatically.

4.6 Stability with Respect to Variations in Supply Voltage. Over the following ranges of variation in supply voltage, (1) 105 to 125 volts, for audiometers designed for a power line of 117 volts; (2) ratios of voltage ranges equivalent to (1), for audiometers designed for power line sources of other than 117 volts, or; (3) limits of voltage recommended by the manufacturer, for battery operated audiometers, the audiometer is to meet the requirements of 4.1.2 and 4.1.3 as to frequency and purity of test tones, and also the acoustic output of the audiometer is to meet the requirements of 4.1.4.3 and shall not vary through a total range of more than 2 dB. However, measurements made at a 70 dB hearing threshold level setting and at the 1000 Hz frequency setting will be considered as sufficient for tests of compliance with the requirements of this section. The requirement of a warm-up time of 30 minutes (see 3.5) shall apply initially and after any change in supply voltage.

4.7 Stability with Respect to Ambient Temperature Variations. Through a range of ambient temperatures of at least from 60°F to 90°F, the audiometer is to meet the requirements of 4.1.2 and 4.1.3 as to frequency and purity of test tones and also the acoustic output of the audiometer is to meet the requirements of 4.1.4.3 and shall not vary through a total range of more than 2 dB. However, measurements made at the nominal rated supply voltage for which the audiometer is designed, with the attenuator set at 70 dB hearing threshold level and the frequency at 1000 Hz, will be considered as sufficient for tests of compliance with these requirements. The audiometer shall be considered stabilized at any ambient temperature after it has operated continuously in that temperature for at least 30 minutes.

4.8 Provisions for Bone-Conduction Measurements. This section applies to those audiometers in which facilities are provided for making bone-conduction measurements.

4.8.1 *Bone Vibrator*. A bone vibrator shall be provided. At any test frequency of 2000 Hz or lower, and as far as possible also at higher test frequencies, the bone vibrator shall not radiate sound to such an extent that the sound reaching the ear by air conduction through the ear canal might impair the validity of the bone-conduction measurement. As judged by an observer with otologically normal ears, the sound radiation from the bone vibrator shall have a sensation level at least 5 dB below the level which the vibrator generates by bone conduction when in contact with the head. Tests for compliance with this requirement shall be made by first: (1) determining the bone conduction threshold in the usual manner, and then (2) determining the auditory threshold with the vibrator in approximately the same position except that its normal contact area is covered with the soft flesh of the operator's finger and with no contact between the finger or the bone vibrator and the skull or the ear. The auditory threshold (2) shall be at least 5 dB below the bone conduction threshold (1). A mean shall be taken of the test results of a jury of at least six persons with otologically normal ears.

4.8.2 *Head Band*. A head band or alternative device shall be provided to hold the bone vibrator in position and to exert the static thrust necessary to make applicable the calibration provided with the audiometer.

NOTE: The mastoid is recognized as a suitable point for contact of the vibrator with the skull, but this does

not preclude the use of other points of contact provided the point be clearly identified and corresponding calibration furnished.

4.8.3 *Test Tones*. Test tones shall be provided in accordance with 4.1.1 and 4.1.2 as to frequencies and accuracy of the frequencies. The purity of these test tones shall be in accordance with 4.1.3, tests for compliance with this to be made electrically pending the availability of other suitable test means.

4.8.4 *Reference Threshold for Audibility for Bone Conduction*. The reference threshold for audibility for bone-conducted sound is the median value of threshold determinations on a large number of otologically normal ears of individuals between 18 and 30 years of age. These reference threshold values, expressed in absolute units, are now in process of determination, as is also the choice of suitable means for storing the data and for transference to other vibrators.

4.9 Masking Sound. All audiometers which have facilities for making bone conduction measurements, shall have facilities for furnishing to the subject a masking sound to be presented to the ear opposite to the ear being tested. Facilities for masking during tests by air conduction shall be provided for wide range audiometers and for speech audiometers. On other audiometers they are optional.

4.9.1 *Frequency Characteristics*. Some suggested frequency characteristics of the masking sound are the following:

(1) A narrow band of noise near the frequency of the test tone.

(2) A wide band of noise covering at least the range from 250 to 4000 Hz.

4.9.2 *Levels and Range*. The masking sound shall be available at levels at least sufficient to mask the tones produced when the dial reading is 40 dB hearing threshold level at 250 Hz, 50 dB at 500 Hz, and 60 dB at 1000 Hz and higher test frequencies, as determined by the median of values obtained on at least six otologically normal ears, by tests with the masking tone and the test tone being applied to the same ear by air conduction.

However, the total output sound pressure level of the masking sound shall not exceed 120 dB referred to 0.0002 microbar as measured with the NBS 9A coupler (see Fig. 1) and an rms meter. The masking sound shall be adjustable over a range of at least 40 dB below the levels listed above, with the dial marked in steps of 5 dB or less. The reference base of the dial markings shall be specified by the manufacturer.

4.10 Audiogram Forms. The results of hearing threshold measurements made with a pure tone audiometer may be recorded as a numerical tabulation or in the graphical form of an audiogram. Insofar as possible, such an audiogram shall be on cross-section paper, with the abscissas being frequencies on a logarithmic scale and the ordinates being hearing threshold level in decibels on a linear scale. It is recommended that one octave on the frequency scale be linearly equivalent to 20 dB on the hearing threshold level scale.

5. Requirements for Speech Audiometers

5.1 Acoustoelectric Source. The primary signals are comprised of spoken material. Using appropriate transducers such as microphones, recording heads and pickups, these signals may be stored on a disc record or on a magnetic or other tape for subsequent use, or may be applied directly to the audiometer amplifier as live voice. A meter is required to verify that the output has a known or predetermined level.

5.1.1 *Reproducers for Recorded Material.* A reproducer for recorded material shall provide turntable or tape speeds and frequency-response equalization consistent with the recordings to be used.

5.2 Monitor. All speech test material shall be so presented as to attain a standard reference level, as shown by a monitoring meter provided in the audiometer. The meter shall be connected ahead of the attenuator. For live voice tests, this shall be a meter with characteristics as described in American National Standard Volume Measurements of Electrical Speech and Program Waves, C16.5-1954 (specifications for a VU meter, Sections 3.2 to 3.5, inclusive). Provision shall be made in the amplifier for close adjustment of its gain to attain the desired reference level, and to accommodate differences of 20 dB in the absolute level of presented acoustic material, either recorded or live. If automatic alternative means are provided for governing the reference level, they shall produce the same result as would be

obtained with the above arrangement of gain on the basis of a meter reading.

5.3 Sound Pressure Level of Speech. For the purpose of this standard, the sound pressure level of a speech signal at the earphone is defined as the rms sound pressure level (as defined in 2.6) of a 1000 Hz signal adjusted so that the VU meter deflection produced by the 1000 Hz signal is equal to the average peak VU meter deflection produced by the speech signal. The level indication of the VU meter for a preliminary carrier phrase may be taken as the level indication of the immediately following speech material when that material is delivered in a natural manner at the same communication level as the carrier phrase.

5.4 Standard Reference Threshold Sound Pressure Level for Speech. The standard reference threshold sound pressure level for speech shall be as given in Table 2. The relationship between the elements of the speech audiometer shall be such that the scale markings of the attenuator will indicate zero hearing threshold level for speech when a calibrating tone of 1000 Hz brings the monitor meter to its standard reference deflection and simultaneously produces a sound pressure level from the earphone equal to the standard reference threshold sound pressure level for speech as given in Table 2.

5.5 Level Adjustment for Live Voice. In a live-voice audiometer, the amplifier gain shall be adjustable so as to attain the standard reference level for the speech material used as indicated by the VU meter, when the operator speaks in a natural conversational voice, the relationship between the microphone and the mouth of the speaker being that recommended by the manufacturer as to distance and orientation.

5.6 Acoustical Fidelity

5.6.1 *Live Voice Audiometer.* The frequency response characteristic of a live-voice audiometer shall be such that with the microphone in an acoustic sine wave field of a given sound pressure level (approximately 74 dB), and in the relationship to the acoustic source which is recommended by the manufacturer as to distance and orientation, the sound pressure level developed by the audiometer at each of the frequencies 200, 300, 400, 700, 1500, 2000,

15

3000, and 4000 Hz does not differ from that at 1000 Hz by more than ±5 dB.

5.6.2 *Recorded Speech Audiometer.* The frequency response characteristic of a recorded speech audiometer shall be such that when used with an appropriate sine-wave recording, as described below, the sound pressure level developed by the audiometer throughout the frequency band from 200 to 4000 Hz shall not differ from that at 1000 Hz by more than ±5 dB, and shall not rise at any frequency outside of this band by more than 10 dB.

Speech audiometers using disc records shall be designed for use with recordings made in accordance with Record Industry Association of America Standards, *Standard Recording and Reproducing Characteristic* and *Dimensional Standards—Disc Phonograph Records for Home Use*, Bulletin No. E-4.

It is implied that the pickup will be provided with an appropriate network, such that the overall system shall have the characteristics specified in the first paragraph of 5.6.2, when used with a record in which the radial velocity level of the modulated groove as a function of frequency has the following relative values:

Frequency, Hz	Relative Groove Velocity Level, dB
100	−13.1
200	− 8.2
300	− 5.5
400	− 3.8
700	− 1.2
1000	0.
2000	+ 2.6
3000	+ 4.8
4000	+ 6.6
5000	+ 8.2
7000	+10.9
10 000	+13.8

5.6.3 *Filtering.* In all speech audiometers, it is permissible to introduce into the circuit a high-pass filter with nominal cutoff at 150 Hz or lower to suppress undesired low-frequency signals.

5.6.4 *Overall Distortion.* In a speech audiometer, with a pure tone input having no harmonic less than 40 dB below the fundamental, the fundamental of the output signal shall be at least 25 dB above the level of any higher

harmonic when the output of the amplifier is 6 dB above the standard reference deflection of the VU meter. Tests for conformance with this requirement shall be made with the attenuator set to its minimum attenuation or so as to produce a sound pressure level of 120 db referred to 0.0002 microbar. The tests shall be conducted either at the set of frequencies of 200, 400, 700, 1000, 2000, and 4000 Hz or at the alternative set of frequencies of 250, 500, 1000, 2000, and 4000 Hz. A recorded speech audiometer shall be tested with a suitable test recording, such as those described by the Record Industry Association of America. A live-voice audiometer shall be tested with pure tones of the above frequencies supplied to the microphone at a sound pressure level of 74 dB referred to 0.0002 microbar.

5.7 Sound Pressure Levels for Speech Audiometers

5.7.1 *Range and Intervals of Hearing Threshold Levels for Speech.* Dial readings of the hearing threshold levels for speech shall extend at least from 0 dB to 100 dB in steps of 2.5 dB or less, with the 0 dB setting corresponding to the reference speech threshold level as given in Table 2. The measured difference between two successive designations shall not differ from the dial-indicated difference by more than 1 dB. Measurements for compliance with this requirement shall be made electrically at the input of the earphone, with the earphone attached to the coupler, using a pure tone signal of 1000 Hz, or the earphone may be replaced by a dummy load which simulates the earphone electrically.

5.7.2 *Accuracy of Sound Pressure Levels.* The sound pressure levels produced by the earphone as referred to the standard reference threshold level shall not differ from the indicated values by more than 3 dB. Measurements for compliance with this requirement shall be made at 1000 Hz, and may be made by combining an acoustical measurement of sound pressure level at a 60 dB dial setting with the results of interval measurements made under 5.7.1. (See 5.3 and 5.4.)

5.8 Noise. The electrical background noise from all sources other than surface noise of the recordings shall be at least 50 dB below the level of the signal. This measurement for noise shall be made in the following manner:

16

(1) The amplifier shall be adjusted so that the meter indicates the reference level when the input is a 1000 Hz signal from a record, or in the case of a live-voice speech audiometer, when there is delivered to the microphone a 1000 Hz signal at a sound pressure level of 85 dB. The output sound pressure level of the audiometer shall be measured with the above input signal and with the attenuator at the 100 dB hearing threshold level setting.

(2) Secondly, the output sound pressure level shall be measured with no signal input to the audiometer, and with the attenuator set at the 100 dB hearing threshold level. In testing an audiometer with a mechanical reproducer, the pickup is placed in the "rest" position, but the turntable is allowed to revolve. In testing with a magnetic-tape playback, the mechanism is activated but no tape is run across the pickup. In testing a live-voice type of audiometer, the microphone shall be protected as completely as is feasible from any acoustic input, or a dummy microphone may be used.

The pressure level measured under condition (2) above shall be at least 50 dB below the pressure level measured under condition (1).

A speech audiometer shall also meet the requirements of 4.4 as far as these are applicable to a speech audiometer.

5.9 Limited Range Speech Audiometer. A limited range speech audiometer shall meet the above specifications for a speech audiometer except that the dial readings of hearing threshold level for speech shall extend from 0 dB to 70 dB, and the attenuator settings for the tests of 5.8 (1) and (2) shall be 70 dB.

5.10 Masking for Speech Tests. Some suggested frequency characteristics of the masking sound to be used with speech tests are the following:

(1) A wide band of noise covering at least the range from 250 to 4000 Hz; or

(2) A noise giving approximately equal masking over the range from 250 to 4000 Hz. One such approximation is a 3 dB per octave rise from 250 to 1000 Hz, and a 12 dB per octave fall from 1000 to 4000 Hz.

The masking sound shall be in accordance with 4.9.2, except that the available level shall be at least sufficient to mask a speech sound of 60 dB speech threshold level.

17

Appendixes

(These Appendixes are not a part of American National Standard Specifications for Audiometers, S3.6-1969, but are included to facilitate its use.)

Appendix A
Description of National Bureau of Standards 9-A Coupler
(Adapted from NBS Report 8658)*

A1. Definition and Purpose

A coupler is a cavity of predetermined shape and volume, which is used for the calibration of earphones in conjunction with a calibrated microphone adapted to measure the pressures developed within the cavity.

The NBS 9-A coupler is a reference coupler for loading an earphone with a specified acoustic impedance, providing a means for standardizing the sound pressure output of audiometer air-conduction earphones in the frequency range of 125 to 8000 Hz. The standard reference zero for audiometers is stored in terms of sound pressures produced at various frequencies in the coupler by an audiometric earphone when voltages corresponding to the standardized threshold of hearing are applied to the earphone.

A2. Construction

A2.1 General. The coupler, shown in Fig. 1 of the standard, is made of a hard, stable, nonporous, nonmagnetic material such as brass, and preferably completely machined from a single block of material. The coupler consists essentially of a cylindrical cavity, the acoustical reactance of which is approximately that of an air volume of 5.6 cm³. (See Fig. 1.) The base of the cylindrical cavity is designed to be terminated by the diaphragm of a microphone of high mechanical impedance, by which the sound pressure level in the coupler is measured.

A2.2 Critical Dimensions. The critical dimensions of the coupler are those defining the volume and shape of the cavity, the capillary leak, the upper edge (lip), and 45 degree slope. Other dimensions depend upon the microphone length and associated apparatus. The volume of the cavity and the critical dimensions should be kept within the tolerances indicated in Fig. 1 of the standard.

A2.3 Calibrated Pressure Microphone. The diameter of the microphone diaphragm and the depth of the recess in front of the diaphragm are those of a number of commercially available condenser microphones. The dimensions of Fig. 1 are specifically based on the Western Electric 640-AA condenser microphone, the mechanical diaphragm impedance of which is equivalent to that of about 0.1 cm³ of air. If a condenser microphone of slightly different configuration is used, care must be taken to preserve the stipulated volume and associated dimensions. This may necessitate the use of an adaptor for the microphone. The acoustical compliance of the microphone diaphragm shall be less than that of a volume of 0.2 cm³ of air. The microphone is to be used without a protective grille.

The microphone should be sealed in the coupler with a thin layer of nonvolatile grease around the circumference near the top of the microphone. On microphones having a pressure-equalizing leak at the side, care should be taken to prevent closing the leak with grease. Also, with such microphones, an additional 0.24-inch hole should be drilled into the coupler at a position to be oriented with the microphone's capillary tube when assembled.

A2.4 The Static-Pressure Equalizer. The capillary tube (with wire inserted into it) which equalizes the static air pressure inside the cavity with the external atmospheric pressure, is held in place in such a way that air leakage occurs only through the inner bore. The sound pressure difference developed by a given voltage on the earphone terminals with the capillary plugged or left open, should not be greater than a few tenths of a decibel at frequencies down to 100 Hz. The capillary tube may be

---
*WEISSLER, P.G.; SMITH, E.L.; and COOK, R.K. Description of National Bureau of Standards 9-A Coupler. *NBS Report* 8658, March 1965.

18

made of glass or metal, or an accurately drilled 0.024-inch hole in the coupler wall.

A2.5 Coupling of Earphone to Coupler. The cap of the earphone being calibrated rests on the upper edge or lip of the coupler with a coupling force equal to the weight of the earphone plus a force, either a weight or spring force, between 400 and 500 grams force. (See Fig. 1a.) Note that the earphone does not rest on the sloping sides of the coupler but only on the upper edge, indicated by "lip" in Fig. 1a.

In the case of earphones with a hard earcap, a flat ring of thin sheet rubber of less than a millimeter in thickness or a thin film of caulking compound such as Mortite or soft red wax should be used on the lip in order to produce an effective seal between the earphone and upper edge of the coupler.

Appendix B

Bone Conduction Standard Reference Threshold Levels

Standards have not yet been established for bone conduction reference threshold levels nor for the most suitable means of storing such information and for transferring it to other vibrators. Work in this field is in progress both in the United States of America and on the international level as a project of the International Organization for Standardization.

Appendix C

Records for Speech Audiometers

The following comments concerning records for use with speech audiometers are not a part of the standard specification of the audiometers themselves. However, in order to insure uniform and proper overall results from the combined use of speech records and speech audiometers the following standards for these records are suggested.

(1) Disc records for use with speech audiometers shall be made in accordance with the bulletins listed in Section 5.6.2 of the standard.

(2) Records for use with a speech audiometer shall include a preliminary signal of 1000 Hz at the same level as the speech material on the record (see 5.3), for the purpose of allowing the amplification of the speech audiometer to be readily adjusted by reference to the monitor meter, to make applicable the calibration of the sound output levels.

(3) The speech material on records for the general testing of the speech threshold level of subjects shall be spondee words, although this does not preclude the use of other speech material for more extensive tests or for other purposes.

(4) It is recommended that disc records be made for a speed of 33⅓ r/min and for use with a 0.001 inch stylus.

19

S3.6

Appendix D

Reference Threshold Levels
for Air Conduction

The standard reference threshold levels given in Table 2 of this standard are those recommended by the International Organization for Standardization (ISO) in 1964. These have been referred to as the ISO-1964 values, but may now be termed the ANS1 values. These values differ from those which have been in use in the United States of America since 1939, officially adopted in 1951 and given in Table 2 of American Standard Z24.5-1951. The latter may conveniently be termed the ASA-1951 values.

The table below gives these two sets of reference threshold values, in terms of the Western Electric 705-A earphone and the National Bureau of Standards 9-A coupler.* The numerical values given in the 1951 specification have been shifted by 74 dB to put them on the reference basis of 0.0002 microbar, and have been rounded off to the nearest 0.5 dB to accord with present methods of representation.

*The associated condenser microphone being used without a protective grille.

Frequency Hz	Reference Threshold Levels re 0.0002 Microbar, (dB)		
	ASA-1951	Current Values	Difference
125	54.5	45.5	0
250	39.5	24.5	15
500	25	11	14
1000	16.5	6.5	10
1500	16.5†	6.5	10†
2000	17	8.5	8.5
3000	16†	7.5	8.5†
4000	15	9	6
6000	17.5†	8	9.5†
8000	21	9.5	11.5

†These figures are interpolations.

References

Standard Reference Zero for the Calibration of Pure Tone Audiometers, ISO Recommendation 389-1964.

WEISSLER, P.G. International standard reference zero for audiometers. *Journal of the Acoustical Society of America*, vol 44, No. 1, July 1968, pp 264-275.

Appendix E

Designations of Audiometers
and Audiograms

It is evident that for a period of time there will be in use some audiometers calibrated to the ASA-1951 values and some calibrated to the current American National Standard values. In order to facilitate an orderly transition from the use of one set of reference levels to the other, it is strongly recommended that the following procedures be followed:

(1) Audiometers calibrated to the current American National Standard levels are to be identified by the designation "Hearing Threshold Level: American National Standard" *for the attenuator dial.*

NOTE: During the course of the development of these audiometer specifications, some audiometers were made with the symbol "150" or "USASI," and are calibrated to what is now termed the American National Standard reference levels.

(2) Each record of an audiometric test is to include a specific indication as to whether it is based on the American National Standard or the ASA-1951 reference levels. For convenience, the following notation may be printed on the record form, either tabulation or audiogram:

Reference levels used:
☐ American National Standard
☐ ASA-1951
(Check one of these squares)

(3) On the audiogram form, the vertical scale is to be designated:

Hearing Threshold Level (Decibels)

APPENDIX   S3.6

The horizontal scale is to be labeled:

Frequency, Hz	Difference, db (ANSI vs ASA-1951)
125	9
250	15
500	14
1000	10
1500	10
2000	8.5
3000	8.5
4000	6
6000	9.5
8000	11.5

This last line of differences is optional, but may be of some convenience. If it is used, the following notation should appear on the audiogram form:

To convert American National Standard values to ASA-1951 values, subtract the appropriate differences in dB at each frequency. A reverse conversion may be made by addition.

(4) For the purpose of comparison of ASA-1951 audiogram values with corresponding American National Standard values, it may be of some convenience to use a suitable plastic transparency that could be laid over an ASA-1951 audiogram to show the corresponding values on the American National Standard scale.

Appendix F

Reference Threshold Levels for Various Earphones

Table 2 of this specification gives reference threshold levels in terms of the Western Electric 705-A earphone. Corresponding reference threshold values in terms of a number of other earphones have been compiled. These values are given below with the recommendation that they be used.

All of the data in the table are based on measurements made on the National Bureau of Standards 9-A coupler;* and with the earphones fitted with the MX-41/AR earphone cushion. (See Figs. 1 and 2 of the standard.)

The reference threshold sound pressure level for intelligible speech from the TDH-39 earphone is 20 dB above 0.0002 microbar, measured in accordance with Section 5.3, and based on 50 percent intelligibility of spondee words.

*The associated condenser microphone being used without a protective grille.

Table F1
Reference Threshold Levels for Various Earphones

Frequency, Hz	Reference Threshold Levels re 0.0002 Microbar, dB			
	Permoflux PDR-1	Permoflux PDR-8	Permoflux PDR-10	Telephonics TDH-39
125	46.5	44	51	45
250	26	25	28.5	25.5
500	11	11.5	10	11.5
1000	7	6.5	6	7
1500	7	5.5	6.5	6.5
2000	9	7.5	6.5	9
3000	10	8	9	10
4000	13.5	9	9	9.5
6000	8.5	17	18.5	15.5
8000	11	13	14	13

21

S3.6

References

WHITTLE, L.S. and ROBINSON, D.W. British normal threshold of hearing. *Nature*, vol 189, 1961, pp 617-618.

COX, J.R., Jr, and BILGER, R.D. Suggestion relative to the standardization of loudness-balance data for the Telephonics TDH-39 earphones. *Journal of the Acoustical Society of America*, vol 32, 1960, p 1081.

WHITTLE, L.S. and DELANY, M.E. Equivalent threshold sound-pressure levels for the TDH-39/MX41-AR earphone. *Journal of the Acoustical Society of America*, vol 39, 1966, pp 1187-1188.

Communications made by Allison Laboratories, Inc; the Subcommittee on Noise, American Academy of Ophthalmology and Otolaryngology; the Maico Company; the National Bureau of Standards; and the Walter Reed Army Medical College have been used in the preparation of this Appendix.

AUTHOR INDEX

Numbers in italics refer to pages on which complete references are cited.